GREEN & TON

HEALTH PROMOTION

GREEN & TONES'

HEALTH PROMOTION

Planning and Strategies

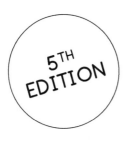

5TH EDITION

RUTH CROSS
JAMES WOODALL

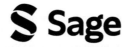

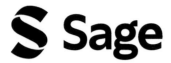

1 Oliver's Yard
55 City Road
London EC1Y 1SP

2455 Teller Road
Thousand Oaks
California 91320

Unit No 323-333, Third Floor, F-Block
International Trade Tower
Nehru Place, New Delhi – 110 019

8 Marina View Suite 43-053
Asia Square Tower 1
Singapore 018960

Editor: Martha Cunneen
Editorial assistant: Sahar Jamfar
Production editor: Sarah Sewell
Copyeditor: Jane Fricker
Proofreader: Martin Noble
Marketing manager: Ruslana Khatagova
Cover design: Sheila Tong
Typeset by: C&M Digitals (P) Ltd, Chennai, India
Printed in the UK

Library of Congress Control Number: 2023930674

British Library Cataloguing in Publication data

A catalogue record for this book is available from the British Library

ISBN 978-1-5297-7061-2
ISBN 978-1-5297-7059-9 (pbk)

At Sage we take sustainability seriously. Most of our products are printed in the UK using responsibly sourced papers and boards. When we print overseas we ensure sustainable papers are used as measured by the Paper Chain Project grading system. We undertake an annual audit to monitor our sustainability.

CONTENTS

HOW TO USE THE ONLINE RESOURCES

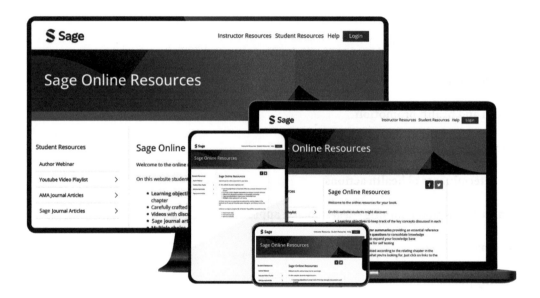

The fifth edition of *Health Promotion* is supported by a variety of online resources for students and lecturers to aid both learning and teaching. Further readings and weblinks provide a solid foundation through which to explore topics in the book in more depth. Using contributors from around the world, we also have nine original case studies that give an insight into practice and evaluation across a variety of different contexts.

All resources are available at https://study.sagepub.com/greentones5e

RESOURCES FOR LECTURERS

Seminar questions

- Seminar questions provide lecturers with general discussion points to use when teaching chapter-specific topics, and drill down into the sub-topics of the subject, with more critical thinking points and questions to explore with students.

RESOURCES FOR STUDENTS

Journal articles

- A selection of free SAGE journal articles that support each chapter to help deepen your knowledge and reinforce your learning of key topics. An ideal place to start for literature reviews/dissertations/assignments. Preceding each article is an annotation from the chapter editors, Ruth Cross and James Woodall, introducing its relevance for practice and/or revision.

International case studies

- International case studies, mapped against each chapter, written by contributors from around the world, map to each chapter and provide a unique insight into the challenges of health promotion across a range of socioeconomic and cultural contexts. Countries represented include Ghana, Jamaica, UK, The Gambia, Norway, Uganda and Zambia.

CASE STUDY SUMMARIES AND CHAPTER MAPPING

Case Study 1: Eve for Life Jamaica Mentor-Mom Programme

Antionette Barton-Gooden, Joy Crawford and Patricia Watson

Figueroa et al. (2020) reported that the Human Immune Virus (HIV) prevalence rate in Jamaican adults was 1.5%. Nevertheless, there are disproportional rates of infection in some at-risk populations. Females are one such group with a greater risk of HIV due to their anatomical features, cultural practices and socioeconomic factors. Globally, it appears that gender inequity is getting greater attention since the *Me-Too Movement*. However, Eve for Life Jamaica, which was established in 2008, has been a champion for gender empowerment, institutional support and advocacy prior to this. This health promotion strategy combines modelling, individual and community empowerment for girls and women infected and affected by HIV.

Relevant to Chapters 1, 5, 6, 7 and 9.

Case Study 2: Cash Transfer Programmes as a Health Promotion Strategy

Ebenezer Owusu-Addo, Sally Baba Owusu-Addo, Andren M.N. Renzaho and Ben J. Smith

A key development in health promotion has been the recognition of how social policy interventions influence population health and health inequities. It has been acknowledged that without appropriate interventions that address the social determinants of health (SDoH), the health of most people particularly in low- and middle-income countries will continue to deteriorate. The World Health Organization (WHO) in 2008 made a strong call for governments across the globe to develop culturally appropriate interventions to address health inequity through action on the SDoH. A particularly promising social intervention that could help in this direction is cash transfer programmes (CTs). The aim of this case study is to show how CTs can be used as a health promotion strategy to address the broader determinants of health and health inequalities.

Relevant to Chapters 2, 3, 4, 6, 9, 10 and 11.

Case Study 3: Employee-driven Shift Scheduling: A Case Study from Norway

Kari Ingstad

In Norway, over 70% of primary healthcare workers have part-time jobs, and staff shortages are expected to increase. A greater need for healthcare workers in combination with high stress levels among staff calls for new thinking around the organization of shift work. This study shows that staff involvement in drawing up shift rotas can lead to more full-time work, which again enhances job continuity and makes more staff take greater responsibility. One challenge of staff involvement in creating their own shift schedule is conflicting preferences. Employee-driven shift generation requires negotiation among staff members involving give and take.

Relevant to Chapters 1, 3, 10 and 12.

Case Study 4: Satellite Healthcare Services: The Jamaican Perspective

Sandra Chisholm-Ford, Sheryl Garriques-Lloyd and Mauvette Waite

The satellite healthcare model is a practical and 'best fit' healthcare service offered to the most vulnerable aggregate populations in various communities in Jamaica. An adapted version of the model is being utilized in the Whitfield Town community resulting in improvements in the immunization coverage, reduction in infant and maternal mortality and morbidity as well as improvements in mental and physical health and life expectancy of community members.

Relevant to Chapters 1, 4, 3, 6 and 9.

Case Study 5: COVID Vaccination: What Did We Miss in Relation to Public Health Messaging to Protect Pregnant Women?

Tendai Nzirawa

The first World Health Organization (WHO) official announcement was made on 31 December 2019, that a cluster of cases of pneumonia of unknown cause had been detected in Wuhan City, Hubei Province, China. Based on the patient samples it was later identified as coronavirus (SARS-CoV-2) (UK Health Security Agency, 2022). A wave of fear, worry and anxiety spread across the world. Little was known at the time on how this virus would affect pregnant women and other vulnerable people. This case study aims to highlight the impact coronavirus can make on a pregnant woman and their family when they are not COVID-19 vaccinated.

Relevant to Chapters 2, 3, 5, 6, 7 and 8.

Case Study 6: Alcohol Investment: A Public Health Risk of Disease Burden in Zambia

Philip Chimponda

In the recent past, increased investment in alcohol, especially in Africa and in particular Zambia by multinational corporation companies coupled with local alcohol industries, has resulted in increased alcohol production, availability and high consumption, subsequently increasing the disease burden and ill health within the general population. Lack of evidence-based policies to inform best practices and poor implementation of existing by-laws impact on prevention of health-related harms at individual level and within the general population.

Relevant to Chapters 1, 2, 3, 6 and 12.

Case Study 7: The Role of Research Officers in Promoting HIV/AIDS Research: A Case of Mbarara University of Science and Technology Grants Management Office

Jacqueline Karuhanga

Although the incidence of HIV/AIDS infection has declined in recent years, it continues to be the leading cause of disease and death in Uganda (Kazibwe et al., 2022); with Mbarara district among 13 HIV high-risk districts in the country; and some suburbs registering a prevalence rate (12.6%) that is twice the general district rate (Uganda Population HIV Impact Assessment, 2017). To avert this trend, Mbarara University of Science and Technology (MUST) and its collaborators remain committed to HIV/AIDS research. To further strengthen HIV research, the MUST UVA project was launched to substantially raise the external research award obtainment success rate for HIV/AIDS research programmes at MUST through human skills development and well-researched technological advances, and in doing this, has become a leader in the field.

Relevant to Chapters 2, 6 and 12.

Case Study 8: The Anglican Communion: Responding to a Health Emergency

Michael Beasley, Luke Pato, Janice Tsang, Rachel Carnegie, Ben Walker and Sally Smith

This case study describes how the Anglican Communion Health and Community Network (AHCN) was established during the COVID-19 pandemic, meeting the needs of its members for accurate information, connection and support during the pandemic, as well as launching advocacy for equitable access to vaccines and promoting COVID-19 vaccine uptake among its membership.

Relevant to Chapters 1, 4, 7, 8, 9 and 10.

Case Study 9: Results-Based Financing to Improve Utilization of Maternal and Child Health Services in The Gambia: A Case of Community Empowerment

Tahir Ahmad Touray and Yusupha Sangyang

Maternal and child health are major public health concerns in The Gambia, with a maternal mortality rate of 289 deaths per 100,000 live births in 2020 and an infant mortality rate of 40 deaths per 1000 live births in 2022 (The Gambia Bureau of Statistics, 2021). The Government of The Gambia has come up with interventions such as the Results-Based Financing (RBF) programme to increase access to and utilization of maternal and child health services in the country. The purpose of this case study is to show how the intervention reflects some values and principles of health promotion.

Relevant to Chapters 2, 3, 4, 7, 8, 9 and 10.

ABOUT THE EDITORS

Dr Ruth Cross is Course Director for Health Promotion in the School of Health at Leeds Beckett University. Ruth has authored and co-authored several books and book chapters on health promotion theory and practice. Ruth was Editor of the *International Journal of Health Promotion and Education* from 2015 to 2021.

Dr James Woodall is a Reader in Health Promotion and Head of Subject in Health, Nutrition and Environment at Leeds Beckett University. James has published work on health promotion theory and practice, but has particular interest in areas related to prison and offender health. James is the current Editor of the journal *Health Education*.

ABOUT THE AUTHORS

Jackie Green is Emeritus Professor and former Director of the Centre for Health Promotion Research at Leeds Metropolitan University – now renamed Leeds Beckett University. She has been President of the Institute of Health Promotion and Education and was Editor-in-Chief of *Promotion and Education*, the journal of the International Union for Health Promotion and Education. She has over 30 years' experience of providing education and training in the field of health promotion and she has also worked in practice as a Health Promotion Specialist.

Keith Tones was Emeritus Professor at Leeds Beckett University, formerly Leeds Metropolitan University. His work has had a seminal influence on the development of Health Promotion as a discipline and a profession.

PUBLISHER'S ACKNOWLEDGEMENTS

The authors and publisher are grateful to all third parties for their kind permission to reproduce the following material:

Table 2.2 Comparison of life expectancies and early mortality in selected countries, United Nations Population Division (UNPD) (2022) *Life Expectancy of the World Population* (*Website*: www.world ometers.info); Juneau, M. (2021) *Why do the Japanese Have the Highest Life Expectancy in the World?* Institut de Cardiologie de Montréal (*Website:* www.observatoireprevention.org); O'Neill, A. (2022) *Infant Mortality in Japan 2009-2019. (Website:* www.statista/com); Nayak, M. (2019) *Ten Facts about Life Expectancy in the Central African Republic.* The Borgen Project (*Website:* www.borgen. org); UNICEF (2021) *Central African Republic: Key Demographic Indicators* (*Website:* www.data. unicef.org).

Table 2.3 Leading causes of DALYs globally, Global Health Observatory (2022a) 'Global health estimates: Leading causes of DALYs'. Geneva: WHO.

Table 2.4 Guidelines for causality, Bonita, R., Beaglehole, R. and Kjellström, T. (2006) *Basic Epidemiology* (2nd edn). Geneva: WHO.

Figure 2.3 Dimensions of well-being and ill health, Downie, R.S., Tannahill, C. and Tannahill, A. (1996) *Health Promotion Models and Values* (2nd edn). Oxford: Oxford University Press.

Table 2.5 Accounts of health – sociopolitical philosophies and cultural bias, Beattie, A. (1993) 'The changing boundaries of health', in A. Beattie, M. Gott, L. Jones and M. Sidell (eds), *Health and Wellbeing: A Reader.* London: Macmillan. Palgrave Macmillan © The Open University.

Figure 2.4 Accounts of health, Beattie, A. (1993) 'The changing boundaries of health', in A. Beattie, M. Gott, L. Jones and M. Sidell (eds), *Health and Wellbeing: A Reader.* London: Macmillan. Palgrave Macmillan © The Open University.

Figure 2.5 The expanded health field concept, Raeburn, J.M. and Rootman, I. (1989) 'Towards an expanded health field concept: conceptual and research issues in an era of health promotion', *Health Promotion, 3* (4): 383–92.

Figure 2.6 The main determinants of health, Dahlgren, G. and Whitehead, M. (1991) *Policies and Strategies to Promote Social Equity in Health.* Stockholm: Institute of Futures Studies, World Health Organization.

Figure 2.7 Some interrelationships in the complex system of lifestyle, environment and health status, Green, L.W., Simons-Morton, D.G. and Potvin, L. (1997) 'Education and life-style determinants of health and disease', in R. Detels, W.W. Holland, J. McEwen and G.S. Omenn (eds), *Oxford Textbook of Public Health*, Vol. 1 (3rd edn). Oxford: Oxford University Press.

Table 2.6 Selected key facts on health inequalities in England, Williams, E., Buck, D. and Babalola, G. (2020) *What Are Health Inequalities?* London: The King's Fund.

Table 2.7 Which health differences are inequitable? Whitehead, M. (1992) *Policies and Strategies to Promote Equity*. Copenhagen: WHO.

Table 2.8 National Statistics Socio-economic Classification (NS-SEC), National Statistics (2007) *National Statistics Socio-economic Classification*. (*Website*: https://webarchive.national archives.gov.uk/20160105232615/http://www.ons.gov.uk/ons/guide-method/user-guidance/social-capital-guide/the-social-capital-project/guide-to-social-capital.html); Babb, P., Martin, J. and Haezewindt, P. (2004) *Focus on Social Inequalities*. London: TSO. (*Website*: www.ons.gov.uk/ons/rel/social-inequalities/focus-on-social-inequalities/2004-edition/a-summary-of-focus-on-social-inequalities.pdf).

Table 2.10 Gordon, R. (2013) 'Unlocking the potential of upstream social marketing.' *European Journal of Marketing*, *47* (9): 1525–47. Emerald Insight.

Table 3.2 Influences on self-efficacy – implications for health promotion, Bandura, A. (1986) *Social Foundations of Thought and Action: A Social Cognitive Theory*. Englewood Cliffs, NJ: Prentice-Hall..

Figure 4.2 Dignan and Carr's Planning Model, Dignan, M.B. and Carr, P.A. (1992) *Program Planning for Health* (2nd edn). Malvern, PA: Lee & Febiger.

Figure 4.5 Bracht et al.'s community organization model, Bracht, N., Kingsbury, L. and Rissel, C. (1999) 'A five-stage community organization model for health promotion', in N. Bracht (ed.), *Health Promotion at the Community Level: New Advances*. Thousand Oaks, CA: Sage.

Figure 4.6 A planning framework for incorporating community empowerment into top-down health promotion programmes, Laverack, G. and Labonte, R. (2000) 'A planning framework for community empowerment goals within health promotion', *Health Policy and Planning*, *15* (3): 255–62. Oxford University Press.

Figure 4.7 French and Milner's view of real planning, French, J. and Milner, S. (1993) 'Should we accept the status quo?', *Health Education Journal*, *52* (2): 98–101.

Figure 4.9 Health Equity Audit Cycle, Office of the Deputy Prime Minister (ODPM) and Department of Health (2005) *Creating Healthier Communities: A Resource Pack for Local Partnerships*. Wetherby: ODPM Publications.

Figure 4.11 Quality dimensions associated with SESAME, Haglund, B.J.A., Jansson, B., Pettersson, B. and Tillgren, P. (1998) 'A quality assurance instrument for practitioners', in J.K. Davies and G. Macdonald (eds), *Quality, Evidence and Effectiveness in Health Promotion*. London: Routledge.

Table 4.3 Proportion (%) of projects that completed tasks, stages and phases, Godin, G., Gagnon, H., Alary, M., Levy, J.J. and Otis, J. (2007) 'The degree of planning: an indicator of the potential success of health education programs', *Promotion & Education*, *14* (3): 138–42.

Figure 4.12 Consequences of inadequate funding, Scriven, A. and Speller, V. (2007) 'Global issues and challenges beyond Ottawa: the way forward', *Promotion & Education*, *XIV* (4): 194–8.

Figure 5.2 A representation of Maslow's hierarchy of needs, Maslow, A.H. (1954) *Motivation and Personality*. New York: Harper.

Table 5.1 Mean ranks of women's psychosocial health needs in Northern Ireland (lowest score = highest priority), Lazenbatt, A. and McMurray, F. (2004) 'Using participatory rapid appraisal as a tool to assess women's psychosocial health needs in Northern Ireland', *Health Education*, *104* (3): 174–87. Emerald Insight.

Figure 5.6 Arnstein's ladder of participation, Arnstein, S.R. (1969) 'A ladder of citizen participation', *Journal of the American Planning Association*, *35* (4): 216–24. Taylor and Francis.

Figure 5.8 Information profile, Annett, H. and Rifkin, S. (1990) *Improving Urban Health*. Geneva: WHO.

Table 5.2 The domains of social capital and community cohesion, Forrest and Kearns (2000), in Home Office Community Cohesion Review Team (2001) *Community Cohesion*. London.

Figure 5.9 Beattie's model of health promotion, Beattie, A. (1991) 'Knowledge and control in health promotion: a test case for social policy and social theory', in J. Gabe, M. Calnan and M. Bury (eds), *The Sociology of the Health Service*. London: Routledge.

Table 5.3 Levels of evidence for studies on the efficacy of public health interventions, National Institute for Health and Care Excellence (NICE) (2005) *Public Health Guidance Methods Manual version 1*. London: NICE.

Figure 6.1 Health promotion – alternative approaches, Beattie, A. (1991) 'Knowledge and control in health promotion: a test case for social policy and social theory', in J. Gabe, M. Calnan and M. Bury (eds), *The Sociology of the Health Service*. London: Routledge.

Figure 6.2 Health education and health promotion, Tones, K. and Tilford, S. (1994) *Health Education: Effectiveness, Efficiency and Equity*. London: Chapman & Hall.

Table 6.1 Health impact assessment, Prashar, A., Abrahams, D., Taylor, D. and Scott-Samuel, A. (2004) *Merseytram Line 1: A Health Impact Assessment of the Proposed Scheme*. Liverpool: The International Health Impact Assessment Consortium. (*Website:* www.liverpool.ac.uk/media/livacuk/instituteof psychology/researchgroups/impact/Merseytram_Line_1_HIA_-_Final.pdf).

Table 6.2 Health impacts on different population groups under transport scenario 1 (low spend) and scenario 3 (high spend), Douglas, M.J., Conway, L., Gorman, D., Gavin, S. and Hanlon, P. (2001) 'Developing principles for health impact assessment', *Journal of Public Health Medicine*, *23* (2): 148–54.

Table 7.1 Targets of change and strategies for different ecological levels, McLeroy, K. (1992) 'Editorial: health education research: theory and practice – future directions', *Health Education Research*, 7: 1–8. Oxford University Press.

Figure 7.3 Motor skills model of social interaction, Argyle, M. and Kendon, A. (1967) 'The experimental analysis of social performance', *Advances in Experimental Social Psychology*, 3: 35–98. Elsevier.

Figure 7.5 The experiential learning cycle, © 2018 Experience Based Learning Systems, Inc.

Table 7.4 Contrasting teaching styles, Ryder, J. and Campbell, L. (1988) *Balancing Acts in Personal, Social and Health Education: A Practical Guide for Teachers.* London: Routledge.

Figure 7.6 Appropriate learning strategies, Belbin, E., Downs, S. and Perry, P. (1981) 'How do I learn?', in J. Anderson (ed.), *The HEA Health Skills Dissemination Project: A Whole School Approach to Life Skills and Health Education.* Leeds: Counselling and Career Development Unit.

Figure 7.11 The OK Corral, Turner, C.M. (1978) *Interpersonal Skills in Further Education.* Blagdon: Further Education Staff College, Coombe Lodge.

Figure 7.13 Life skills and community action, Hopson, B. and Scally, M. (1980–2) *Lifeskills Teaching Programmes 1–5.* Leeds: Lifeskills Associates.

Table 8.1 Advantages and disadvantages of selected media channels, National Cancer Institute (undated) *Making Health Communication Programs Work.* National Cancer Institute. (*Website*: www.cancer.gov/pinkbook).

Figure 8.1 Elements of social marketing, French, J. and Blair-Stevens, C. (2007) *Big Pocket Guide to Social Marketing* (2nd edn). London: National Consumer Council.

Table 8.2 Cost–benefit assessment, Hastings, G. (2007) *Social Marketing: Why Should the Devil Have All the Best Tunes?* Oxford: Butterworth-Heinemann.

Table 9.1 Key differences between community-based and community development approaches, Boutilier, M., Cleverly, S. and Labonte, R. (2000) 'Community as a setting for health promotion', in B.D. Poland, L.W. Green and I. Rootman (eds), *Settings for Health Promotion: Linking Theory and Practice.* Thousand Oaks, CA: Sage., based on Felix, M., Chavis, D. and Florin, P. (1989) 'Enabling community development: language, concepts and strategies', Presentation sponsored by Health Promotion Branch, Ontario Ministry of Health, Toronto, May 16–18.

Figure 9.1 Community-centred approaches for health and well-being, Public Health England (2018) 'Health matters: community-centred approaches for health and wellbeing' (2018) (*Website*: www.gov.uk/government/publications/health-matters-health-and-wellbeing-community-centred-approaches/health-matters-community-centred-approaches-for-health-and-wellbeing).

Figure 9.3 Pathways from community participation, empowerment and control to health improvement is from Popay, J. (2010) 'Community empowerment and health improvement: the English experience', in A. Morgan, M. Davies and E. Ziglio (eds), *Health Assets in a Global Context: Theory, Methods, Action.* New York: Springer, pp. 183–197. Republished with permission of Jennie Popay.

Figure 9.4 Pathways from community participation, empowerment and control to health improvement, National Institute for Health and Care Excellence (NICE) (2008) *Community Engagement to Improve Health. NICE Public Health Guidance 9.* London: NICE.

Table 9.2 Good practice for community development and health work, Henderson, P., Summer, S. and Raj, T. (2004) *Developing Healthier Communities.* London: Health Development Agency.

Table 10.1 Moving from traditional school health education to the health-promoting school, Young, I. and Williams, T. (1989) *The Healthy School.* Edinburgh: Scottish Health Education Group.

Figure 11.3 An overview of constructivist evaluation, Pawson, R. and Tilley, N. (1997) *Realistic Evaluation.* London: Sage.

Figure 11.7 A Theory of Change for work with traveller children, Barnes, M. (ed.), Allan, D., Coad, J., Fielding, A., Hansen, K., Mathers, J., McCabe, A., Morris, K., Parry, J., Plewis, I., Prior, D. and Sullivan, A. (2004) *Assessing the Impact of the Children's Fund: The Role of Indicators. National Evaluation of the Children's Fund.* Birmingham: NECF.

INTRODUCTION

The fact that health follows a social gradient is no longer contested (Bambra et al., 2010); a lot of robust evidence demonstrates this – people who are better off (economically and socially) fare better health-wise (Marmot, 2010; Marmot et al., 2020). In the wake of the global COVID-19 pandemic the world is further witness to this pattern of outcomes. New infectious diseases pose new challenges for everyone, yet the least well-off and most socially marginalized fare worst. Since late 2019 we are all living with the continued impact of COVID-19; however, it has not affected everyone equally. Contemporary public health problems are all too frequently attributed to individual behaviour such as poor diet, lack of exercise, unsafe sex and smoking, drinking alcohol and using other addictive substances. In the case of COVID-19 individual behaviour was again under focus – social distancing/isolating, handwashing, wearing a face covering, getting vaccinated. Interpretations of this sort tend to be associated with a biomedical discourse and a deficit model of health that equates it with the absence of disease, rather than more holistic interpretations of health that encompass positive well-being. Such attributions are clearly overly simplistic. Nonetheless, they are still potentially damaging with regard to public health practice as responsibility for unhealthy behaviour, and therefore by implication health, becomes delegated to the individual. Health promotion has challenged such a narrow focus on behaviour and has supported a more comprehensive analysis of the factors that influence health and well-being. In particular, it recognizes the fundamental importance of environmental influences on health and the complex interplay between these factors and health-related behaviour. Environmental factors are taken to include not only the physical environment, but also psychosocial aspects and, importantly, the socioeconomic environment. Acknowledging the importance of these wider determinants moves the primary focus of health promotion towards creating the conditions supportive of health and health behaviour. It also effectively involves the state in the responsibility for tackling the so-called upstream determinants of health and draws attention to the essentially political nature of health promotion. Returning to the example of COVID-19, all countries were impacted but some, due to political choices or ideologies, faced more extensive mortality and morbidity. Rather than being a matter of individual responsibility, health therefore becomes an issue of social justice. The key to addressing health inequalities is to tackle the root causes, including economic inequality.

The 'big issues' that are a threat to health at the global level include poverty and deprivation, discrimination and exploitation, and violence in all forms including terrorism. Additionally, there is the rise of 'wicked' or 'super wicked' health promotion problems and contemporary challenges to health such as climate change, environmental degradation, war and conflict, and emerging infectious diseases. Inequalities in health persist between high- and low-income countries and within countries too. A child born in Japan or Sweden can today expect to live to over 80 years of age whereas in some African countries life expectancy is still less than 50. The effects of global recession and climate change are being experienced disproportionately by poorer countries – despite the fact that the most affluent nations carry the major share of blame for the problem. Tackling global health inequalities demands international commitment and coordinated action but this response is not always forthcoming.

At the national level, there are also major inequalities: 'life expectancy at birth for males living in the most deprived areas in England was 73.9 years in 2016–18 compared with 83.4 years in the least deprived areas; the corresponding figures for females were 78.6 and 86.3 years' (Marmot et al., 2020: 11). However, it is not only the poorest in society who experience worse health. There are gradations in health at all levels of the socioeconomic scale. This appears to be the case in all countries.

Attempts to improve public health may fail to be effective for a number of reasons – notably by focusing on individual behaviour rather than the social and environmental determinants of health and ill health. Clearly, inadequate understanding of the key determinants will risk interventions addressing inappropriate variables. In some instances, they are a knee-jerk reaction to addressing an emerging issue. They may, therefore, be poorly planned with insufficient attention to relevant theory and existing research and evaluation evidence. Interventions may also be under-resourced with unreasonable expectations of what might be achieved within the time frame.

Responses to tackling contemporary health problems are often driven by the political imperative to be seen to be doing something – regardless of whether or not it is the most appropriate means of achieving significant and sustainable improvements in health. They are often concerned with demonstrating early high-profile wins to fit in with political time frames dictated by electoral cycles rather than achieving long-term sustainable change. Furthermore, there is a marked reluctance to adopt unpopular measures that might risk alienating the electorate; for example, by requiring the majority to make cutbacks or major changes to their behaviour – hence the muted (some would argue wholly inadequate) response to tackling world poverty or climate change. We are advised to switch off the standby light on our televisions rather than take any serious action to reduce energy expenditure. Efforts to reduce health inequality tend to focus downstream on mitigating the effects of poverty and unequal life chances rather than upstream on tackling disadvantage itself through redistributive policy.

Health promotion has been characterized by a concern to create supportive environments for health through healthy public policy. Effectively, this shifted the emphasis away from health education. For many, health education had become associated with attempts to persuade individuals to change their behaviour and was criticized for failing to take account of the wider influences and, therefore, being victim-blaming in orientation. However, health promotion has been encapsulated as the synergistic interaction between health education and healthy public policy summed up as:

health promotion = health education × healthy public policy

The marginalization of health education effectively stifled debate about its continuing relevance to health promotion (Green, 2008). Yet a broader conceptualization of health education recognizes its potential for contributing to the major goals of health promotion – equity and empowerment. This broader conceptualization is concerned with enabling individuals and communities to gain control over their health and is, therefore, more radical and political in intent. We use the term 'new health education' to distinguish it from more traditional forms.

A basic premise of this text is that the new health education can be a major driver within health promotion with the capacity to:

- develop the knowledge, values and skills required for individual decision-making and voluntary action and, importantly, contribute to individual empowerment
- raise awareness of the need for environmental and policy change to support health and health choices
- develop critical awareness among communities about factors influencing their health and the skills and motivation required to take collective action – thereby contributing to critical consciousness-raising and community empowerment
- be part of professional education and training to enable professionals across a range of sectors to contribute to the health and well-being of their client groups and engage in advocacy on their behalf.

Green and Tones's rationale for producing the first edition of this book was that in order to be effective health promotion must be systematically planned. Their second edition updated this argument by drawing on contemporary examples and revisiting the various debates. The third and fourth editions, edited by Ruth Cross and James Woodall, retained Green and Tones's contention that planning should be more than a mere technical exercise. The fourth edition included a new chapter focusing on evidence-based health promotion and the necessity for health promotion to legitimize its approach and strategy. This fifth edition, again edited by Ruth Cross and James Woodall, provides a framework that allows initiatives to be grounded in the core values and principles of health promotion. Accordingly, it begins by identifying these values and principles to establish a foundation for detailed discussion of planning and its application to practice. Throughout, the importance of theory is emphasized. This is demonstrated by its application through the use of examples, research and case studies from a range of international contexts.

Notwithstanding the inclusion of contemporary research and case studies from around the world, no apology is given for including references to older 'classic sources' and seminal work; rather, this is viewed as a major strength of the book. Green and Tones argued in the introduction to the second edition that health promotion is in danger of losing sight of its roots and that there is an emerging tendency to 'reinvent the wheel' – not always as well as the first time round! It therefore remains the aim to maintain the visibility of some of the early innovative and radical thinking, which continues to be of relevance to contemporary health promotion.

Since the publication of the fourth edition of the book in 2019, the world has changed considerably and has highlighted further that tackling complex public health problems requires a multidisciplinary response. Health promotion has an essential and pivotal role in orchestrating that response. However, if it is to make a significant contribution to tackling contemporary health issues, it needs to re-engage with its radical agenda and core values and maintain its distinctive identity and purpose. This edition continues to examine the relationship between health promotion and modern multidisciplinary public health and establish its unique contribution.

The fifth edition maintains the overall coherence of the text as it has evolved through four iterations. The core themes underpinned by a commitment to equity and empowerment are retained. Like Jackie Green and Keith Tones, we consider these to be absolutely central and have, therefore, adhered to the principles set out in the earlier editions. As the editors of this new edition, our approach has again been to update and refresh the text by introducing new material on selected topics in order to maintain the book's currency and relevance to health promotion practice. Readers familiar with previous editions will note that key sections remain unchanged; this is purposefully the case. We have also broadly kept the book's structure, albeit with the addition of a new chapter on evidence-based health promotion in the previous edition, and adopted the same style and approach while drawing on more international examples and instances.

As in the previous editions, a number of key themes run throughout the whole text. These are:

- the need to adopt a systematic approach to planning
- the importance of theory and other forms of evidence
- support for an empowerment model of health promotion
- health education as a major driving force within health promotion
- acknowledgement of the upstream social determinants of health – the 'causes of the causes'
- the complex interplay between agency and structure – between individuals and their environment
- the need to tackle health inequalities.

In addition, we have identified a number of more contemporary issues for health promotion and introduced or expanded on these in subsequent editions as follows:

- assets-based approaches, including the latest thinking on salutogenesis
- understandings of mental health promotion and well-being
- concepts of healthy communities
- nudge theory and choice architecture
- social media, social networks and the role of the Internet in health promotion
- new perspectives and debates in public health evidence
- developing debate on inequalities, equity and social exclusion
- health in all policies agenda
- ethics in health promotion
- evidence-based health promotion
- contemporary threats to health in the form of new infectious diseases
- climate change and sustainability.

Health is a nebulous and contested concept, meaning different things to different people. Clearly, those working to promote health should have a clear view of what they are aspiring to. The book begins by considering alternative conceptualizations of health and a simple working model is developed. This includes physical, mental and social dimensions. It also recognizes the existence of health – or its absence – at individual and societal levels. It acknowledges the split between negative approaches to conceptualizing health that focus on the absence of disease and positive approaches that incorporate well-being. However, it is contended that empowerment should be central to definitions of health and, further, that an emphasis on empowerment supports the achievement of both disease prevention and positive health goals.

The term 'health promotion' has variously been used to refer to a social movement, an ideology, a discipline, a profession and a strategy or field of practice delineated by commitment to key values.

Chapter 1 discusses the ideology of health promotion and seeks to identify its core values. It also reviews the major World Health Organization (WHO) documents that have contributed to shaping its development right up to the 10th Global Health Promotion Conference hosted online from Geneva in late 2020 and, in particular, the Ottawa Charter (WHO, 1986). It identifies different models of health promotion and argues on ethical, ideological and even pragmatic grounds that health promotion should subscribe to an empowerment model. Empowerment approaches recognize the reciprocal relationship between individuals and their environment and the complex interplay between agency and structure – one of the themes of this text. This chapter references the importance of mental health and well-being and contemporary agendas around these areas.

Following on from the discussion of health and health promotion, Chapter 1 then locates health promotion within the context of modern multidisciplinary public health and identifies its distinctive contribution to the public health endeavour. It also considers the importance of maintaining a separate identity for health promotion and discusses competency and professional standards for health promotion capacity including a section on ethics and ethical practice. It concludes by examining the relationship between health education and health promotion. It is argued that the '"new" critical health education' is the driving force in health promotion – another of the major themes that run through the book.

Chapter 2 focuses on identifying the determinants of health and various ways of assessing them. Importantly, it looks at the value of incorporating lay perspectives and distinguishes salutogenic from pathogenic explanations of health and ill health, focusing on well-being and assets-based approaches. It concludes by considering inequality and social exclusion and social capital.

Chapter 3 begins by looking at the uptake of new ideas and practices at the community level. It then goes on to consider, at the micro level, how various factors interact to influence decisions and behaviour. In order to do so, it draws on a number of psychosocial theories and particularly the health action model (HAM). In line with supporting an empowerment model of health promotion, it pays particular attention to the dynamics of empowerment. It considers issues associated with power and control and the reciprocal determinism between individuals and their environment. Revised content around choice architecture and nudge theory is included.

Chapter 4 sets out the argument supporting systematic planning and introduces a number of planning models. It emphasizes the central importance of developing clear objectives. It also recognizes that partnerships across different sectors are needed to tackle the multiple and complex determinants of health. This chapter also looks at what is involved in developing successful partnerships and collaborations.

Chapter 5 focuses on the first stage of the planning cycle – identifying health needs. It looks at different conceptualizations of need. Consistent with the values of health promotion, it supports participatory approaches to identifying and prioritizing health needs.

We continue to emphasize throughout the book the importance of environmental determinants of health. Chapter 6 explores in detail the role of healthy public policy in establishing supportive environments for health. It considers the process of policy development and identifies the important contribution of health education and advocacy. Clearly, policies across a whole range of areas – including, for example, education, agriculture, planning and transport – will potentially influence health. The chapter therefore focuses discussion on Health in All Policies, a concept vehemently espoused in recent WHO charters and declarations. The chapter concludes by discussing the use of health impact assessment to assess the potential effects on health of policies at all levels, from the macro level down to local policies.

One of the major themes of the book is the central importance to health promotion of what Green and Tones termed the 'new' health education. Chapter 7 specifically focuses on the role of health education. It begins by examining the communication process and the design of messages before looking at different models of health education and types of learning. It then looks at methods of facilitating learning and specifically at the use of peer education and creative arts. It briefly discusses the use of health education for persuasion and attitude change – recognizing the potential conflict with empowerment. The chapter concludes by looking at health education as a strategy for social and political change, including reference to Freirean approaches.

Health education has, in the past, been associated with mass media campaigns. Chapter 8 analyses the potential and limitations of mass media interventions. It discusses relevant theories and also the technical issues involved in mass media campaigns. It also considers the more general influence of mass media on behaviour. A separate section revisits the contribution of social marketing, which has been receiving considerable attention. The role of social media, social networking and the use of mobile technologies are discussed. The chapter concludes by considering the use of mass media for advocacy purposes to shape public opinion and influence policy-makers.

Chapter 9 focuses on working with communities and in particular on community development and empowerment approaches. It identifies key aspects of good practice in working with communities and considers some of the challenges of putting the rhetoric of community development into practice. In particular, it draws attention to the need to ensure that disadvantaged and socially excluded groups are able to participate.

Chapter 10 looks at the settings approach and its potential for improving health. By focusing on the conditions that are supportive of health, the approach shifts the emphasis away from individual behaviour and towards organizations and structural factors. Having examined the principles of the approach, it goes on to consider in detail the health-promoting prison as an example, as well as making observations about a range of different settings.

Evaluation is an essential element of health promotion practice and the development of an evaluation strategy is clearly integral to systematic programme planning. Chapter 11 distinguishes between formative evaluation that contributes to the development and quality of programmes and summative evaluation to assess their overall effectiveness. It emphasizes that, in addition to measuring outcomes and the extent to which the goals of a programme have been achieved, evaluation should also comment on the process and identify those factors that may have contributed to the success and sustainability of programmes – or equally have resulted in failure. Chapter 11 considers the methodological debates about evaluation in order to make recommendations about appropriate methodology – that is, a methodology that is capable of identifying the range of potential health promotion outcomes and unpicking the complex pathways that lead towards them. Importantly, it must also be consistent with the values of health promotion and conform with ethical principles.

Following on from the discussion of evaluation, Chapter 12 considers the contribution of evaluation and empirical research findings to the evidence base for health promotion and the use of systematic reviews to synthesize the evidence. It also argues that the development of the evidence base should include practitioner expertise and insights and, importantly, should also incorporate theory. Indeed, theory should constantly be updated and refined in the light of emergent empirical evidence as part of a continuing cycle of development. Finally, the chapter considers how evidence can be put into practice. By looking at how evidence can be used in systematic planning, we effectively come full circle.

Health promotion has been referred to as an idea whose time has come. It has the potential to make a major contribution to tackling contemporary health problems and improving the health of individuals and communities. The purpose of this book is to demonstrate how that potential can be maximized through systematic planning, with due regard to evidence, theory and values at each stage of the planning cycle.

In this fifth edition each chapter contains select abstracts that are indicative of how the concepts within in the chapter are operationalized, discussed and debated in the wider research literature. Key concepts are also indicated throughout the text by the light bulb icon.

The key concepts deemed central to health promotion, as the authors understand it, are empowerment, equity, participation, partnership and ethics. Each time a key concept is considered in some detail readers will see the icon in the margin to indicate this. Finally, a critical reflection section is included at the end of each chapter that offers readers an opportunity to think about how the contents of the chapter may relate to their health promotion practice. We trust you will find these features helpful in your reading and would welcome any feedback.

1 HEALTH AND HEALTH PROMOTION

OVERVIEW

This chapter focuses on three broad areas – the concept of health, setting out the distinctive features and values of health promotion, and establishing the position of health promotion vis-à-vis modern multidisciplinary public health and health education. It will:

- explore alternative conceptualizations of health
- develop a working model of health
- consider the ideology and core values of health promotion
- identify different models of health promotion
- set out the rationale for an empowerment model of health promotion
- locate health promotion within modern multidisciplinary public health
- propose a new 'critical' health education as the major driver and distinctive voice of health promotion.

INTRODUCTION

The primary concern of this book is to provide insight into the factors that contribute to the effective and efficient design of health promotion programmes. The way in which health is conceptualized has major implications for planning, implementing and evaluating programmes. Equally, the approach adopted at each of these stages will be influenced by the values of those working to promote health.

HEALTH AS A CONTESTED CONCEPT

Developing clear goals will depend on how health is defined. Yet, it is acknowledged that health is, as Gallie (1955) famously described, a contested and elusive concept, a notion which is widely accepted (Duncan, 2007). Its many, often conflicting, meanings are socially constructed. Lowell S. Levin likened the task of defining health to shovelling smoke. It is difficult, to say the very least, to provide precise definitions, largely because health is one of those abstract words, like love and beauty, that mean different things to different people, a point reiterated by Warwick-Booth et al. (2021). However, we can confidently say that health is, and apparently always has been, of significant value in people's lives. If we do not acknowledge the contentious nature of health and have a sound understanding of the determinants of our preferred conceptualization, it is unlikely that we will be able to develop incisive strategies for promoting it.

Defining health: contrasting and conflicting conceptualizations

A number of tensions emerge in defining health. These include the relative emphasis on:

- disease or well-being
- holistic or atomistic interpretations
- the individual or the collective
- lay or professional perspectives
- subjective or objective interpretations.

One of the most persistent distinctions between definitions of health has been whether the focus is on wellness or on the absence of disease.

As Cross et al. (2021: 17) argue, it is very difficult, if not impossible, to reach a consensual definition of what health *is*. Probably the best known definition of health comes from the Constitution of the World Health Organization (1946, 2006a): 'Health is a state of complete physical, mental and social well-being and not merely the absence of disease or infirmity.' While this definition has been criticized because of its utopian nature, the use of the word 'complete' (Oleribe et al., 2018) and therefore as impossible to achieve (Blaxter, 2010), it extended the boundaries of health beyond the absence of disease to include positive well-being and firmly acknowledged the multidimensional, holistic nature of health. The Constitution further asserts that:

> The enjoyment of the highest attainable standard of health is one of the fundamental rights of every human being without distinction of race, religion, political belief, economic or social condition.

This assertion, also enshrined in numerous United Nations human rights treaties such as the International Covenant on Economic, Social and Cultural Rights (Office of the High Commissioner for Human Rights [OHCHR], 1966) and the Universal Declaration on Human Rights (UN, 1948), politicizes health and places pressure on governments to create the conditions supportive of health (WHO, 2007a). Furthermore, this emphasis on health as a fundamental human right focuses the attention of those seeking to promote health on equity and empowerment.

We have seen understandings about subjective health turn more towards notions of happiness, well-being, mental health, resilience and assets. This potentially makes the limits to health boundless, leading to all problems becoming 'health' problems and possibly unleashing unlimited demands for health services. It could arguably, therefore, undermine health and human rights arguments. Some argue for more attention to be paid to notions such as quality of life and, as seen in more recent trends, well-being (Ruggeri et al., 2020).

Lay interpretations of health

Notwithstanding the undoubted difficulties associated with measurement, from a health promotion perspective, the subjective element – health as it is experienced in people's lives – is of central importance. Buchanan (2006), who has defined health as synonymous with the 'good life' ('a life worth living, with the means to flourish and thrive' – Komduur et al., 2009: 307), emphasizes the importance of subjective, autonomous interpretations:

> we should shift the emphasis in the field from the rather narrow focus on producing specimens of physical fitness, to a broader concern for human wellbeing, here understood in terms of enhancing moral judgment, promoting greater self-understanding, liberating people from scientistic assumptions (perpetuating the belief that human behavior is determined by antecedent causes that only highly trained scientists can divine), advancing the cause of social justice, and promoting respect for the diversity of understandings of the good life for human beings. (2006: 302)

This draws attention to lay interpretations of health that will be considered more fully in Chapter 2. However, for now it is relevant to observe that lay interpretations are complex and multidimensional. The absence of disease is central to lay views, but resilience – the ability to cope with life – and functional capacity are also important (see Abstract 1.1). Social class differences have also been noted (Blaxter, 2010; Calnan, 1987; Hu et al., 2021), with a greater emphasis on the ability to function in lower social classes, a more multidimensional conceptualization including positive well-being in higher social classes as well as differences in perceptions of the ability to self-manage health (this increases with social class). Lay interpretations of health inequalities also differ (Garthwaite and Bambra, 2017). While lay interpretations are often taken to be different from more systematized 'professional' accounts, commonalities do exist. Lay accounts – particularly public as opposed to private accounts – tend to incorporate knowledge and understandings developed in expert paradigms (Shaw, 2002). One of the difficulties that we have in establishing lay beliefs about health is that much of the research that claims to explore these actually focuses on ill health and disease rather than on more positive notions of health (Hughner and Kleine, 2004).

ABSTRACT 1.1

Do conceptualisations of health differ across social strata? A concept mapping study among lay people. Stronks, K., Hoeymans, N., Haverkamp, B., den Hertog, F.R.J., van Bon-Martens, M.J.H., Galenkamp, H., Verweij, M. and van Oers, H.A.M. (2018)

Objectives: The legitimacy of policies that aim at tackling socioeconomic inequalities in health can be challenged if they do not reflect the conceptualizations of health that are valued in all strata. Therefore, this study analyses how different socioeconomic groups formulate their own answer regarding: what does health mean to you?

Design: Concept mapping procedures were performed in three groups that differ in educational level. All procedures followed exactly the same design.

Setting: Area of the city of Utrecht, the Netherlands.

Participants: Lay persons with a lower, intermediate and higher educational level (+/−15/group).

Results: The concept maps for the three groups consisted of nine, eight and seven clusters each, respectively. Four clusters occurred in all groups: absence of disease/disabilities, health-related behaviours, social life, attitude towards life. The content of some of these differed between groups; for example, behaviours were interpreted as having the opportunities to behave healthily in the lower education group and in terms of their impact on health in the higher education group. Other clusters appeared to be specific for particular groups, such as autonomy (intermediate/higher education group). Finally, ranking ranged from a higher ranking of the positively formulated aspects in the higher education group (e.g. lust for life) to that of the negatively formulated aspects in the lower education group (e.g. having no chronic disease).

Conclusion: The results provide indications to suggest that people in lower socioeconomic groups are more likely to show a conceptualization of health that refers to (1) the absence of health threats (vs positive aspects), (2) a person within his/her circumstances (vs quality of own body/mind), (3) the value of functional (vs hedonistic) notions and (4) an accepting (vs active) attitude towards life.

Adaptation, actualization, ends and means

Utopian visions of health, while aspirational and even inspirational, are ultimately unattainable. Humanity rarely, if ever, achieves stasis. People are constantly engaged in an often-problematic process of adaptation to their environments – to their physical, material, economic and social circumstances. The dynamic interaction between individuals and their environments is recognized in definitions of health promotion as enabling people to gain control over their lives and their health (WHO, 1984). Dubos's (1979) influential perspective on health supposes that positive health is a mirage. As reiterated by Blaxter (2010) – health is evanescent and unattainable, but worth pursuing. If health means anything, it resides in the pursuit, in engaging with these constantly changing and typically unpredictable environmental forces.

Aspects of Maslow's (1970) notion of self-actualization resonate with Dubos's perspective on the nature of health. Maslow defines it as follows:

> Self-actualization … refers to man's [*sic*] desire for self-fulfilment, namely, to the tendency for him to become actualized in what he is potentially. This tendency might be phrased as the desire to become more and more what one idiosyncratically is, to become everything that one is capable of becoming … In other words, 'What a man *can* be, he *must* be.' (1970: 46)

Self-actualization is encapsulated as the full realization of one's creative, intellectual and social potential (Selva, 2021). Apart from providing a useful operational definition of psychological health and his emphasis on the importance of self-esteem, Maslow's work has considerable relevance for the empowerment imperative of health promotion. Furthermore, it raises the issue of whether health is an end in itself – a terminal value – or whether it is instrumental for the achievement of other valued goals. The latter interpretation is encapsulated in the Ottawa Charter conceptualization of health as a 'resource for everyday life, not the objective of living' (WHO, 1986) and in the Declaration of Alma Ata (WHO, 1978) as a means of achieving a 'socially and economically productive life'. Whether desired goals in this context are defined by individuals themselves or by society generates further questions about the respective emphasis on self-actualization or collective responsibility.

Coherence, commitment and control: health as empowerment

In an article published posthumously, Antonovsky (1996) declared his concern about the dominant paradigm common to both medicine and health promotion. This, he argued, is based on the dichotomous classification of people into those who have succumbed to disease as a result of exposure to risk factors, and those who have not. He urged health promoters to move away from this obsession with risk factors and adopt a 'salutogenic model' that views health and disease as a continuum and focuses on the conditions leading to wellness.

'Salutogenesis' is a key concept that focuses on the 'salutary' – that is, health enhancing – rather than 'pathogenic' – that is, disease causing aspects of health. It incorporates Antonovsky's main theory about the factors that determine the extent to which people become healthy and experience well-being. Central to this theory is the challenge posed by coping with 'the inherent stressors of human existence' (1996: 15) – encapsulated in the notion of 'entropy' that refers to the level of disorder within systems. At a psychological level, it refers to *perceptions* that disorder exists. People's worlds may be more or less chaotic. Such 'chaos' is held to be undesirable, whether it exists in reality or only in people's perceptions. The salutogenic approach is, therefore, designed to reduce entropy and perceptions of entropy and, in so doing, generate a sense of coherence, which it identifies as a central attribute of a healthy person.

Antonovsky defines coherence as:

> a global orientation that expresses the extent to which one has a pervasive, enduring though dynamic feeling of confidence that one's internal and external environments are predictable and that there is a high probability that things will work out as well as can reasonably be expected. (1979: 123)

The three main elements are comprehensibility, manageability and meaningfulness. These are concerned with how we make sense of the world around us and what we experience; how we feel about this and the extent to which we are able to manage or cope with the challenges of life (Sidell, 2010). Mittelmark and Bauer (2022: 11) note that 'in its most general meaning, salutogenesis refers to a *salutogenic orientation* … focusing attention on the origins of health and assets for (positive) health, contra to the origins of disease and risk factors'. Salutogenesis has received increasing international attention in health promotion research and health policy over the past two decades led by work by the International Union of Health Promotion and Education (IUHPE). This has resulted in the second edition of *The Handbook of Salutogenesis* (Mittelmark et al., 2022). In the foreword to this book Margaret Barry, President of the IUHPE, writes 'an understanding of the nature of positive health, how it is created and can be sustained at a population level, is critically important to provide a theoretical base for health promotion and its implementation in practice' (Barry, 2022: v).

Health and empowerment

The concept of empowerment will receive further consideration throughout this book. For now, we will confine the discussion to the relationship between empowerment and health. If we accept that having control is central to definitions of health, a number of alternatives follow. First, empowerment could be seen as synonymous with (positive) health. In other words, to be healthy is to be empowered! Alternatively, empowerment could be seen as instrumental – that is, as a means to achieving (positive) health. A third conceptualization is also possible. Empowerment could be viewed as both a terminal and an instrumental value. The standpoint here is that empowerment will necessarily be a key component of positive health as an end. At the same time, it will be a means, if not the most important means, to achieving disease prevention and management goals that are components of holistic interpretations of health.

The Commission on Social Determinants of Health (2007) emphasizes the importance of empowerment as a means to achieving health equity. It identifies three key dimensions of empowerment – material, psychosocial and political – and focuses attention on the structural factors necessary for empowerment. It particularly notes the disadvantaged position of women. A health equity perspective on empowerment is highlighted further by Popay (2021: 2), who argues that community empowerment should be understood as a sociopolitical process which disrupts power dynamics in order that 'people bearing the brunt of social injustice [can] exercise greater collective control over decisions and actions that impact their lives and health'.

We might make two further observations on empowerment in the context of salutogenesis. First, two of the three key requisites of a sense of coherence – notably, comprehensibility and manageability – are concerned with beliefs about control and these also figure prominently in conceptualizations of empowerment. Second, there is potential conflict between empowerment and the sense of meaningfulness, which is the third element of a sense of coherence. In short, while the feeling that 'all is for the best in the best of all possible worlds' will doubtless make people feel better, and that life, from a salutogenic perspective, is more meaningful, it may well be delusory and hence disempowering.

HEALTH: A WORKING MODEL

As may be seen in Figure 1.1, for all practical purposes, health is defined as having both positive and negative aspects. The term 'well-being' is used as shorthand for the positive dimension. Rather than seeing well-being and disease as opposite ends of a single spectrum, they are represented as coexisting. Furthermore, although each may influence the other, they can vary independently. For example, although well-being may be affected by the presence of negative disease states, it is possible, even desirable, to have high levels of well-being regardless of disease being present. Conversely, there may be high or low states of well-being in the absence of disease. We are quite clear that preventing and managing disease and disability is a laudable goal in its own right and a central concern of those who are professionally involved in healthcare and health promotion. However, it is equally clear that the more positive dimensions must also figure prominently in the formulation of a satisfactory definition of health. In the first place, those involved in public health and health promotion cannot ignore its

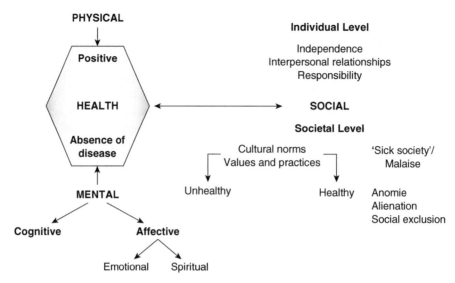

Figure 1.1 A working model of health

importance. But also, those measures that result in the achievement of positive goals are frequently more effective in achieving preventive outcomes than the more limited tactics employed by espousing a narrow disease prevention model.

Being all that you can be

The three components that make up WHO's holistic conception of health are featured in the model. Following Maslowian self-actualization principles, it is tempting to argue that maximal health status involves 'being all that you can be'. Healthy individuals would thus be those who had fulfilled their mental, physical and social potential. As we have argued, the attainment of complete mental, physical and social health is logically and practically impossible. Furthermore, it would be feasible to achieve high levels of potential in relation to one component of health at the expense of others. For example, the degree of commitment required to achieve maximal physical fitness might not only militate against social health and, possibly, be inconsistent with cultural norms, it might also be viewed as evidence of obsessional neurosis! Equally, a lifestyle characterized by sloth and self-abuse might lead to considerable happiness and a very successful social life, but result in an early death.

Accordingly, health must involve some kind of balance between mental, physical and social components. How, though, is such a balance to be determined? Do individuals themselves make the decision or should society decide for them? As the second option is inconsistent with the principles of empowerment (which are intrinsically healthy), only the first option is a serious contender. We will, however, emphasize later in this book the importance of healthy individuals being guided by commitment to a considerate way of life. Thus, individuals should be in a sufficiently empowered position to enable them to choose a course of action, provided only that the rights of other people are not damaged and, ideally, take action to support those who may be disadvantaged.

Mental, social and spiritual health

The definition of physical health is comparatively straightforward. On the one hand, it is associated with minimizing disease and disability; on the other hand, it may involve having a sufficient level of fitness necessary for achieving other (more important) life goals and/or the experience of high-level wellness or, more realistically, the feelings of well-being (allegedly) associated with a high degree of physical fitness. Well-being may thus be associated with fitness, but is by no means an identical dimension of health. A person might, for example, exhibit high levels of fitness, but limited feelings of well-being or, alternatively, high levels of well-being but minimal fitness!

Defining mental health is rather more complicated and problematic. We will confine the current discussion to making just two observations. First, it is useful to consider mental health as having both cognitive and affective dimensions. The affective dimension includes emotions and feelings and most discourse on mental health centres on this aspect. The cognitive dimension rarely features in definitions of mental health, but might be incorporated in a holistic model. 'Being all you can be' in cognitive terms refers to the extent to which individuals fulfil their intellectual potential. The reasons for failure to fulfil intellectual potential have been a source of considerable study and evidence of inequity in this regard has provoked concern. It is thus intimately associated with broad-based health promotion initiatives designed to address general social inequalities and break cycles of deprivation. Second, many people have asserted that any serious consideration of positive health must include the spiritual dimension. This is itself open to several interpretations, but features in Figure 1.1 in the context of mental health and well-being. It has both a cognitive element, consisting of the doctrinal aspects of, for instance, a religious system, and the emotional commitment associated, in this case, with the value system central to the notion of faith which can be integral to meaningfulness and the sense of coherence that is central to salutogenesis. Furthermore, religious values can underpin personal health choices and a sense of responsibility towards upholding the rights of others to health. Spiritual health, while variously defined (Jaberi et al., 2019), receives increasing attention, as does spiritual health promotion. Spiritual health is viewed by many as an important aspect of human health alongside physical, mental and social health (Nunes et al., 2018). However, the ambiguities and vagueness of the term spiritual health have been noted and a comprehensive definition is lacking (Ghaderi et al, 2018). Hanrieder (2017) noted the shift to discourses around religious health assets and the 'faith factor', recognizing the value, benefits and advantages that these bring to subjective health experience and general well-being in a range of different global contexts.

The importance of mental health and well-being was highlighted by the publication of the *Perth Charter for the Promotion of Mental Health and Wellbeing* (2012), which resulted from the 7th World Conference on the Promotion of Mental Health and the Prevention of Mental and Behavioural Disorders. While acknowledging the importance of the holistic stance of the Ottawa Charter for Health Promotion, the Perth Charter argues that 'health promotion in practice has largely been confined to physical health promotion' and that therefore the Perth Charter should be viewed as 'a first step towards the eventual integration of physical and mental health promotion' (*Perth Charter for the Promotion of Mental Health and Wellbeing*, 2012). It sets out seven key principles as follows:

- *Principle 1*: Mental health is more than the absence of mental illness. Mental health promotion includes both preventing illness and increasing well-being.

- *Principle 2*: The foundations of social and emotional well-being develop in early childhood and must be sustained throughout the lifespan.
- *Principle 3*: Mental health promotion must be integrated with public health and requires a cross-sectional approach.
- *Principle 4*: Mental health and illness are constructed, experienced and viewed as different to physical health and illness.
- *Principle 5*: Mental health and mental illness are a dynamic balance.
- *Principle 6*: Destigmatization of mental illness and addressing discrimination are essential components of mental health promotion.
- *Principle 7*: Mental health promotion must take place at the individual and societal levels.

Lay interpretations of mental health are also central to the promotion of mental health. In a Danish study exploring lay understandings of mental health a participant defined mental health as 'what makes life worth living' (Nielsen et al., 2017: 26). This points to the importance of mental health for subjective health experience.

Social health: individual and society

The social dimension of health is equally complex. As can be seen from Figure 1.1, there are two categories. The first of these refers to the social health of the individual; the second is concerned with the health of society itself. Three main aspects of individual social health have been identified.

Independence: a socially mature individual acts with greater independence and autonomy than a relatively immature individual.

Interpersonal relationships: a socially healthy individual is characterized by the capacity to relate to a number of significant others and cooperate with them.

Responsibility: a person who is socially mature accepts responsibility for others.

The distinction between the social health of individuals and the health of society is recognized in everyday parlance with references to 'sick societies' and 'social malaise'. We will make further reference to this dimension of social health later in this chapter and at a number of points in this book when we consider the concerns in health promotion with powerlessness, meaninglessness, normlessness, isolation and self-estrangement that are characteristic of 'sick societies' and contribute to social exclusion.

PROMOTING HEALTH: COMPETING IDEOLOGIES

No science is immune to the infection of politics and the corruption of power.

Dr Jacob Bronowski, *The Ascent of Man*, BBC2, 1973

Defining health promotion

A key issue in defining health promotion is whether it is viewed as an umbrella term, covering the activities of a range of disciplines committed to improving the health of the population, or as a discipline in its own right. Bunton and Macdonald (2002: 6) suggest that 'recent changes in the knowledge base and the practice of health promotion are characteristic of paradigmatic and disciplinary development'. They take a discipline to involve an ordered field of study embracing associated theories, perspectives and methods. A discipline would be expected to have its own ideology that would also inform standards of professional practice. Prior to our analysis of the ideology of health promotion and the values integral to different models, we will briefly clarify the distinction between health education and health promotion.

Although the generic use of the term 'health promotion' to describe any activity that improves health status can be traced back earlier, Terris (1996) noted that in 1945 Henry Sigerist described the four tasks of medicine as the promotion of health, prevention of illness, restoration and rehabilitation of the sick (cited by French, 2000). However, it was not until the late 1970s that this term began to be applied in a more specific way to a concept, movement, discipline and, indeed, profession. While a systematic account of the history of health promotion is beyond the scope of this text, we should note that the roots of contemporary health promotion are in health education.

The earliest examples of health education in the context of public health would now be described as health propaganda. This typically took the form of pamphleteering, which was intended to generate political change in support of a variety of environmental health measures designed to combat squalor and provide clean water supplies. Early health education was thus seen as an adjunct to public health efforts. Indeed, Wills (2023: 56) notes that, by the 1920s, health education had become associated with 'diarrhoea, dirt, spitting and venereal disease!' With this increasing focus on personal rather than public health, health educators continued their adjuvant role in support of the medical profession. Their activity during this period essentially involved giving information and persuading people using mass communication strategies.

The dominant themes in the early health education journals of the 1950s and 1960s centred on methods of delivering information in ways that would attract attention and interest people in the substantive content of health messages. The primary concern was very much with the technicalities of delivering information. The assumption was that if people were given the 'right' knowledge, they would act appropriately. As we will see in Chapter 3, this grossly underestimated the complexity of the task.

Two broad paths can be traced in the subsequent development of health education. One, the *preventive approach*, sought ever more sophisticated ways of achieving behaviour change by means of the application of psychological theory. The other, which was more in tune with progressive educational philosophy, was concerned with enabling people to make informed choices, the so-called *educational approach*.

In the period following the Lalonde Report (Lalonde, 1974) on the health status of the population of Canada, a renewed interest in the importance of the social and environmental influences on health status – both directly and indirectly by shaping behaviour – brought health education under fierce critical scrutiny (see, for example, Navarro, 1976; Ryan, 1976). Of particular concern were the emphasis on individual responsibility and the failure to recognize constraints on individuals' behaviour – most notably their economic and material circumstances. Health education was accused of 'victim-blaming' – a term attributed to Ryan. The essence of victim-blaming lies in attempts to persuade individuals to take responsibility for their own health while ignoring the fact that they are victims of social and environmental circumstances. It is now several decades since these criticisms were levelled at health education yet we still often see the focus on individual responsibility at the expense of taking into account the social and structural determinants of health (Lee, 2019). The emergence of health promotion was in response to the need to address the environmental as well as the behavioural determinants of health – the so-called upstream determinants. In effect, it marked a shift from being concerned with healthy choices to making 'the healthy choice the easy choice'.

Health promotion includes efforts to tackle the social and environmental determinants of health by means of healthy public policy. The scope of health promotion can, therefore, be summed up in a simple formula:

health promotion = health education × healthy public policy

We will review different models of health promotion later in this chapter. At this point, we will consider the influence of the WHO on the development of health promotion.

The contribution of the World Health Organization (WHO) to the definition of health promotion

The evolution of health promotion has been accompanied by considerable debate about its nature and purpose – debate that has exposed its core underlying values. The WHO has been a major voice in shaping the development of health promotion. Not only have its documents been a source of reference for health promotion practice, but they have also been assimilated into professional training courses – that is, they have become part of the doctrine of health promotion.

As mentioned above, the WHO has taken a holistic view of health from its inception. The 'Health for All' movement was launched at the 30th World Health Assembly in 1977. The following year saw the *Declaration of Alma Ata* (WHO, 1978), which identified primary healthcare (PHC) as the principal means to attaining 'Health for All' targets. Primary healthcare – as distinct from primary medical care – was envisaged as embracing all the services that impact on health, including, for example, education, housing and agriculture.

A number of key issues in the *Declaration* have informed subsequent thinking. In addition to emphasizing the importance of a holistic view of health, the following assertions figure in many WHO publications and declarations:

- health as a fundamental right
- the unacceptability of inequality in health within and between nations
- health as a major social goal
- the reciprocal relationship between health and social development
- the need to involve a number of different sectors in working towards health

- the rights and duties of individuals to participate individually and collectively in their own healthcare
- education as the means of developing communities' capacity to participate.

In January 1984, the WHO set up a new programme on 'health promotion'. A discussion document on health promotion (WHO, 1984) saw it as a 'unifying concept', bringing together 'those who recognize the need for change in the ways and conditions of living, in order to promote health'. It defined health promotion as 'the process of enabling people to increase control over, and to improve, their health'.

Income, shelter and food were acknowledged to be primary requisites for health. Importance was also attached to the provision of information and life skills, the creation of supportive environments providing opportunities for making healthy choices and the creation of health-enhancing conditions in the economic, physical, social and cultural environments.

The document outlined the key principles of health promotion as:

- the involvement of the whole population in the context of their everyday life and enabling people to take control of, and have responsibility for, their health
- tackling the determinants of health – that is, an upstream approach, which demands the cooperative efforts of a number of different sectors at all levels, from national to local
- utilizing a range of different, but complementary, methods and approaches – from legislation and fiscal measures, organizational change and community development to education and communication
- effective public participation, which may require the development of individual and community capacity
- the role of health professionals in education and advocacy for health. (WHO, 1984)

Action was, therefore, seen to require an integrated effort to encourage individual and community responsibility for health along with the development of a health-enhancing environment. The document reflected a commitment to voluntarism and formally acknowledged the risk of dictating how individuals should behave. This has been referred to as 'healthism' – a notion that we will return to later. Other potential problems included an overemphasis on individual behaviour rather than the social and economic determinants of behaviour and the possibility of increasing social inequality if the varying capacity of different social groups to exercise control over their health was not tackled. A further concern was that health promotion might be appropriated by particular professional groups to the exclusion of others and lay people.

A series of major international conferences followed. The Ottawa Charter, developed at the 1st International Conference on Health Promotion (WHO, 1986), built on many of the key principles set out in the WHO discussion document and has been a constant source of reference. It identified three broad strategies for working to promote health:

- **advocacy** to ensure the creation of conditions favourable to health
- **enabling** by creating a supportive environment, but also by giving people the information and skills that they need to make healthy choices
- **mediation** between different groups to ensure the pursuit of health.

The Ottawa Charter listed five main action areas that have been central to the conceptual framework of health promotion:

- build healthy public policy
- create supportive environments
- strengthen community action
- develop personal skills
- reorient health services.

There is potentially some tension between individual and societal responsibility for health, between individual and collective responsibility, and between voluntarism and control. The Ottawa Charter handled this by seeing individuals as having responsibility for their own health, but also a collective concern for the health of others. However, there is an overriding societal responsibility to create the conditions that enable people to take control of their health. Recognition that health is created where people 'learn, work, play and love' heralded the 'settings approach' to health promotion.

The 2nd International Conference on Health Promotion in Adelaide (WHO, 1988) focused on healthy public policy as a means of creating supportive environments that would be health-enhancing in themselves and would also – in the words of the much-used phrase – contribute to making the healthy choice the easy choice. In particular, it acknowledged the importance of addressing the needs of underprivileged and disadvantaged groups and emphasized the responsibility of higher-income countries to ensure that their own policies impacted positively on lower-income countries. It saw healthy public policy as 'characterized by an explicit concern for health and equity in all areas of policy and an accountability for health impact'. The Adelaide Conference identified the need for strong advocates and also saw community action as a major driving force.

The Sundsvall Conference (WHO, 1991) addressed the issue of supportive environments for health. In addition to the physical environment, it recognized the importance of the social environment and the influence of social norms and culture on behaviour. It also noted the challenge to traditional values arising from changing lifestyles, increasing social isolation and lack of a sense of coherence. The need for action at all levels and across sectors was recognized and, in particular, the capacity for community action.

The key elements of a 'democratic health promotion approach' were seen to be empowerment and community participation. The importance of education as a means of bringing about political, economic and social changes was recognized as well as its being a basic human right.

The Jakarta Declaration on Leading Health Promotion into the 21st Century (WHO, 1997) was developed at the 4th International Conference on Health Promotion. It viewed health both as a right and as instrumental to social and economic development. It envisaged the 'ultimate goal' of health promotion as increasing health expectancy by means of action directed at the determinants of health in order to:

- create the greatest health gain
- contribute to reduction in inequities
- further human rights
- build social capital.

The Jakarta Declaration built on the commitments of the previous documents and provided clear endorsement of the value of comprehensive approaches and involving families and communities. It called for strong partnerships to promote health including – for the first time – the involvement of the private sector.

Overall, the priorities set out for the twenty-first century were to:

- promote social responsibility for health
- increase investments for health development
- consolidate and expand partnerships for health
- increase community capacity and empower the individual
- secure an infrastructure for health promotion.

The first resolution on health promotion, which was passed at the 51st World Health Assembly in May 1998 (WHO, 1998a), incorporated the thinking of the Jakarta Declaration.

As it moved into the twenty-first century, the WHO (1998b) identified the following key values underpinning the 'Health for All' movement:

- providing the highest attainable standard of health as a fundamental human right
- strengthening the application of ethics to health policy, research and service provision
- equity-orientated policies and strategies that emphasize solidarity
- incorporating a gender perspective into health policies and strategies. (1998d: v)

The 5th Global Conference on Health Promotion held in Mexico City in 2000 focused on 'bridging the equity gap'. It issued a Ministerial Statement signed by some 87 countries, including the United Kingdom (WHO, 2000a), that acknowledged that 'the promotion of health and social development is a central duty and responsibility of governments that all sectors of society share' and concluded that 'health promotion must be a fundamental component of public policies and programmes in all countries in the pursuit of equity and health for all'. The Mexico City conference emphasized the need to 'work with and through existing political systems and structures to ensure healthy public policy, adequate investment in health, and facilitation of an infrastructure for health promotion' (WHO, 2000b: 21).

The Bangkok Charter for Health Promotion in a Globalized World (WHO, 2005) responded to emerging global issues by focusing attention on increasing inequalities between countries, commercialization and new patterns of consumption and communication, and also global environmental change and urbanization. It identified the following required actions:

- advocate for health based on human rights and solidarity
- invest in sustainable policies, actions and infrastructure to address the determinants of health
- build capacity for policy development, leadership, health promotion practice, knowledge transfer and research, and health literacy
- regulate and legislate to ensure a high level of protection from harm and enable equal opportunity for health and well-being for all people

- partner and build alliances with public, private, non-governmental and international organizations and civil society to create sustainable actions.

It further demanded four key commitments, to make health promotion:

- central to the global development agenda
- a core responsibility for all of government
- a key focus for communities and civil society
- a requirement for good corporate practice.

While the primary concern of these documents has been with identifying appropriate action, they are underpinned by clear values. Indeed, it could be said that unless activity is consistent with these values, it should not be regarded as 'health promotion'. These values include equity and empowerment – the twin pillars of health promotion – along with health as a right, voluntarism, autonomy, participation, partnerships and social justice. Consideration of rights and responsibilities, power and control generates some interesting paradoxes in relation to health education and policy interventions, which we discuss more fully later.

The 7th and 8th WHO conferences on health promotion were held in Nairobi in 2009 and Helsinki in 2013, respectively. Importantly, the Nairobi conference was the first to be held on the continent of Africa. The Nairobi Call for Action specifically addresses action needed to close the implementation gap in health and development through health promotion (Catford, 2010; WHO, 2009). One of the key themes of this conference was mainstreaming health promotion in health policy (Eriksson, 2010). Empowerment remained central. The key urgent responsibilities were outlined as follows:

- strengthen leadership and workforces
- mainstream health promotion
- empower communities and individuals
- enhance participatory processes
- build and apply knowledge. (WHO, 2009)

The importance of policy was again highlighted in the Helsinki conference. Intersectoral action and healthy public policy were identified as key requirements for health promotion. The conference statement emphasizes the 'Health in All Policies' approach, calling for cross-governmental action and political will (WHO, 2013e).

The significance of non-communicable diseases was emphasized at the Nairobi conference in 2009 and this was picked up in 2011 at the UN High-Level Meeting of the General Assembly on the Prevention and Control of Non-Communicable Diseases (NCDs). NCDs kill three in five people globally (UN, 2011) and are becoming much more of a challenge in lower-income countries. A political declaration ensued from this meeting specifically aimed at tackling NCDs. In the same year, the WHO held a world conference in Brazil on the Social Determinants of Health (WHO, 2011). This resulted in the adoption of the *Rio Political Declaration on Social Determinants of Health* (WHO, 2012). The declaration upholds the core principles established by the Alma Ata conference in 1978 and the

Ottawa Charter (WHO, 1986) that have been reinforced by the subsequent WHO conferences on health promotion as detailed previously.

The 9th Global Conference on Health Promotion took place in Shanghai in late 2016. The resulting declaration focuses on promoting health in the 2030 Agenda for Sustainable Development in recognition that 'health and well-being are essential to achieving the United Nations Development Agenda and its Sustainable Development Goals and reinforces the importance of structural factors and of the wider determinants of health' (see Box 1.1).

BOX 1.1 THE SHANGHAI DECLARATION

We reaffirm health as a universal right, an essential resource for everyday living, a shared social goal and a political priority for all countries. The UN Sustainable Development Goals (SDGs) establish a duty to invest in health, ensure universal health coverage and reduce health inequities for people of all ages. **We are determined to leave no one behind.**

Call to action

We recognize that health is a **political choice and we will counteract interests detrimental to health and remove barriers to empowerment** – especially for women and girls. We urge political leaders from different sectors and from different levels of governance, from the private sector and from civil society to join us in our determination to promote health and wellbeing in all the SDGs. Promoting health demands coordinated action by all concerned, it is a shared responsibility. With this Shanghai Declaration, we, the participants, pledge to accelerate the implementation of the SDGs through increased political commitment and financial investment in health promotion.

Source: WHO (2016a)

The 10th Global Conference on Health Promotion took place in December 2021 – *Health Promotion for Well-being, Equity and Sustainable Development* – 'marking the start of a global movement on the concept of well-being in societies' (WHO, 2021a: npn). Given the global impact of the COVID-19 pandemic the conference met virtually for the first time. The conference resulted in the *Geneva Charter for Well-being*, which highlights the importance of well-being, not just for people and society but for the planet itself. Five key action areas were identified, as follows (WHO, 2021a):

- design an equitable economy that serves human development within planetary boundaries
- create public policy for the common good
- achieve universal health coverage
- address the digital transformation to counteract harm and disempowerment and to strengthen the benefits
- value and preserve the planet.

The charter re-emphasized the importance of many of the themes of the preceding WHO conferences, such as intersectoral working, the importance of partnership and political will. Planetary health and sustainability were key concerns and there was a call to reframe health as 'an investment in our common future' (WHO, 2021a: npn).

Ideology, social construction and competing discourses

Defining ideology

The original meaning of 'ideology' was merely the scientific study of human ideas. It has been transformed over time into a concept that includes cognitive, affective and action dimensions. Although ideologies are value laden – and it is not unusual for the term to be used synonymously with value systems – the contemporary construction of the word 'ideology' is much more complex.

De Kadt, discussing the ideological dimensions involved in implementing WHO's 'Health for All' agenda, states that ideologies are an amalgam of fact and unsubstantiated assertion. He observes that 'comprehensive ideologies (as opposed to partial ideologies) are commitment-demanding views about societies, their past history and present operation, which contain a strong evaluative element and hence provide goals for the future' (de Kadt, 1982: 742).

In order to clarify the central meaning of 'ideology', Eagleton contrasts the emotionally charged nature of ideology, which has a 'partial and biased view of the world', with an 'empirical' or 'pragmatic' approach. There is, of course, a tendency for those espousing political causes to describe their 'pragmatic' construction of reality as rational and based on common sense whereas opponents' views are characterized by ideological zealotry involving, as Eagleton notes, their:

> judging a particular issue through some rigid framework of preconceived ideas which distorts their understanding. I view things as they really are; you squint at them through a tunnel vision imposed by some extraneous system of doctrine. There is usually a suggestion that this involves an over-simplifying view of the world – that to speak or judge 'ideologically' is to do so schematically, stereotypically, and perhaps with the faintest hint of fanaticism. (1991: 3)

Ideology, values and ethics

Belief systems and doctrine are major parts of the territory of ideology. However, values and value systems feature with equal prominence. Rokeach defines values as 'an enduring belief that a specific mode of conduct or endstate of existence is personally or socially preferable to an opposite or converse mode of conduct or endstate of existence' (1973: 10). Following Guttman's (2000) review, the major ethical values assumed to underpin health promotion (or, more specifically, 'public health communication interventions') are:

- beneficence, or 'doing good'
- non-maleficence, or 'doing no harm'
- respect for personal autonomy

- justice or fairness
- utility and the public good
- (possibly) community involvement and participation.

These central ethical values have stood the test of time even though they, arguably, 'favour a biomedical paradigm with an individualistic focus' rather than 'a relational paradigm with a collective focus' (Smith et al., 2015: 232). As we will see, the extent to which these values are actually central to the ideology of health promotion will depend on the preferred model. At this point, it is interesting to note the remarkable degree of resonance between the empowerment model of health promotion and the stewardship model (see Box 1.2) developed by the Nuffield Council on Bioethics. It sets out the ethical principles that should underpin the development of healthy public policy and achieve a balance between individual and government responsibility.

BOX 1.2   THE STEWARDSHIP MODEL

Acceptable public health goals include:

- reducing the risks of ill health that result from other people's actions, such as drinking and smoking in public places
- reducing causes of ill health relating to environmental conditions, for instance provision of clean drinking water and setting housing standards
- protecting and promoting the health of children and other vulnerable people
- helping people to overcome addictions that are harmful to health or helping them to avoid unhealthy behaviours
- ensuring that it is easy for people to lead a healthy life, for example by providing convenient and safe opportunities for exercise
- ensuring that people have appropriate access to medical services
- reducing unfair health inequalities.

At the same time, public health programmes should:

- not attempt to coerce adults to lead healthy lives
- minimize the use of measures that are implemented without consulting people (either individually or using democratic procedures)
- minimize measures that are very intrusive or conflict with important aspects of personal life, such as privacy.

Source: Nuffield Council on Bioethics (2007)

The centrality of power

Given the emphasis on empowerment in this book, it is axiomatic that individual and community power are pivotal issues in the ideology of health promotion and central to the design of health promotion programmes. Questions of power feature prominently in discussions of ideology. Giddens and Sutton are quite explicit about this:

> Ideology refers to the influence of ideas on people's beliefs and actions … [it] is about the exercise of symbolic power – how ideas are used to hide, justify or legitimate the interests of dominant groups in the social order. (2021: 789)

Eagleton provides a comprehensive account of the mechanisms whereby a dominant group exerts its power and creates 'false consciousness':

> A dominant power may legitimate itself by *promoting* beliefs and values congenial to it; *naturalizing* and *universalizing* such beliefs so as to render them self-evident and apparently inevitable; *denigrating* ideas which might challenge it; *excluding* rival forms of thought, perhaps by some unspoken but systematic logic; and *obscuring* social reality in ways convenient to itself. (1991: 5–6)

The relevance of ideology is not only measured in terms of the ways in which the power of dominant social groups is legitimized. More significant for health promotion are the ways in which subordinate groups are 'de-powered' by dominant groups. Indeed, the radical ideology underpinning the model of health promotion proposed in this book is substantially concerned with empowering subordinate and oppressed social groups. Pursuing the matter of false consciousness, Eagleton reminds us of the subtle and potentially insidious ways in which people may be de-powered:

> The most efficient oppressor is the one who persuades his [*sic*] underlings to love, desire and identify with his power; and any practice of political emancipation thus involves that most difficult of all forms of liberation, freeing ourselves from ourselves. (1991: xiii)

He does, however, caution against exaggerating the power of this 'hegemonic' process and optimistically notes that nobody is ever wholly mystified. Despite a capacity for self-delusion, human beings are at least moderately rational and, unless the process of domination provides sufficient gratification over time, the dominated will rebel. If this were not true, health promotion's emancipatory strategies for critical consciousness-raising would be seriously compromised.

Ideology and discourse

Although, as Wodak (2008) argues, the term 'discourse' is used in various ways, there is general agreement that it is concerned with a set of 'connected sentences or utterances' (Litosseliti, 2006: 47) and patterns or systems of language (Lock and Strong, 2010). The notion of discourse has its roots in linguistics. It is more than mere language – rather, the thought underlying language. Accordingly, 'discourse analysis' involves penetrating beneath the surface of language or images and seeking out subtexts and meanings relating to wider beliefs and value systems – often their social and political contexts. As Parker (2005) argues, discourse analysis enables scrutiny of how language is mobilized to maintain (or challenge) power relations.

Discourse analysis has relevance for health promotion by providing insight into the way in which people's ideas about health – or indeed health promotion messages – are constructed, along with their underpinning values and motivations. The concern with challenging structures of power also renders it directly relevant. It can equally be applied to professional discourse to identify the underlying ideology.

Scott-Samuel and Springett draw attention to the interrelationship between discourse and power. Increase in the prominence of discourse may increase the power of groups that it represents and conversely power relations among different groups may shape the level of influence of discourse. They assert that the dominance of public health medicine has influenced the public health discourse and led to 'hegemonic suppression of the radical element within the public health agenda' (2007: 212).

Critical discourse analysis focuses on power and dominant ideologies and the way these are both reflected in and perpetuated by language (Lupton, 1992; Wood and Kroger, 2000). Fairclough has referred to it as 'discourse analysis "with an attitude"' (Fairclough, 2001, cited by Porter, 2006) reflecting critical examination of social cultural processes as well as the scrutiny of structures within society and issues of power/control (Litosseliti, 2006; Wodak, 2001; Wood and Kroger, 2000). Porter (2006) examined the Ottawa and Bangkok Charters using critical discourse analysis. She identified a shift from a '"new social movements" discourse of ecosocial justice in Ottawa to a "new capitalism" discourse of law and economics in Bangkok' (2006: 75). She also contends that while the Bangkok Charter proposes actions to tackle the problems of a globalized world, its discourse may serve to perpetuate the structural determinants of those very problems. The importance of analysing how discourse shapes, creates and maintains power is also emphasized by Garneau et al. (2019), who contend that 'attention to discourses that sustain inequities … is required to mitigate health inequalities and related power differentials' (p. 746).

Medical discourse and the preventive model

The history of health promotion has been marked by a struggle to distance itself from the medical model that has dominated twentieth-century discourse on health and illness. Some would contend that this break is more evident in the rhetoric than in the practice of health promotion (Kelly and Charlton, 1995). Although the medical model has been alluded to earlier, it is worthwhile considering – in the context of our discussion about ideology, power and control – the nature of the model and the origins of concern about its applicability to health promotion. The key features of the medical model have been variously seen as including:

- a mechanistic view of the body
- mind–body dualism
- disease as the product of disordered functioning of the body or a part of it
- a focus on pathogenesis – that is, the causes of disease
- the pursuit of the causal sequences of disease and an emphasis on micro-causality
- specific diseases having specific causes.

The medical model is, therefore, very much in tune with modernist rational thought and characterized by a reductionist view of the causes of ill health, together with a mechanistic focus on micro-causality.

The medical model is inextricably linked with medical practice and, more generally, with bio-medicine. It shares common ideological origins and has acquired added authority as a result of its association with the power and authority of the medical profession. The dominance of medicine has itself been the subject of an extensive sociological critique – for example, its role in supporting a cap-italist value system (Doyal and Pennell, 1979; Navarro, 1976); the monopolization of healthcare (de Kadt, 1982); the commodification of health and appropriation of authority over the areas that influ-ence health (Illich, 1976); and maintaining gendered power structures in society (Doyal and Pennell, 1979; Ehrenreich and English, 1979). Deborah Lupton offers a critique that carefully explicates the social and cultural construction of modern medicine and healthcare (Lupton, 2012).

The medical model belongs to a group that Rawson has termed 'iconic models' – that is, 'simplified descriptions of some aspect of known reality, portraying a literal or isomorphic image of nature' (1992: 210). It is possible, in principle, to identify a number of different models within medical practice and, equally, the medical model can be recognized within a range of different types of professional practice. It is also worth noting, in passing, that the ascendancy of high-tech medicine in the twentieth century and marginalization of preventive medicine has not gone unchallenged within medicine itself. The work of McKeown is well known in this regard (see, for example, McKeown, 1979). The emergence of 'The New Public Health' has been an attempt to retreat from an emphasis on individual responsi-bility for health and health actions and refocus on the factors that collectively influence health status. However, critics such as Petersen and Lupton (1996) contend that 'The New Public Health' has not entirely freed itself from the ethic of individual responsibility. Nor has it mounted an effective chal-lenge to the increasing disparity in wealth and power within many societies.

Application of the medical model to health promotion leads to an emphasis on prevention. This association with prevention effectively 'rebadges' the medical model as the preventive model.

The dominant concept is that of risk, whether viewed as a 'property of individuals or as an external threat' (Petersen and Lupton, 1996: 174). Furthermore, the conceptualization of risk is often narrow, ignoring the wider social and environmental determinants of health. The emphasis is on individual responsibility, which – as noted above in our comments on 'victim-blaming' – places the onus on individuals to reduce their exposure to risk by avoiding risky behaviour and contact with risks in the environment. The individual is increasingly held to account for managing risk and uncertainty (Arnoldi, 2009). Attempts to improve health primarily take the form of health education interven-tions to persuade individuals to adopt healthy behaviours and lifestyles, and avoid risk.

The preventive model has a number of consequences. As we noted above, it results in an essentially 'victim-blaming' approach in its disregard for the social, environmental and political factors that shape and, indeed, constrain behavioural choices.

Illich's (1976) critique of the extension of medical control beyond legitimate concern with disease to include ordinary aspects of human experience – so-called 'social iatrogenesis' or medicalization of life – is well known. Including exposure to risk within the medical remit and, along with it, a whole range of behavioural and lifestyle factors, extends the notion of medicalization even further and brings substantial areas of life under expert, rather than autonomous, control. Kelleher et al. note that, along with the decline in organized religion, this has led to:

doctors being cast more and more in the role of secular priests whose expertise encompassed not only the treatment of bodily ills but also advice on how to live the good life, and judgements on right and wrong behaviour. (1994: xii)

Moreover, the acknowledgement of expert authority over areas of life normally managed by individuals, families and communities erodes confidence in their own capacity to take responsibility for their health. By undermining self-reliance, communities and cultures are disempowered. Illich refers to this as 'cultural iatrogenesis', which he sees as 'destroy[ing] the potential of people to deal with their human weaknesses, vulnerability, and uniqueness in a personal and autonomous way' (1976: 42).

Horrobin's (1978) riposte to Illich accepts the existence of some undue dependence on the medical profession in matters of sickness, but notes the remarkable resistance of the healthy to accept medical advice and the over-exaggeration of the power of medicine to influence people.

Furthermore, he contends that Illich's portrayal of society as 'an ignorant and unwilling victim of medical imperialism' (1976: 29) is a misrepresentation. Here in 2022 we are witnessing something of a shift in power relations as noted by Eric Topol (2015) in his book *The Patient Will See You Now: The Future of Medicine is in Your Hands*, where he discusses the democratization of medicine that has occurred with rapidly changing technology centring on the increasing use of mobile devices (such as smartphones) to monitor, test and diagnose.

Notwithstanding these arguments, medicine is still accorded considerable expert power, a point endorsed by Lupton (2012). Healthy lifestyles/healthy behaviours are prescribed by experts (Ayo, 2012). Deference to such authority provides further legitimation. It reinforces the dominance of the medical model and *ipso facto* the preventive model, even when the view espoused is at odds with the experiences of individuals.

What, then, is the source of this medical authority? De Kadt suggests that:

Expertise and the 'life and death' responsibilities of the physician are used to provide ideological justification for physician dominance in the doctor–patient (healing) context. (1982: 746)

Parsons's (1958) concept of the 'sick role' throws further light on the doctor–patient interaction. When people are ill, they are unable to fulfil their normal social roles and everyday activities. Diagnosis will medically legitimate their adoption of the sick role that exempts them from their normal social obligations. However, there is a concomitant obligation to attempt to get better, by seeking and complying with medical advice. The sick role, therefore, requires submission to medical authority and compliance with a therapeutic regimen.

Formalization of the 'at-risk' role within the preventive model makes equivalent demands in terms of an obligation to modify behaviour and exposure to risk (Barić, 1969). Individuals are held responsible for their exposure to risk and failure to act accordingly may be attributed to ignorance at best or deliberate fecklessness at worst. Unlike the sick role, the at-risk role does not confer any rights. The outcome of this is twofold. On the one hand, it labels as deviant those who cannot or choose not to comply with admonitions on how to live their life, and holds them responsible for the consequences. The categorization of more and more areas of life as healthy or unhealthy effectively creates its own dogma about ways of living, coupled with the associated moral sanction of disapproval if unhealthy options are chosen. As Petersen and Lupton note:

The idealization of the 'normal', 'healthy' subject as one endowed with certain 'natural' capacities and inclinations fails to recognize the multiplicity of possible subject positions, and can serve to coerce, marginalize, stigmatize and discriminate against those who do not or cannot conform with the ideal. This ideal denies difference – whether this is based on social class, gender, sexuality, 'race' ethnicity, physical ability, or age – and the kinds of personal commitments and demands that are required of those who are called upon to conform to it. (1996: 178)

On the other hand, it creates a remorseless pressure to improve health. The responsibility for health lies with the individual (Bolam et al., 2003; Katainen, 2006). The identification of a number of lifestyle 'risk factors' linked to chronic ill health results in an emphasis on individual responsibility (Brown et al., 2019). As a result it has become a requirement, or moral imperative, for the contemporary citizen to strive for health (Nettleton, 2020; Petersen et al., 2010).

An overemphasis on keeping healthy has been referred to as 'healthism' – a term attributed to Crawford, who defines it as:

the preoccupation with personal health as a primary – often the primary – focus for the definition and achievement of wellbeing; a goal which is to be attained primarily through the modification of lifestyles, with or without therapeutic help. (1980: 368)

Despite healthism's emphasis on positive health, its focus on individual responsibility can be seen to have some parallels with victim-blaming. The no-fault principle enshrined in the notion of the sick role does not apply and is replaced by a 'your fault dogma'. Those, therefore, who fail, or refuse, to seek health-promoting ways of life become 'near pariahs' (Crawford, 1980: 379). Furthermore, preoccupation with health elevates it in status to a super value – health becomes an end in itself rather than a means of achieving other values, and positive health behaviour acts as a hallmark of good living. Crucially, the emphasis at the individual level draws attention away from government and social responsibility for health (Cross and O'Neil, 2021; Room, 2011).

 Reference to our earlier discussion of health promotion will indicate that the preventive model and healthism are both inconsistent with the two central tenets of health promotion – equity and empowerment. The emphasis on individualism and lack of attention to the social and environmental factors that impinge on health – both directly and indirectly as a result of their influence on behaviour – could, in fact, increase rather than decrease the health gap in society. Health gains will inevitably be greatest in those who are most able to make changes by virtue of their relatively advantaged position.

However, even though we have argued that a preventive model is inconsistent with the values position of health promotion, we should finish on a word of caution. Rejection of the preventive model does not necessarily imply rejection of the need for biomedical knowledge or appropriate preventive action. Furthermore, evidence about cause is necessary to much health promotion practice – indeed, any attempts to influence behaviour in the absence of evidence that this will be beneficial would be unethical. The problem lies not so much with a biomedical interpretation *per se*, but with too exclusive a reliance on it and dismissal of other perspectives – that is, with the imbalance of power and the dominance of medical expert authority. Our discussion of empowerment in Chapter 3 also draws attention to the importance of knowledge and the ability to access and interpret accurate knowledge as key components of empowerment. Such knowledge and understanding can give people greater control over their own lives. It also enables them to enter into a circle of shared understanding with professionals, thereby breaking down power structures and facilitating dialogue.

Education and the discourse of voluntarism

Health education is a key component of health promotion. We propose the following 'empirical' definition, which centres on the process of learning:

> health education is any planned activity designed to produce health- or illness-related learning.

'Learning' has frequently been defined as a relatively permanent change in capability or disposition – that is, the change produced is not transitory and, after the educational intervention, people are capable of achieving what they were not capable of achieving before the intervention and/or feel differently about ideas, people or events. Accordingly, effective health education may result in the development of cognitive capabilities such as the acquisition of factual information, understanding and insights. It may also provide skills in problem-solving and decision-making and the formation or development of beliefs. It might also result in the clarification of existing values and the creation of new values – and, quite frequently, in attitude change. Health education also aims to foster the acquisition of health-related psychomotor or social interaction skills. It may even bring about changes in behaviour or lifestyle or create the conditions for the adoption of healthy public policy.

One of the most important and enduring sources of ideological argument centres on the question of rationality and voluntarism. For example, Hirst (1969) asserted unequivocally that the central purpose of *all* education should be rationality. The educational philosopher Baelz contrasts education with manipulation and with indoctrination:

> The educator encourages his [*sic*] pupil to develop the capacity to think for himself, while the indoctrinator wishes to make it impossible for his pupil ever to question the doctrine that he has been taught. (1979: 32)

The concept of doctrine is equated with the notion of dogma and typically refers to some creed or body of religious, political or philosophical thought that is offered for acceptance as truth. The purpose of indoctrination is, therefore, to present a body of ideas in an appealing way such that the ideas are accepted. The distinction between indoctrination and education is, therefore, fundamental.

Health education, voluntarism and choices for health

For many health educators, voluntarism is an ideological *sine qua non*. Note, for instance, Green and Kreuter's influential definition:

> Health education is any combination of learning experiences designed to facilitate *voluntary* actions conducive to health ... *Voluntary* means *without coercion* and with the full understanding and acceptance of the purposes of the action. (1999: 27)

Faden and Faden (1978) made the point even more forcibly in their discussion of the ethics of health education. They cited the Society of Public Health Education (SOPHE) *Code of Ethics* (1976), noting its affirmation of the importance of voluntary consumer participation:

> Health educators value privacy, dignity, and the worth of the individual, and use skills consistent with these values. Health educators observe the principle of informed consent with respect to individuals and groups served. Health educators support change by choice, not by coercion.

According to the educational model of health education, coercive strategies and techniques are, therefore, unacceptable. Coercion occurs when an individual's or group's freedom of action is constrained. It frequently results from externally imposed sanctions or other barriers.

It is important, then, to recognize the existence of two varieties of coercion. The first of these is externally imposed. For instance, it involves the implementation of policy measures imposing a potentially wide range of restrictive regulations, in the form of legislation, fiscal measures and environmental engineering. Examples of such 'healthy public policies' would include banning smoking in public areas; redesigning roadways and traffic calming measures; the inclusion of vitamins in popular food products; regulation of the food industry to reduce the fat content of products; increase in the price of alcohol; and so on. The attraction of these various coercive strategies is doubtless self-evident, but McKinlay summarized it succinctly as follows:

> One stroke of effective health legislation is equal to many separate health intervention endeavours and the cumulative efforts of innumerable health workers over long periods of time. (1975: 13, in Guttman, 2000: 85)

The second form of coercion is perhaps less obvious and may be designated as psychological rather than environmental manipulation. It involves the use of certain techniques to create a particular kind of learning that lacks the element of genuine informed choice that characterizes the principle of voluntarism. Figure 1.2 locates these techniques on a continuum ranging from high degrees of coercion to maximal potential for facilitating 'free' choice. Accordingly, 'brainwashing' is seen as highly coercive while 'facilitation' is, by definition, seeking to assist learners to achieve their own goals. 'Persuasion' is generally viewed as an intervention concerned with achieving the goals of the persuader rather than helping the persuadees to make up their own minds.

In the case of psychological coercion or 'persuasion', personal choice is modified in some way without the knowledge of the person in question. In proposing this latter description, Faden and Faden (1978) had in mind Warwick and Kelman's (1973) definition of persuasion as a 'form of interpersonal influence, in which one person tries to change the attitudes or behaviour of another by means of argument, reasoning, or, in certain cases, structured listening'. In fact, it is somewhat misleading to define coercion of this kind solely in terms of the persuadee's lack of knowledge of what is going on. 'Insight' might be a better term as it is clear that, in many instances, individuals are well aware that someone is trying to influence them. Indeed, the most blatant form of psychological coercion, brainwashing, leaves the unfortunate recipient under no illusion that some fairly dramatic coercive techniques are being applied!

It may at first glance seem surprising that brainwashing has been partnered with primary socialization. This represents both an expression of doubt about the power of brainwashing to fundamentally

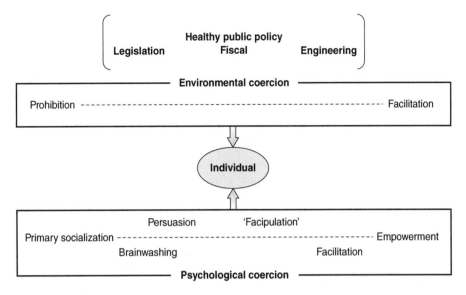

Figure 1.2 A spectrum of coercion

affect firmly grounded values and, at the same time, seeks to acknowledge the potentially greater power of the processes of 'shaping', conditioning and modelling that are part and parcel of the child-drearing experience.

At a more mundane level, people exposed to persuasive advertising also know that the advertiser is seeking to influence them. They may, however, lack insight into the influence process – for instance, why the advertiser is manipulating certain images or using certain presenters. This lack of insight into the psychodynamics of the attempt to influence militates against the principle of voluntarism, albeit in a rather more subtle way than the deliberate presentation of misleading information or the partial presentation of evidence supporting the attitude or behaviour change the persuader is seeking to induce.

Limits to freedom of choice

One of the avowed aims of an empowerment model of health promotion is to remove obstacles to rational decision-making and freedom of choice. In some instances, overcoming such barriers is relatively simple – for example, the barrier created by ignorance. Others are more substantial – consider, for example, the case of addiction or other compulsive behaviours that sap freedom of choice. As McKeown pointed out:

> it is said that the individual must be free to choose [whether they wish to smoke]. But he [*sic*] is not free; with a drug of addiction the option is open only at the beginning. (1979: 125)

Environmental barriers to voluntaristic action have received considerable recognition and, in part, have contributed to the formulation of the contemporary ideology of health promotion. Indeed, probably the greatest progress in health promotion in recent years has been acknowledgement of the fact that material, social and cultural environments can both damage health and limit people's capacity to take action to promote their own health and the health of their communities. It is quite apparent that various natural disasters, such as famine and war, may damage health both directly and indirectly by removing the possibility of making empowered health-related decisions. Climate change and environmental degradation also pose major challenges (WHO, 2021a) and their effects are likely to be experienced disproportionately by the most disadvantaged in society.

Poverty and social inequality damage individuals' and communities' capacity for action and are now recognized as being major determinants of public health. On a smaller scale, lack of access to affordable healthy food will largely nullify the effects of health education initiatives about the importance of a healthy diet. Less obviously, the complementary effects of culture and childrearing may effectively block choice and genuine decision-making. For instance, in the process of socialization, cultural values may result in certain foods being classified as 'taboo', thus creating a moral imperative against consumption, regardless of the nutritional value of the food in question.

In the face of these many and varied psychological and environmental obstacles to the achievement of health, the emphasis on 'healthy public policy' is hardly surprising. Policy measures typically involve fiscal, economic and legislative measures and associated environmental change. On the one hand, they can create the conditions that support health and individual health choices. On the other hand, as is apparent from Figure 1.2, other more draconian measures that have been proposed can militate against freedom of choice. The Nuffield Council on Bioethics suggests that individual consent may not be required if measures are not 'very intrusive' or 'prevent significant harm to others'. Further, collective approval through democratic processes can replace individual consent when there is only limited interference with individuals' liberty (2007: paras 2.22–2.26). Although it is argued that healthy public policy makes the healthy choice the easy choice, it may effectively make the healthy choice the only choice! How can such attacks on freedom be reconciled with the discourse of voluntarism, which characterizes an 'educational model'?

The fact is, of course, that unbridled freedom is only the prerogative of the despot and, possibly to a lesser extent, of certain privileged groups. There are inevitably and appropriately limitations on freedom of choice. The national lockdowns across the world during the COVID-19 pandemic illustrate this. It could well be argued that 'true' education should encourage people to think in a systematic way about what is of most importance to them in their lives so that they might consistently act in accordance with the values they have clarified. It is also important that educated individuals should be helped to make decisions rather than uncritically absorb dogma. There are, however, obvious limitations to freedom of choice. As noted elsewhere (Tones, 1987), all values are not equally acceptable in a given society: antisocial behaviour would not normally be considered acceptable.

Health promotion would certainly not subscribe to unfettered freedom of choice. It is avowedly committed to certain major values to which most nations subscribe (or to which they at least pay lip service) and that have been incorporated into the various doctrines and discourse propagated by the WHO. This position is, or should be, non-negotiable. While cultural sensitivity is part of a concern for people in general, where cultural practices are inconsistent with the overriding values of health promotion, they must be challenged – take, for example, the issue of female genital mutilation or cutting. In the context of the principles of voluntarism, we must therefore observe two major qualifying principles. People should have a right to self-fulfilment, provided that this does not impede others' right to fulfilment and/or otherwise damage the well-being of the community at large. A good deal of consideration has, in fact, been given to the question of imposing limitations on liberty. The resulting ideological principles are most usefully expressed in terms of utilitarianism and paternalism. These principles provide support for the occasional overriding of personal liberty, either for the greater good or because some people seem incapable of exercising choice.

Utilitarianism, paternalism and the justification of coercion

There are two broad approaches to defining the ethics of interventions. One of these supports the principle that the integrity of a moral principle should be of prime consideration, whatever the consequences. For example, it is always wrong deliberately to provide inaccurate information, even if this might seem to be in the interests of the recipient of that information. The alternative view is that it is the results of actions that are most important (Guttman, 2000). This latter moral principle is generally described as utilitarianism.

There is an obvious and generally acceptable rationale underpinning actions based on the principle of utilitarianism. In short, people's freedom of action should be respected, so long as it does not interfere with the general good (for example, Mappes and Zembary, 1991). Indeed, it provides a simple baseline value for health education that legitimately espouses the imperative of self-actualization. However, personal gratification should not limit others' equal right to self-actualization.

It follows logically, therefore, that it is quite legitimate to use many of the varieties of coercion identified in Figure 1.2 where individuals' actions can be shown to damage others. The restriction on smoking in public places, for example, is therefore entirely justifiable in that smoking is not merely a public nuisance, but puts non-smokers at risk as a result of passive smoking.

Less clear-cut perhaps is the argument that seeks to restrain self-destructive behaviour on the grounds that the prudent in society should not have to pay for the excesses of the imprudent. More generally, economic arguments have indicated how self-inflicted illness damages the economy in terms of reduced productivity due to working days lost and increases the burden on already hard-pressed health services. Legislation can, therefore, be justified. For instance, in the UK, legislation enforcing seatbelt use and the wearing of protective headgear by motorcyclists has been in place for some time and is demonstrably effective. The situation regarding smoking is more equivocal. Certainly, many arguments have been used to demonstrate that smokers cover the cost of their morbidity and early mortality as a result of the finances levied by taxation and should actually be treated as social benefactors.

The cost–benefit analysis of smoking is a matter for health economics and so will not be debated here. However, a serious point is frequently made that those indulging in high-risk activities should be allowed to do so, providing that this does not damage the well-being of others and that possible social and medical costs are covered by insurance. The financial argument would not, of course, apply to those who impose a financial burden on the state because of illness for which they cannot be blamed.

The principle of utilitarianism, then, does not prove as unambiguous as it first appears. The question of limitations to free choice again proves problematic and leads us to consider the second principle, which may justify coercive methods. If people are not really responsible for their actions, then society must make decisions on their behalf, for their own good. These decisions will inevitably involve the restriction of liberties and involve some degree of coercion. This principle of paternalism (Nikku, 1997), though, proves even more difficult to justify than the appeal to utilitarianism. Beauchamp cites John Stuart Mill's (1961) treatise on liberty and his assertion that utilitarianism is the only justification for coercion:

> The only purpose for which power can be rightfully exercised over any member of a civilized community, against his [sic] will, is to prevent harm to others. His own good, either physical or moral is not a sufficient warrant. He cannot rightfully be compelled to do or forbear because it will be better for him to do so, because it will make him happier, because in the opinion of others, to do so would be wise, or even right. These are good reasons for remonstrating with him, or reasoning with him or persuading him or entreating him, but not for compelling him. (Beauchamp, 1978: 244)

However, as Daniels indicates:

> Even a view that holds the individual to be the best architect of his [sic] ends and judge of his interests rests on important assumptions about the information available to the agent, the competency of the agent to make these decisions rationally, and the voluntariness of the decisions he makes. It is because these assumptions are not always met that we require a theory of justifiable paternalism. (1985: 157, in Guttman, 2000: 52)

Pollard and Brennan (1978), in discussing the basis for governmental intervention in cases of self-regarding behaviour – that is, behaviour affecting only the individual but not others – cite Dworkin's justification of paternalistic behaviour on the grounds that some adults may not be capable of rational thought because 'at some point in the future the individual will see the wisdom of the paternalistic intervention, even though at present he or she is not aware of its value' (1972: 71).

The intervention thus, in some way, protects the 'real' will of the individual. At first glance, such a proposition looks distinctly dubious. However, it is undoubtedly true that most societies routinely take responsibility for certain categories of individual. For instance, the very young and those having a substantial degree of mental impairment would routinely be protected in many societies. Again, the notion of protecting someone's real will is not as Machiavellian as it might appear. For instance, it would seem fairly clear that a substantial majority of smokers would prefer not to smoke and it is appropriate to recall McKeown's observation that 'the critical decision to smoke is taken not by consenting adults but by children below the age of consent' (1979: 125). Paternalistic intervention to limit people's freedom to choose to smoke might make some sense ethically. Furthermore, even if suicide were legal, a depressed person might be legitimately prevented from taking his or her life on the reasonable supposition that, when no longer depressed, (s)he would not wish to do so.

Choice architecture positions itself as being 'libertarianism paternalism' (Thaler and Sunstein, 2008). While at first glance this combination appears to be a contradiction in terms, Thaler and Sunstein (2008) argue that the meaning of the word paternalism changes when preceded by the word 'libertarianism' in that the focus becomes about preserving liberty. Choice architecture and the concept of 'nudge' are discussed further in Chapter 10.

The question of choice versus coercion in the interest of public health is very real. On the one hand, the principle of voluntarism urges freedom of choice unless good reason can be provided for coercive measures on the basis of utilitarianism, paternalism or 'social justice'. On the other hand, it seems particularly difficult to reach consensus about when, where and to what extent these principles can be used to justify coercive interventions in the interest of public health. Those of a left-wing orientation might object to any infringement of liberty of disadvantaged people, but wholeheartedly support paternalistic (or should it be 'maternalistic'?) measures by the nanny state on the grounds of social justice and equity. Equally, the more tough-minded advocates of market forces would vocally object to interventions that restricted their own freedom of action, but might well subscribe to the utilitarian restriction of the liberty of people of a different political persuasion! Public attitudes about individual versus government responsibility for health were explored by the British Social Attitudes Survey (NatCen Social Research, 2017) (see Box 1.3).

BOX 1.3 PUBLIC OPINION ON THE DETERMINANTS OF, AND RESPONSIBILITY, FOR HEALTH

- The vast majority of the people surveyed (96%) considered 'free health care' to have a 'large' or 'quite large' impact on health.
- 93% of those surveyed thought that individual behaviours have an impact on health.

The support of family and friends, safety in the local area, area quality, inherited characteristics, being employed, education and friendly neighbourhood/community were also viewed as having an impact on health but to a lesser extent than the previous two factors.

In terms of responsibility for health:

- 61% thought that individuals had a greater responsibility for health than the government.
- Only 9% thought that the government had more responsibility than individuals.
- Young people, and those with poorer health, were more likely to view the government being more responsible for health (36% of those surveyed over the age of 75 years thought that individuals were entirely responsible for health compared to 9% of 18–24 year olds).

Source: Holt-White (2019) Health Foundation analysis of NatCen Social Research's British Social Attitudes Survey 2017.

The debate about who is responsible for health continues and is inextricably tied up with ideological and political perspectives. In 2011, England saw the introduction of the 'Responsibility Deal', a voluntary agreement designed to encourage healthier lifestyles relating to four key areas – physical activity, food, alcohol and health at work. By 2015, 776 companies, including manufacturers and supermarkets, had signed up. Since the end of the Coalition government in 2015 the Public Health Responsibility Deal has not been driven forward. Nevertheless, this light-touch approach contrasts somewhat with that taken in the USA, where a healthcare law was passed in 2010 requiring calorie counts to be put on menus and vending machines. Despite some cities having enforced this (led by

New York City in 2010), there have been significant delays in its implementation in some sectors for a number of complex reasons.

The stewardship model described in Box 1.2 (see p. 25) provides a framework for considering the balance between individual freedom and state responsibility in relation to public health. We may be able to move some way towards resolving the dilemma by promoting self-empowerment. However, we should take account of Beauchamp's noteworthy observation that 'Public health should – at least ideally – be suspicious of behavioural paradigms for viewing public health problems since they tend to "blame the victim" and unfairly protect majorities and powerful interests from the burdens of preven-tion' (Beauchamp, 1976, reprinted in Beauchamp and Steinbock, 1999: 106). Accordingly, our analysis later in this chapter and discussion of empowerment will emphasize the importance of *community* participation and *community* empowerment.

Ethics and ethical practice

Guttman (2017) contends that the debate on ethics in health promotion practice can be summarized in two key questions: first, does it indeed promote people's health and second, whom does it actu-ally benefit? These two questions relate respectively to evidence of what works (discussed in more detail in Chapter 12) and issues of fairness and equity. Underpinning these questions are some of the well-known biomedical ethical principles that Beauchamp and Childress (2019) espouse: namely beneficence, non-maleficence and justice. Beauchamp and Childress's (2019) final principle is respect for autonomy or the rights of the individual. Arguably, being able to exercise such rights is the literal outworking of empowerment (at an individual level at least) but there are limits to the extent to which this might be possible; for example, when the rights of others are impinged upon. In addition, as Parker et al. (2007) argue, health promotion interventions should achieve positive outcomes and avoid, where possible, any negative unintended outcomes that might harm the things that people value. Robust evaluation strategies can help in this regard (see Chapter 11 for further details).

The biomedical ethics model has value in health promotion, as discussed. In contrast, however, Sindall (2002) points out that the social model of health necessitates a broader macro-ethical frame-work, which moves away from the individual responsibility and accountability for behaviour change inherent in a lot of public health policy. Communitarian ethics 'moves beyond the principles derived from bioethics, to incorporate theories from social and political philosophy' (Sindall, 2002: 202). Communitarianism recognizes that the individual cannot be separated from their social context and, therefore, rejects the privileging of the individual promoting the notion of common good and the necessity for collective action to achieve this. In keeping, but notwithstanding the challenges of col-laborative and facilitative methods for promoting health, Tengland (2012) illustrates how the ethical dilemmas of the behaviour change approach can be countered by using an empowerment approach since it respects and promotes autonomy.

Wills (2023: 86) asserts that health promotion 'raises many questions over its ends and means' such as:

- Good health is a relative concept, so whose definition should take precedence? Is it ethical for a practitioner to persuade someone to adopt their perception of a healthier lifestyle?

- What means are justifiable to promote good health in the population? Should the interests of the majority always prevail?
- Since most ill health is avoidable, should those who knowingly adopt unhealthy behaviours be refused treatment?

Questions such as these can, and should, guide and influence health promotion practice. More generally, Gardner (2014) outlines a further three questions about key ethical issues for health promotion, which can serve as a general prompt for reflective practice:

1. What are the ultimate goals for public health practice, i.e. what 'good should it achieve'?
2. How should this good be distributed in the population?
3. What means may we use to try to achieve and distribute this good?

It is not possible to address questions such as these without considering the sociological concepts of agency and structure, as reflected in debates about responsibility for health – namely, individual responsibility for health versus state responsibility. Indeed, 'the growing public-health threats of non-communicable diseases, including those caused in part by unhealthy behaviours such as smoking, poor diet or lack of exercise, have raised the question of the extent to which (public-health) authorities should interfere with personal choices on health' (Coleman et al., 2008: 578). However, Coleman et al. (2008) also contend that the structural context needs to be considered in terms of the factors that create healthy communities and societies, which is a principle embedded in health promotion's overriding concern with the wider social determinants of health.

Several authors point to ethical concerns in health promotion interventions, many of which are raised in this chapter and throughout this book. For example, Guttman (2017, npn) notes that 'interventions can have repercussions in multicultural settings since members of diverse populations may hold beliefs or engage in practices considered by health promoters as "unhealthy" but which have important cultural significance'. In addition, Cross et al. (2017a) outline a number of ethical dilemmas in health promotion such as the use of persuasive communication, emotional appeal, shock tactics, and the tension that arises between personal freedom (the right for an individual to behave in an autonomous way) and the greater good tenet of utilitarianism.

There is increasing recognition that ethics and evidence in health promotion are inextricably linked (Carter, 2012; Carter et al., 2011b). Tannahill (2008: 388) proposed an 'ethical imperative' for health promotion – 'to make decisions based on the explicit application of ethical principles, using available evidence and theory appropriately to inform judgements'. Ethical practice, therefore, has to relate to the evidence about what works, the point reiterated by Guttman (2017) earlier. Carter et al. (2011b) propose five principles for planning and evaluating health promotion based on these two central and important features of health promotion practice (ethics and evidence), as follows:

1. Recognize that health promotion thinking must be responsive to particular situations – it cannot be universal.
2. Formally recognize and implement two iterative systems of reasoning, an evidence-based system and an ethical system, each containing explicit values.

3. Clearly specify the evidential and ethical concepts that are valued or devalued in each situation, and the dimensions along which these vary. Use both existing theory and detailed empirical study of the practice of health promotion in the situation.
4. Be specific about trade-offs occurring along the identified dimensions – consider how valued or devalued concepts interact.
5. Prioritize procedural transparency: be certain that processes used for reasoning, defining and trading off can be explained clearly.

For further exploration of this framework and an application of it to a specific health promotion campaign, please see Carter et al. (2011b, p. 468).

There is currently no specific or universal code of ethics for health promotion, although a number of frameworks or guidelines have existed. In preparation of developing a code of ethics, the International Union of Health Promotion and Education (IUPHE) carried out a survey of IUPHE members regarding the need for a code of ethics for health promotion (Bull et al., 2012). The findings supported the development of a code of ethics, based on the evidence that ethical dilemmas were frequently encountered in health promotion practice (Bull et al., 2012). The subsequent IUPHE core competencies and professional standards for health promotion (IUPHE, 2016: 6) are underpinned by a set of ethical values and principles – namely, 'a belief in equity and social justice, respect for the autonomy and choice of both individuals and groups, and collaborative and consultative ways of working'. For a more in-depth exploration of ethical considerations in health promotion please see Guttman (2017).

Health promotion and the discourse of empowerment

The assertion that the main concern of health promotion should be that of empowerment is becoming increasingly acceptable, although this acceptance often takes the form of lip service rather than practice and policy! Certainly, as noted above, most of the key documents published by the WHO since the inception of 'Health for All by the Year 2000' placed emphasis on individuals gaining control over their lives and their health and on the importance of active participating communities. In his Harveian Oration, Marmot (2006: 2081–2) recognized the central importance of the social environment and empowerment, asserting that: 'Failing to meet the fundamental human needs of autonomy, empowerment and human freedom is a potent cause of ill health.' In subsequent work led by Sir Michael Marmot, *Fair Society, Healthy Lives* (Marmot, 2010), a key theme was to create conditions in which people could take control over their lives – prioritizing empowerment. In *Health Equity in England: The Marmot Review 10 Years On* (Marmot et al., 2020) the importance of community control and empowerment was still at the forefront.

It is axiomatic from our earlier discussion that empowerment is based on the principles of voluntarism. The key issue for health promotion is how people who lack power can become more powerful and actually gain a reasonable degree of control over their lives. How can they compete with, and resist coercion by, those who already have power?

ABSTRACT 1.2

Behavior change or empowerment: on the ethics of health promotion goals. Tengland, P. (2016)

One important ethical issue for health promotion and public health work is to determine what the goals for these practices should be. This paper tries to clarify what some of these goals are thought to be, and what they ought to be. It specifically discusses two different approaches to health promotion, such as behaviour change and empowerment. The general aim of this paper is, thus, to compare the behaviour-change approach and the empowerment approach, concerning their immediate (instrumental) goals or aims, and to morally evaluate the strengths and weaknesses of these two goal models, in relation to the ultimate goals of health promotion. The investigation shows that the behaviour-change approach has several moral problems. First of all, it is overly paternalistic and often disregards the individual's or group's own perception of what is important – something that also increases the risk of failed interventions. Furthermore, it risks leading to 'victim-blaming' and stigmatization, and to increased inequalities in health, and it puts focus on the 'wrong' problems, i.e. behaviour instead of the 'causes of the causes'. It is thereafter shown in the study that the empowerment approach does not have any of these problems. Finally, some specific problems for the empowerment approach are discussed and resolved, such as, the idea that empowering some groups might lead to power over others, the objective that the focus is not primarily on health (which it should be), and the fact that empowered people might choose to live lives that risk reducing their health.

Further reflections on power

Empowerment, by definition, has to do with people acquiring a degree of power and control. Self-empowerment describes the extent to which individuals have power and control over their interactions with their physical and social environment. Further, an empowered community is an identifiable group of people that also possesses power and control. It is a matter of some importance to understand the different circumstances under which people acquire power, wield it and yield to it.

Definitions of power and related concepts

The notion of power may manifest itself at macro, meso and micro levels. All three levels have some degree of relevance for health promotion. Studies of power at the micro level are concerned with influences on, and exerted by, individuals or small groups; meso-level power might refer to the power exerted by organizations or communities; the influence of national policy would be a macro-level influence – as would the kinds of ideological controls discussed above.

The classic Weberian analysis identifies three forms of power:

- **social power** based on such factors as prestige, family status, lifestyle and patterns of consumption
- **economic power** based on a group's relationship to the mode of production, its position in the labour market and general life chances
- **political power** based on affiliation to parties, bureaucracy and legal structure.

Naturally, there are a number of different ideas associated with power. For instance, concepts such as 'control', 'authority' and 'influence' may be used almost interchangeably with power.

Bachrach and Baratz (1970) acknowledge the variations in the nomenclature and meaning of these various terms and offered a useful typology of influence that still has currency (see Box 1.4).

BOX 1.4 A TYPOLOGY OF INFLUENCE

Force The individual or group is obliged to comply by removing all choice.

Coercion Compliance is achieved by the threat of deprivation where conflict exists regarding values or courses of action.

Manipulation This is a 'subconcept' of force. Compliance results in the absence of recognition by those who comply or the source of nature of the demand made.

Influence This term is used when an individual or organization succeeds in causing others to change their intended actions, but without overt or tacit threat of deprivation.

Authority This form of power operates when people comply because they accept that commands are reasonable in terms of their own values or because an appropriate and acceptable procedure has been adopted.

Source: Bachrach and Baratz (1970: 28)

Lukes (2021) reminds us that dominant groups shape people's needs and wants – by means of mass media, 'indoctrination' at school or, more powerfully, by socialization. Lukes's analysis is clearly consistent with our earlier discussion of the often-subtle means whereby dominant ideologies are perpetuated, including the creation of false consciousness. These observations are not only relevant to our discussion of ideologies in general, but, as we noted earlier in this chapter, more particularly to questions of utilitarianism and paternalism. They also have an important bearing on our later examination of the assessment of health needs. Moreover, these two notions underpin thinking about empowerment, bearing in mind Kindervatter's definition of empowerment as: 'People gaining an understanding of and control over social, economic and/or political forces in order to improve their standing in society' (1979: 62). A clear understanding of the different constructions of power also has special significance in, for example, determining the success or failure of lobbying and advocacy for the implementation of healthy public policy at macro and meso levels.

Notwithstanding the relevance of these macro- and meso-level influences on the development of healthy public policy, at this juncture we will focus on the individualistic perspective and the micro-level exercise of power. After all, continuing pressure is placed on individuals from a variety of sources, both explicitly and implicitly, to modify their behaviours in ways that may – or equally may not – be healthy.

Five varieties of power: an individual perspective

One of the classic, and still valid, analyses of power at the micro level was provided by French and Raven (1959), who distinguished five varieties of power. This scheme (which has similarities to Weber's analysis of charismatic, traditional and rational–legal power) is frequently used to illuminate interactions when analysing small group dynamics and discussing leadership functions. Their analysis comprises the following five varieties of power:

- **Legitimate power**: authority is derived from legitimate status formally bestowed by a given social system.
- **Expert power**: authority derives from the actual and perceived expertise of the individual in question. It may or may not be associated with legitimate authority or be an informal adjunct of referent power (see below).
- **Reward power**: authority derives from the individual's capacity for providing rewards.
- **Coercive power**: authority derives from the individual's capacity to sanction.
- **Referent power**: authority derives from the referent's individual characteristics, which, for some reason, are valued by the person who is influenced.

Stardom and charisma

Alberoni (1962, in McQuail, 1972) also discusses the characteristics of individuals who, despite lacking legitimate authority, can nonetheless exert quite a powerful influence over other people. He describes this 'powerless "élite"' as 'stars'. Their 'institutional power is very limited or nonexistent, but [their] doings and way of life arouse a considerable and sometimes even a maximum degree of interest'. He likens their personal characteristics to Weber's notion of charisma:

> By charisma we mean a quality regarded as extraordinary and attributed to a person … The latter is believed to be endowed with powers and properties which are supernatural and superhuman, or at least exceptional even where accessible to others; or again as sent by God, or as if adorned with exemplary value and thus worthy to be a leader. (Weber, 1968: 241)

It is sometimes said, with a degree of acrimony, that many celebrities in contemporary society are 'famous for being famous'! It is certainly the case that these charismatic characters may well exert a quite dramatic degree of influence on people. They may influence taste and preferences and act as models. This phenomenon will be revisited in Chapter 7, when we consider the influence of source credibility and attractiveness in persuading individuals to adopt healthy or unhealthy courses of action.

We might legitimately conclude that empowered individuals would be more able and willing to resist pressure and not submit to unreasonable demands, particularly those that run counter to their existing values.

While analyses such as French and Raven's are undoubtedly useful in designing health promotion programmes, it is essential to ask how someone comes to wield legitimate authority, how they are in a position to reward, how they acquire the power to coerce, how they acquire expert authority or come to be treated as referents by their communities. As we noted earlier, power does not rely only on the crude application of force and coercion, but can also be exerted by the ideological control of culture and the hegemony of political and state institutions.

Self-empowerment, community empowerment and reciprocal determinism

Earlier in this chapter, we emphasized the dramatic effects an oppressive environment can have on individuals' health and their capacity to make choices.

It is, therefore, self-evident that empowerment – people's opportunities to make genuinely free choices – is not possible unless physical, socioeconomic and cultural circumstances are favourable. Thus, it is imperative that empowerment policy and the ensuing strategies must engage with the thorny question of environmental change. However, it is clear that individuals are, in many situations, capable in principle of making choices even when the environment is not especially conducive to individual action. Three different perspectives on human agency can be identified (see Figure 1.3).

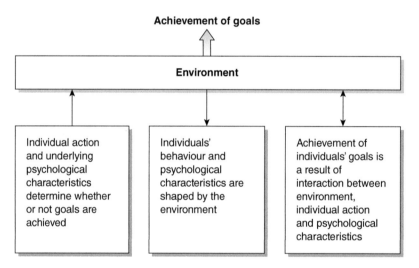

Figure 1.3   Three perspectives on human agency

In the first situation, the focus of attention is centred on individuals and those characteristics that explain their behaviour. The theorist may be interested only in psychological phenomena or even be effectively blind to the existence of the environment. Some forms of counselling may be characterized by this approach. In the second instance, individuals are viewed as being largely controlled by their circumstances – directly or indirectly.

The third formulation of human agency asserts that humans (and animals) interact with their environments. They are, on the one hand, affected by environmental forces but, on the other, typically capable of having at least some impact on the various physical, socioeconomic and cultural factors that influence them. The ideology and practice of empowerment ultimately derives from this last standpoint and has been a central feature of social learning theory. Its major exponent and advocate is Bandura (1986), who described the interactive process as 'reciprocal determinism' and contrasted it with the Skinnerian assertion that 'A person does not act upon the world, the world acts upon him [*sic*]' (Skinner, 1971: 211). Bandura argues that a process of 'triadic reciprocality' operates when humans engage with life. In short, there is an often complicated system of interaction between psychological factors (such as beliefs and attitudes), behaviour and the environment. A more comprehensive account of this system is given and discussed in Chapter 3.

We should also note that this archetypal psychological analysis of human agency is by no means inconsistent with the broader perspectives of sociology. For instance, Giddens (1991: 204) observes that 'actors are at the same time creators of social systems yet created by them'.

Individual and community dimensions of empowerment

The logic of reciprocal determinism for an empowerment model of health promotion is inescapable. If empowerment is about facilitating voluntaristic decision-making and achieving free choices (or those that are consistent with moral imperatives), then it must operate at both the level of the environment and at the level of the individual. Furthermore, it is important to recognize that the environment itself has many levels – from macro to meso, from the level of national policy to the level of regional organizations and institutions, down to the level of the neighbourhood or village. At each level, individuals exist within a web of social systems. At the neighbourhood level, the community is a social system that has particular significance for health promotion. Figure 1.4 gives an indication of this complexity within the context of commenting on both individual and community empowerment. These, as South and Woodall (2010) argue, should be viewed as inextricably linked. Indeed, in terms of approaches, there is evidence that the two are connected. For further discussion about community empowerment and health equity please see Popay (2021).

As may be seen from Figure 1.4, the community may mediate individual agency in relation to the general physical, socioeconomic and cultural environment. The community is an especially important social system within the lexicon of empowerment and health promotion. Following the doctrine of the Ottawa Charter, an active, empowered community is perhaps seen as the most important of the desirable empowerment outcomes of health promotion activities. In short, it enables people to take an active part in influencing policy. Three key features of an empowered community are also shown: namely, a sense of community – that is, a therapeutic feeling of identification with fellow community members; an active commitment to achieve community goals; and what is increasingly termed 'social capital' (see Chapter 2 for more about this).

Individual or self-empowerment, however, comprises a cluster of attributes related to a personal capacity for voluntaristic action:

> Self-empowerment is a state in which an individual possesses a relatively high degree of actual power – that is, a *genuine* potential for making choices. Self-empowerment is associated with a number of beliefs about causality and the nature of control that are health promoting. It is also associated with a relatively high level of realistically based self-esteem together with a repertoire of *life skills* that contribute to the exercise of power over the individual's life and health. (Tones and Tilford, 2001: 40)

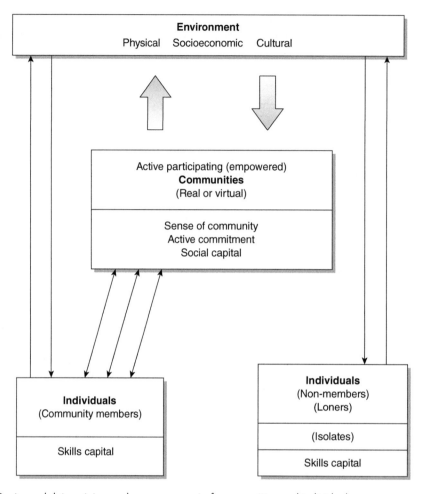

Figure 1.4 Reciprocal determinism and empowerment of communities and individuals

Clearly, a community is composed of its membership – and it is arguable whether or not a community is more than the sum of the individuals making up this membership. In all events, a community is generally considered to be beneficial for its individual members, and the characteristics and capabilities of these individuals will contribute to the power of the community as a whole.

Figure 1.4 makes a distinction between 'real' and 'virtual' communities. The former represents a traditional idea of community as a group of people within a relatively small geographical area having a sense of identity and a network of relationships. A virtual community may lack the narrow geographical dimension of a real one, but otherwise has a shared identity. For instance, we can realistically talk about the LGBTQIA+ community or about communities comprising of people connected through social media. A virtual community may actually have more power at its disposal than a real community and, moreover, with technology such as the Internet, may benefit from different kinds of interaction.

Although often ignored in discussions of communities, Figure 1.4 reminds us that some individuals may not be part of any community – real or virtual. We have labelled as 'non-members' individuals who exist in relative isolation because no community exists. By contrast, and borrowing terminology from the domain of sociometry, we have used the term 'loner' to distinguish people who do not wish to belong to a community from those whose felt need is to belong, but who are not accepted or rejected – so-called 'isolates'. Figure 1.4 also notes that individuals are affected by, and in turn affect, their environments at different levels without the mediation of community groups.

We might also note that environments do not exert their effects in a unidimensional way. It is more realistic to consider any given environment as exerting both facilitative and inhibitory influences of different strengths on communities and individuals. The sum total of both positive and negative pressures might be described in terms of these macro or meso influences 'making the healthy choice the easy choice' or, alternatively, being fundamentally oppressive. The specific, technical, detailed aspects of both community and individual empowerment will be explored at some length in Chapter 3.

One of the factors most closely associated with empowerment – with respect to both ideological and technical aspects – is that of participation. The WHO has frequently commented on the importance of an active, participating community and the desirability of individual involvement in decision-making is virtually taken for granted as a healthy development. We will also note in Chapter 5 the centrality of participation to the needs assessment process. How does participation actually contribute to empowerment? It is almost a matter of common sense! A community that takes action – that is, participates in action to influence policy or practice at local or national level – feels that it has actually achieved something, even if the outcome is not dramatic. Similarly, individuals who are actively involved are likely to experience at least some degree of control. Obviously, there are many different degrees of involvement and Figure 1.5 indicates an assumed relationship between degrees of participation/involvement and empowerment. It draws on the classic analyses of Arnstein (1969) and Brager and Specht (1973).

It should be noted that Figure 1.5 applies equally not only to communities but also to settings such as health-promoting hospitals and health-promoting schools and, at the micro level, to interactions between individuals, such as doctor and patient.

Empowerment and health and well-being

A review by Woodall et al. (2010) assessed the evidence in relation to empowerment and its effect on health and well-being. Based on the available literature, the review suggested that there are five key areas where empowerment strategies or interventions had improved individual health-related outcomes. These areas were identified as:

- improved self-efficacy and self-esteem
- greater sense of control
- increased knowledge and awareness
- behaviour change
- a greater sense of community, broadened social networks and social support.

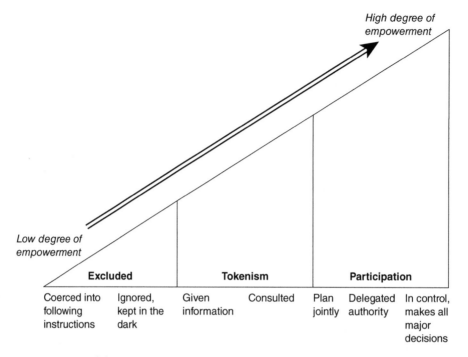

Figure 1.5   Participation and the empowerment gradient

The review found fewer instances where empowerment approaches had made a difference to the actual health and well-being of communities, although there was good evidence showing that community engagement was beneficial for social cohesion, social capital and strengthening relationships and trust among participants. The authors suggested that further research is needed to establish the evidence for links between empowerment and improvements in the health status of communities. Since the publication of the review numerous studies from around the world have reported associations between the empowerment of communities and benefits to health. More recent examples include Abbas et al. (2021) for Pakistan, Coan et al. (2020) for the UK and Guli and Geda (2021) for Ethiopia.

An empowerment model of health promotion

We have considered the medical discourse associated with public health and a preventive model of health promotion or, rather, health education. We have also explored ideas related to the discourse of voluntarism, which might be said to give rise to an educational model of health promotion. Both of these models are limited in that they are inconsistent with the ideological thrust of health promotion. They are also technically limited in their capacity to explain what would be involved in achieving the empowerment goals of health promotion. Figure 1.6 sets out the main components of an empowerment model of health promotion and their interrelationships.

The central dynamic of the empowerment model is the interplay of education and healthy public policy. The development and implementation of policy are the essential precursors to the creation of health-promoting environmental influences. The relationship is multiplicative, as we noted earlier in the 'formula': health promotion = health education × healthy public policy. The empowering function of education not only strengthens individual capabilities for health-related action, but also makes a major contribution to the establishment of healthy public policy.

Action to achieve healthy public policy

We discussed the five action areas of the Ottawa Charter earlier in this chapter, including the imperative to reorientate health services. Accordingly, Figure 1.6 shows how policy initiatives are necessary to improve service provision to meet the health needs of particular populations. More importantly, it identifies the significance of policy initiatives to address physical, socioeconomic and cultural circumstances. This position is reinforced in the Health in All Policies thrust of subsequent WHO international health promotion conferences (WHO, 2009, 2013e, 2016a). The focus is more on reframing than on reorientation. In tune with modern multidisciplinary public health, it recognizes the contribution to health of a range of services whose primary *raison d'être* may not be health in any formal sense; for example, transport, housing, economic development. However, all of these have a major impact on health and, indeed, on disease.

Two major action strategies are included in the model. One is the traditional means of seeking to influence policy, such as lobbying. Advocacy is defined here as lobbying those who exercise power by those who have power but who are doing so on behalf of the relatively powerless. The term 'mediation', which was incorporated into the Ottawa Charter list of major actions, refers to the process of mediating between competing interests. By way of illustration, we might consider the different concerns of the owners and producers of mass media programmes and health professionals. On the one hand, the main goal of the former is to entertain the public and advertise products in order to make profits. On the other hand, the interests of the health promoters are to control advertising and any representation of health issues in ways that are considered to be damaging to the public health.

The second – and ultimately the most powerful – means of producing policy change is to create a sufficient level of public pressure so that decision-makers and politicians at the national or local level feel obliged to change. In a democracy, this might, in the final analysis, result in change by means of the ballot box.

The catalyst for change is health education, but emphatically not the variety of health education that has been tarred with the same brush of victim-blaming! Rather, following the precepts of critical theory, it might usefully be called 'critical health education' and its purpose is radical and political. Again, the nature of education and its technology will be reviewed in Chapters 7 and 8 and particular attention will be devoted to its radical and critical manifestations.

Health education and individual empowerment

Figure 1.6 includes an analysis of the essential contribution made by education to individual action. A training function has also been included in the model to demonstrate the continuing importance of providing skills – not only to communities, but also to the professionals who work in the various

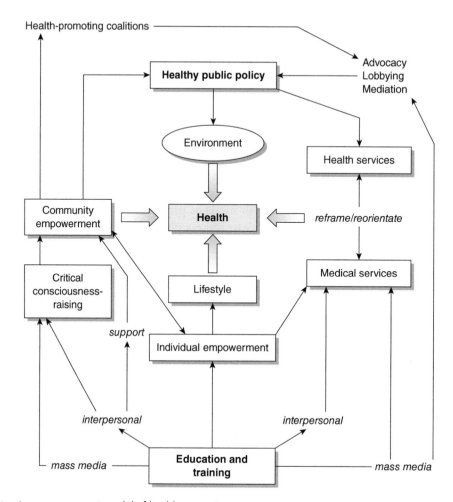

Figure 1.6 An empowerment model of health promotion

services to which reference was made above. This training would include awareness-raising of the health-promoting role of the organizations, as well as making available the competences needed to communicate with clients and the general public, providing appropriate education and analysing the impact of policy on health – and making appropriate adjustments in the interest of effectiveness and efficiency.

We earlier reviewed the traditional health education function. We noted that its purpose was to persuade individuals to adopt behaviours that would result in the prevention of disease, with regard both to lifestyle and making proper use of medical services. The role of critical health education is not primarily that of persuasion (which is both ethically dubious and of limited effectiveness), but one of empowerment and support. Empowered individuals are more likely to make an effective contribution to community action, which, in turn, contributes to their empowerment, as we mentioned earlier.

They are also more likely to engage with the various services contributing to health in an assertive and productive fashion. They are almost certainly more likely to adopt a lifestyle conducive to achieving the objectives of preventive medicine than if they were not empowered! Indeed, one of our more forceful assertions here is that the successful adoption of an empowerment model of health promotion is not only more likely to achieve positive health outcomes in an ethical fashion, but also to be more efficient in attaining the important outcomes associated with the prevention and management of disease and disability.

The empowerment model: critiques and reservations

The empowerment model of health promotion is not without its critics. For instance, some might reasonably argue that empowerment is a fashionable term, distinguished by its lack of clarity in conceptualization and use (the same criticism could, of course, be levelled at health promotion itself and even the notion of public health). A second objection derives from the assertion that empowerment lacks a theoretical base. This assertion is fundamentally incorrect, as we are in the process of demonstrating!

What is undoubtedly more problematic is translating the rhetoric into action.

Unresolved challenges are also seen to exist in terms of the definition and operationalization of empowerment (Woodall et al., 2012a). A lack of consensus around defining empowerment leads to challenges in its measurement at whatever level it occurs (Cross et al., 2017a; Popay, 2021). In a paper that posits a critical stance on whether empowerment has, in fact, lost its power, Woodall et al. (2012a) contended that the concept of empowerment has become diluted in contemporary health promotion and has somewhat lost touch with its radical social roots. Christens (2013) was in agreement with Woodall et al.'s (2012a) conclusions that empowerment needs to be defined more precisely, that multilevel approaches are needed and that research is required that links changes at structural levels to changes at individual levels. However, Christens (2013) also added to the debate, pointing out some potential oversights in Woodall et al.'s arguments. He asserts the need to distinguish carefully between the use of the terms 'individual' and 'psychological' empowerment and argues that critical consciousness is crucial to bringing empowerment back to its radical, liberationist roots, noting that this first takes place at the individual level. Christens et al. (2016: 15) note that empowerment and critical consciousness are 'concepts with shared roots' as 'both are associated with attempts at overcoming oppression and fostering human development, community participation, and wellbeing'. In his 2019 book *Community Power and Empowerment* Christens analyses collective empowerment in detail, addressing previous limitations in the literature such as the overemphasis on psychological empowerment and the relative lack of attention given to processes of community empowerment.

It should hopefully be clear from the observations made in this chapter that power and politics are central to health promotion. It would be a mistake to underestimate the difficulties of challenging power structures. Nonetheless, we believe that sophisticated analysis grounded in sound theory can result in the development of empowering strategies that can achieve results. The empowerment model of health promotion is advocated here on grounds of both ideological soundness and practical effectiveness. Moreover, it stands up well to ethical scrutiny.

PUBLIC HEALTH, HEALTH PROMOTION AND HEALTH EDUCATION

Health promotion and modern multidisciplinary public health

We have considered at some length the ideology of health promotion and have argued in favour of an empowerment model that recognizes the primacy of the broader social, cultural, economic and environmental determinants of health. To conclude this chapter, we will briefly examine the relationship between health promotion and modern multidisciplinary public health and the position of health promotion as a profession. We will also consider the future role of health education.

For some, there is no distinction between health promotion and public health. Kickbusch (2007) reminds us of the subtitle to the Ottawa Charter for Health Promotion – *the move towards a new public health*. Indeed, the Ottawa Charter has been hailed as heralding the third public health revolution. Potvin and McQueen (2007) have characterized revolutionary change as affecting three fundamental dimensions of systems:

- the direction or finality of the system – the target, objectives and goals
- knowledge base – including the conditions that support the production of knowledge as well as substantive knowledge itself
- actions – including design, implementation and evaluation.

Terris (1983) identified the first public health revolution as concerned with tackling communicable disease and the second with non-communicable disease. Breslow (1999, 2004, 2006) puts the case that the emphasis on health as a resource for living constitutes the third revolution.

However, for some authors, health promotion and public health, although related, are not synonymous. Raeburn and MacFarlane refer to some governments seeing public health as health protection plus health promotion, where health protection comprises 'the more regulatory, centralized and reactive aspects of public health' (2003: 245) and health promotion is more self-determined, community-based and developmental. In this interpretation, public health is the umbrella term and health promotion a defined sphere of activity within it.

The Bangkok Charter refers to health promotion as a 'core function of public health' (WHO, 2005). Potvin and McQueen see health promotion as 'a strategy for public health that reflects modernity' (2007: 14). They note that subsequent to its emergence in the 1970s and more formal adoption in the 1980s, health promotion rapidly spread through public health organizations and institutions internationally. However, latterly, while the principles and strategies remain relevant, the term 'health promotion' appears to be becoming 'outmoded' in some parts of the world. Here in England between 1980 and 2000 specialist health promotion declined and attempts at professionalization failed during the period (Duncan, 2013). However, in other contexts, health promotion is thriving, for example in Canada and Australia. In addition, in the African context, Zambia and Ghana's changes in government in the second decade of this century saw a renewed focus on health promotion as a means to achieving sustainable development. There was a renewed interest in health promotion in the UK with the creation of the new Office for Health Promotion in early 2021, which was tasked with leading improvements in the public's health through healthy public policy and cross-governmental working. Subsequently however, the name was changed to the Office for Health Improvement and Disparities. Its primary purpose is to tackle health inequalities as well as focusing on prevention (Department of Health and Social Care [DHSC], 2022).

Potvin and McQueen argue that while some countries may have a cadre of health promotion professionals, health promotion activity involves a wide range of groups, including lay people, and that health promotion is 'not a discipline, nor an institution, nor a profession' (2007: 16). They see health promotion as embracing a 'structured discourse and a set of practices' and identify its two characteristic features as 'a distinctive perspective on health; and a critical orientation towards action' (2007: 16).

However, our position, set out earlier in this chapter, is that health promotion is a discipline with its own ideology and we will at later points in this book identify the theories, perspective and methods that characterize it as an 'ordered field of study'. A study of the views of key informants in the UK by Tilford et al. (2003) found that they associated health promotion with a clear set of values as well as a set of activities. These included instrumental values associated with ways of working as well as terminal values, notably a holistic conceptualization of health, equity, empowerment, autonomy/ self-determination and justice/fairness. While there was felt to be some degree of consensus between the values of public health and health promotion, there was a much stronger emphasis for health promotion on empowerment and autonomy with the associated instrumental values of involvement and participation. Prevention and protection featured more prominently in relation to public health, along with a clear population focus and greater attention to 'ends'. In contrast, health promotion was more concerned about means and had a broader focus that included individuals as well as communities. Tilford et al. (2003) conclude that within the context of the move to multidisciplinary public health, health promotion makes a distinctive contribution through its core values (see Box 1.5). By virtue of its more radical orientation, health promotion has in the past been described as the militant wing of public health. The emphasis on attention to process might also lead to it being seen as the critical conscience of public health.

BOX 1.5 VALUES AT WORK

Values influence the ways that health issues are understood, the ways that knowledge and theoretical bases are developed and the nature of strategies identified for health improvement. Values also influence the selection of activities that are undertaken to promote health and the priorities accorded to actions, the balance between activities at individual and population levels, the relationships with individuals and communities who participate in initiatives, the goals which are being sought, and decisions about means and ends in achieving goals.

Source: Tilford et al. (2003: 120)

As we noted above, the early emergence of health promotion was characterized by a struggle to distance itself from public health, held to be associated with the preventive medical model of health. Furthermore, it also sought a separate identity from health education – viewed as the 'handmaiden of public health' and tainted by association with approaches deemed to be victim-blaming in orientation. The move towards 'The New Public Health', which subscribed to a social model of health, brought about greater alignment with health promotion. The social model of health reflects, as we have seen, an attendant emphasis on issues such as inequality and sustainability (Duncan, 2013). Most of those who claim to be 'health promoters' would see commonalities with the broad statement of purpose used for public health:

- to improve health and well-being in the population
- to prevent disease and minimize its consequences
- to prolong valued life
- to reduce inequalities in health. (Skills for Health and Public Health Resource Unit, 2009)

Within England, the origins of modern multidisciplinary public health can be traced back to the Acheson Report, which defined public health as: 'the science and art of preventing disease, prolonging life and promoting health through the organized efforts of society' (Department of Health, 1988). The report also recognized that public health:

> works through partnerships that cut across disciplinary, professional and organizational boundaries and exploits this diversity in collaboration, to bring evidence and research based policies to *all areas* which impact on the health and well being of populations. (1988)

The specialist health promotion workforce in the UK has depleted over the past three decades. Duncan (2013) argues three key reasons as to why this is the case. First, he points to a lack of a collective identity and a unified purpose among the health promotion workforce; second, the lack of a permanent organizational 'place' from which health promotion could sustainably operate; and, finally, the powerful dominance of medicine, or more specifically public health medicine. The structure of public health in England has subsequently undergone rapid change in the last few years. At the beginning of April 2013, Public Health England (PHE) came into being, established to 'protect and improve the nation's health and wellbeing, and to reduce inequalities' (Department of Health, 2012). In 2021 Public Health England was replaced by two new organizations – the Office for Health Improvement and Disparities and the UK Health Security Agency. Nowhere in the PHE structure was the term 'health promotion' actually used, rather 'health protection', 'health improvement' and 'population health'. The new title of the Office for Health Improvement and Disparities has been criticized for losing 'public health' and for using the term 'health disparities' rather than health inequalities (Scally, 2021). Nevertheless, the use of terms in the finer detail such as 'levelling up', acting on the wider factors that impact on health, and a commitment to working in partnership perhaps remains indicative of a health promotion ethos.

Towards a competent health promotion workforce

Where does health promotion feature in this? Should health promotion have a separate identity and should there be distinct career pathways for those engaged in health promotion? As observed, towards the end of the old millennium, the term 'health promotion' started being used less frequently in both policy documents and job titles, despite the fact that the sphere of activity that had hitherto been described as health promotion was receiving more attention. Scott-Samuel and Springett (2007: 212) refer to this as the 'semantic eclipse of health promotion'. Further, health promotion courses began to disappear from universities' portfolios of provision to be replaced by a variety of titles, including Public Health and Public Health Promotion (Scriven, 2007). In many instances, this was merely a rebadging exercise rather than a significant change in content, but still generated concerns about the future of health promotion as a discipline and a profession. A review of specialist health promotion practice in England and Wales conducted by Griffiths and Dark concluded that: 'Specialised health promotion is a discipline integral to public health' but 'has been eroded in recent years' (2005: 6). They recommended that the specialist health promotion workforce requires recognition and advocacy along with systematic skills and competency development. A collaborative programme, 'Shaping the Future of Health Promotion', was set up in 2006 to implement these recommendations and:

- achieve recognition and identity for specialized health promotion
- develop an agreed career pathway for specialized health promotion staff.

Specification of core competencies and systems for professional registration can serve to define areas of professional practice and ensure standards. A statement on priorities for action issued by the International Union for Health Promotion and Education (IUHPE) and the Canadian Consortium for Health Promotion Research identified a specialist health promotion role as well as the need for a multisectoral response. It emphasized the importance of building a competent health promotion workforce. A number of countries have developed their own competency standards. In Australia there has been considerable work on the professionalization of the health promotion workforce (Shilton et al., 2008). The Australian Health Promotion Association has produced a national competencies framework aimed at a graduate level of competency. Five broad areas of competency are identified, as follows:

1. Programme planning, implementation and evaluation.
2. Partnership building.
3. Communication and report-writing.
4. Technology.
5. Knowledge.

There is some debate about the use of a competency-based system. Wills (2023), for example, argues that the narrow mechanistic focus of competencies is not an adequate basis for assessing professional practice because it overlooks not only the theoretical base but, importantly, the values which underpin critical reflective practice. An international review of the literature in this area pointed to the uneven progress that has been made in developing competency frameworks for health promotion and health education (Battel-Kirk et al., 2009). For example, in relation to the African context, Onya (2009) writes about the slow and inconsistent development of health promotion competencies and, with specific reference to South Africa, Wills and Rudolph (2010) point to a lack of occupational standards or competencies. In South East Asia, there has been work around developing competencies in health promotion specifically in academic education programmes for health promotion and a call for a consistent approach across the region (Van der Putten et al., 2012).

There are also dissenting views about maintaining a separate identity for health promotion. Ashton, for example, is concerned that it is inconsistent with 'an inclusive, holistic and integrated approach to public health practice' and risks 'health promotion apartheid' (2007: 207). The alternative position is that 'health promotion has been the subject of hegemonic absorption by an increasingly individualistic public health discourse' (Scott-Samuel and Springett, 2007: 211). The consequence of not acknowledging the distinctive contribution of health promotion will be failure to nurture – and risk losing – the specific set of skills and values that it brings to modern multidisciplinary public health. It will also result in the suppression of what has long been regarded as the more radical and militant wing of public health. Responding to contemporary challenges to health, both nationally and internationally, has never before put so much emphasis on the importance of health promotion. For many, it is seen as an idea whose time has come (Scriven, 2007). Rising to this challenge requires recognition of the distinctive contribution of health promotion; the development of proper career pathways; and support for the professional development of a specialist cadre of health promotion staff – that is to say, those who see their role as entirely concerned with health promotion.

The Galway Consensus Conference aimed to encourage 'global exchange and understanding concerning domains of core competency in the professional preparation and practice of health promotion and health education specialists' (Barry et al., 2009: 5). The identification of core competencies, standards and quality assurance systems was seen to be essential for developing and strengthening the capacity to improve public health in the twenty-first century. Eight domains of core competency were identified:

- Catalysing change
- Leadership
- Assessment
- Planning
- Implementation
- Evaluation
- Advocacy
- Partnerships.

A European-wide project led by Professor Margaret Barry established a framework of core competencies for health promotion in Europe (Barry et al., 2012). The CompHP Core Competencies Framework for Health Promotion sets out the key requirements for effective health promotion practice and is intended as a resource for workforce development in health promotion in Europe.

Reflecting a European commitment to health promotion, it identifies nine professional standards for health promotion underscored by 'a core base of professional and ethical values integral to the practice of health promotion' (Speller et al., 2012: 15). The nine standards are as follows:

Standard 1: Enable change

Standard 2: Advocate for health

Standard 3: Mediate through partnership

Standard 4: Communication

Standard 5: Leadership

Standard 6: Assessment

Standard 7: Planning

Standard 8: Implementation

Standard 9: Evaluation and research.

In 2016, the International Union of Health Promotion and Education published the IUHPE Core Competencies and Professional Standards for Health Promotion, which reflects these nine domains of competency (IUHPE, 2016). It will be clear from our earlier discussion that defining a competent health promotion workforce should go beyond skills to include the values and ethical principles integral to health promotion – in short, it must be shaped by the discourse of health promotion and more specifically, by an empowerment model of health promotion. For a broader critique of competency frameworks in health promotion as a whole please see Cross et al. (2017a).

The 'new' critical health education

We have touched on health education at a number of points in this chapter. To bring the chapter to a close, we will briefly summarize our position on the role of health education vis-à-vis health promotion. The emergence of health promotion effectively marginalized health education by shifting attention towards the broader determinants of health and the need for a policy response. Yet this begs the question of how change is to be instigated and what processes should be put in place to improve the health of populations and, indeed, individuals. Our contention here is that the primary driver has to be health education. While it is acknowledged that health education requires a supportive environment to achieve its goals, the converse is all too often overlooked. The development of healthy public policy to create a supportive environment is dependent on health education. As Figure 1.6 makes clear, the development of healthy public policy requires some form of learning – and *ipso facto* education – be it among policy-makers themselves, advocates or communities seeking change.

Critiques of health education have centred on its individualistic, victim-blaming orientation. However, what the critics are actually attacking is the preventive medical model of health education. Alternative, coexisting models of health education – especially the more radical, empowering models – are overlooked. Health education has a key role in tackling the structural determinants of health. Even at the individual and community level, health education can have an empowering and emancipatory function. It can also facilitate the voluntary adoption of health-enhancing behaviour. The review by Tilford et al. of the values of health promotion supports the continued relevance of health education that is empowering and in tune with the precepts of critical theory:

> We have also concluded that health education, especially using a critical empowerment model, still has an important part to play in health promotion and public health. (2003: 120)

Health education can thus be a major driver within an empowerment model of health promotion – shedding its behaviourist, victim-blaming associations. To emphasize the distinction, we refer to health education that incorporates this wider vision as the 'New Health Education'. Subsequent chapters, which address planning and strategies for health promotion in more detail, will provide the opportunity to examine its potential more fully.

KEY POINTS

- There are alternative conceptualizations of health. A working model is proposed that includes physical, mental, social and spiritual health and incorporates positive well-being as well as the absence of disease.
- Although health is influenced by human agency, structural factors have a major influence on health and health-related behaviour.
- Health promotion is a discipline with its own ideology and core values. These include equity and empowerment along with health as a right, social justice, voluntarism, autonomy, participation and partnerships.
- Ethical health promotion practice requires attention to these core principles along with the more general principles of beneficence, non-maleficence and the pursuit of the public good.
- Power is a key factor in relation to individuals' health behaviour and health choices. Power also shapes discourse about health and health promotion.
- While different models of health promotion exist, the case is put forward for an empowerment model.
- Health promotion should generally uphold the principle of voluntarism, but the use of more coercive methods may exceptionally be justified on the grounds of utilitarianism, paternalism or social justice.
- Health promotion has a specialist role within a wider, multidisciplinary response to improving public health.
- Critical and empowering, the 'New Health Education' is a major driver within health promotion.

CHAPTER 1: INTERNATIONAL CASE STUDIES

The following case studies on the online resources website are relevant to the content of this chapter: 1, 3, 4, 6 and 8.

CRITICAL REFLECTION AND APPLICATION TO PRACTICE

This chapter discusses a range of concepts that are key to health promotion including ethics. What, in your opinion, are the key ethical issues in health promotion? Can you identify any specific ethical challenges in your practice? How might you address these using the principles that have been discussed in this chapter? Brown (2018) argues that health promotion can moralize people's lifestyles. Reflect on your own morals and values. Where do they come from? How might they influence your practice? Which of the ethical frameworks in this chapter have most utility in terms of your practice?

ONLINE RESOURCES

Please visit https://study.sagepub.com/greentones5e for all the online resources for the book, including recommended further reading on each chapter subject, useful weblinks (both introduced by the authors), as well as the abovementioned case study material.

2 ASSESSING HEALTH AND ITS DETERMINANTS

In questions of science, the authority of a thousand is not worth the humble reasoning of a single individual.

Galileo Galilei (1564–1642)

OVERVIEW

This chapter considers approaches to assessing the health of communities and identifying the range of factors which impact on health and health inequalities. It will:

- identify the contribution of epidemiology to understanding health and its determinants
- establish the need for alternative perspectives including the lay perspective
- consider salutogenic as opposed to pathogenic explanations of health and ill health
- consider lifestyle and environment as determinants of health
- focus on inequality, social capital and social exclusion, with particular reference to issues of definition and measurement
- examine asset-based approaches to assessing health needs.

INTRODUCTION

Green and Kreuter (1991, 2005) trace their initial motivation to develop a planning model for health education to their observation that, in practice, they could frequently discern no apparent reason for choosing the health issue to be addressed, nor the target population to be reached. Furthermore, the intervention strategy selected was also often simply a preferred method of working rather than the most strategic option to achieve defined outcomes. They assert that 'the systematic and critical analysis of priorities and presumed cause–effect relationships can start the planner on the right foot in health promotion today' (1991: 25). What is required, therefore, is:

1. An analysis of health issues/problems
2. Prioritization
3. Analysis of the determinants.

We are said to be living in an increasingly target-driven culture. It is paramount, therefore, that we remain critically aware of how targets are defined and, indeed, given our earlier discussion of ideology, whether they are appropriate. Health promotion, as noted in Chapter 1, is characterized by its multisectoral nature and the involvement of a variety of different professional groups. Furthermore, a central tenet of health promotion is the importance of involving individuals and communities. The differing ideological positions and values among various professional and lay groups will inevitably influence the way in which the determinants of health and causal factors are defined, the evidence that is accepted to support their existence and the ways in which priorities are identified and framed. We will begin by looking at epidemiological perspectives before considering alternative or complementary approaches.

EPIDEMIOLOGICAL PERSPECTIVES

Epidemiology has been viewed as a 'primary feeder discipline' for health promotion by virtue of its contribution to setting the agenda and its role in driving the system (Macdonald and Bunton, 2002; Tannahill, 1992). As we shall see, there is considerable criticism of over-reliance on epidemiological perspectives, which are often equated with a biomedical interpretation of health. However, for now, we will confine discussion to consideration of its scope and potential contribution.

Epidemiology has typically been defined as 'the study of the distribution and determinants of disease in human populations' (Barker and Rose, 1984: v). While this draws attention to the focus of epidemiology on populations rather than individuals, it will be immediately apparent that this interpretation conforms to a negative model of health. More recent definitions signal some move towards including a positive dimension – for example, 'the study of the distribution and determinants of health-related states or events in specified populations, and the application of this study to control of health problems' (Last, 1988, in Bonita et al., 2006: 2). This particular example also emphasizes the action-orientated role of epidemiology.

Unwin et al. (1997) identify three categories of information needed as a basis for planning interventions to improve the health of populations and communities:

- basic demographic information
- the health status of communities
- determinants of health in the community.

Kroeger (1997) further lists nine key epidemiological questions that can inform the planning process. These can be organized under four headings, as shown in Box 2.1.

BOX 2.1   NINE EPIDEMIOLOGICAL QUESTIONS

Identification

1.   What are the main health problems?

Magnitude and distribution

1.   How common are they?
2.   When do they generally occur?
3.   Where do they occur?
4.   Who is affected?

Analysis

1.   Why does the problem occur?

Action and evaluation

1.   What measures could be (were) taken to deal with the problem?
2.   What results were anticipated (achieved)?
3.   What else could be done?

Source: Derived from Kroeger (1997)

Descriptive epidemiology

As we demonstrated in Chapter 1, health is both a contested concept and a subjective state. It is not without difficulty, then, that epidemiology seeks to measure health objectively. Descriptive epidemiology is essentially concerned with charting the disease burden of communities, together with the patterns of distribution of diseases – classically in relation to time, place and persons. There is frequently a heavy reliance on the use of routinely collected official health data, such as mortality and morbidity statistics, together with basic population data.

Mortality rates

The collection of data on vital events has its origins in the civil registration of births, marriages and deaths. Because of the legal requirement to register deaths, mortality data are regarded as providing a complete representation. Deaths are recorded by underlying cause – confirmed either by a medical practitioner or an inquest. The death certificate requires identification of the immediate cause of death together with any underlying cause, defined as 'the disease or injury which initiated the train of events leading to death' (Unwin et al., 1997: 12). Other significant conditions contributing to death can also be recorded. The production of mortality statistics is based on coding of the underlying cause of death according to the *International Classification of Diseases* (ICD). Since 1948, the World Health Organization has been responsible for 10-year revisions of the ICD (WHO, 2013a); ICD-11 was released in June 2018. Distinguishing between the immediate cause of death and underlying cause can be a source of error. Death rates are expressed in a number of different ways, as summarized in Table 2.1.

Table 2.1   Mortality rates

Actual rates	
Crude mortality rate	Number of deaths per 1000 people
Age-specific mortality rate	Number of deaths per 1000 people in a specific age group
Infant mortality rate	Number of deaths in the first year of life per 1000 live births
Under-5 mortality rate	Number of deaths in the first five years of life per 1000 live births
Sex-specific rates	Number of deaths per 1000 women/men
Cause-specific rates	Numbers of deaths from a specific cause per 1000 people
Constructed rates	
Age-standardized mortality rates	The death rate that would exist in a population if it had the same age structure as a standard population (e.g. national population, European standard population, Segi World Population, WHO World Standard Population; Ahmad et al., 2001)
	A direct method of standardization
Standardized mortality ratio (SMR)	The ratio of the actual number of deaths in a population to the number of deaths that would be expected if that population had the same levels of mortality as a reference population. The ratio is multiplied by 100. An SMR greater than 100 indicates a level of mortality higher than the reference population
	An indirect method of standardization

Clearly, each of the various mortality rates will create a different overall picture. The actual rates provide insight into the burden of mortality, but, given that the level of mortality is influenced by the age structure of the population, they are of little use when comparing populations with different age structures. The standardized rates, although artificial constructs, compensate for variations in age structure and can be used for comparative purposes. It is important, therefore, that appropriate rates are selected according to the intended purpose.

Morbidity rates

An important distinction in morbidity rates – and indeed health-related behaviour – is between incidence and prevalence. *Incidence* represents the number of new cases within a particular time period. *Prevalence*, in contrast, includes all the cases – either at a point in time (point prevalence) or over a defined period in time (period prevalence). Prevalence is often depicted as a pool, its overall magnitude being determined by the balance between factors filling and emptying the pool, as shown in Figure 2.1.

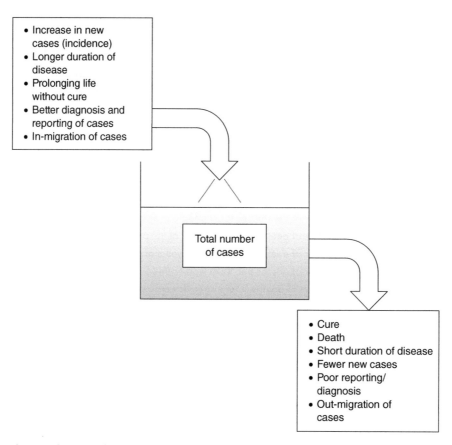

Figure 2.1   The prevalence pool

Morbidity data, unlike mortality data, are not complete in the sense that only those who come into contact with the health services will be routinely recorded. They are regarded as representing the tip of the clinical iceberg (Last, 1963) and below the surface are those who are self-medicating, using alternative therapy, with subclinical symptoms or just putting up with their symptoms. Last (1963) estimated that as much as 94% of ill health remained 'undetected' by professionals. This still rings true in 2023. For example, during the global COVID-19 pandemic the number of people hospitalized with infection only signified a small proportion of the infections in the wider population. The volume under the surface is likely to be greater the less serious – and *ipso facto* the more common – the condition. It will also be influenced by the availability of services and cultural factors associated with their usage.

Countries such as India and China, for example, use sample registration systems that rely on lay reports of causes of death. Given that the majority of day-to-day illnesses never bring people into contact with formal healthcare systems, they will go unreported or under-reported. The 'iceberg' concept is helpful again here. As Donaldson and Rutter (2017: 22) assert, the number of people who actually

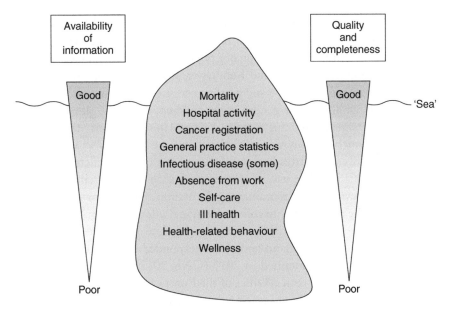

Figure 2.2   The data iceberg

make contact with formal healthcare services is 'often referred to as the tip of the iceberg'. Figure 2.2 applies the notion of the clinical iceberg to the availability of data and their completeness in what might be referred to as a 'data iceberg'.

Relatively little routine information is available on minor illnesses, states of well-being or health-related behaviour. Obtaining data on these is, therefore, usually dependent on surveys. In Great Britain, the General Household Survey, for example, used to ask each year about:

- long-standing illness, disability or infirmity and the extent to which this limits activities
- acute sickness or restricted activity during the preceding two weeks
- use of health services
- general health during the preceding year.

It also included questions about health-related behaviour such as smoking and drinking and other issues on a more occasional basis (see Office for National Statistics [ONS], 2005). The General Household Survey was subsumed under the Integrated Household Survey (IHS) in 2007. One of the key themes within the IHS is 'Health and Disability' and the survey includes questions about sexual identity, perceived general health, education, housing and employment (ONS, 2016).

Population data

Bonita et al. (2006) note that the central tool of epidemiology is the comparison of rates:

Rate = number of events in a population (numerator) ÷ size of the population (denominator)

In order to calculate rates, it is essential to know the size of the population and, for comparative purposes, the characteristics of that population. Such information is typically obtained by a census, which has been defined as 'a complete count or enumeration of a population conducted under the auspices of some governmental authority' (Ginn Daugherty and Kammeyer, 1995: 293). The United Nations Statistics Division also notes that national population and housing censuses provide valuable information on vulnerable groups, such as those affected by gender issues, children, youth, the elderly, those with impairment or disability, and the homeless and migrant populations (United Nations Statistics Division, 2002).

The first complete modern census was carried out in Sweden in 1749 (Ginn Daugherty and Kammeyer, 1995). The UK census dates back to 1801 and has been conducted every 10 years since then, with the exception of 1941. The nature of a census is such that it attempts to count the entire population. It therefore provides the denominator information required for the calculation of rates. The census also provides the opportunity to collect additional information on a range of demographic and socioeconomic factors – those selected tend to vary over time and between countries. It was estimated that 97% of households in England and Wales responded to the 2021 census (ONS, 2021), an increase on the 90.4% coverage attained in 2011 (ONS, 2012). The United Nations Economic Commission for Europe and the Statistical Office of the European Communities (undated: 7) suggest that the topics included in a census should result from a balanced consideration of:

- the needs of the country, national as well as local, to be served by the census data
- the achievement of the maximum degree of international comparability, both within regions and on a worldwide basis
- acceptability of questions to respondents and their ability to provide the required information without an undue burden being placed on them
- the technical competence of the enumerators (if any) to obtain information on the topics by direct observation
- the total national resources available for enumeration, processing, tabulation and publication, which will determine the overall feasible scope of the census.

The UN provides a list of recommended areas and topics to be included in a country's census. A list of the areas included in Jamaica's 2011 census is provided in Box 2.2. Jamaica's 2021 census was postponed due to the COVID-19 pandemic and took place in late 2022/early 2023.. Data collected included age, sex, marital status, educational attainment, religious affiliation, household composition, family characteristics, household size, as well as access to facilities such as water, electricity, waste disposal and the Internet (Linton, 2022). At the time of writing this chapter the data were not available.

BOX 2.2 AREAS INCLUDED IN JAMAICA'S 2011 CENSUS

Topics included based on UN recommendations:

- Geographical and Internal Migration Characteristics
- International Migration Characteristics

- Household and Family Characteristics
- Demographic and Social Characteristics (sex, age, marital status, religion, ethnicity)
- Fertility and Mortality (number of living children, household deaths, etc.)
- Educational Characteristics
- Economic Characteristics (occupation, time worked, income, etc.)
- Disability Characteristics.

Additional topics included:

- Usual Mode of Transportation
- Individual Use of Information and Communication Technology Devices
- Social Welfare Benefits
- Union Status – Consensual (Non-legal) Unions.

Source: Adapted from Nam (2013)

Kerrison and Macfarlane (2000) draw attention to two potential limitations of health data obtained by census processes. First, the precise wording of the questions is important in relation to the response elicited. Second, it relies on the accuracy of self-reporting, which will be subject to a whole range of potentially contaminating or distorting factors. In relation to using census data to estimate home-lessness the Australian Bureau of Statistics (ABS) (2012) point to two key limitations. First, under/over-estimation – whereby 'people are enumerated in the Census but the data collected about them is not sufficient to be certain about whether or not they were homeless on Census night'; second, under-enumeration – 'people who were not enumerated in the Census' (ABS, 2012). Skinner (2018) argues that, worldwide, census taking encounters a number of difficulties including 'cost pressures, concerns about intrusiveness, privacy and response burden, reduced cooperation, difficulties in access-ing secure apartments and enumerating unsafe areas, more complex living arrangements, and timeli-ness concerns' (p. 49).

Life expectancy, HALE, DALYs and QALYs

Life expectancy is frequently used as a general indicator of a population's health status. It is the average number of years that individuals of different ages can be expected to live if current mortality rates apply (Bonita et al., 2006). It is included as a measure in the Health Profile for England – life expectancy at birth in England in 2019 was 79.9 years for men and 83.6 years for women but, due to the COVID-19 pandemic, this fell in 2020 to 78.6 years for men and 82.6 years for women (Raleigh, 2021). However, not all those years are likely to be lived in full health (Department of Health, 2007a). The notion of healthy life expectancy or health-adjusted life expectancy (HALE) makes allowance for this. It is the: 'average number of years that a person can expect to live in "full health" taking into account years lived in less than full health due to disease and/or injury' (WHO, 2013b). HALE therefore 'summarises mortality and non-fatal outcomes in a single measure of average population health' (Salomon et al., 2012). A systematic review by Salomon et al. (2012: 2144) examining HALE in 187 countries over two decades concluded that HALE 'differs substantially between countries' and that 'as life expectancy has increased, the number of healthy years lost to disability has also increased in most countries'. Table 2.2 provides a comparison of life expectancy, healthy life expectancy and early life mortality rates in three countries – the country with the lowest, the Central African Republic, the country with the highest, Japan, and the country with the lowest life expectancy in South America, Guyana.

Table 2.2   Comparison of life expectancies and early mortality in selected countries

Indicator	Value (year) Guyana	Value (year) Japan	Value (year) African Central Republic
Life expectancy at birth (years) both sexes	70.26 (2022)	85.03 (2022)	54.36 (2022)
Life expectancy at birth (years) males	67.22 (2022)	81.91 (2022)	52.16 (2022)
Life expectancy at birth (years) females	73.53 (2022)	88.09 (2022)	56.58 (2022)
Healthy life expectancy (HALE) at birth (years) males	52.0 (2007)	72.68 (2021)	51.7 (2018)
Healthy life expectancy (HALE) at birth (years) females	55.0 (2007)	75.38 (2021)	54.4 (2018)
Probability of dying (per 1000 live births) under 5 years of age (under-5 mortality rate)	28.4 (2020)	2.3 (2020)	103 (2020)
Infant mortality rate (per 1000 live births)	24.2 (2020)	1.8 (2019)	77 (2020)

Sources: Derived from UNPD (2022); Juneau (2021); O'Neill (2022); Nayak (2019); UNICEF (2021)

Mortality can be considered premature if individuals do not survive to an expected age and this shortfall can be regarded as years of life lost. The total number of premature years of life lost (PYLL) due to different causes of mortality can be calculated. The use of PYLL as a measure of disease burden and for comparative purposes clearly attaches more weight to deaths occurring in younger age groups.

The concept of PYLL is extended and refined by the notion of disability adjusted life years (DALYs), which, in addition to premature loss of life, includes loss of healthy life, broadly referred to as disability:

> One DALY can be thought of as one lost year of 'healthy life'. The sum of these DALYs across the population, or the burden of disease, can be thought of as a measurement of the gap between current health status and an ideal health situation where the entire population lives to an advanced age, free of disease and disability. (WHO, 2013d)

The severity of the disability is graded on a scale from 0 (perfect health) to 1 (dead).

DALY = YLL + YLD

The DALY was introduced in the *World Development Report 1993* (World Bank, 1993) as a means of measuring the global burden of disease. Effectively, it is a measure of the health gap between the current situation and the ideal in which everyone lives to an old age in full health. In most countries, disability becomes more significant as death rates go down (Institute for Health Metrics and Evaluation, 2013) and disability is an increasingly large portion of the global disease burden (Vos et al., 2020). Whereas assessing disease burden had formerly been overly reliant on mortality statistics, the DALY provided a broader view of disease burden by including conditions that affect health status. The use of DALYs, for example, has revealed the magnitude of the contribution of neuropsychiatric conditions to the global disease burden. By way of example, the Global Burden of Disease Study 2017 determined that depressive disorders were one of the four leading causes of years lived with disability (YLDs) (James et al., 2018). Globally we have seen a shift towards non-communicable diseases in adults from communicable diseases in children. In 2019 the leading risk factors for attributable deaths were high systolic blood pressure and tobacco use whilst the leading risk factor for DALYs was maternal and child malnutrition (GBD 2019 Risk Factor Collaborators, 2019). It should be noted that this varies with geographical location and age. For example, with regard to age, 'iron deficiency was the leading risk factor for those aged 10–24 years, alcohol use for those aged 25–49 years, and high systolic blood pressure for those aged 50–74 years and 75 years and older' (GBD 2019 Risk Factor Collaborators, 2019: 1223). Risk is not evenly distributed. During the COVID-19 pandemic data from several different countries showed that being older, male, a smoker and having two or more comorbidities increased the likelihood of death (Tazerji et al., 2022), and in the United Kingdom being poor or from an ethnic minority also increased the risk of mortality (Whitehead et al., 2021).

Table 2.3 shows how the leading causes of DALYs globally have changed in the years between 2000 and 2019.

According to WHO (2022a) by the year 2019, compared to 2000, there was a global decline of 50% in DALYs due to communicable diseases such as HIV/AIDS and diarrhoeal diseases. However,

Table 2.3 Leading causes of DALYs globally

Ranking	2019	2000
1	Neonatal conditions	Ranked 1
2	Ischaemic heart disease	Ranked 4
3	Stroke	Ranked 5
4	Lower respiratory infections	Ranked 2
5	Diarrhoeal diseases	Ranked 3
6	Road injury	Ranked 8
7	Chronic obstructive pulmonary disease	Ranked 9
8	Diabetes mellitus	Ranked 14
9	Tuberculosis	Ranked 6
10	Congenital anomalies	Ranked 11

Note: There are substantial differences in rankings of leading causes in different global regions.

Source: Global Health Observatory (WHO, 2022a)

DALYs from diabetes increased by 80% over the same period of time and DALYs from Alzheimer's disease were twice as many in 2019 as in 2000. Road injuries remain in the top 10 leading causes of DALYs in the world, ranked 8th in 2000 and in 2010 (Murray et al., 2012) and 6th in 2019 (see Table 2.3).

The well-known health promotion maxim of adding life to years not just years to life draws attention to the issue of *quality* of life. Although, in principle, quality of life embraces 'emotional, social and physical well-being, and ability to function in the ordinary tasks of living' (Donald, 2001), quality of life measures tend to focus on disease states. The notion of quality adjusted life years (QALYs) was developed as a means of assessing the benefits of interventions in terms of the number and quality of years gained. 'QALYs combine mortality and morbidity into a single metric, reflect [individual] preferences, and can be used to assess health gains across a wide range of treatments and healthcare settings' (Neumann and Cohen, 2018: 2). The QALY was primarily developed to provide a utility rating to compare the health benefits of different interventions. It is a way of assigning a numerical value to a health state, based on the premise that, if a year of good-quality life expectancy is given the value of 1, then a year of poor-quality or unhealthy life must be worth less than 1. It therefore combines the length and quality of life into a single index (Bowling, 1997a).

Quality in this context is generally taken to be the absence of negative health states (that is to say, disease and disability) rather than positive well-being, which we discuss below. The EuroQol Group developed the EQ-5D as a standardized instrument for measuring health outcome (EuroQol, undated). It uses five dimensions of health (mobility, self-care, usual activities, pain/discomfort, anxiety/depression), and each dimension comprises three levels (some, moderate or extreme problems). Given the subjective nature of quality of life and the various philosophical interpretations of health and well-being referred to in Chapter 1, it will come as no surprise that there is considerable debate about attempts to measure these factors objectively.

This use of QALYs has been much criticized. The criticisms are both technical, on account of their method of construction, and ethical. Reed Johnson (2009) points out that, although the simplicity of the QALY has led to its widespread use, there are several limitations including empirical and conceptual ones. Concerns have been raised about an integral part of the assessment of QALYs – an evaluation of health status – which varies significantly from person to person (Kocot et al., 2021). The use of QALYs as a means of prioritization of healthcare has been viewed as unjust because it is essentially ageist – systematically favouring interventions that improve the health status of the young by virtue of their longer life expectancy. It also arbitrates on the basis of capacity to benefit rather than on the basis of actual need – a point that we will return to in Chapter 5. However, arguments in defence of QALYs refer to the need for a single index of health with which to compare the outcomes of different interventions in order to deploy limited resources to achieve maximum benefits for the community (Williams and Kind, 1992) and that can help 'to guide healthcare decisions while maintaining consistency and transparency' (Neumann and Cohen, 2018: npn).

The allocation of resources based on DALYs is surrounded by similar arguments to those about QALYs. In addition, the greater value attached to adult life as opposed to that of children or the elderly in the construction of DALYs attracts particular criticism (Abbasi, 1999), a point reiterated more recently by Kocot et al. (2021).

Positive health

Much of the foregoing has focused on mortality and morbidity. The application of this information to the assessment of health is predicated on the assumption that the absence of disease is indicative of health. Yet, we noted in Chapter 1 that health is more than just the absence of disease. Catford's (1983) early attempt to identify positive health indicators provides examples of individual behaviour and health knowledge, socioeconomic conditions and aspects of the physical environment. However, the analysis is still located within a disease causation continuum. The factors identified can only be deemed healthy by virtue of their contribution to prevention of disease and do not, of themselves, constitute positive well-being. Surveys such as the Health Survey for England collect data about the nation's health and exposure to selected risk factors (Department of Health, 2007a). The survey was established in 1991 to monitor trends and progress towards national health targets (Mimas, 2001) and has run every year except 2020 (due to the impact of COVID-19). It includes a questionnaire as well as objective measures such as physical measurements and the analysis of blood samples. As well as a Well-Being Module added in 2011, the survey has a 'core' that is repeated annually (physical health; mental health and wellbeing; lifestyle behaviours such as smoking, drinking, dietary habits; social care; and physical measures such as height, weight and blood pressure – NHS, 2022), plus additional modules on topics of special interest such as cardiovascular disease and accidents that can change year on year.

Kemm (1993) notes the relative ease of defining negative rather than positive health states and the greater success of epidemiology in handling the former rather than the latter. Bowling (1997a: 5) suggests that positive health:

> implies 'completeness' and 'full functioning' or 'efficiency' of mind and body and social adjustment. Beyond this there is no one accepted definition. Positive health could be described as the ability to cope with stressful situations, the maintenance of a strong social support system, integration in the community, high morale and life satisfaction, psychological well-being, and even levels of physical fitness as well as physical health.

Both authors are in agreement that the components of well-being require both precise definition and the formulation of criteria. A key issue is whether positive and negative states are opposite ends of the same dimension with some neutral midpoint or, as argued by Downie et al. (1996), they occupy different dimensions. These alternative conceptualizations are shown in Figure 2.3. Kemm (1993) asserts that there is little evidence to support positive health being viewed as a distinct dimension, although there may be theoretical reasons for doing so. Furthermore, positive and negative health may occupy the same dimension for some aspects, such as objective physical health, but different dimensions for subjective health.

A number of devices and scales exist for assessing aspects of quality of life and well-being. These include:

- SF-36
- Health Assessment Questionnaire
- Sickness Impact Profile

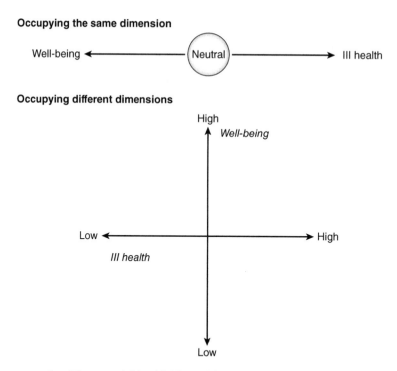

Figure 2.3   Dimensions of well-being and ill health (derived from Kemm, 1993; and Downie et al., 1996)

- Missoula-VITAS Quality of Life Index
- European KIDSCREEN.

There is considerable variation in the conceptual underpinnings of the various instruments and their validity and reliability. (For a more detailed discussion, see Bowling, 1997a, 1997b; Donald, 2001; Edgar et al., 1998.) Some of these scales derive from professional perspectives; some have incorporated lay views in their development.

Health and happiness

A number of measures have been developed in order to measure happiness. For many, happiness is inextricably linked to health. As Borghesi and Vercelli (2010) point out, the causal relationship between health and happiness is well documented and 'many international institutions, national governments and communities are promoting and measuring happiness in various ways' (Iriarte and Musikanski, 2019: 115). When asked about happiness, people often refer to their current health status; conversely, health status impacts on perceived levels of happiness. There have been several attempts, at an international level, to develop measures of happiness (Cross et al., 2021). Happiness can be measured using subjective (that is to say, self-reporting) or objective (that is to say, observing physiological states) means. A number of factors are assumed to impact on levels of personal happiness, such as income. However, the relationship between health and happiness is not straight-forward. For example, people have an amazing capacity to adapt to very difficult life circumstances, including significant challenges to health. Some research shows that living in poverty or being unemployed has adverse effects on happiness (Yiengprugsawan et al., 2012). However, survey data from Australia, the USA, Britain and Indonesia show that the quality of people's social relationships and their health (mental and physical) affect well-being and happiness more than their economic situation (Clark et al., 2017). Another study on health and happiness carried out in four countries (Australia, Britain, Germany and the USA) concluded that 'human misery is due not to economic factors but to failed relationships and physical and mental illness' (London School of Economics [LSE], 2016) and where you live makes a difference too – a Guyanese study exploring the determinants of subjective health and happiness found significant differences between those living in urban areas as compared with rural, especially among young women, whereby those living in urban areas reported better health and happiness (Wang et al., 2020). The World Happiness Report (WHO, 2022b) has been in existence for the past 10 years (as of 2022). The 10th report, published in the context of the global pandemic, revealed that alongside the significant challenges faced by people across the world, which include a general rise in stress and worry, there was also a reported increase in benevolence and social support (WHR, 2022). The report notes that, over the past 10 years, there has been a trend towards measures of happiness compared with the previous focus on income and GDP (Helliwell et al., 2022). For further, more detailed discussion on some of the paradoxes in the relationship between health and happiness, see Borghesi and Vercelli (2010).

Analytic epidemiology

While the patterns of distribution of disease revealed by descriptive epidemiology may generate tentative hypotheses about causation, analytic epidemiology focuses specifically on exploring cause-and-effect relationships. One of the best known early examples is the work of John Snow, who, by meticulously mapping cholera outbreaks in London during 1848–9 and 1853–4, was able to demonstrate that the disease was spread by contaminated water (Chave, 1958). Although derided by the miasmatists, who favoured the view that such diseases were caused by the miasma emanating from filth and putrefying material, and well in advance of Koch's discovery of the micro-organism that causes cholera in 1884, Snow's work provided evidence to support the general introduction of public health measures, such as improved water and sanitation – over and above the renowned removal of the handle of the Broad Street water pump to halt an outbreak of cholera in the vicinity.

The evidence for causality is subject to epistemological debate. Furthermore, many contemporary health problems are not the product of simple cause-and-effect relationships. Analysis is often concerned with multiple causes and, in some instances, multiple effects. Frequently, therefore, the focus is on complex multifactorial webs. Moon and Gould (2000) identify three main conditions that must be present if observed associations are to be judged as causally linked. First, do the levels of exposure and disease vary in the same way – that is, co-variation? Second, does cause precede the effect – that is, temporal precedence? Third, have other possible explanations and confounding factors been eliminated?

A number of different types of epidemiological studies are used to explore causality. These range from observational studies, such as ecological and cross-sectional studies, which are regarded as relatively weak in their capacity to demonstrate causality, to the more robust case control and cohort studies. Intervention or experimental studies are more able to control for confounding variables and may take the form of randomized controlled, field or community trials. Bonita et al. (2006) provide a useful set of guidelines for assessing causality and these are listed in Table 2.4.

Table 2.4 Guidelines for causality

Temporal relation	Does the cause precede the effect?
Plausibility	Does it make sense in the light of existing knowledge and mechanisms of action?
Consistency	Do other studies produce similar findings?
Strength	Is there a strong association?
Dose-response relationship	Does increase in exposure produce increased effect?
Reversibility	Does the risk decrease when the possible cause is removed?
Study design	Is the evidence robust and derived from strong studies?
Judging the evidence	How many lines of evidence lead to the conclusion?

Source: Derived from Bonita et al. (2006: 90)

We will give further consideration to the complexity of causal relationships in health promotion programmes when we discuss evaluation in Chapter 11. However, returning to the subject of disease causation, Bonita et al. (2006: 83) define the cause of a disease or injury as:

> an event, condition, characteristic or a combination of these factors which plays an important role in producing the health outcome. Logically a cause must precede an outcome. A cause is termed *sufficient* when it inevitably produces or initiates an outcome and is termed *necessary* if an outcome cannot develop in its absence. [Emphasis in the original]

It therefore follows that, in many instances, well-recognized causal factors are neither necessary nor sufficient. Take smoking, for example. Some people who have never smoked will develop lung cancer, so smoking cannot be seen as necessary, and some people who smoke do not develop lung cancer, hence smoking is not sufficient. There is, however, indisputable evidence that smoking is an important causal factor that increases the probability of developing lung cancer and, conversely, that this will be reduced by the cessation of smoking. Thus, it becomes important to think in terms of probability and risk. The term 'risk factor' is applied to those factors that are associated with the development of a disease, but not sufficient in themselves to cause it – often with the underlying intent of identifying factors that can be modified to prevent disease occurring. 'Relative risk' is the ratio of the rate of the disease in those exposed to a particular factor to the rate in those not exposed (see Box 2.3 on risk). It indicates the number of times that it is *more likely* that an individual exposed to the factor will develop the disease. It is useful in establishing the strength of the association and also in graphically encapsulating the levels of additional risk incurred by individuals.

In contrast, the notion of 'attributable risk' acknowledges the fact that many diseases develop independently of exposure to risk factors. In order to assess the amount of disease that is actually attributable to exposure, the rate in those not exposed to the risk factor (that is, those who would have developed the disease regardless of exposure) is subtracted from the rate in those exposed (see Box 2.3 for formula).

A related concept is the 'population attributable risk' (see Box 2.3). This indicates the amount of disease that would be avoided in a population if exposure to the risk factor was completely eliminated.

BOX 2.3 ASSESSMENT OF RISK

Relative risk (·)	= rate of the disease in those exposed to the risk factor · rate of the disease in those not exposed
Attributable risk (rate)	= rate of the disease in those exposed to the risk factor - rate of the disease in those not exposed
Population attributable risk	= attributable risk · proportion of the population exposed to the risk factor

Establishing the potential and feasibility for prevention rests on the capacity to identify modifiable risk factors. Conventionally, different levels of prevention are distinguished:

- **primary prevention** is concerned with preventing the development of disease by reducing exposure to risk factors – environmental and behavioural
- **secondary prevention**, in contrast, focuses on early diagnosis – for example, by screening – to improve the prospects of treatment
- **tertiary prevention** includes measures to reduce the consequences of illness and is often seen as integral to a rehabilitation programme.

A fourth level of prevention has also been recognized (Bonita et al., 2006):

- **primordial prevention** aims to prevent the emergence of social, economic and cultural patterns known to be associated with disease in cultures that already have healthy traditional ways of life.

More recently, recognition is also given to an additional level of prevention:

- **quaternary prevention**, which aims to mitigate or avoid the results of unnecessary or excessive interventions (Cook, 2012) or over-medicalization (Starfield et al., 2008).

A further issue is whether it is preferable to target preventive interventions at the population in general or high-risk groups (Rose, 1992). Arguments in favour of the high-risk approach include its greater cost-effectiveness and the fact that people who are known to be at high risk may be more motivated to change. However, it presupposes that it is both possible to identify those at risk and that the disease will not occur in those who do not fall within this category. Nor would such an approach contribute to changing general norms, so it might be more difficult for individuals to make changes. Furthermore, health and health behaviour are influenced by a broad range of social and environmental factors that can only be tackled at the population level. Even when focusing on specific behaviour, the whole population approach has the capacity to achieve a significant reduction in disease. Nevertheless, although major change may be achieved at the population level, it requires many individuals to make changes and relatively few of them will gain any personal benefit – referred to by Rose (1992) as the 'prevention paradox'.

THE NEED FOR ALTERNATIVE PERSPECTIVES

Two key questions are often asked when assessing the utility of health information:

- Is it necessary?
- Is it sufficient?

Both are pertinent to the selection of information to identify priority health issues and assess health needs. Furthermore, the answers to both will be influenced by issues of ideology, epistemology (concerned with the nature of knowledge and how it is acquired) and, not least, practicality.

Fundamentally, much epidemiology is about association rather than cause (Smith, 2001). Epidemiological approaches to assessing health status and identifying the determinants of health are consistent with a modernist emphasis on rationality and faith in the scientific method. De Kadt (1982) suggests that perspectives on health are informed by the dominant conceptions of medicine. Of particular relevance is its mechanistic nature, together with its focus on micro-causality. As a consequence, attention is directed towards individuals who become sick and, by inference, their unhealthy lifestyles, rather than the social, economic and environmental factors that are responsible for these lifestyles. Krieger (2001) states that the early epidemiology and public health of the mid to late nineteenth century clearly recognized that population health is shaped by both social and biological processes. However, increased interest in personal preventive measures in the late nineteenth and early twentieth centuries signalled a shift in emphasis for mainstream modern epidemiology which takes little account of the structural factors that influence people's lives.

The emergence of 'social epidemiology' in the 1950s was distinguished by its explicit focus on the *social* determinants of health – a position reflected in the 'New Public Health' movement. 'Critical epidemiology', furthermore, 'places an emphasis on the social and power relations that shape disease definition and disease causation' (Moon and Gould, 2000: 7).

Issues of micro-causality are undoubtedly relevant to understanding the factors that impact on health status, such as is the case with exposure to the *tubercle bacillus* and the development of tuberculosis. However, they are not sufficient. They need to be understood in the context of the social and environmental factors – such as overcrowding, social class, poverty and urbanization – that are also associated with the development of the disease. Furthermore, Kelly and Charlton (1995) caution against reification of the social system and a simple deterministic view of the relationship between social factors and ill health, which merely replicates the type of thinking integral to a biomedical approach – albeit further upstream. They note the tension in health promotion discourse between free will and determinism – that is, between *agency* and *structure* – and call for an understanding of the reciprocal relationship between the two.

The application of science and rationality to the analysis of the determinants of ill health, or even positive health states, assumes that there is an objective reality. A postmodern understanding, in contrast, views reality as both contextual and contingent. Rather than one objective reality, there are multiple perspectives and interpretations of reality. For example, young women's risky health practices such as binge-drinking are often viewed as problematic by health professionals, yet young women tend to frame such practices in more positive, agentic ways (Cross et al., 2013).

Furthermore, contrary to the customary view that science and the scientific method are concerned with the objective pursuit of truth, in fact, science itself is socially constructed – both in its focus and its methods. The construction of problems – the ways in which they are framed and the determinants explored – are all socially shaped (Lupton, 2006; Petersen and Lupton, 1996). How far upstream will, or should, the quest for determinants go? What risk factors are regarded as legitimate areas of enquiry? What evidence will be accepted?

Official statistics form the basis of much epidemiological and, indeed, sociological enquiry. It is appropriate at this point to consider the nature of official data.

Official health data – reality or myth?

The characteristics of official health statistics are that they generally include large data sets that have been collected regularly by official agencies over long periods of time. It is a truism that data do not exist in their own right, but are constructed. There are clearly issues concerning the technicalities of data collection, its representativeness and completeness. As we have already noted, official health data will only include those who have come into contact with services, registered vital events or been included in official surveys. Consulting a doctor or taking time off work will inevitably be influenced by a range of social and cultural factors. The collection of some official data – such as mortality and census data – attempts to include all cases, whereas surveys will only involve a sample.

The way in which data are classified and categorized is also socially constructed. For example, in relation to certification of death, 'old age', which featured prominently as a cause of death in the late nineteenth century, becomes an inadequate descriptor in our more biomedically enlightened times – more specific causal explanations are required. There is a well-known tendency towards under-reporting of emotionally charged issues, such as suicide and AIDS. Furthermore, at what point in the temporal sequence of causality do we identify a single cause? For a child dying in one of the least developed parts of the world, is it measles, malnutrition or poverty? For a man dying prematurely in a rundown inner-city area, is it lung cancer or smoking or unemployment? Interestingly, the 10th revision of the *International Classification of Diseases* introduced a set of codes for factors that influence health status and contact with health services. When even ostensibly objective issues such as mortality and morbidity can be seen to be socially constructed, assessing 'quality of life' becomes even more problematic. Classifying people by gender, ethnic group and socioeconomic status provides further evidence of social construction.

Official data, then, are not facts in their own right, but are constructed. The ways in which they are constructed will be influenced by both technical and ideological issues. There are several questions to consider when assessing the quality of official health data (see Box 2.4 for examples – this is by no means an exhaustive list).

BOX 2.4 KEY ISSUES ON THE QUALITY OF POPULATION HEALTH DATA

- Accuracy – to what extent are the data correct?
- Precision – have appropriate measures of uncertainty been included?
- Completeness – how many of the data are missing?
- Timeliness – what period do the data refer to? Is it relevant to the current position?
- Coverage – is the whole population of interest represented?
- Accessibility – who has access to the data?
- Confidentiality/suppression/disclosure control – what restrictions/regulations are being followed?
- What was the original purpose of collection/collation of the data? (May be a source of bias.)
- Who undertook the data collection? – This may not be available.
- How were the data collected? – This may not be available
- Whether what is included in the data set is the actual requirement, or whether it will have to act as a proxy for the real item.
- Is the data set comparative, what are the comparators and are they appropriate?
- If the data set presents rates or ratios, have appropriate techniques been used to control for differing population structures?

Source: Adapted from Goodyear and Malhotra (2007)

Goodyear and Malhotra (2007) have listed a number of issues and questions worth applying to any information data set on public health. Their list is by no means exhaustive, and arguably not necessarily specific to public health data, but it does raise a number of important considerations with which to interrogate such information. Using the acronym CAT, the Centers for Disease Control and Prevention identifies three main characteristics of high-quality data in population (public) health – Completeness, Accuracy and Timeliness (CDC, 2020).

May (1993) identifies three schools of thought in relation to official statistics:

- **realist** – considers official statistics to be objective indicators of phenomena
- **institutionalist** – sees official statistics as artificial constructs revealing more about an institution's priorities in collecting data than the phenomena they purport to represent
- **radical** – extends the institutionalist view to include discretionary practices embedded within and replicating the power structure and dynamics of society.

By way of example, let us take the use of waiting lists for hip replacement surgery as an indicator of prevalence and need. A realist interpretation would presuppose that individuals have equal access to general practitioners, who would refer them to hospital for treatment and the length of the waiting lists would simply be the product of the number of individuals requiring treatment and the period required for throughput. An institutionalist view would question the way in which the hospital constructed the waiting list for treatment. For example, have treatment waiting lists been kept short by having a long waiting period prior to consultation? A radical view would locate this last question within the context of any national imperative to reduce waiting lists and political pressure to demonstrate more efficient services. Changes in these contextual factors would inevitably influence the comparability of data over time. Conspiracy theorists would subscribe to the view that statistics are deliberately manipulated to suit an agenda rather than being the unconsciously biased products of systems and practices.

The danger in seeing official data merely as social constructs is that it can lead us to reject them as having no inherent value. We then have a limited capacity to assess health status and identify problem issues. The evidence that initially exposed, and continues to document, the effects of social inequality, for example, drew substantially on official health data. Without this insight, it would have been difficult to mount an argument in favour of tackling social inequality. What is needed is the *critical* use of health data that takes full account of the ways in which they have been constructed.

The lay perspective

The lay perspective introduces a completely different dimension. Lay knowledge is rooted in the direct and vicarious experience of individuals and communities and their cultural understandings. It is interpreted within the context of people's real lives and day-to-day experiences. The earlier reference to the 'clinical iceberg' would indicate that most of our individual and collective experiences of ill health and health occur below the surface. There, it is effectively hidden from the reaches of routine data-collection systems and, hence, does not feature in most official accounts of health.

Faith in the value of lay knowledge about health and ill health has been central to the development of the self-help movement – a movement that challenged medical, and, indeed, expert hegemony. Furthermore, community activists have used their own insights, derived by means of what has been termed popular or lay epidemiology, to mount campaigns to tackle what they perceive to be the cause of local health problems. Lay epidemiology can support the case for local measures, such as improved housing and traffic-calming measures.

Allmark and Tod (2006: 460) assert that lay epidemiology is a term 'used to describe the processes through which lay individuals understand and interpret health risks'. Moon and Gould (2000: 7) note that, although critics have challenged this approach as being 'anecdotal, uninformed and even dangerous', it provides direct insight into the ways in which health and ill health are commonly experienced, understood and managed. In an exploration of lay epidemiology and cancer, possible causes were attributed to behavioural, environmental, biological and psychological factors; however, the participants also emphasized the 'randomness' of cancer (Macdonald, 2011). Clearly, as Allmark and Tod (2006) argue, an appreciation of lay epidemiology is relevant for planning preventive (and more effective) health promotion interventions. Likewise, establishing the meaning that certain so-called risky health practices hold for people is important in designing health communication messages aimed at reducing risk (Cross et al., 2017a).

Lay interpretations of health are complex and multidimensional. Far from being trivial, they demonstrate coherent and sophisticated understandings. A number of major studies have explored these understandings (for example, Blaxter and Patterson, 1982; Cornwell, 1984; Herzlich, 1973; Stainton Rogers, 1991; Williams, 1983). Blaxter (2007) identified five categories of responses given when people are asked about what health is, as follows:

- health as not ill
- health as physical fitness, vitality
- health as social relationships
- health as function
- health as psychosocial well-being.

Lay recognition of the absence of disease, illness and pain as integral to health is noteworthy as the professional discourse on well-being does not always explicitly address this issue.

There is some interplay between professional and lay accounts of health, though. Lay perspectives often encompass knowledge and understandings developed within expert paradigms (Shaw, 2002). For example, the germ theory is fully integrated into most Western lay interpretations of disease. It is interesting to note, however, that lay accounts might include such reductionist explanations, but they also go further, addressing issues associated with meaning, such as 'Why me?' and 'Why now?' (Williams and Popay, 1994). A full understanding of health and ill health will necessarily seek to incorporate these hitherto often private accounts.

The premise underpinning our earlier discussion of risk was that, from an epidemiological perspective, it can be measured objectively. In the same way that health and illness are not simple biological states, but are socially constructed, lay interpretations and perceptions of risk are also complex. As we will explore more fully in Chapter 3, they derive from the interplay of a plethora of psychosocial and cultural factors.

Frankel et al. (1991) noted that lay perceptions of risk are often in tune with mainstream epidemiological analyses. For example, with regard to coronary heart disease, there is lay understanding of an association with both hereditary factors and adverse social circumstances – issues that rarely feature in health education campaigns. Frankel et al. raise the interesting question as to why there was a rapid and dramatic reduction in egg consumption in the UK in the late 1980s in response to concerns about salmonella infection when years of warning about the harmful effects of the cholesterol content of eggs brought about little change. They propose that there are different lay conceptualizations of risk. At one end of the spectrum, the risk is both immediate and easily imagined and therefore to be avoided – encapsulated as 'bad/poisonous behaviour'. At the other end of the spectrum, risks are perceived to be less immediate and less specific. Some behaviours associated with this type of risk, such as smoking, are acknowledged to be harmful, but may also have desirable aspects – hence, they are termed 'bad/desirable behaviour'. They suggest that the advertising industry attempts to keep behaviour away from the bad/poisonous end of the spectrum by emphasizing the desirable elements.

The biomedical model has often been criticized because of its expert-led, top-down orientation. However, even interpretive approaches – which purport to provide greater insight into the experiences of lay people – may still remain an essentially expert-led analysis of that experience. A true commitment to including the lay perspective involves going beyond seeing people merely as research subjects. It requires an egalitarian approach to seeking their active involvement at all stages of the research process – not least in formulating the priority issues to address.

Pathogenesis or salutogenesis

Regardless of whether or not they conform to a reductionist, biomedical or more interpretive position, the majority of studies of the determinants of health and ill health are located within a pathogenic paradigm. As Kelly and Charlton (1995: 82) note:

> The social model of health is, in this regard, no different to the medical model. In the medical model the pathogens are microbes, viruses or malfunctioning cellular reproduction. In the social model they are poor housing, unemployment and powerlessness. The discourse may be different but the epistemology is the same. The social model is not, in our view, an alternative to the discredited medical model. It is a partner in crime and a very close modernist relative.

Antonovsky (1984) asserts that the fundamental assumption of this paradigm is that individuals are in a state of balance or homeostasis and that when this state is challenged by microbial, physical or chemical factors or psychosocial stressors, regulatory mechanisms come into play to restore homeostasis. He identifies a number of consequences of this thinking:

- the tendency to think dichotomously about people, classifying them as healthy or diseased
- a focus on disease states or risk factors
- the search for cause or multifactorial causes
- the assumption that stressors are bad
- mounting wars against specific diseases
- ignoring the factors associated with wellness.

In proposing a salutogenic paradigm, Antonovsky advocates a radical change in perspective concerning what is involved in staying healthy. This shifts the focus away from specific diseases and towards those general factors involved in health, and in moving along what he terms the 'health-ease/dis-ease continuum' (Antonovsky, 1984: 117). He does not, however, totally abandon the pathogenic paradigm, but offers salutogenesis as an *additional* perspective.

> I am not proposing that the pathogenic paradigm be abandoned, theoretically or institutionally. It has immense achievement and power for good to its credit. I have attempted to point to its limitations, to the blinders involved in any paradigm.

Salutogenesis focuses on the factors associated with successful coping, which are envisaged as buffers mitigating the effects of stressors. While there are numerous individual coping variables, Antonovsky (1987: 19) proposes the 'sense of coherence' (SOC) as an overarching explanatory variable.

The sense of coherence is a global orientation that expresses the extent to which one has a pervasive, enduring, although dynamic feeling of confidence that:

1. The stimuli deriving from one's internal and external environments in the course of living are structured, predictable and explicable;
2. The resources are available to one to meet the demands posed by these stimuli; and
3. These demands are challenges, worthy of investment and engagement.

These three components of the SOC are called comprehensibility, manageability and meaningfulness.

In considering how a strong SOC helps people to cope with stressors, Antonovsky (1987) attempts to identify generalized and specific resistance resources. The features that such resistance resources have in common are:

- **consistency** – the greater the consistency of life experiences, the more they will be comprehensible and predictable
- **underload–overload balance** – demand is appropriate to capability
- **participation in decision-making** – the emphasis here is on active participation rather than control.

Early formulations of the SOC suggested that it was the product of early life experiences and that, by adulthood, it was more or less a fixed part of a person's makeup. Such a view offers little to those seeking to improve health. However, Antonovsky subsequently accepted that movement along the SOC can occur even in adulthood, albeit within fairly narrow limits. While he still subscribes to the view that macrosocial change is the only way to achieve substantial change in SOC for most people, he accepts that changes in everyday life can make some difference (Antonovsky, 1984). Antonovksy (1996) argued for the importance of a salutogenic orientation in health promotion. For more on salutogenesis see Mittelmark et al. (2022).

ABSTRACT 2.1

Rethinking sense of coherence: perceptions of comprehensibility, manageability, and meaningfulness in a group of Palestinian health care providers operating in the West Bank and Israel. Veronese, G., Dhaouadi, Y. and Afana, A. (2021)

Drawing on a salutogenic perspective, the authors explored sense of coherence (SOC) in a group of Palestinian mental healthcare providers living and working in Israel and the occupied Palestinian territories (West Bank). Specifically, they conducted a qualitative exploration of the cultural characteristics of SOC and its components (*comprehensibility, manageability* and *meaningfulness*) in two groups of Palestinian Muslim helpers. It was found that context-specific features of SOC can mobilize generalized resistance resources for coping with traumatic and stressful experiences, even in an environment characterized by political instability, military violence and social trauma. Ten main themes emerged from the thematic content analysis: *acceptance, reacting to adversity, acknowledging human insecurity* (comprehensibility), *self-control, talking to family, education as a resource* for survival, connecting to the severity of the event, responsibility as a source of control (manageability), religiosity and a sense of belonging (meaningfulness). The Islamic faith, as expressed through the concepts of *Sumud* and *Taslim*, seemed to permeate individuals' ability to attribute meaning to historical and transgenerational trauma, as well as to their ongoing traumatic conditions, thus acting as their ultimate source of health and well-being. A holistic, spiritual and collectivist outlook helped respondents to approach their lives with optimism. The authors discuss the implications for mental healthcare providers and future research directions.

Whose voice counts?

The validity of different accounts of health is the subject of debate, caught up in epistemological questions concerning ways of knowing and what constitutes truth. Beattie (1993) provides a useful analysis of 'different ways of knowing' based on modes of thought and the focus of attention. Modes of thought are seen as ranging from 'hard' mechanistic approaches consistent with the natural sciences to 'soft' humanistic approaches associated with sociological enquiry. Similarly, lay perspectives are often regarded as pre-rational and trivial in contrast to the rational, and therefore supposedly serious, view of the so-called experts. The focus of attention ranges from individuals to collectives. Figure 2.4 provides an overview of the relationship between these and identifies four models.

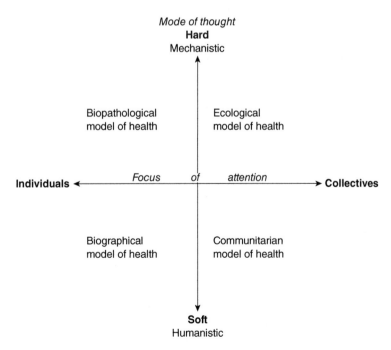

Figure 2.4 Accounts of health (Beattie, 1993)

One of the characteristic features of health promotion is its concern with holism – a view of health that includes positive well-being in addition to the absence of disease, a broad conceptualization of the determinants of health and an emphasis on participation. Its information needs, therefore, are necessarily broad and include a range of different professional interpretations deriving from different disciplinary bases and including the lay perspective.

Table 2.5   Accounts of health - sociopolitical philosophies and cultural bias

Account of health	Sociopolitical philosophy	Cultural bias
Biopathological	Conservative	Subordination
Biographical	Libertarian	Individualism
Ecological	Reformist	Control
Communitarian	Radical pluralist	Cooperation

Source: Beattie (1993)

Much of the literature on lay perspectives draws on a discourse of conflict, couched in such terms as 'mounting a challenge' to biomedical interpretations and 'struggle over meaning'. Sociological accounts are also frequently expressed in this vein (please see Table 2.5.) Debate about the relative merits of the contributions of different research disciplines and perspectives is helpful insofar as it exposes the strengths and limitations of the various approaches and their respective utility – particularly when this results in positive attempts to redress shortcomings by seeking complementary approaches. It becomes damaging when it is merely a contest between different epistemological positions and methodologies in laying claims to the truth and different accounts of health are afforded different status.

A narrow and partial analysis of health problems cannot provide a secure basis for identifying priority issues and their determinants. Green and Kreuter (1991: 50) suggest that priorities are 'generally based on an analysis of data indicating the pervasiveness of the problems and their human and economic cost'. Mainstream epidemiological diagnoses, as we have noted, are concerned with objectively assessing the magnitude and distribution of diseases and health states together with the factors that contribute to them. Green and Kreuter strongly argue that a wider view is needed and problems should be defined from the outset in broad social terms. They offer two main reasons for

this. Involving communities helps to ensure that their priority social and quality of life concerns are addressed and so avoids missing the mark in relation to social targets. It also contributes to encouraging community participation. They see the relationship between social and epidemiological diagnoses as complementary, operating in what they term either a 'reductionist' or an 'expansionist' way. Starting with an analysis of social problems, a reductionist approach would analyse the health and non-health factors that contribute to, or cause, the problem. The expansionist approach, in contrast, starts with an epidemiologically defined issue and works towards identifying the way this 'fits' into the larger social context. Green and Kreuter suggest that this avoids any tendency towards oversimplification.

While recognizing its contribution, Tannahill (1992) also cautions against an overemphasis on epidemiology as a driver in health promotion programme planning. He suggests that it neglects methodological issues by focusing on 'what to' rather than 'how to', creates an incomplete view of health, takes a narrow view of outcomes and leads to unsound programme planning. Of particular concern is the translation of single-issue problems into single-issue programmes, which ignores, on the one hand, the broader determinants and, on the other, that there may be factors common to a number of different conditions. For example, tobacco would be a common issue in relation to coronary heart disease, cancers and addiction, and all three are influenced by socioeconomic status. Programmes that address single issues in isolation – so-called 'vertical programmes' – therefore risk duplication of messages and inefficiency. Our position is that we need multiple complementary perspectives to identify priority health issues and their determinants.

DETERMINANTS OF HEALTH

Major improvements in health in the latter part of the nineteenth century have been attributed to improvements in the environment and general living and working conditions. The development of the germ theory and the improved possibility for immunization towards the end of the nineteenth century shifted the emphasis towards personal preventive services. The introduction of insulin and sulphonamide drugs in the 1930s heralded the dawn of the therapeutic era (Ashton and Seymour, 1988). The numerous subsequent technological developments in the biomedical field and faith in their capacity to improve health led to the rise of high-tech medicine. An increasingly technological view of health resulted in a shift in emphasis away from public health and community-based services and towards hospitals – so-called 'disease palaces'. Green (1996) noted that, in North America, towards the end of the twentieth century, over 90% of expenditure on health was on medical care and less than 10% on promoting healthy behaviour, lifestyles and environments, even though these accounted for between 50 and 71% of all preventable premature mortality before the age of 75.

The Lalonde Report (Lalonde, 1974) is frequently cited as the seminal document challenging the narrow, technically focused emphasis on disease and advocating a broader, social model. It recognized the need for a simple conceptual framework to bring order to the many and various factors influencing health:

> to organize the thousands of pieces into an orderly pattern that was both intellectually acceptable and sufficiently simple to permit a quick location, in the pattern, of almost any idea, problem or activity related to health; a sort of map of the health territory. (Lalonde, 1974: 31)

This was achieved using the 'health field concept', which identified four main elements – human biology, environment, lifestyle and healthcare organization (see Box 2.5).

BOX 2.5 ELEMENTS OF THE 'HEALTH FIELD CONCEPT'

- Human biology includes all those aspects of health, both physical and mental, which are developed within the human body as a consequence of the basic biology of man [sic] and the organic makeup of the individual.

(Continued)

- The environment includes all those matters related to health which are external to the human body and over which the individual has little or no control.
- Lifestyle consists of the aggregation of decisions by individuals which affect their health and over which they more or less have control.
- Healthcare organization consists of the quantity, quality, arrangement, nature and relationships of people and resources in the provision of healthcare.

Source: Lalonde (1974: 31–2)

The health field concept, therefore, marked a radical break from the increasing emphasis on high-tech medicine, elevating the other three categories to equal standing. The concept itself is both simple and comprehensive. It was designed to provide insight into the factors associated with sickness and death and identify courses of action to improve health. The health field concept was also expected to encourage an analysis of any health problem in relation to all four categories. It could, therefore, be used to identify areas for research and guide policy and planning.

Some 15 years after the publication of the health field concept, Raeburn and Rootman (1989) noted that the development of health promotion within this framework had focused particularly on lifestyle with insufficient attention being given to the influence of the environment, a concern echoed by others such as Morgan (2006) and Cross and O'Neil (2021). They also suggested that it was implicitly concerned with reduction of morbidity and mortality. To address these limitations, they proposed an expanded model that includes both inputs and explicit outputs (see Figure 2.5). The output side moves beyond morbidity and mortality to include functional capacity, positive health indicators and subjective perceptions. The input side is derived from the five action areas of the Ottawa Charter. With the exception of human biology, the other elements of the original health field concept are present. The reasons offered for its omission are that it is both a 'given' and an issue that falls under the aegis of health services rather than within the wider domain of policy, planning and research to promote overall health and well-being.

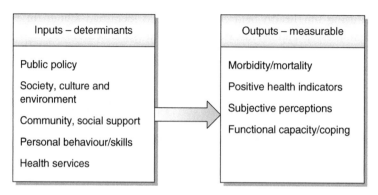

Figure 2.5   The expanded health field concept (derived from Raeburn and Rootman, 1989)

Lifestyle and environment

The relative importance of lifestyle and environment as determinants of health has been the subject of much debate – a debate that has contributed to defining health promotion as a discipline.

Lifestyle

The recognition of chronic diseases as the major cause of death in the more highly developed parts of the world in the mid twentieth century – against a backdrop of escalating healthcare costs – brought renewed interest in the role of prevention. Lifestyle is identified as a key factor in improving health status. Non-communicable diseases (NCDs) (cardiovascular diseases, cancers, respiratory diseases and diabetes) account for 41 million deaths per year: 71% of all deaths globally (WHO, 2021b). These NCDs share four 'lifestyle' risk factors: tobacco use, physical inactivity, alcohol misuse and unhealthy diet (WHO, 2021b).

Despite widespread recognition of the importance of lifestyle factors, there is little agreement about the meaning of the term. The concept of lifestyle generally refers to behavioural practices and ways of living (Fugelli, 2006; Korp, 2008) and to the behaviour/s that people engage in as they go about their daily lives (Ioannou, 2005).

The way in which the construct has become blurred over the years is succinctly encapsulated by Sobel (1981: 1, in O'Brien, 1995: 197): 'If the 1970s are an indication of things to come, the word lifestyle will soon include everything and mean nothing, all at the same time.' O'Brien's analysis of the appropriation of 'lifestyle' identifies three major influences:

- new systems of product marketing that segment the population into groups on the basis of lifestyle characteristics and consumption patterns (see Box 2.6 for examples)
- counterculture movements and alternative lifestyles as markers of ideological commitments
- critiques of modernization and a re-emphasis on self-determination.

Green and Kreuter (1991: 12) draw on anthropological, sociological and psychological interpretations to define lifestyle as:

> patterns of behaviour that have an enduring consistency and are based in some combination of cultural heritage, social relationships, geographic and socio-economic circumstances, and personality.

They are critical of the widespread and erroneous use of the word 'lifestyle' for any kind of behaviour and note that it has even been applied to temporary behaviour or single acts. A cursory glance at the literature reveals a plethora of papers about lifestyle factors and various risks of disease and ill health. There has been a focus on the clustering of unhealthy behaviours or 'multiple lifestyle risk' (Buck and Frosini, 2012: 4). Research in the UK revealed that nearly 70% of the adult population engaged in two or more unhealthy behaviours (drinking excess alcohol, poor consumption of fruit and vegetables, little physical activity and smoking) (Buck and Frosini, 2012). Latterly reference has been made to the 'Big 6' lifestyle risk behaviours in adolescents – physical inactivity, consumption of sugar sweetened beverages, alcohol use, smoking, poor sleep and excessive recreational screen time, many of which often occur concurrently and alongside poor fruit/vegetable consumption (Gardner et al., 2023). Crucially, these are all linked to the development of chronic disease in adulthood (Thornton et al., 2021).

One example of an attempt to classify different categories of lifestyle is provided in Box 2.6.

BOX 2.6   EXAMPLES OF LIFESTYLE CATEGORIES

Superprofiles use census and other data to distinguish 10 lifestyles. The categorization was principally developed for marketing purposes but has also been used within the context of health inequality:

- affluent achievers
- thriving greys
- settled suburbans
- nest-builders
- urban venturers
- country life
- senior citizens
- producers
- hard-pressed families
- have-nots
- unclassified.

See: Carr-Hill and Chalmers-Dixon (2005); Local Government Data Unit – Wales (2003)

'Millennials' is a term in common use to categorize people born between 1981 and 1996. They are identified as digital natives, who are engaged in social media, driven by causes, and conscious of sustainability, and personal health and wellness issues (Boufides et al., 2019; Lo et al., 2020), all of which points to potentially shared characteristics and a typified lifestyle. Green and Kreuter (1991: 13) suggest that the term 'lifestyle' should be used only to describe 'a complex of related practices and behavioural patterns, in a person or group, that are maintained with some consistency over time'. They argue that greater precision in the distinction between behaviour and lifestyle supports a more holistic and comprehensive approach to promoting health. If behaviour is understood within the context of the complex web that makes up a lifestyle, it immediately becomes evident that attempts to change that behaviour will need to have regard for the social, environmental and cultural circumstances that sustain that lifestyle. Furthermore, it demands sensitivity to possible knock-on effects for other aspects of the lifestyle. They also suggest that the use of the terms 'behaviour', 'action' or 'practice' to describe targets signals greater realism than the more aspirational term 'lifestyle', which is notoriously difficult to influence independently of the wider environmental context. This raises the issue of the relationship between lifestyle and environment, which we will explore more fully below along with a consideration of environmental factors.

Much of the literature on lifestyle is located within a pathogenic paradigm and focuses on the association between risk behaviours and disease (Antonovsky, 1996). In contrast, the focus within a salutogenic paradigm would be on the identification of those aspects of lifestyle that actively promote health – so-called 'salutary factors' – rather than the absence of risk factors. The recent interest in 'social capital' makes some move towards incorporating this salutogenic perspective.

Environment

The health field concept's interpretation of 'environment' placed considerable emphasis on the *physical* aspects of the environment with only passing reference being made to the *social* environment. Its central defining criteria for environmental factors are that they are external to the body and outside our immediate control. More recently, there has been much greater emphasis on social, cultural and economic aspects, particularly in the context of inequality. The Health in All Policies agenda recognizes the influence that political environments have on health (see Chapter 6 for more discussion).

Environmental factors can influence health either directly or indirectly. Simple examples of direct effects include exposure to toxic materials, shortage of food, lack of safe drinking water and overcrowding. Other factors will operate in a more indirect way. For example, lack of facilities for exercise in the environment will be associated with lower levels of physical activity and poorer heart health, while poor access to health services will be associated with low levels of uptake and so on. The latter example points to the role that politics plays in health.

Environmental factors may also interact – in some instances creating vicious circle effects. Poverty is associated with poor housing, diet, education and healthcare for example, leading to fewer life chances overall. Again, the influence of the political environment is salient here. Even ostensibly random occurrences, such as natural disasters, disproportionately affect poorer communities. Lower-income countries experience greater (relative) loss of life due to disasters than higher-income countries do (Centre for Research on the Epidemiology of Disasters, 2017). Equally, climate change disproportionately impacts the disadvantaged. Islam and Winkel (2017) argue that this is for three reasons:

- increase in the exposure of disadvantaged groups to the adverse effects of climate change;
- increase in the susceptibility of disadvantaged groups to damage caused by climate change; and
- decrease in the ability of disadvantaged groups to cope and recover from damage.

Our earlier discussion of the term 'lifestyle' indicated that it is heavily influenced by the environment. The Lalonde Report discusses the validity of using free choice as the basis for distinguishing between lifestyle and environmental factors in the health field concept. The premise is that individuals can make choices about their lifestyle, but can do little about the environment. The Lalonde Report (Lalonde, 1974: 36), while accepting that the environment does affect lifestyle, concludes that: 'the deterministic view must be put aside in favour of faith in the power of free will, hobbled as this power may be at times by environment and addiction'. However, there has been increasing doubt about whether or not behaviour can legitimately be seen to be under autonomous control. Green and Kreuter (1991: 12) see it as 'socially conditioned, culturally embedded and economically constrained'.

O'Brien (1995: 192) draws on earlier sociological interpretations of lifestyle to identify two main elements in its construction – political, economic and cultural resources and the psychosocial characteristics of the individual or group – that is, a combination of environmental and personal factors, with the former having the major influence: '"Lifestyle" implied "choice" within a constrained context and the contexts were held to be more important than the choices.'

There is clearly tension between recognizing humans as autonomous free agents and taking a deterministic view of environmental factors. This tension between agency and structure is also evident in decisions about the relative merits of environmental or lifestyle approaches to health promotion. Clearly, the two are inextricably linked. The Precede planning model (Green and Kreuter, 1991, 2005) (see Chapter 4) recognizes the interrelationship between behaviours and environment. It identifies factors in the environment and conditions of living that facilitate actions by individuals or organizations – i.e. 'enabling factors'.

Diagrammatic representation of the health field concept – which has typically shown the four elements of lifestyle, environment, human biology and healthcare organization as discrete entities – has perhaps reinforced the tendency to see them as independent variables. Nesting the main determinants within each other, as depicted by Dahlgren and Whitehead (1991), is more indicative of their broad interrelationships and the respective positioning of macro and micro determinants, as shown in Figure 2.6. Green et al. (1997) provide a more detailed analysis of the complex interrelationships, as shown in Figure 2.7.

An alternative approach acknowledges the relative importance of the various major determinants of health at different stages of the lifespan – for example, the powerful early influence of primary

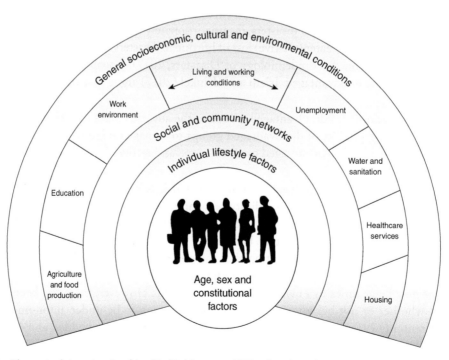

Figure 2.6   The main determinants of health (Dahlgren and Whitehead, 1991)

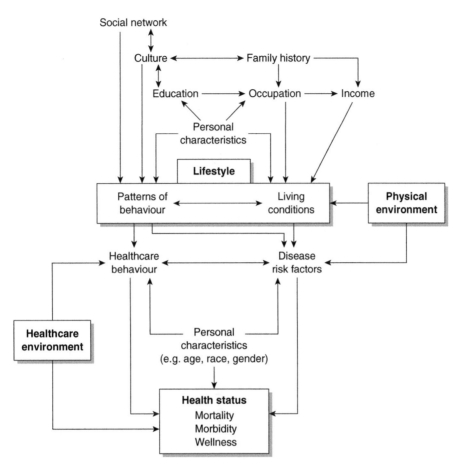

Figure 2.7 Some interrelationships in the complex system of lifestyle, environment and health status (Green et al., 1997)

socialization. This conceptualization is central to the notion of the 'health career', which charts individuals' progress through the lifespan and the ways in which different factors come into play over time (Tones and Tilford, 2001). The focus is on individuals and their cumulative experience rather than a more general overview of determinants. Figure 2.8 represents the health career as a coaxial cable, with the central core being made up of an individual's values, attitudes and beliefs. The health career analysis can assist in ascertaining the key influences on individuals at different stages in their life and also in identifying opportunities for intervention.

Social capital

There is an increasing body of evidence suggesting that social relationships and social support are protective against ill health, while social isolation and exclusion are associated with higher levels of ill health. For example, much is already known about how social support protects people against mental

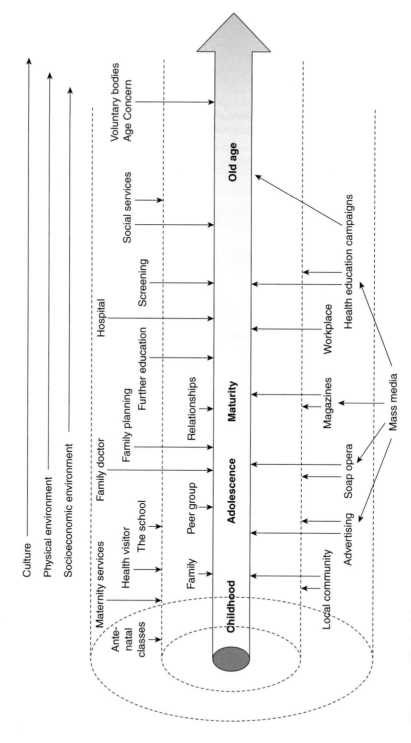

Figure 2.8 The health career

health problems such as depression, enhances self-esteem and how it generally increases quality of life (Alshammari et al., 2021). We also know that a lack of social support is detrimental to health, for example, it is associated with increased mortality in older adults (Chambers et al., 2022).

Stansfield (1999) makes the important distinction between social networks and the functional aspects of support. A measure of social networks would include the number and frequency of contacts – taking account of the closeness of the contacts – and the density of the network. The quality of the support would include positive emotional and practical support and also any negative, undermining aspects of close relationships. Over and above offering direct support and encouraging health-enhancing behaviour, social connectedness, in itself, has been shown to have a positive effect on health status, possibly by acting as a buffer for stressors. As Evans and Fisher (2022: 20) point out, 'social isolation is a powerful predictor of poor mental and physical health, while social support has been shown to be protective'; however, the *type* of social support also seems to make a difference to health outcomes, for example in reducing anxiety and depression in people who are socially isolated.

Mittelmark (1999: 447) suggests that the anticipated benefits of strengthening social ties are 'better-functioning individuals, families, neighbourhoods and work groups, and improved physical and mental health'. He also summarizes the various pathways that have been proposed to explain how social ties affect health. These include:

- sources of information to help avoid high-risk or stressful situations
- positive role models
- increased feelings of self-esteem, self-identity and control over the environment
- social regulation, social control and normative influences
- sources of tangible support
- sources of emotional support
- perceptions that support is available
- buffering actions of others during times of stress.

The conceptual model developed by Berkman et al. (2000) locates social networks within the upstream social and cultural context that shapes them. It then identifies four primary pathways through which social networks operate downstream at the behavioural level:

1. Provision of social support
2. Social influence
3. Social engagement and attachment
4. Access to resources and material goods.

While the emphasis in the literature is on the health-enhancing consequences of social ties, Mittelmark draws attention to the emerging evidence (spearheaded by fields such as gerontology) that they may also be a source of social strain. Such strain would derive from actions by persons in an individual's social network, such as excessive demands, criticism, invasion of privacy and meddling, that 'intended [or] unintended, cause a person to experience adverse psychological or physiological reactions' (Mittelmark, 1999: 448). There is evidence to suggest that membership of certain social networks may actually be detrimental to health. For example, research in North America by Christakis and Fowler (2007) shows that obesity seems to spread through social networks.

Furthermore, Mittelmark contends that social support and social strain are not opposite ends of the same continuum – and so not mutually exclusive – but separate constructs. It follows, then, that there can be four permutations – high support/high strain, high support/low strain and so on.

The notion of 'social capital' has been applied to the social resources within a community and has been given a lot of attention in the literature in relation to being a potential determinant of health (Eshan et al., 2019; Rodgers et al., 2019). The concept was first explored by Bourdieu (1980) and further developed by other authors such as Coleman (1988, 1990) and Fukuyama (1999). However, the term is particularly associated with Putnam and his early work on local government in Italy (Putnam, 1993). For Putnam (1995: 67), social capital:

> refers to features of social organization such as networks, norms and social trust that facilitate coordination and cooperation for mutual benefit … life is easier in communities blessed with a substantial stock of social capital … networks of civic engagement foster sturdy norms of generalized reciprocity and encourage the emergence of social trust. [They] facilitate coordination and communication … and allow dilemmas of collective action to be resolved. Finally, dense networks of interaction probably broaden the participants' sense of self, developing the 'I' into the 'we' …

This interpretation encompasses more than just the existence of community networks and the resources available. It also includes the social norms of trust and reciprocity, a sense of belonging and willingness to engage in civic activity. While the density of networks is of general relevance to social capital, the notion has been extended to include different forms based on the characteristics of networks:

- **bonding social capital** – refers to the ties between people in closely linked similar situations such as families or closely knit neighbourhoods
- **bridging social capital** – refers to looser connections between people which may cross-cut boundaries, for example workmates and wider friendships
- **linking social capital** – refers to links between people occupying different hierarchical and power positions, i.e. those who are not on an equal footing. (National Statistics, 2007; Performance and Innovation Unit, 2002; Woolcock, 2001)

Fukuyama (1999), writing from the perspective of an economist, provides an interesting interpretation of social capital. He notes that the usual definitions of social capital actually refer to *manifestations* of social capital rather than to its basic constructs. Thus, his definition is as follows:

> social capital is an instantiated informal norm that promotes cooperation between two or more individuals. The norms that constitute social capital can range from a norm of reciprocity between two friends, all the way up to complex and elaborately articulated doctrines like Christianity or Confucianism. They must be instantiated in an actual human relationship: the norm of reciprocity exists *in potentia* in my dealings with all people, but is actualized only in my dealings with *my*

friends. By this definition, trust, networks, civil society, and the like which have been associated with social capital are all epiphenomenal, arising as a result of social capital but not constituting social capital itself. (Fukuyama, 1999: 1–2)

According to Fukuyama (1999: 2), the norms that constitute social capital are 'related to traditional virtues like honesty, the keeping of commitments, reliable performance of duties, reciprocity, and the like'. Notwithstanding the potential for cooperation, which can extend beyond the immediate group, social capital can have negative effects (just as 'physical capital can take the form of assault rifles or tasteless entertainment, human capital can be used to devise new ways of torturing people'). Moreover, a group's internal cohesion may be achieved by treating outsiders with suspicion, hostility or even hatred. According to the author, organizations such as the Ku Klux Klan and the Mafia, because they have shared norms and cooperate, actually have social capital, but they produce 'abundant negative externalities for the larger society'. Furthermore, if a group's social capital produces positive externalities, the 'radius of trust' will extend beyond the group itself. Fukuyama sees modern society as a series of overlapping radii of trust – from friends, family and cliques up to large organizations and religious groups. Small radii of trust and within-group solidarity reduce the capacity for cooperation with outsiders and may be typical of more traditional social groupings. As Campbell (2011: 5965) argues, 'different forms of social capital may serve to advance or exclude different social groups'. In this respect, Villalonga-Olives and Kawachi (2017: 105) note that social capital is a 'double-edged phenomenon', which, at times, has a harmful or negative effect.

The large variety of overlapping social groups in modern societies may make it easier to transmit information, have greater resources and be readier to innovate than was the case in the past. Fukuyama asserts that social capital is an important feature of modern economies and underpins modern liberal democracy.

There has been considerable interest in the notion of social capital as a means of improving health prospects and particularly as a response to the adverse effects of social exclusion, which we will discuss below. A review of reviews on social capital and health found good evidence suggesting that social capital predicts better health and helps protect against mortality; however, the authors concluded that it remained unclear how different aspects of social capital affected different outcomes for different people (Ehsan et al., 2019). Research in the global north tends to dominate knowledge about social capital and health, and Gundewar and Chin (2020) argue that context, macro-/micro-level and structural factors need to be taken into account. Whilst a casual influence between social capital and health are demonstrated in many studies, for example, in relation to health development in children (Klocke and Stadtmüller, 2019), the links between social relationships and health are highly complex and the exact nature of the effect is difficult to determine. In addition, social capital is hard to research for many different reasons, as will now be discussed.

Assessing levels of social capital is challenging because of the nebulous nature of the concept and its cultural sensitivity (Babb, 2005). Eriksson (2011) also asserts that social capital is highly context-specific – as are the potential health impacts. Campbell et al. (1999) describe an exploratory qualitative study in the UK to assess the applicability of Putnam's conceptualization of social capital to the UK context as well as the variations in social capital between different communities with comparable socioeconomic status but different health experiences. They conclude that:

- the social capital constructs of trust and civic engagement may be particularly relevant to health status
- sources of social capital may cross the geographically defined boundaries of communities
- some network types (diverse and geographically dispersed) might be more health-enhancing than others
- Putnam's typology of social networks needs to be expanded to include informal networks
- the provision of community facilities does not constitute social capital – the processes by which such facilities are established and run require consideration
- Putnam's notion of community cohesion should be reconsidered in the light of the high levels of mobility and plural nature of contemporary communities
- there are major differences within communities in the ways in which social capital is created, sustained and accessed.

Commonly used measures of social capital are the levels of civic participation and social trust (Cooper et al., 1999). For example, Kawachi (1997) reports high levels of trust being associated with both lower mortality rates and higher levels of reported good health in the USA. Furthermore, bowling league membership (used by Putnam [1995] as indicative of levels of social participation) also correlates with lower mortality rates.

Fukuyama (1999) distinguishes two broad approaches to measuring social capital:

- a census of the groups and group membership in a given society
- a survey of levels of trust and civic engagement.

Putnam, for example, draws on group membership (derived from the number of groups, bowling leagues, sports clubs, political groups and the membership of groups) as an indicator of the level of civic engagement and social capital in society. He is sceptical about the contribution of 'mailing list' organizations to social connectedness on the grounds that the members do not actually meet and their ties are to a common ideology rather than to each other (Putnam, 1996), and he is cautious about the impact of the Internet:

> I think strong social capital has to have a physical reality – a purely virtual tie is a pretty thin reed on which to build anything; it's highly vulnerable to anonymity and spoofing and very difficult to build trust. (Putnam interviewed by Bunting, 2007)

Nonetheless, the increased role of virtual communities in contemporary society is beginning to receive attention (see Chapter 9 for further discussion).

Fukuyama identifies a number of additional relevant variables:

- the internal cohesion of groups
- the radius of trust and the extent to which this encompasses the whole group plus or minus outsiders
- group affiliation and the extent to which this engenders distrust of outsiders.

Coulthard et al. (2002: 1) suggest that the main indicators of social capital are:

- social relationships and social support
- formal and informal social networks
- group memberships
- community and civic engagement
- norms and values
- reciprocal activities, such as childcare arrangements
- levels of trust in others.

Within the UK, there has been considerable interest in developing a harmonized approach to measuring social capital in official surveys. For this purpose, the definition adopted by National Statistics was: 'networks together with shared norms, values and understandings that facilitate cooperation within or among groups' (Cote and Healy, 2001, cited by Babb, 2005). The following five key constructs were identified and modules of questions developed for each:

- civic participation
- social networks and support
- social participation
- reciprocity and trust
- views about the local area.

However, it is acknowledged that cultural specificity and national characteristics may limit its use for international comparison (Babb, 2005). Furthermore, the way in which social capital has been conceptualized may fail fully or adequately to address the experience of specific groups such as young people, who tend to have more informal social networks and less involvement in political and civic activity (Deviren and Babb, 2005). In a study in Brazil examining the relationship between social capital and health-related behaviours (Loch et al., 2015) the following indicators were used:

- number of friends
- number of people they could borrow money from when in need
- extent of trust in community members
- number of times members of the community help each other
- community safety
- extent of membership in community or civic activities.

Research carried out in India by Gundewar and Chin (2020: 44) conceptualized social capital as having two domains: structural ('social support – informational, instrumental, and emotional accessed through one's social networks') and cognitive (community characteristics such as 'trust, sense of safety, shared norms of behaviour, and … reciprocity') – see Abstract 2.2 for further details.

Harpham et al. (2002) point out that there are several important issues when measuring social capital, such as establishing a measure of social capital that captures the latest theoretical developments and at what level measurement should take place (individual, community, and so on). The majority of research on social capital is carried out, and reported from, high-income countries. Agampodi et al. (2015) carried out a systematic review on the measurement of social capital in relation to health in low- and middle-income countries. They point out how many of the tools used to measure social capital are developed in high-income contexts and therefore 'cultural adaptation [and] validation and assessment of [the] reliability of the tool … are important in [the] measurement of social capital' in low- and middle-income countries (Agampodi et al., 2015: 102).

ABSTRACT 2.2

Social capital, gender, and health: an ethnographic analysis of women in a Mumbai slum. Gundewar, A. and Chin, N.P. (2020)

Objective: Quantitative studies have demonstrated that social capital can positively impact on community health, but qualitative explorations of the factors mediating this relationship are lacking. Furthermore, while the world's poor are becoming increasingly concentrated in the cities of lower-middle income countries, most of the existing literature on social capital and health explores these variables in Western or rural contexts. Even fewer studies consider the impact of social constructs like race, gender, or class on the creation of social capital and its operationalization in health promotion. This study aimed to address these gaps in the literature through an ethnographic exploration of social capital among women living in Kaula Bandar (KB) – a marginalized slum on the eastern waterfront of Mumbai, India. The authors then sought to identify how these women leveraged their social capital to promote health within their households.

Methods: This was a mixed-method, qualitative study involving participant observation and 20 in-depth, semi-structured, individual interviews over a nine-month period. Field notes and interview transcripts were manually analysed for recurring content and themes.

Results: The authors found that women in KB relied heavily on bonding social capital for both daily survival and survival during a health crisis, but that the local contexts of gender and poverty activity impeded the ability of women in this community to build forms of social capital – namely bridging or linking social capital – that could be leveraged for health promotion beyond immediate survival.

Conclusions: These findings illustrate the context-specific challenges that women living in urban poverty face in their efforts to build social capital and promote health within their households and communities. Community-based qualitative studies are needed to identify the macro- and micro-level forces, like gender and class oppression, in which these challenges are rooted. Directly addressing these structural inequalities significantly increases the potential for health promotion through social capital formation.

INEQUALITY AND SOCIAL EXCLUSION

Exposure to a plethora of different determinants throughout the course of life will inevitably result in some variations in health experience. A central concern of health promotion – one that is driven by a vision of health as a basic human right, together with a commitment to the fundamental value of social justice – has been to reduce inequality in health, both within and between nations (see Table 2.6 for examples). There is a vast body of literature on inequality that addresses the key issues of social class, gender, ethnicity, age, disability and unemployment – many of which are interrelated and mediated through poverty and social exclusion. However, we will confine ourselves here to key definitional issues.

While some variation in health experience is unavoidable, much of it can be attributed to unequal opportunities – that is, social inequality. The use of the term 'equity' introduces greater precision here. The World Health Organization (2011) defines health inequities as:

> differences in health status or in the distribution of health resources between different population groups, arising from the social conditions in which people are born, grow, live, work and age. Health inequities are unfair and could be reduced by the right mix of government policies.

The important point to note here, therefore, is that health inequities are amenable to change. Table 2.7 below provides a simple checklist for assessing which differences in health are inequitable. However, in many industrialized countries, the term 'inequalities in health' is often taken to be synonymous with inequity (Leon et al., 2001).

There is considerable evidence that social class is a key determinant of health status. For example, Erikson and Torssander (2008) analysed mortality data in Sweden in relation to social class and

Table 2.6 Selected key facts on health inequalities in England (derived from Williams et al., 2020)

Type of inequality	Examples
Inequalities in life expectancy (LE)	- In the least deprived areas, men can expect to live 9.4 years longer; women 7.4 years longer - LE is lower in the north of England where there is a higher concentration of deprived communities
Inequalities in long-term health conditions	- People in lower socioeconomic groups are more likely to have long-term health conditions - Deprivation increases the likelihood of having more than one long-term condition at the same time
Inequalities in the prevalence of mental ill-health	- People who identify as lesbian, gay, bisexual or transgender experience higher rates of poor mental health including depression, anxiety and self-harm - One in five women report symptoms of mental health disorder compared to one in eight men
Inequalities in access to and experience of healthcare services	- More deprived areas tend to have fewer GPs than less deprived areas - Different social groups have different experiences of the services they use and whether they feel they are treated with dignity and respect
Inequalities in housing	- Households from minority ethnic groups are more likely than White households to live in overcrowded homes and experience fuel poverty

Table 2.7   Which health differences are inequitable?

Determinant of differentials	Potentially avoidable?	Commonly viewed as unacceptable?
Natural biological variation	No	No
Health-damaging behaviour if freely chosen	Yes	No
Transient health advantage of groups who take up health-promoting behaviour first (if other groups can easily catch up)	Yes	No
Health-damaging behaviour where choice of lifestyle is restricted by socioeconomic factors	Yes	Yes
Exposure to excessive health hazards in the physical and social environment	Yes	Yes
Restricted access to essential healthcare	Yes	Yes
Health-related downward social mobility (sick people move down social scale)	Low income – yes	Low income – yes

Source: Whitehead (1992: 4)

found that the risk of dying for any cause of death was double for men in the unskilled working class as compared with men in the higher professional and managerial occupations. As seen in this study, social class has typically been measured as occupational class. Erikson and Torssander (2008) used the following classifications:

Social Class

I Higher managerial and professional occupations

II Lower managerial and professional occupations

IIIa Intermediate occupations

VI Lower supervisory and skilled manual occupations

IIIb Routine non-manual occupations

VII Unskilled manual occupations

IVcd Employers and own account workers in agriculture

IVab Employers and own account workers not in agriculture

(Note: 'the roman numerals correspond to the categories in the class schema suggested by Erikson and Goldthorpe' [Erikson and Torssander, 2008: 474].)

In the UK, the main government classification system – the social class based on occupation (Registrar General's Social Class) – was based on grouping occupations according to the levels of skill involved. Using this system, the population could be divided into six classes, as shown in Box 2.7

below. This broad pattern of categorization was introduced in 1921 and, apart from subdividing class III into manual and non-manual in 1971, has remained substantially unchanged.

A new social classification system was introduced in 2001 to reflect the changing patterns of work – the National Statistics Socio-economic Classification (NS-SEC) – see Table 2.8. Although still based on occupation, it focuses on employment conditions and, particularly, the amount of control that people have over their own and other people's work rather than on skill. It also includes a category for the long-term unemployed and those who have never had paid work.

BOX 2.7   SOCIOECONOMIC CLASSIFICATIONS

Social class based on occupation

I   Professional occupations

II   Managerial and technical occupations

III   Skilled occupations:

(N) non-manual

(M) manual

IV   Partly skilled occupations

V   Unskilled occupations

Table 2.8   National Statistics Socio-economic Classification (NS-SEC)

1	Higher managerial and professional occupations	Professional and managerial
1.1	Large employers and higher managerial occupations	
1.2	Higher professional occupations	
2	Lower managerial and professional occupations	
3	Intermediate occupations	Intermediate
4	Small employers and own account workers	
5	Lower supervisory and technical occupations	Routine and manual
6	Semi-routine occupations	
7	Routine occupations	
8	Never worked and long-term unemployed	

Source: Derived from National Statistics (2007); and Babb et al. (2004).

Much of the evidence on health inequality is based on occupational class. However, there has been some debate about its relevance for groups such as women, the unemployed, the elderly and children, and concern that occupational class may not fully reflect their circumstances. For example, married women have often been classified by their husband's occupation. This conceals their own employment status and may fail to fully recognize the effects of paid employment and working conditions on women's health.

A further issue concerns what occupational class actually measures. Family members are usually classed according to the occupation of the head of the household and, although they may not be directly exposed to occupation-linked factors, share the variation in health associated with social class – for example, children from lower social classes are at greater risk of injury through road traffic accidents and dying in a house fire (Errington and Towner, 2005). Occupational class, therefore, clearly encompasses a whole constellation of factors over and above different occupational conditions. These would include levels of income, housing, area of residence, education and lifestyle. In the UK, the landmark Black Report analysed possible explanations for variation in health status with social class and concluded that, although genetic and cultural factors might make some contribution, the major underlying factor was material inequality and deprivation (Department of Health and Social Security [DHSS], 1980). This has been picked up by the work of others such as Sir Michael Marmot.

The increasing emphasis on health and social inequalities has resulted in critiques of existing measures of social class that have traditionally been biased towards categories of employed men to the exclusion of many minority groups. Savage et al. (2013) proposed a new model for social class. Based on data from a large-scale survey carried out by the BBC in the UK in 2011, Savage et al. have devised an alternative seven-category classification system that does not solely rely on occupational status. This is a much more nuanced model that, the authors argue, better reflects a multidimensional picture, recognizing 'social polarisation in British society and class fragmentation in its middle layers … and the interplay between economic, social and cultural capital' (Savage et al., 2013: 219). See Table 2.9 for details.

The average number of social contacts is selected here as an indicator of social capital. Interestingly, the precariat does not have the worst mean for this indicator; it is second lowest to the 'technical middle class'. The average household income has also been included here as an indicator of economic capital. The differences (inequalities) between the classes are striking. Out of interest, the average income in the UK at the time of editing this chapter (mid 2022) was £31,772.

Income has frequently been identified as a key determinant of social variation in mortality. Dorling et al. (2007) distinguish different levels of income (see Box 2.8). They note that over the previous 15 years there were more poor households in Britain, but fewer were very poor and there had been an increased polarization between different areas – wealthy areas became wealthier and poor areas poorer. Globally income levels have been conceptualized according to four different levels (Gapminder, 2022):

Level 1: People in extreme poverty living on less than $2 per day

Level 2: People living on $2–$8 per day (almost half of the world's population)

Level 3: People living on $8–$32 per day

Level 4: People living on more than $32 per day (the richest billion on earth)

Wilkinson and Pickett (2009) noted that societies with a smaller gap between the least well-off and the most well-off fare better on a range of health-related indicators than societies with larger gaps. Notably, it is not just the people at the lower end of the scale who fare badly in more unequal societies but everyone along the social gradient.

Table 2.9   Summary of social classes

Social class	Description	Average household income (£)	Average number of social contacts*
Elite	Very high economic capital (especially savings), high social capital, very high highbrow cultural capital	89,082	16.2
Established middle class	High economic capital, high status of mean contact, high highbrow and emerging cultural capital	47,184	17.0
Technical middle class	High economic capital, very high mean social contacts, but relatively few contacts reported, moderate cultural capital	37,428	3.6
New affluent workers	Moderately good economic capital, moderately poor mean score of social contacts, although high range, moderate highbrow but good emerging cultural capital	29,252	16.9
Traditional working class	Moderately poor economic capital, although with reasonable house price, few social contacts, low highbrow and emerging cultural capital	13,305	9.8
Emergent service workers	Moderately poor economic capital, although with reasonable household income, moderate social contacts, high emerging (but low highbrow) cultural capital	21,048	14.8
Precariat	Poor economic capital and the lowest scores on every other criterion	8,253	6.7

Note: *Average number of social contacts refers to a number derived from a possible 34 types. For further information, see Savage et al. (2013).

BOX 2.8   LEVELS OF INCOME

- Core poor: people who are income poor, materially deprived and subjectively poor
- Breadline poor: people living below a relative poverty line, and as such excluded from participating in the norms of society
- Non-poor, non-wealthy: the remainder of the population classified as neither poor nor wealthy
- Asset-wealthy: estimated using the relationship between housing wealth and the contemporary Inheritance Tax threshold
- Exclusive wealthy: people with sufficient wealth to exclude themselves from the norms of society.

Source: Dorling et al. (2007)

Absolute and relative poverty

Poverty influences physical health as it limits access to good-quality nutrition and housing, but also has an effect on mental health (Shaw et al., 1999). The Marmot Review Team (Marmot, 2020) highlighted this again more recently. Yet, against a backdrop of overall improvement in general prosperity and health status, differentials seem to be widening – a pattern not untypical of industrialized nations, as established in Wilkinson and Pickett's (2009) work. A key factor would seem to be income inequality (Davey Smith, 1996). Indeed, Wilkinson (1994) states that life expectancy has increased most in industrialized nations where income differences have narrowed and mortality is more closely related to income inequality *within* countries than absolute differences in income *between* countries (Wilkinson, 1997).

This raises the issue of absolute and relative poverty. *Absolute* poverty exists when insufficient resources are available to provide the basic essentials of life, such as food and shelter. The World Bank, for example, has used the notional US$1 per day as an absolute minimum survival budget. However, this measure of extreme poverty has little meaning in the context of advanced industrialized societies. Some countries, such as the USA, have defined an official poverty line based on the cost of a basic food basket. The Canadian Council on Social Development (2001) provided an analysis of different ways of defining poverty and noted the debate over which items should be regarded as necessities. A key issue concerns whether a poverty line should be set in relation to a basic survival budget or a level of income that would enable people to participate in society.

Relative poverty, in contrast, is defined by the European Commission (2004: 2) as follows:

> People are said to be living in poverty if their income and resources are so inadequate as to preclude them from having a standard of living considered acceptable in the society in which they live. Because of their poverty they may experience multiple disadvantage through unemployment, low income, poor housing, inadequate health care and barriers to lifelong learning, culture, sport and recreation. They are often excluded and marginalised from participating in activities (economic, social and cultural) that are the norm for other people and their access to fundamental rights may be restricted.

An article by Frank (2000) in the *New York Times Magazine* drew attention to the importance of relative poverty/affluence in people's lives:

Consider a choice between the two scenarios:

- World A: You earn $110,000 per year and others earn $200,000.
- World B: You earn $100,000 per year and others earn $85,000.

The figures for income represent real purchasing power. Although in absolute terms individuals would be better off in Scenario A, a majority of Americans chose Scenario B.

There are several different ways of establishing relative poverty levels: for example, the proportion of income needed to cover the basic necessities of life, the proportional relationship to the median income and measures based on 'market baskets', which would include items in line with community norms.

A national survey of poverty and social exclusion in Britain (Gordon et al., 2013) used a variety of measures of poverty. These included not being able to afford what are generally perceived to be 'necessities'. Table 2.10 gives a list of the top eight items that adults and children respectively regard as necessities. It is clear that the interpretation of what constitutes a necessity goes beyond the basic survival needs of subsistence diet, shelter, clothing and fuel to include participating in social customs, fulfilling obligations and taking part in activities.

Table 2.10   Items perceived as necessities

Item	% considering item 'necessary'
For adults:	
Heating to warm living areas of the home	96
Damp-free home	94
Two meals a day	91
Visit friends or family in hospital or other institutions	90
Replace or repair electrical goods	86
Washing machine	82
Celebrations on special occasions	80
Attend weddings, funerals and other such occasions	79
Telephone	77
For children:	
Warm winter coat	97
Fresh fruit and vegetables once a day	96
New, properly fitting shoes	93
Three meals a day	93
Garden or outdoor space to play safely	92
Books at home suitable for their age	92
Child celebration on special occasions	91
Suitable place at home to study or do homework	89
Child hobby or leisure activity	88

Source: Derived from Gordon et al. (2013)

The Joseph Rowntree Foundation has attempted to develop a Minimum Income Standard for Britain. This goes further than thresholds based on relative income, measures of deprivation or budget standards calculated on baskets of goods and services to establish a level of income which is sufficient to support 'having what you need in order to have the opportunities and choices necessary to participate in society' (2008: 1). While there is inevitable disagreement about what constitutes poverty there does seem to be consensus that it is concerned with not being able to live a decent life, and the inability to 'purchase goods and services that it is widely believed are necessary in order to do so' (Niemietz, 2011: 15).

The United Nations Development Programme (UNDP), recognizing the complex relationship between economic indicators such as per capita income and human well-being, uses the Human Development Index (HDI) for international comparison. The HDI measures life expectancy, educational attainment and income and combines these to create a single statistic by which social and economic development are measured and compared across countries (UNDP, 2013). In 2019, Norway was ranked highest and Niger and the Central African Republic were ranked lowest. (For further information see: hdr.undp.org/en/statistics/hdi)

Whereas absolute poverty is a central issue in the developing world, poverty in urban, industrialized countries has been defined (Supplementary Benefits Commission, 1979, cited in Dahlgren and Whitehead, 1991: 15) as:

> a standard of living so low that it excludes and isolates people from the rest of the community. To keep out of poverty they must have an income which enables them to participate in the life of the community.

This definition focuses on social exclusion, which is currently receiving considerable attention. Although social exclusion is defined in a number of different ways, common components are 'disadvantage in relation to certain norms of social, economic or political activity pertaining to individuals, households, spatial areas of population groups: the social economic and institutional processes through which disadvantage comes about: and the outcomes or consequences for individuals, groups or communities' (Percy-Smith, 2000: 4). Therefore, this disadvantage is not solely restricted to economic factors, but would also include other forms of cultural and social discrimination. Major groups of socially excluded people are the unemployed, ethnic minorities, refugees, the elderly, lone parents and their children and those, especially children, with disability.

Clearly, social exclusion exerts a powerful psychosocial influence and there are obvious links with the notion of social capital. Kawachi (1997) demonstrates lower levels of social trust in states with a higher 'Robin Hood Index' – a measure of income inequality based on the proportion of aggregate income that would have to be redistributed to level up earnings. Similar findings are obtained for participation in voluntary associations. However, Lynch et al.'s (2000) analysis of income inequality and mortality cautions against an exclusive emphasis on psychosocial effects and the lack of social cohesion, which, they allege, is akin to victim-blaming at the community level. They propose that the main causes of health inequality are material – including access to both private and social resources, such as education, healthcare, social welfare and work. Raphael's (2001: 30) analysis of social inequality and heart disease in Canada provides a concise summary of the interaction between these various elements:

> Social exclusion is a process by which people are denied the opportunity to participate in civil society; denied an acceptable supply of goods or services; are unable to contribute to society, and are unable to acquire the normal commodities expected of citizens. All of these elements occur in tandem with material deprivation, excessive psycho-social stress, and adoption of health-threatening behaviours shown to be related to the onset of, and death from, cardiovascular disease.

Composite indicators of deprivation

The concept of deprivation can apply to both individuals and areas and includes material and social elements (Krieger, 2001). There is some evidence that, independently of an individual's level of deprivation, living in a deprived area has an adverse effect on health (Shaw et al., 1999). Subsequently deprivation is understood to be compromised of three concepts: deprivation, multiple deprivation and urban deprivation (Jones, 2017).

There are composite indicators of deprivation that can be used to assess the overall levels of deprivation within different areas. The Jarman and Townsend indices have been used widely in the UK and draw on census data (see Box 2.9). Indices of deprivation can be criticized for only using relative measures of deprivation rather than absolute measures, and for not giving light to detailed, local-level information, which can reduce the ability to make comparisons between places (Dymond-Green, 2021).

BOX 2.9 THE JARMAN AND TOWNSEND INDICES OF DEPRIVATION

Jarman underprivileged area score (UPA)

Derived from GPs' views about factors that influence their workload.

- Percentage of children under five
- Percentage of unemployment
- Percentage of ethnic minorities
- Percentage of single-parent households
- Percentage of elderly living alone
- Overcrowding factor
- Percentage of lower social classes
- Percentage of highly mobile people
- Percentage of unmarried couple families
- Poor housing factor.

The above 10 items were originally included in the Jarman UPA score, but the last two are omitted from the Jarman UPA8 score.

Townsend combined deprivation indicator

- Percentage of economically active residents aged 16–59/64 who are unemployed
- Percentage of private households that do not possess a car
- Percentage of private households that are not owner occupied
- Percentage of private households with more than one person per room.

Source: Derived from Whitehead (1987)

Attempts to measure levels of deprivation on a large geographic scale often obscure smaller pockets of deprivation. There is considerable interest, therefore, in small area analysis. In England, the government uses seven dimensions of deprivation as follows:

- income deprivation
- employment deprivation
- education, skills and training deprivation
- health deprivation and disability
- crime deprivation
- barriers to housing and services
- living environment deprivation. (McLennan et al., 2019)

Carr-Hill and Chalmers-Dixon (2002) emphasize that these various indices are artificial constructs and only partial or proxy measures of phenomena such as deprivation. They caution against reification, which can occur when operational constructs used as approximate measures become substituted for the actual meaning of the concepts they purport to measure. While their argument focuses on the measurement of deprivation, it would apply equally to other indicators of health status.

Childhood poverty

Childhood poverty, particularly when persistent over a number of years, is of concern not only because of its immediate effects on this vulnerable group but also because of longer-term effects and its contribution to sustaining cycles of deprivation. Within the UK, by 2019/20 it was estimated that almost a third of children were living in poverty with predictions that this was still on the rise given patterns seen since 2013 (Joseph Rowntreee Foundation, 2022). International comparison clearly presents challenges in terms of selection and comparability of indicators. UNICEF's (2013) comparison of children's material well-being among 29 industrialized nations ranked the Netherlands the highest and Romania the lowest. For educational well-being, the rankings were the same for the Netherlands and Romania; for health and safety, Iceland was ranked highest and Romania, again, the lowest. There is a great deal of evidence that investing in childhood has huge repercussions for adult life. It is clear that early intervention at this stage of the life course is an important health and social investment that has the potential to impact on health and social inequalities. The highest priority policy recommendation in the Strategic Review of Health Inequalities in England Post-2010, *Fair Society, Healthy Lives*, was that every child is given the best start in life (Marmot, 2010); however, child poverty actually increased over the subsequent decade (Marmet et al., 2020) despite the cross-party governmental commitment to tackling the issue as demonstrated by the Child Poverty Act of 2010. The aim was to eradicate child poverty by the year 2020. Clearly this has not been achieved.

As a result of an analysis of international examples of effective approaches in reducing child poverty, the National Children's Bureau (NCB) produced a set of guidelines that included increasing free early years education and reducing childcare costs. Specifically, the NCB recommended that the following be embedded in any strategy designed to tackle child poverty:

- having a robust mechanism for taking forward a cross-government child poverty strategy holding all government departments to account
- introducing a package of measures to promote maternal employment
- supplementing families' incomes for engaging in activities that promote child well-being
- taking forward evaluated neighbourhood-based approaches to tackling child poverty and promoting health well-being. (Fauth et al., 2013: 4)

The three policy areas believed to have the greatest potential for tackling child poverty are:

- prioritizing education and childcare in early childhood;
- reducing the risk of poverty (such as increasing wages and employment opportunities) among those families in employment; and
- effective income support benefits for those on very low incomes. (Gábos, 2013, cited in Cheung, 2018: 33)

Tackling inequality

Measuring inequality within and between nations is not an abstract exercise but serves to expose social injustice and highlight the need for action (see, for example, Acheson, 1998). Marmot (2005: 1099) drew attention to the inequitable 'spread of life expectancy of 48 years among countries and 20 years or more within countries' in his call for political action to address inequality. The need to measure and understand the problem was recognized in the priorities for action set out in the final report of the Commission on Social Determinants of Health (CSDH) (2008) – see Box 2.10.

BOX 2.10 PRINCIPLES OF ACTION FOR CLOSING THE HEALTH GAP

1. Improve the conditions of daily life – the circumstances in which people are born, grow, live, work and age
2. Tackle the inequitable distribution of power, money and resources – the structural drivers of those conditions of daily life – globally, nationally and locally
3. Measure the problem, evaluate action, expand the knowledge base, develop a workforce that is trained in the social determinants of health, and raise public awareness about the social determinants of health.

Source: CSDH (2008: 2)

The central arguments in this section point to the importance of policy-level interventions in tackling the determinants of health. Health public policy is discussed in detail in Chapter 6. An effective policy response clearly depends on tackling the cause of inequality. Only at a policy level is it possible to tackle the conditions that give rise to certain sets of behaviours. While the extreme effect of poverty and deprivation may be self-evident, Marmot emphasizes the importance of understanding the social determinants of health inequalities – which he refers to as the 'causes of the causes'. The CSDH report (2008) notes the need to tackle the unequal distribution of power, money and resources.

Looking at inequality within countries, Wilkinson and Marmot (2003) identified the following key areas:

- the social gradient
- stress
- early life
- social exclusion
- work
- unemployment
- social support
- addiction
- food
- transport.

Further work led by Sir Michael Marmot highlights how health inequalities are linked to a person's social position – for example, where they live and the type of employment they are engaged in (Marmot, 2010). The Marmot Review concluded that we need to focus more on inequalities in well-being rather than health; that examining the 'causes of the causes' is of paramount importance; that mental health is extremely important in determining physical health and life chances; and, finally, that there should be a focus on resilience (personal and community). The notion of resilience is receiving increasing attention and it links to more salutogenic approaches to understanding health. Ten years on, against a backdrop of increasing inequality, Marmot et al. (2020) again reiterated the importance of the recommendations made in the initial review and concluded that the following six policy actions were still necessary:

- giving every child the best start in life
- enabling all children, young people and adults to maximize their capabilities and have control over their lives
- creating fair employment and good work for all
- ensuring a healthy living standard for all
- creating healthy and sustainable places and communities
- strengthening the role and impact of ill-health prevention

In order for this to happen it was recommended that the following was needed:

- develop a national strategy for action on the social determinants of health with the aim of reducing inequalities in health
- ensure proportionate universal allocation of resources and implementation of policies
- early intervention to prevent health inequalities

- develop the social determinants of a healthy workforce
- engage the public
- develop whole systems monitoring and strengthen accountability for health inequalities.

Clearly, to be effective, any efforts must be based on an understanding of the *unequal distribution* of the determinants of health.

Asset-based approaches

Asset-based approaches to health promotion and public health are integral to addressing health inequalities. Asset-based approaches counter deficit-based approaches to assessing health promotion need (Morgan and Ziglio, 2007: 17). They focus more on the positive aspects of health and what makes us healthy rather than on what makes us sick (Foot, 2012). Assets are defined as 'the collective resources which individuals and communities have at their disposal, which protect against negative health outcomes and promote health status' (Glasgow Centre for Population Health, 2011: 2). The key premise of asset-based approaches is that people can attain better health outcomes when they have the opportunity and capacity to manage and control their own lives (De Andrade, 2016). To adopt an assets-based approach is to recognize the experience, skills, strengths, knowledge and potential that already exist in a group or community and how these (may) contribute to the support of health and well-being. There is an obvious connection here to salutogenic and resilience-building approaches and, in fact, Morgan and Ziglio (2007: 17) set out the case for using 'salutogenic indicators' in a key paper on asset-based approaches. There are clear links here to capacity and issues such as social capital.

There are a number of challenges in using and developing asset-based approaches, such as how assets are measured, establishing the relationship between assets and well-being and issues to do with how we measure and assess positive health and well-being in a culture that has been more concerned with measuring ill health and disease (Glasgow Centre for Population Health, 2012). In addition De Andrade (2016) highlights the difficulties in demonstrating the efficacy of such approaches. However, the focus on empowerment and on health gain is key and there is, therefore, a central place for asset-based approaches in tackling health inequalities despite the challenges faced. Nevertheless, Friedli (2013) adopts a more cautionary approach and is more critical, arguing that they focus attention away from economic, material and structural issues onto psychosocial factors; and De Andrade (2016) highlights the important differences between meaningful community engagement and undertaking tick box exercises. Notwithstanding such critiques, asset-based approaches form an important part of Joint Strategic Asset Assessments (JSAAs). JSAAs are a refocusing of Joint Strategic Needs Assessment and promote an asset-based approach to needs assessment (Tobi, 2013). Such approaches are often drawn on in UK-wide efforts to promote public health. For further discussion of Joint Strategic Needs Assessment, see Chapter 6.

THE CONTRIBUTION TO PROGRAMME PLANNING

It is axiomatic that planning interventions to promote health requires understanding of the current health status of populations and the factors that influence it. We have considered different approaches to assessing health and its determinants.

Rather than engage in sterile debate about the relative superiority of biomedical or interpretivist approaches, we would contend that they offer complementary insights. Tension arises from the unequal power positions of those subscribing to different methodologies and the dominance of biomedicine. This has been challenged from both professional and lay quarters. In that health is essentially a subjective experience, the lay perspective is particularly relevant. Furthermore, understanding a complex multidimensional concept such as health necessarily needs to draw on multiple perspectives – including salutogenic as well as pathogenic perspectives.

The emergence of health promotion as a discipline placed an emphasis on environmental influences on health – both directly and in terms of shaping behaviour and lifestyle. Notwithstanding the debate about the primacy of agency or structure, it is clear that there is a reciprocal relationship between the two elements. The complexity of the interrelationship has become more evident as our conceptualization of the environment has broadened. While the contribution of social and socioeconomic aspects of the environment has been recognized for some time, the recent resurgence in interest in social capital focuses attention on social connectedness and opportunities for civic engagement.

The measurement of health and quality of life and their determinants is undoubtedly challenging. To conclude this chapter, we should note that the capacity to assess the health of communities and identify key determinants underpins rational planning processes. Clearly, the way in which such an assessment is approached should reflect the ideology and values of health promotion and pay particular attention to factors associated with health inequalities.

KEY POINTS

- Measuring health and its determinants is of fundamental importance to efforts to improve health.
- Epidemiological measures contribute to our understanding of health and its determinants – particularly in relation to mortality and morbidity.
- Multiple perspectives, including the lay perspective, are needed for a more complete understanding of health, including positive well-being.
- Salutogenic as well as pathogenic explanations of health should be considered.
- Both environment and lifestyle factors influence health and are themselves interrelated.
- Social aspects of the environment, including social connectedness and social capital, have an impact on health status.
- Poverty and material deprivation are major causes of health inequality.
- Understanding the wider social determinants of health inequality and social exclusion are of central importance in developing initiatives to tackle inequality.

CHAPTER 2: INTERNATIONAL CASE STUDIES

The following case studies on the online resources website are relevant to the content of this chapter: 2, 5, 7 and 9.

CRITICAL REFLECTION AND APPLICATION TO PRACTICE

This chapter has considered a range of approaches to assessing health and determinants of health. What type of data do you use in the context that you work? How do you use the data? How might you view the data more critically? (Where do the data come from? How are the data generated? Who 'owns' the data?) Are you assessing health or ill health? Do you use a positive or negative view of health? How could you incorporate more salutogenic perspectives? Why are lay perspectives important in assessing health experience and determinants? How might you draw on lay perspectives to inform your work? What will you do differently as a result of reading this chapter?

ONLINE RESOURCES

Please visit https://study.sagepub.com/greentones5e for all the online resources for the book, including recommended further reading on each chapter subject, useful weblinks (both introduced by the authors), as well as the abovementioned case study material.

3 THE DETERMINANTS OF HEALTH ACTIONS

The truth is rarely pure and never simple.

Oscar Wilde (1854–1900), *The Importance of Being Ernest*

OVERVIEW

The purpose of this chapter is to consider the factors that influence the adoption of health-related behaviour. More specifically, it will:

- consider the factors influencing the adoption of health behaviours at the community level
- identify the major influences on individual health decisions using the health action model as a framework
- examine the factors that affect whether health intentions are put into practice
- analyse those factors that contribute to control and empowerment.

INTRODUCTION

The emphasis of this chapter is on understanding at the individual, or micro, level how various factors interplay to influence behaviour by drawing on explanatory theory. Given the central importance of empowerment to health promotion, particular attention will be given to the dynamics of empowerment. The health action model (Tones, 1979, 1981) forms the basis of the majority of discussion in this chapter. The variables in the health action model are signposted at key points throughout by **bold type** in the relevant sub-headings and content. The health action model is systemically applied to COVID-19 in a detailed case study later in the chapter. Various influences on individuals are nested within, and are themselves the product of, meso- and macro-level social systems. Detailed discussion of social change is beyond the scope of this chapter. However, we will begin by locating our discussion of individual change in the context of the adoption of innovations in social systems using a theoretical analysis that has frequently been applied to the adoption of health innovations – diffusion of innovations theory.

THE ADOPTION OF INNOVATIONS IN SOCIAL SYSTEMS

Diffusion of innovations theory

Diffusion of innovations theory was originally known as communication of innovations theory (Rogers and Shoemaker, 1971) and has subsequently been developed and regularly updated. The latest version was published in 2010 (Rogers, 2010). Diffusion theory is concerned with the factors relating to the adoption of innovations within social systems. An 'innovation' is defined as 'an idea, practice or object perceived as new by an individual or other unit of adoption' (Rogers, 2003: 12). The theory can be applied to organizations as well as individuals, but for the purpose of this chapter we will focus on the latter. Adoption is 'the decision to make full use of the innovation as the best course of action available' (Rogers, 1995: 21). The core principle of the theory is that the adoption of innovations by individuals within a relatively fixed social system follows a consistent pattern. There is a slow initial rate of adoption, the *lag* phase. The process then gathers momentum (*take-off* phase) to involve the majority and then tails off as *saturation* is reached. Cumulative adoption therefore follows an 'S'-shaped curve as shown in Figure 3.1.

The overall shape remains the same regardless of the intervention. However, the gradient of the slope will be steeper for innovations that are relatively 'attractive' and taken up rapidly. The various adopter categories and their typical characteristics are:

Initiators (2.5%) – venturesome

Early adopters (13.5%) – opinion leaders, successful, respected within their social circle

Early majority (34%) – deliberate before adopting new ideas

Late majority (34%) – cautious and sceptical

Laggards (16%) – traditional.

It is estimated that when between 10 and 20% are involved, a 'critical mass' is reached when diffusion becomes self-sustaining through social networks.

The theory identifies the pathway leading to adoption. Initial *awareness* is followed by *interest* and seeking more information. Then *evaluation* involves mentally applying the intervention and deciding whether or not to try it out. This may lead to a *trial* involving full use of the innovation and the ultimate decision about whether to continue, that is to say *adoption*.

The innovation–decision process itself has five stages (Rogers, 2003):

1. Knowledge – development of awareness and understanding
2. Persuasion – the formation of an attitude to the innovation
3. Decision – engagement in activities leading to choice, possibly including trying out the innovation
4. Implementation – putting the innovation into practice
5. Confirmation – reinforcement based on experience of the outcomes.

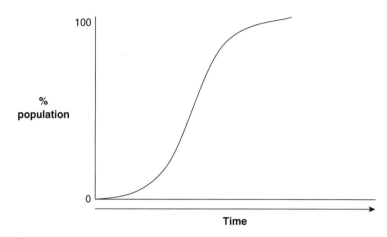

Figure 3.1   The classic 'S'-shaped curve

From a health promotion perspective, identifying the factors associated with the uptake of practices conducive to health is essential for effective programme planning. Furthermore, attention also needs to be given to the final stage if initial adoption is to be sustained. The classical diffusion model identifies four key elements associated with uptake:

- the characteristics of the innovation
- communication channels
- time
- the social system.

The characteristics of the innovation

It is well recognized, and indeed common sense, that people's perceptions about the nature and implications of the innovation they are being asked to adopt will be a highly significant factor in determining whether or not they are willing to try it out. Adoption is influenced by the following key features:

- relative advantage – offered by the innovation compared with current practice
- compatibility – with values, previous experience and current needs
- complexity – the extent to which the innovation is felt to be difficult to understand or implement
- trialability – the possibility of testing out before making a more permanent commitment
- observability – the extent to which the results are visible to others.

Communication channels

According to Rogers (2003), the main elements of the communication process are held to be the innovation, an individual (or unit) that knows about the innovation or has experience of it, an individual (or unit) without such knowledge and a channel of communication between the two. It might be assumed that communities having extensive and sophisticated mass media would be inclined to change more rapidly than those without. Certainly, on the one hand, mass media offer potential as the most rapid means of creating awareness but, on the other hand, interpersonal influence is known to be more effective in changing attitudes and developing skills.

The role of the change agent is of importance to the diffusion process. Change agents frequently differ from the population in general because of greater technical competence and other characteristics such as education and social status, that is to say they are heterophilous. Leadership characteristics will parallel our earlier comments on power in Chapter 1 and, in particular, French and Raven's (1959) analysis on page 43. They also relate to the notion of credibility of the source, to which further reference will be made in later discussions about attitude change theory.

The powerful principle of 'homophily' suggests that people are more likely to be influenced by those with whom they identify. Rogers and Shoemaker (1971: 14) define it as follows:

> Homophily is the degree to which pairs of individuals who interact are similar in certain attributes, such as beliefs, values, education, social status and the like. A further refinement of this proposition includes the concept of empathy … the ability of an individual to project himself [*sic*] into the role of another.

Echoing Bandura's (1986) ideas around 'role modelling', Rogers (2003) notes that individuals depend to a great extent on the experience of 'near peers' in making decisions and that this is at the heart of the diffusion process. Ideally, then, change agents would collaborate with opinion leaders, who share characteristics more closely with the community and act as referents and models.

Time

The time factor is an important element of the diffusion process and reflected in the relative steepness of the diffusion curve. Rogers (2003) specifies its relevance to three areas: the innovation–decision process, the innovativeness of the individual and the rate of adoption within the system. The level of innovativeness will vary between the various adopter categories identified above – indeed, it is the basis of their classification. Innovators, for example, will be quick to adopt and can cope with higher levels of uncertainty about the innovation. At an aggregate level, however, the rate of adoption is concerned with the proportion of individuals in a social system who take up the innovation.

The social system

Diffusion is a social process (Weil, 2018) and the social system influences diffusion in a number of ways: first, through the type of relationships, including both the more formal elements of social structure and the informal (and more homophilous) interpersonal relationships; and, second, through the norms and level of resistance to new ideas. Rogers (2003) notes that the most innovative members of a social system may be perceived as 'deviant' and, therefore, have limited capacity to influence others. Opinion leaders on the other hand are, by definition, accepted and respected.

The most striking characteristic of opinion leaders is their unique and influential position in their system's communication structure: they are at the center of interpersonal communication networks. (Rogers, 2003: 30)

Typically, they are more exposed than their peers to external communication, have higher socioeconomic status and tend to be more innovative. As argued by Li et al. (2013: 327), 'when a "critical mass" of popular opinion leaders in a social group begin to model a new behaviour, they alter the perception of what is normative'.

A further factor in the adoption of an innovation is of particular importance – not least because of its centrality to the ideological commitments of health promotion. In short, it concerns the extent to which the community is involved in defining its own needs (a point to which we will return in the context of needs assessment) and in identifying ways of meeting those needs. Table 3.1 sets out the relationship between this degree of participation and the anticipated rate of adoption of a given innovation.

As highlighted by Steury (2013), diffusion of innovations theory has practical application to health issues. Specifically, Steury argues that 'Rogers's Diffusion of Innovations Model can be used to plan and implement community-focused interventions into the cultures of developing nations' (p. 189). She illustrates this with reference to using transcultural nurse educators in malaria in Zambia, arguing that concepts from the model are transferable to other similar cultures or communities. Further explication of the application of diffusion of innovations theory and, indeed, other models of social system change is beyond the scope of this chapter (for more information, see Bartholomew et al., 2001; Goodman et al., 1997; Oldenburg et al., 1997; Parcel et al., 1990). Our concern now is to shift the focus from the macro to the micro level, to examine influences on individual health actions.

Table 3.1   Participation by rate of adoption

Level of community participation	Anticipated rate of adoption of the innovation
Community spontaneously recognizes that it has a problem	Very rapid change
Community identifies solution to problem	
External agency considers that community has a problem	Very slow – or never!
External agency prescribes solution	

CHANGE AT THE INDIVIDUAL LEVEL – INFLUENCES ON INDIVIDUAL HEALTH INTENTIONS

It is the purpose of this next part of the chapter to provide a detailed examination of the various psychological, social and environmental determinants of health- or illness-related choices and behaviour.

The health action model

A plethora of models and theories is available to those wishing to understand individual decision-making. While they have many features in common – even though the terminology may differ – they vary in emphasis and their own particular orientations. Many were developed for general use, but have been found to have special relevance for health behaviour, while others were constructed with health education, health promotion and public health in mind. They include:

- the health belief model
- the theory of reasoned action
- the theory of planned behaviour
- the transtheoretical model of change
- the social learning theory
- the protection motivation theory.

(For further details, see Hayden, 2022; Nutbeam et al., 2010; Prestwich et al., 2017.)

It is not possible here to review all the models listed above. Accordingly, one particular model will be used to identify the constructs that are central to understanding health- and illness-related behaviour and particularly relevant to planning health promotion programmes. The variables in this model form the basis of the discussion in this chapter and are explicated in detail. The model in question is the health action model (HAM), which was initially devised by Tones in the early 1970s to provide a theoretical base for the emerging specialist professional practice of health education (Tones, 1979, 1981). It was subsequently modified to take account of the shift in emphasis that took place with the emergence of health promotion (with its emphasis on healthy public policy and related macro influences). As will be apparent, it draws eclectically, pragmatically (and unashamedly!) on a number of key models and theories. It is reproduced as Figure 3.2. The HAM identifies key psychological, social and environmental influences on individuals adopting and sustaining health- or illness-related actions. It comprises two major sections – the **systems** that contribute to 'behavioural intention' (see the bottom half of Figure 3.2) and the **factors** that determine the likelihood of that behavioural intention being translated into practice (see the top half of Figure 3.2).

In short, four interacting systems – concerned with beliefs, motivation, normative influences and the self – all determine the likelihood of an individual developing an *intention* (labelled '**behavioural intention**' in Figure 3.2) to adopt a particular course of health- or illness-related action. Whether this happens or not will depend on a number of enabling or facilitating factors, including the **knowledge** and **skills** necessary to adopt the health action. Of special importance – as should now be apparent – is the availability of a supportive **environment** that 'makes the healthy choice the easy choice' (also see the later discussion in this chapter on choice architecture and nudge theory). An alternative way of expressing the importance of these enabling factors is to assert that health promotion is charged with removing those psychological, behavioural and environmental barriers that militate against people making healthy choices.

The **health action/s** in question may include actions related to positive health outcomes and/or actions designed to prevent disease. In both cases, the actions are not necessarily confined to individual health, but may also contribute to the health of the community – for instance, by empowering individuals to undertake political actions that contribute to healthy public policy. The HAM acknowledges the difference between single time, discrete health actions and routines. A discrete health action might be involved when, for example, only one visit is necessary to a clinic to have a child immunized, or when a potential political activist writes a letter of complaint to a Member of Parliament. Usually, though, benefits only accrue when health actions become part of a **routine** – for instance, when individuals routinely build exercise into their lifestyle or the political activist continues to stir up public indignation at breaches of human rights.

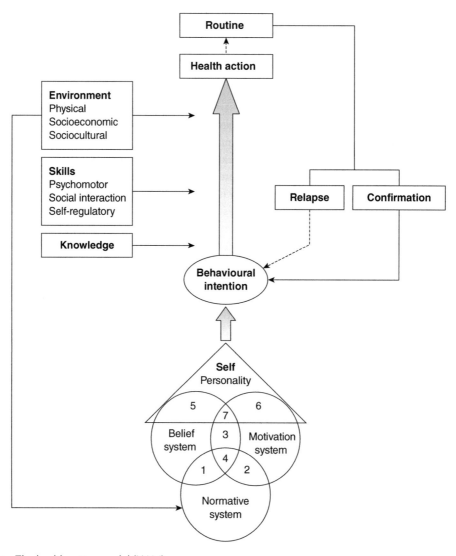

Figure 3.2   The health action model (HAM)

When a single-time choice has been made or, more commonly, when a routine has been established, two outcomes are possible. The first is that the health action in question is not problematical and results in confirmation of the **behavioural intention**. Alternatively, the innovation may be rejected and the individual **relapses**. The notion of relapse is traditionally associated with addictive or quasi-addictive behaviour, such as giving up smoking or other drugs. However, it could equally be applied to those actions that involve discomfort or inconvenience. The transtheoretical model, which we will consider more fully later, is especially concerned with questions of maintenance and relapse. Usefully, it notes how those who initially relapse will frequently try again (and even again and again!) before finally being confirmed in a healthy way of life (Prochaska and DiClemente, 1984; Prochaska et al., 1997).

The belief system

The K-A-P formula

One of the simplest attempts to explain the adoption of particular behaviour is encapsulated in the K-A-P 'formula'. It is based on the reasonable assertion that knowledge alone does not lead to behaviour – it is usually necessary, but rarely sufficient. Accordingly, the provision of knowledge (K) has to be supplemented by persuasive techniques designed to bring about a change in attitude(s) (A) before the target person or population will adopt appropriate practices (P).

The model has significant limitations but so-called K-A-P surveys are still in evidence. They might, for example, ask people whether they have heard of a certain disease or illness – as in an Australian study exploring midwives' K-A-P in relation to gum disease (Ngu-yen et al., 2020). They might check whether people are aware of associated risks, as Beckwith (2020) did in Ecuador in relation to sexual and reproductive health. K-A-P surveys are often used to evaluate the knowledge, attitudes and practices of healthcare personnel: for example, K-A-P relating to female sexual health among obstetricians and gynaecologists in China (Li et al., 2021), and K-A-P of primary care physicians in Greece during the COVID-19 pandemic (Symvoulakis et al., 2022).

Despite the continued use of the K-A-P approach, as will be apparent from Figure 3.2, a much more sophisticated analysis involving a constellation of constructs is necessary if behaviour is to be understood and influenced. One of the most important of these is the concept of belief, which in the HAM is presented as part of a belief system – that is, a complex of interacting elements.

Beliefs defined

To understand how beliefs operate, it is essential to make some conceptual distinctions, particularly in relation to knowledge, beliefs and attitude. As with knowledge, beliefs are cognitive constructs, whereas attitudes are affective – that is, they refer to a person's evaluation of some object, person or activity. Attitudes, therefore, refer to feelings in favour of or against the object in question – be it exercise, smoking, sun exposure or immunization. Fishbein (1976) classically defined a belief as:

> a probability judgement that links some object or concept to some attribute. The terms 'object' and 'attribute' are used in a generic sense and both terms may refer to any discriminable aspect of an

individual's world. For example, I may believe that Pill A (an object) is a depressant (an attribute). The content of the belief is defined by the object and attribute in question, and the strength of the belief is defined by the person's subjective probability that the object–attribute relationship exists (or is true).

In relation to attitudes, Fishbein (1976: 103) notes:

> An attitude is a bipolar evaluative judgement of the object. It is essentially a subjective judgement that I like or dislike the object, that it is good or bad, that I'm favourable or unfavourable towards it. [The term 'object'] … is used in a generic sense. Thus I may have attitudes towards people, institutions, events, behaviours, outcomes, etc.

Beliefs are, thus, subjective probabilities and will frequently operate in parallel with objective probabilities. By way of example, epidemiological data might suggest that cancer is a major cause of mortality – a statistical observation mirrored by individuals' beliefs about seriousness. However, subjective and objective interpretations might operate independently. For example, there may be no objective/scientific evidence that the fumes from a local industrial site contribute to lung disease in an adjacent neighbourhood. Moreover, statistical analysis might also reveal that the prevalence of lung disease in the neighbourhood is neither more nor less than in the population at large. The members of the community, nevertheless, are convinced that they have a real problem of 'chesty coughs' (their non-specific lay version of lung disease) and consider it as self-evident that these are due to the fumes from the incinerators in the factory.

The health belief model

The health belief model (HBM) is probably the most frequently used model of all those purporting to explain health-related decision-making. Originated by Hochbaum (1958), based on pioneering work by Lewin (1951) and developed by Rosenstock (1966, 1974), the model was devised to explain variations in the utilization of preventive medical services.

In its early manifestation, it was essentially a model of the expectancy–value/value–expectancy variety. In other words, it argues that decision-making depends on individuals believing that a particular course of action will result in the likelihood of a valued outcome being achieved. While it is not possible to provide a full review of this model (for more details, see Abraham and Sheeran, 2015; Becker, 1984; Prestwich et al., 2017), it is useful to specify the four major beliefs that it identifies:

- belief in personal susceptibility to a negative event
- belief that the event is serious
- belief that the recommended preventive measure will be effective in reducing the threat of the negative event
- belief that the recommended measure will not entail too heavy a cost.

The formulation is eminently logical as common sense suggests that individuals would not take action to avoid an unpleasant event if they did not believe it was likely to happen to them or, if it did, it would be insignificant. Again, it might well be assumed that people would not follow advice if they did not believe it would work and if the disadvantages outweighed the benefits.

The HBM has been modified over time to include additional elements such as 'cues to action', 'health motivation' and 'self efficacy'.

The originators of the model considered that the four beliefs alone might need some additional trigger to jolt into action those who were already predisposed to certain courses of action by their beliefs. A general factor – health motivation – was included in a later version of the model. It was considered that the explanatory value of the HBM might be improved if a measure of people's general health motivation were to be included.

As Abraham and Sheeran (2005: 65) rightly observe in their thorough analysis of the model:

> The HBM has provided a useful theoretical framework for investigators of the cognitive determinants of a wide range of behaviours for more than thirty years. The model's common sense constructs are easy for non-psychologists to assimilate and can be readily and inexpensively operationalized … it has focused researchers' and healthcare professionals' attention on modifiable psychological prerequisites of behaviour and provided a basis for practical interventions across a range of behaviours.

How effective are the HBM beliefs in explaining health-related behaviour? A completely comprehensive model that incorporates every social, psychological and environmental influence on health choices would account for 100% of the difference in people's health actions (the variance). The evidence suggests that the HBM explains *some* of the variance, but not a lot! A meta-analysis of the HBM found that the 'benefits' and 'barriers' were the strongest predictors of behavioural outcomes; however, based on the weakness of the predictive power of the HBM overall, the conclusion was that 'the continued use of the direct effects version of the HBM is not recommended' (Carpenter, 2010: 661). However, it is argued that the HBM still has 'positive explanatory value' (Ritchie et al., 2021: 482).

Belief hierarchies and the notion of salience

One of the particularly useful formulations in Fishbein and Ajzen's (1975) seminal work is the demonstration that beliefs may be either 'salient' or 'latent'. The phenomenon of salience is relevant for health education strategies. Translating latent beliefs into salient beliefs, say in the course of group discussion or face-to-face interaction, might alter the belief–attitude dynamic, reduce uncertainty and result in commitment to adopting a healthy course of action. Figure 3.3 provides an example of a typical hierarchy of beliefs associated with stopping smoking. These beliefs may be salient or latent.

There are several lessons for health promotion. For instance, it is inefficient, even pointless, addressing higher-order beliefs without first ensuring that necessary precursor concepts and subordinate beliefs have already been acquired. It is also apparent that a kind of mental balance sheet is operating and that the outcome will depend on the ultimate balance and relative strengths of the beliefs about the positive and negative outcomes of giving up smoking. This will reflect the relative strengths of the various motivational forces that determine action.

The motivation system

Whereas the belief system is cognitive, the motivation system is affective – it is concerned with feelings. 'Motivation' refers to goal-directed behaviour and its psychological underpinning. It defines the

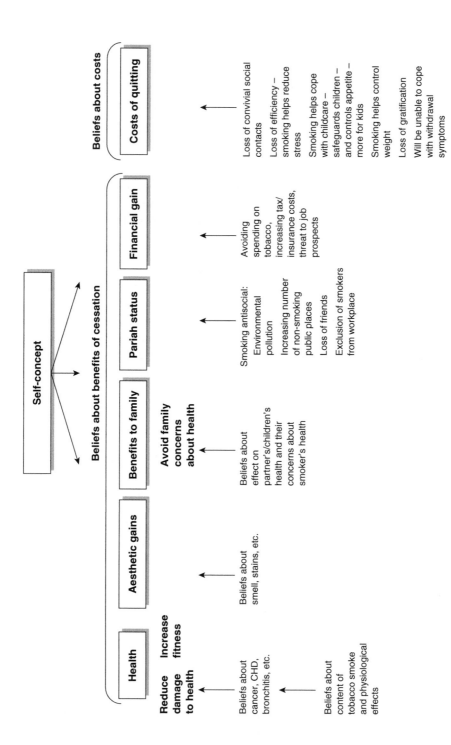

Figure 3.3 Example of a belief system concerning stopping smoking

push and pull forces that impel individuals towards the achievement of pleasure and away from undesirable outcomes.

Different kinds of motivation can be identified and operate at different levels. One of the most widely used psychological theories of behaviour change is the theory of planned behaviour (TPB), which developed from the theory of reasoned action (Ajzen, 1991; Conner and Norman, 2015). The TPB assumes that behavioural intention is predicated on three factors that combine to form motivation to take action. These are attitude towards the behaviour, subject norms (whether or not we think our significant others want us to take action) and perceived behavioural control (whether or not we think we have control over the said behaviour). While the TPB is commonly utilized in behavioural research it does have limitations. The HAM goes further in providing an explanation of what motivates us to take action or change behaviour. It has more complexity and, therefore, more variables. Four kinds of motivation are distinguished in the HAM motivation system: values, attitudes, drives and emotional states.

The values dimension

There is a reasonably clear consensus in psychology about the definition of values and their origin. Rokeach (1973: 3) made five assertions about the nature of human values:

- the total number of values is relatively small
- everyone possesses the same values to different degrees
- values are organized into value systems
- values are created and influenced by culture, society and its institutions and personality
- values play a part in virtually all phenomena investigated by the social sciences – psychology, sociology, anthropology, psychiatry, political science, education, economics and history.

In relation to other psychological and social constructs – all of which are of importance in explaining health- and illness-related decisions – values have a transcendental quality, insofar as they energize attitudes and underpin behaviour. In Rokeach's words, 'values are guides and determinants of social attitudes and ideologies on the one hand and of social behaviour on the other' (1973: 13).

As with beliefs, values typically occupy hierarchies having superordinate and subordinate levels. Rokeach, for example, usefully distinguishes 'terminal values' from 'instrumental values'. Moreover, he links these with self-esteem – that major, higher-order value that has special prominence in empowerment theory and health promotion generally (1973: 14):

Terminal values are motivating because they represent the supergoals beyond immediate, biologically urgent goals. Unlike the more immediate goals, these supergoals do not seem ... to satiate – we seem to be forever doomed to strive for these ultimate goals without quite ever reaching them ... there is another reason why values can be said to be motivating. They are in the final analysis the conceptual tools and weapons that we all employ in order to maintain and enhance self-esteem. They are in the service of what McDougall (1926) has called the master sentiment – sentiment of self-regard.

There are also two kinds of instrumental values: moral values and competence values. Interestingly, one of the examples of an intrapersonal competence value that figures prominently in Rokeach's discussion has to do with self-actualization, which, as we noted earlier, can be viewed as a healthy state in its own right or as the peak of a hierarchical motivational structure.

The attitude dimension

The concept of attitude is central to social psychology. Reference was made earlier to Fishbein's definition of attitude, but a number of alternative and influential formulae can also be found. Perhaps the most common of these makes reference to disposition or readiness for action. Occasionally, the term is used to describe a psychological construct having not only affective but also cognitive and conative elements. The cognitive dimension involves 'beliefs', the affective dimension is concerned with feelings and the conative aspect with the action implications of a given attitude. In the HAM, we follow Fishbein and Ajzen in limiting the conative element to 'behavioural intention'. As we will see, this is viewed as the product of the belief, motivation and normative systems and, depending on the availability of 'empowering' knowledge, skills and environment, may or may not be translated into actual behavioural outcomes or health actions.

Again, attitudes operate within a hierarchical system based on values and may be more or less salient or latent. Figure 3.4 provides a review of the values associated with stopping smoking and thus complements the belief hierarchy presented in Figure 3.3 above.

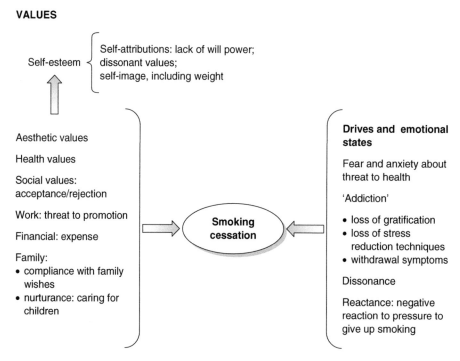

Figure 3.4   Motivations and smoking cessation

Inspection of Figures 3.4 and 3.5, however, reveals that the combined force of values and beliefs ought to generate an overwhelmingly negative attitude to smoking and a resoundingly positive attitude to stopping. The fact that this does not always happen is due to the third key element in the motivation system – that cluster of often primitive feelings that are here variously described as drives and emotional states.

Drives, acquired drives and emotional states

In addition to values and attitudes, a third motivational category is identified in the HAM. This includes the concepts of drive and emotional state. At the risk of being simplistic, we could sum up the term 'drive' as a kind of primary motivation that is considered to be innate or instinctive. It energizes readily recognized behaviour that frequently has survival value. The most instinctive of these are hunger, thirst, sex and the avoidance of pain.

It is assumed that drives typically exert a greater influence over behaviour than motivation derived from values and attitudes. Indeed, Maslow's (1954) pyramid viewed physiological needs for 'air, food, water, sleep, etc.' as providing a foundation for his motivational hierarchy. Although self-actualization and the achievement of various values were located at the top of the hierarchy, the physiological needs required satisfying before higher-order needs could be fully achieved (see Chapter 1 and Chapter 5 for more on Maslow's theory).

Whereas there is clearly evidence that the achievement of valued goals might, for some people, override the need for food or sex, it would be unwise to rely on this! As the WHO has observed, the need for peace, safety and security must be satisfied before people consider adopting behaviour that will improve their health.

The term 'acquired drive' is used to refer to what are normally termed 'addictions'. Again, we must avoid oversimplification, but the power of dependence on various substances generally has more in common with the traditionally defined innate drives than it does with values.

The term 'emotional state' cannot be accorded a precise definition. For instance, on the one hand, while fear is undoubtedly an emotional state, it could equally qualify as a drive, both in respect of its innate qualities and its effects on the individual experiencing it. On the other hand, anxiety would not normally be considered a drive, although it has been defined as a 'fractionated fear response' – that is, a watered-down version of pure fear. In all events, emotional state can exert a powerful effect on decision-making and behaviour and should be considered as qualitatively different from a value.

Consider, for example, the case of breastfeeding. Taylor and Wallace (2011) argue that both formula-feeding and breastfeeding mothers experience shame; in both cases this is based on value-related factors. Mothers who use formula feed report feeling that they fail to live up to the ideals of womanhood and motherhood, while mothers who breastfeed go against cultural expectations regarding feminine modesty. Definitions of emotions such as shame and embarrassment are by no means un-complex, and emotional states, of course, vary. Nevertheless, affective states have an important role to play in health behaviour. Indeed, Gerend and Maner (2011) argue that the effectiveness of health communication messages depends on a person's emotional state. This, in turn, may influence information accessibility and processing, and decision-making processes (Nabi, 2021).

Perceptions about the threat posed by actions (or, indeed, failure to act) coupled with beliefs about personal vulnerability may well generate some degree of autonomic arousal ranging from mild concern to panic. Such perceptions may be the product of the individual's own thought processes or, alternatively, be externally induced by shock-horror attempts to influence behaviour. Regardless of their origin, the resulting emotional state will be a factor in determining an individual's response and their confidence in their ability to change behaviour or perform an action (Tapper, 2021).

One final example of an emotional state that frequently contributes to intention to act is that of 'cognitive dissonance' (Festinger, 1957). It is best described as a state of unease that results from simultaneously holding two or more cognitions (beliefs) that are psychologically inconsistent. The theory posits that individuals experiencing the uncomfortable emotional state of dissonance will be motivated to act to remove it. The dissonance phenomenon has been extensively researched and some further comments will be made in our discussion of attitude change in Chapter 7. However, the position adopted here is that dissonance is but one of many different emotional states that may contribute to behavioural intentions. Its impact can be demonstrated in laboratory situations but, in real-life situations, it will typically compete with a highly complicated system of drives and values in its effect on behavioural intention. One such competitor is encapsulated in the notion of social pressure, to which we now turn.

The normative system

The normative system describes the network of social pressures that might be brought to bear on an individual's intention to adopt or reject health actions. As may be seen from Figure 3.5, it is conceived as a hierarchical set of influences ranging from the proximal impact of close family and friends to the increasingly distal effects of community and the further reaches of the social system. It is assumed that the effect of significant individuals, close family and friends will typically be more powerful than community pressure, which, in turn, will have more influence than national norms.

Interpersonal influences

The potential power of interpersonal pressure exerted face to face needs little further explication here. Those individuals who exert a direct effect are commonly described as 'significant others'. In addition to close friends or partners, individual professionals might well play an important part in influencing attitudes and behaviour (our earlier discussion of the nature of leadership has already suggested the characteristics that might result in the 'other' being considered 'significant'). The relative importance of family and significant friends will, of course, depend on the nature of existing relationships. However, at the levels of both research and anecdote, the impact of a passionately antismoking partner is well documented!

Peer pressure

While the peer group is generally held to exert an influence on its members, this effect is often portrayed as being disproportionately powerful in the case of adolescents and young people. For example, peer pressure has been shown to be one of the strongest predictors of alcohol consumption in university students (Grazia Monaci et al., 2013), and of smoking in adolescence (Vitoria et al., 2020).

This influence is typically assumed to be negative or unhealthy, supporting the view that young people need to be skilled up to resist social pressure. However, there is evidence that the peer effect is more complex (see, for example, a South African study by Rencken et al. [2021] showing that adolescent peer support encouraged adherence to HIV medication) and that peer pressure occurs throughout the lifespan not just adolescence, particularly in relation to alcohol use (Morris et al., 2020). However, young people recognize a number of different groups among their peers and tend to align themselves with friends on the basis of shared interests and behaviour. This raises the question of whether individuals may actively prefer to conform with, rather than resist, the persuasive influence of their peers. Furthermore, it is important to recognize that peers can have a positive influence both directly and by providing a group identity and protection for those who feel they differ from other groups. Indeed, harnessing this positive potential is integral to peer education, which will be discussed more fully in Chapter 7.

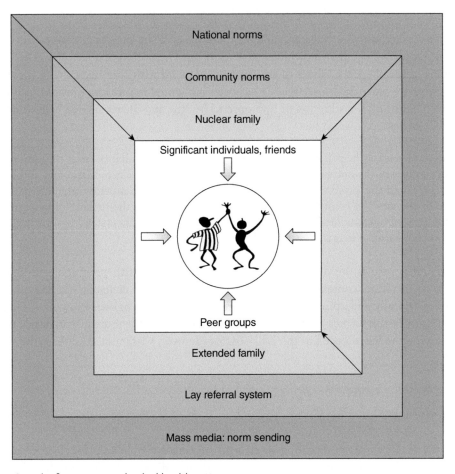

Figure 3.5　Social influences on individual health actions

Social norms and the community

As noted above, the assumption reflected in Figure 3.5 is that the influence of norms will be greater the more proximal groups are to the individual. Nonetheless, the more distal national and community norms will have some effect – both directly and by shaping the norms of families and peer groups. As we comment elsewhere, a genuine community, by definition, has common norms and a network of contacts and relationships, which traditionally include extended families. Where such a community exists, the extent of its social influence will be substantially greater than in a social system character-ized by anomie (normlessness).

Due to the effects of socialization, it is likely that community norms will be reinforced by families and adopted by individuals. In fact, following earlier observations about the subtle and powerful effect of dominant ideologies and following the assumptions inherent in the notion of false consciousness, normative pressures may reinforce the status quo and, thus, the social power structure.

The lay referral system and pressure to comply

Over and above their norm-setting function, communities and the various groups within them are a repository of lay knowledge that individuals may draw on. The notion of a lay referral system (LRS) has its origins in sociological analyses of the factors associated with compliance with medical advice and the appropriate use of health services. It has been influential in providing insight into the effects of community norms on the adoption of 'appropriate' health- and illness-related behaviour. Freidson (1961: 146–7) writes:

> the process of seeking help involves a network of potential consultants from the intimate and informal confines of the nuclear family through successively more select, distant and authoritative lay-men [*sic*] until the 'professional' is reached. This network of consultants which is part of the structure of the local lay community, and which imposes form on the seeking of help, might be called the 'lay referral structure'. Taken together with the cultural understandings involved in the process we may speak of it as the 'lay referral system'.

The lay referral system is, by definition, distinct from formal health provision and systems vary according to sociocultural context. Lay involvement in health is, of course, not a new phenomenon and such roles typically underpin formal healthcare provision albeit in different guises. Consider the use of community health workers in countries like Sierra Leone, or the more recent 'health trainer' and 'health champion' models adopted in the UK (see, for example, Visram et al., 2015; Warwick-Booth et al., 2021).

Label and libel the nature of stigma

It is appropriate at this point to refer to a particularly important effect of social pressure on individual health – the question of stigma.

One of the major barriers preventing individuals seeking available help for curable and prevent-able conditions is the cultural conceptualization of particular diseases and the emotional reactions to these. To the extent that diseases are associated with culpable or antisocial actions or are considered to be due to the intervention of supernatural forces, anticipated public disgrace – which may even take the form of violence – may militate against help-seeking behaviour. Such diseases as leprosy, TB and AIDS will immediately spring to mind in this regard, as will certain diagnoses of mental ill-health. Following the observations about the power of social pressure discussed above, the existence of a close-knit community will increase the perceived threat of disclosure.

The results of a meta study of qualitative research into the experiences of people diagnosed with bipolar disorder are illustrative of the effect of stigma (Russell and Moss, 2013). This meta study analysed reported research from several countries, including Sweden, Australia, Canada, New Zealand and the USA, focusing on the experience of symptoms and receiving a diagnosis. One participant provides a flavour of the anticipated effects of stigma as a result of a diagnosis of bipolar disorder: 'I guess they just think about what they see on TV … They just assume … that you're crazy and you're nuts and you're psycho and you're dangerous' (p. 653). The discourse in another paper is summarized as follows: 'They described being isolated from the community around them and their families and view the community around them as rejecting them' (p. 653). Stigma is, of course, not confined to diagnoses of mental ill-health. Many studies across the world point to the stigma that people living with HIV experience on a day-to-day basis; for example, in Indonesia (Waluyo et al., 2022), in Georgia and California (Kim et al., 2021) and Brazil (Catelan et al., 2022).

Mass media pressures

More detailed analysis of the nature and effectiveness of mass media will be provided in Chapter 8. For the present, we will merely assert that the impact of the mediated norms of the larger culture transmitted in this way are likely to be considerably less effective than the other social influences discussed above.

Beliefs, motivations and normative pressures – interaction effects

Reference to Figure 3.2 indicates that several points of overlap exist between these separate systems and that the nature of the interaction is signalled by the various 'segments' numbered from 1 to 7.

Normative beliefs and motivation to comply

There is a point of distinction between the actual norms within communities and an individual's perception of those norms based on their subjective assessment. The normative system discussed above actually exerts its effect on behavioural intention via the mediation of both the belief and motivation systems. The HAM follows the practice adopted by Fishbein and Ajzen (1975) as it is both theoretically satisfying and practically useful to separately identify beliefs about normative pressures and motivation to conform to those pressures. According to Fishbein, individuals have a set of (salient and latent) beliefs about the likely reactions of key individuals to their intentions to act. However, this anticipated approval or disapproval by significant others will only affect their intention to act if they are also concerned about their reaction. If the others are not actually significant, they will have no influence. Segment 1 indicates beliefs about the reactions of others and segment 2 indicates motivation to comply.

In the HAM, Fishbein and Ajzen's formulation has been extended to the remaining potential influences included in the motivation system. Accordingly, beliefs about the likely reactions of peer groups, awareness and beliefs about the nature of social norms and national norms transmitted by mass media will also contribute to intention to act, provided that the individual in question is also motivated to conform to these various social pressures.

According to the 'pressure gradient', the motivational effect of mass media norm sending is unlikely to be as powerful as interpersonal pressures, and any effect is likely to result from the individual's evaluation of the information content of the message.

Interaction of belief and motivation systems

The above discussion of the normative system describes a *particular* case of the mutual effects of beliefs and motivation. The belief and motivation systems in general routinely interact as a two-way influence process. As we emphasized earlier, beliefs represent subjective probabilities. These internalized probabilities may then trigger emotional states or generate attitudes to particular courses of action as a result of becoming 'affectively charged' by personal values. The strength of the ensuing intention to act will depend on the combined strength of beliefs and motivations that interact in a multiplicative fashion.

The most common health education interventions probably operate in a manner designed to influence people's beliefs in order to generate a level of motivation that will result in some approved action or actions. However, it is important to recall that, although beliefs influence motivation, motivation also influences beliefs. In short, people typically believe what it is comfortable to believe. When faced with uncomfortable facts and experiences, they may well selectively attend to information that confirms their prejudices or is otherwise less threatening. They may reinterpret and distort messages or avoid/deny them. In relation to dissonance, discussed above, people may resort to autistic thinking in order to reduce the discomfort experienced when beliefs about self and behaviour are in conflict.

We should also note that individuals may not only hold beliefs that *generate* motivation, but may actually have beliefs *about* motivation. This phenomenon is represented by segment 3 in the health action model (see Figure 3.2 above). For instance, in Marsh and Matheson's (1983) classic survey of adult smoking attitudes and behaviour, one of the most important factors determining whether or not smokers intended to quit smoking in the future was the belief that they held about the unpleasant withdrawal symptoms that they expected to experience and their anticipated loss of gratification. Thus, beliefs about effects significantly reduced their intention to act.

Segment 4 in the HAM (see Figure 3.2) also refers to individuals' beliefs about affect. In this case, it indicates their beliefs about the level of their motivation to comply with (or resist) normative pressures – for example, the degree of discomfort they expect to experience if they do not comply with a partner's wishes or choose to confront the smoking norms of their workmates.

Segments 5 and 6 in the HAM (see Figure 3.2) indicate the relationships of belief and motivation systems, respectively, with the self. Segment 5 refers to what is normally described as the 'self-concept' – that is, the sum total of individuals' beliefs about themselves as persons interacting with other persons and living in a given environment. Segment 6 describes what elsewhere we term 'self-sentiment', which is the sum total of feelings individuals might have about themselves as people.

This key motivational component is more commonly described as self-esteem. As we will see, it plays a central part in the principles and practice of health promotion.

The final segment in the HAM (see Figure 3.2) – segment 7 – acknowledges the fact that individuals will typically be able to articulate their beliefs about the feelings they have about themselves – for example, acknowledging that their self-esteem is unrealistically low.

The triangle in the model (see Figure 3.2) describes the totality of the individual self, including objectively defined elements of personality as well as the more subjective beliefs and values about self already referred to. This final influence on individual intentions to act will be subjected to scrutiny in the context of consideration of empowerment later in this chapter.

The health action model takes into account the key elements of the self that contribute to behavioural intention. These appear in the model as a triangle (see Figure 3.2), representing the concepts of self and personality and they interact with the motivation and belief systems represented in the model by the overlapping segments. The self-concept includes aspects such as self-esteem, self-efficacy and health locus of control. The concepts of self and personality warrant more in-depth exploration and this is done with respect to a critical review of the dynamics of empowerment in the following section.

EMPOWERMENT: A CRITICAL REVIEW OF THE DYNAMICS

In Chapter 1, we discussed ideological issues underpinning the definition and practice of health promotion. We examined the discourse of empowerment and argued that an empowerment model of health promotion should govern theory and practice. Empowerment is, of course, one of the key values of health promotion as highlighted by the Ottawa Charter (WHO, 1986). We now consider what might be involved in operationalizing empowerment so that we understand how philosophy might be translated into practice. Therefore, we will focus on what could be called the anatomy and dynamics of empowerment. We will do so within the framework of the HAM, which locates self-empowerment within the interlocking systems of beliefs, motivations and normative influence. Recognizing the facilitating or inhibiting effects of the physical, social and economic environment, our focus then shifts on to the systems that determine whether or not 'empowered' intentions can be translated into practice.

However, before considering the various constructs of empowerment in detail, reference to Figure 3.6 will indicate how they interact.

Defining the self-concept

As we observed above, segment 5 in the HAM (see Figure 3.2) refers to the self-concept. A number of beliefs about self have particular significance for health status. For instance, body image can influence the self both positively and negatively. Moreover, low self-esteem may result in mental and physical illnesses, such as those associated with eating disorders. However, mental illness may create low self-esteem. Other beliefs contribute indirectly to health and our emphasis here will be on beliefs about susceptibility to negative outcomes and, more particularly, on beliefs about control, which are central to the process and state of empowerment. Nonetheless, given the importance of the notion of the self and the considerable amount of research, past and present, it is appropriate to give further consideration to this construct.

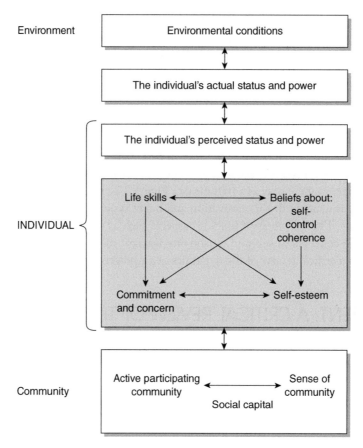

Figure 3.6 Elements of empowerment

Defining the self

It is important to make the distinction between the self as perceived by the individual and that perceived by an external observer or delineated in more objective fashion by a psychometric test. Segment 5 in Figure 3.2 refers to the former and represents the personal formulation of self.

From the perspective of health promotion theory and practice, there are two key issues. The first of these is the extent to which the self-concept is a global construct rather than comprising an aggregate of different component parts (such as sexual attractiveness or intelligence). The second issue concerns the relationship between the self-concept and self-esteem – including the possible tension between the formulation of an ideal self and an actual, perceived self.

The increased interest in the self-concept in recent years – and the varieties of subordinate concepts – are revealed by the number of instruments designed to measure these. The most commonly used measure is the Self-Concept Clarity Scale (SCCS) (Campbell et al., 1996, cited in Cicero, 2020). However, as Ferro and Boyle (2013) point out, although the notion of self-concept has received a lot of research attention, findings are not consistent. In all events, the contemporary view is that the self-concept has a structure that is derived from the substantial body of information that people have accumulated about themselves. This structure is multidimensional and hierarchical. It becomes increasingly differentiated over time as a result of age and experience. Shavelson and Marsh (1986), Song and Hattie (1984) and Hattie (1992) have produced influential taxonomies that illustrate both the differentiation and the hierarchical structure. Figure 3.7 summarizes this structure and, in relation to the 'academic' category, emphasizes not only the importance of school-related achievement but also general intellectual competence and skills. It also indicates the importance of the interpersonal context (note, for instance, our earlier observations about peer group influence) and, of course, the prime importance of body image and the associated attributes of confidence and self-esteem. It is doubtless self-evident that taxonomies of this kind are essentially culturally constructed and, because of the origins of most of the research, tend to reflect North American values and ideals. An exception to this is the development of the Nigerian Children's Self-Concept Scale developed by Ojo and Akinsola (2012) at the University of Lagos.

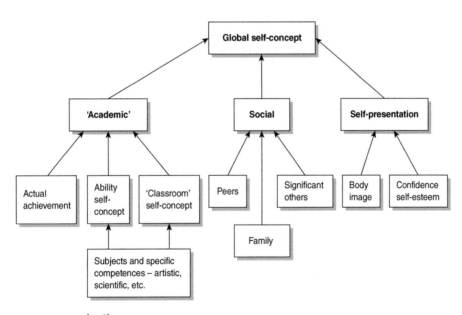

Figure 3.7 A taxonomy of self

The self-concept, susceptibility and risk-taking

As mentioned earlier, beliefs about susceptibility to disease are a key feature of the HBM. Beliefs about susceptibility when associated with beliefs about the seriousness of disease generate a level of perceived threat (in HAM terms, an emotional state associated with the fear drive). This, in turn, is anticipated to lead to preventive action, provided beliefs about the benefits of that action are considered to outweigh the costs. Perception of susceptibility thus signals a specific belief about the self. The belief in question relates to risk. However, as with other beliefs, it reflects – and, quite frequently, may distort – objective reality. Accordingly, the unthinking use of this belief about vulnerability to predict cautious, preventive decision-making may very well lead to dramatically inappropriate conclusions. First of all, a substantial amount of productive research effort has been devoted to the description of *objective* risk – that is, to the use of statistical techniques to accurately record the probabilities of particular activities and circumstances resulting in negative consequences. Second, it is clear from equally sound research that individuals' perceptions of risks and beliefs about vulnerability are only imperfectly related to objective risk. For instance, there is a clearly demonstrated tendency to overestimate the likelihood of the unlikely and underestimate the real frequency of relatively common threats (Kasperson et al., 1988; Lichtenstein et al., 1978; Slovic et al., 1982; Weinstein, 1982, 1984) and for people commonly to employ a strategy of 'selective focus' (Weinstein, 1984). These factors are largely accounted for using a 'deficit' model that assumes that people take risks because they do not understand the nature of risk, they cannot make sense of it or they are simply irrational (Mitchell Turner et al., 2021; Tulloch and Lupton, 2003). They might also, however, result from the so-called 'availability heuristic', whereby risk appraisal is biased by frequently reported, but not necessarily frequently occurring, events.

Again, affective factors often influence the interpretation of risk. The intuitive observation that young people consider themselves immortal is supported by academic research demonstrating that there is a tendency for people to underestimate the extent of their personal vulnerability to harm. Weinstein (1984) has proposed the terms 'Optimistic Bias' and 'Unrealistic Optimism' in an attempt to account for the ways in which people underestimate personal risk when comparing themselves with other people.

By contrast, when frequent reporting of dangerous situations and disasters is accompanied by, for example, extensive media coverage in full and gory Technicolor, the availability heuristic can introduce the dread factor into beliefs about personal vulnerability. A further discussion of the inflation of perceptions of risk and associated feelings of threat is to be found in 'social amplification of risk' theory. Social amplification relates to the way in which risk is magnified through social processes such as media reporting (Kasperson and Kasperson, 2005; Kasperson, 1992; Pidgeon et al., 2003).

An additional problem with a naive interpretation of susceptibility is the fact that some individuals actively pursue risk. They would, by definition, not pursue it unless they believed that they were susceptible to some negative outcome. There are various explanations of the motivation for deliberate risk-seeking. One suggestion is that some individuals enjoy the physiological effects. To put it somewhat crudely, it would seem that they become addicted to these. This might well explain the attractions of theme park and fairground rides that produce adrenaline arousal accompanied by a belief that there is no real danger. However, it would not account for other circumstances where risks are taken only when there is genuine danger. Based on research with people who engage in extreme sports, Lyng (1990, 2005) offers an interesting explanation of this phenomenon that is clearly linked to discussions around empowerment and control (Arnoldi, 2009). Lyng employs the term 'edgework', which concerns negotiating the boundaries in high-risk practices (McGovern and McGovern, 2011).

Lyng's analysis could be said to have a certain authority as it is based on participant observation as a jump pilot! He asserts that all edgework involves:

> a clearly observable threat to one's physical or mental wellbeing or one's sense of an ordered existence. The archetypal edgework experience is one in which the individual's failure to meet the challenge at hand will result in death or, at the very least, debilitating injury. (Lyng, 1990: 856)

Edgework narratives include personal skill, personal fulfilment, control and self-efficacy and are linked to constructions of personal identities (Lyng, 2005).

Lyng argues that many features of drug-taking and even binge drinking do not involve self-destructive behaviour as such but, rather, an attempt to demonstrate mastery and control – both concepts that are central to the notion of empowerment, as we will demonstrate later. Thus Kidder (2022) argues that the meaning of voluntary risk-taking (in whatever form) can be best understood by taking into account the way that people discursively frame their (risk-taking) actions.

The psychological analysis of susceptibility and risk-taking described above poses a serious challenge for the HBM. It may also create a dilemma for those who espouse a narrow preventive model of public health. The paradoxical pursuit of control in hazardous circumstances can result in serious casualties, even when a damage-limitation approach is used and individuals are taught about safety procedures, including how to use drugs 'safely' and deal with an overdose. It poses no difficulty for an empowerment model, provided that there is evidence that risk-takers are making empowered decisions. Clearly, if the casualty rate is so high as to impose too heavy a burden on society or risk-takers put other people at risk, then, following the principle of utilitarianism, coercive measures may prove necessary. However, in the vast majority of circumstances, empowerment is healthy – both in positive and preventive terms.

Empowerment and health

Self-esteem and health

As we noted above, self-esteem is the affective counterpart of the self-concept in the HAM. Indeed, a number of instruments to which reference was made in the discussion of the self-concept above focus on self-esteem, such as Coopersmith's self-esteem inventories, the culture-free self-esteem inventories and Rosenberg's self-esteem scale.

It seems obvious that self-esteem has a significant effect on health – both directly and indirectly. Mann et al. (2004) argue that self-esteem is critical to the improvement of both mental and physical health. Self-esteem is typically considered a key feature of mental health and, therefore, worth pursuing in its own right. For example, based on research with university students in Iran, Mahdavi et al. (2013) found a strong relationship between self-esteem and mental health. Self-esteem may also have an indirect influence through its contribution to intentions to undertake healthy or unhealthy actions. For instance, at a common sense level, individuals who respect and value themselves will, other things being equal, seek to look after themselves by adopting courses of action that prevent disease. Research in the USA by Samuels and Dale (2022) revealed a strong association between higher self-esteem and lower likelihood of depression in Black women living with HIV. Self-esteem is also strongly linked to health-related behaviours. For example, people with higher levels of self-esteem are more likely to engage in behaviours that protect and maximize health (Brann et al., 2022).

It is also worth noting that various aspects of the self-concept contribute differentially to self-esteem. It is generally considered that a discrepancy between the ideal self and actual self is likely to generate low self-esteem (unless, of course, the individual has a sufficient belief in his or her capability to remedy that discrepancy – in which case, successfully bridging the gap will actually enhance self-esteem). For example, the relationship between body image and self-esteem is well recognized. One need not look too far to find a plethora of literature on young women's body image and self-esteem. However, not surprisingly, the research findings are not always consistent or transferable given that the construct of self-esteem reflects prevailing personal, social and cultural values and norms.

Self-esteem is influenced in various ways, one of the most important of which is a belief about being in control.

The case of learned helplessness and hopelessness

The phenomenon of learned helplessness was demonstrated by Seligman (1975: 9): 'Helplessness is the psychological state that frequently results when events are uncontrollable.' Even if something pleasurable happens to an individual, the sense of uncontrollability and the consequent helplessness will result if this 'reward' is not contingent on an individual's own actions:

> Organisms, when exposed to uncontrollable events, learn that responding is futile. Such learning undermines the incentive to respond, and so it produces profound interference with the motivation of instrumental behaviour. It also proactively interferes with learning that responding works when events become uncontrollable, and so produces cognitive distortions. The fear of an organism faced with trauma is reduced if it learns that responding controls trauma; fear persists if the organism remains uncertain about whether trauma is controllable; if the organism learns that trauma is uncontrollable, fear gives way to depressions. (Seligman, 1975: 74)

Lack of control, therefore, has three main effects:

- **cognitive** – it disrupts the ability to learn
- **conative** – it saps the motivation to take action
- **affective** – it produces emotional disturbance.

Seligman speculated on the physiological mechanisms affected by learned helplessness. At the time, this speculation seemed somewhat fanciful, but more recently interest has grown in the notion of 'biological transition'. For instance, Brunner (in Blane et al., 1996) argued for a quite direct link between the lack of control experienced by the lower grades of civil servants in the second Whitehall Study and specific physiological effects, postulating the existence of a pathway linking:

> the chronic stress response of the hypothalamic pituitary adrenal system with resulting elevated levels of corticosteroids to central obesity, insulin resistance, poor lipid profile and increased tendency for the blood to clot. (Marmot, in Brunner, 1996: 290)

In all events, the general notion of helplessness is convincing. However, its original formulation was criticized, largely on the grounds that, clearly, individuals do not always subside into helplessness when they experience uncontrollability, even after frequent exposure to circumstances in which there is little consistency in the relationship between behaviour and the outcomes of that behaviour. Accordingly, a modification of the theory was suggested by Seligman and other researchers (Abramson et al., 1978; Miller and Norman, 1979). The modification involved an emphasis on an individual's 'attribution of causality' – that is, their beliefs about what causes particular outcomes.

The above comments relate in general to individual health. However, as will be apparent from the reference above to false consciousness, the pathological effects of disempowerment can be applied to notions of social health and, conversely, to social malaise. We will, therefore, return to this theme in the context of later discussions of *community* empowerment.

Indirect effects of empowerment on health – beliefs about control

As we have noted before, empowerment can be viewed as a health state in its own right – for both individuals and communities. A lack of empowerment can be seen as unhealthy and/or have direct negative physiological effects. More commonly, however, empowerment is considered to have an indirect effect on health by influencing individual and community action. In this context, it is viewed as involving both *actual* possession of power and *beliefs* about having power. Different kinds and levels of beliefs have been identified (see, for instance, Lewis, 1987; Sarafino and Smith, 2021). The hierarchy below exemplifies these different levels:

- **Informational control** refers to the possession of information necessary for taking action.
- **Cognitive control**, according to Lewis, relates to the acquisition of information that allows the intellectual management of an event and, thus, possibly reduces its threatening properties.
- **Decisional control** refers to having opportunities to make decisions.
- **Behavioural control** indicates the possession of skills necessary for translating decisions into action. It can also be applied to the possession of skills to enhance 'cognitive control'.
- **Existential control**, a term employed by Lewis in the context of patient education, refers to a belief about the meaningfulness of circumstances rather than control proper.
- **Contingency control** refers to individuals' beliefs that the outcomes of decision-making and action are actually under their own control – that is, are contingent on their decision-making. This approximates to the concepts of 'locus of control' and 'self-efficacy'.
- **Locus of control** is perhaps the best known and most influential conceptualization of control. It was developed by Rotter (1966) in the context of social learning theory. He named it 'perceived locus of control' (PLC) to emphasize the fact that it referred to a *subjective* probability rather than the *actual* degree of control possessed by individuals.

The purpose of empowerment strategies is, of course, to foster internality. Perhaps the most important aspect of this notion is the fact that beliefs or expectancies are generalized: they refer to a general tendency to believe that one is in charge of one's life (internal PLC) or, by contrast, generally powerless (external PLC). We should also note that there are two varieties of externality: first, a belief that one is controlled by chance, luck or fate; and, second, that one's life is controlled by 'powerful others'.

Health locus of control

Of particular interest to health promotion is a variant on the notion of PLC in the form of 'health locus of control' (HLC). This originated with the work of Kirscht (1972), who developed measures of PLC specifically orientated towards health, and Wallston et al. (1976), who subsequently developed a more sophisticated version in the form of the 'multidimensional health locus of control scale (MHLC)'. Parcel and Meyer (1978) also produced a special version of MHLC for children.

The concept of perceived locus of control has been subjected to considerable scrutiny and, in 1982, Wallston and Wallston reported that, at the time of writing, there had been over a thousand published papers, in addition to 'a myriad of unpublished theses, dissertations and studies investigating the construct'. Researchers have examined the relationship between PLC and HLC and a range of health-related topics (such as health knowledge, smoking, birth control, weight loss, information-seeking and compliance, seatbelt use and so on). Some results were encouraging, although Wallston and Wallston considered that their (1982) review of *health* locus of control was disappointing.

A thorough review by Norman and Bennett (1996) also concluded that the predictive power of HLC is weak. Wallston concurs with this opinion but, with a touch of irritation, voices the opinion that critics 'do not properly understand or appreciate the theoretical underpinnings of the construct' (1991: 251). Wallston makes the very important point that it is essential to consider HLC together with individuals' health values and other important constructs in any prediction equation, such as specific measures for 'self-efficacy', for example. In short, 'An individual's health behaviour is multi-determined; there is no sense kidding oneself that HLC is the most important determinant.' That said, Jacobs-Lawson et al. (2011) assert that 'health locus of control has been shown to influence how individuals approach their health and health-related decisions'. Wallston et al. (1999) later developed the God Locus of Health Control Scale in order to examine perceptions of external sources of control in more detail, although there is a relative dearth of research exploring this specific construct. A final point to note is that, as Cheng et al. (2013) argue, the concept of external locus does not carry the same negative connotations across cultures. Like all the variables in the MHLC, it has inevitable bias, as do the vast majority of psychological constructs, having been developed and 'tested' within a specific sociocultural context.

Self-efficacy – specific beliefs about control

The concept of self-efficacy is one of the most useful, and applicable, notions in social psychology. It is attributed primarily to Bandura (1977, 1982, 1986, 1992). Its relevance can be appreciated from Bandura's (1982: 122–3) own definition:

> Perceived self-efficacy is concerned with judgements of how well one can execute courses of action required to deal with prospective situations … Self-percepts of efficacy are not simply inert estimates of future action. Self-appraisals of operative capabilities function as one set of proximal determinants of how people behave, their thought patterns, and the emotional reactions they experience in taxing situations. In their daily lives people continuously make decisions about what course of action to pursue and how long to continue those they have undertaken. Because acting on misjudgements of personal efficacy can produce adverse consequences, accurate appraisal of one's own capabilities has considerable functional value. Self-efficacy judgements, whether accurate or faulty, influence choice of activities and environmental settings. People avoid activities that they believe exceed their coping capabilities, but they undertake and perform assuredly those that they judge themselves capable of managing.

Self-efficacy is one of the most valuable and practical features of social cognitive theory (SCT) – an extension and elaboration of social learning theory (SLT). Its importance is reflected in the fact that it has been added to Fishbein and Ajzen's theory of reasoned action as a kind of bolt-on extra. Their revised model was rebranded as the *theory of planned behaviour* (Ajzen, 1991; Conner and Sparks, 2005).

As noted earlier, SLT/SCT offers a simple but effective model of successful human agency. It includes the formula: action is the product of response efficacy and self-efficacy where response efficacy is the belief that a particular course or courses of action will result in the achievement of some desired outcome. It follows that self-efficacy refers to the individual's conviction that he or she is actually capable of undertaking the actions necessary to achieve the outcome. Self-efficacy, like PLC, is therefore what was described earlier as a contingency belief, although self-efficacy differs from PLC in its specificity. Perhaps due to this specificity, it is clear that single measures of self-efficacy can correlate substantially with behavioural outcomes. It is, as Zlatanovi (2017: 17) argues, 'one of the key factors in the exercise of personal control, including control over the state of one's own health'. Research findings corroborate this – for example, a meta-analysis of associations between self-efficacy and sedentary behaviours found that higher levels of self-efficacy were associated with lower incidence of sedentary behaviour (Szczuka et al., 2021), whilst Peker et al.'s (2021) research into self-efficacy and cyber-bullying behaviour showed that a decrease in the former led to an increase in the latter. The following study highlights the link between self-efficacy and health literacy (discussed in more detail later in this chapter).

ABSTRACT 3.1

Self-efficacy, health literacy, and nutrition and exercise behaviors in a low-income, Hispanic population. Guntzviller, L.M., King, A.J., Jensen, J.D. and Davis, L.A. (2017)

Public health goals have emphasized healthy nutrition and exercise behaviours, especially in underserved populations. According to social cognitive theory (SCT) self-efficacy and capability (e.g. health literacy) may interact to predict preventative behaviours. The authors surveyed 100 low-income, native Spanish-speakers living in the United States who were low in English proficiency and predominately of Mexican heritage. Participants reported their nutritional and exercise self-efficacy, Spanish health literacy, and nutrition and physical activity behaviours. Consistent with SCT, the interaction of self-efficacy and health literacy significantly predicted fruit and vegetable consumption and weekly exercise, and marginally predicted avoidance of high fat food. For all three interactions, higher health literacy levels strengthened the positive relationship between self-efficacy and health behaviours. The results offer support for the tenets of SCT and suggest – for low-income, Spanish-speaking adults – that a combination of behavioural confidence and literacy capability are necessary to enact appropriate health behaviours.

The notion of 'reciprocal determinism' is also central to the formulation. In other words, there is a reciprocal relationship between the environment and the individual – each influences the other and outcomes depend on the results of that interaction. The interaction is expressed diagrammatically in Figure 3.8.

In addition to having beliefs about the nature of a health action and the likelihood of being able to perform it, individuals also have beliefs about the extent to which they possess the skills and capabilities they need to achieve the health action goals. Self-efficacy beliefs can be influenced by, and also create, emotional states, such as shame or anxiety at the prospect of failure, or failing to take any action because of lack of confidence.

As we mentioned above, response efficacy is also an affective factor related to an acceptance that the health action is a worthwhile goal. Active goal-setting will occur to the extent that individuals believe that they are capable of achieving those goals. Furthermore, they will have beliefs about the relationship between the environment and the health action. They must accept that there is a reasonable probability of their being able to overcome any environmental barriers before they commit themselves to action. Typically, it will be necessary to have certain capabilities and skills related to the attainment of the desired outcome, including decision-making skills. If individuals do not believe that they possess these competences, their commitment to change will be reduced.

Self-efficacy beliefs will depend substantially on past experience of mastery – of success or failure. The role of health promotion is threefold. First, it aims to influence efficacy beliefs directly. Second, it aims to exercise an indirect influence by providing the competences and skills needed to carry out a health action and/or cope with environmental barriers. Third, it aims to remove those environmental barriers that militate against the formation of efficacy beliefs.

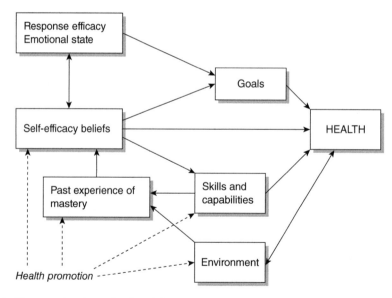

Figure 3.8 Self-efficacy and reciprocal determinism

Self-efficacy – implications for health promotion

Bandura argues that there are four general factors influencing self-efficacy beliefs. They are (in descending order of power): direct experience, vicarious experience, verbal persuasion and physiological state. These are listed in Table 3.2 in conjunction with implications for health promotion.

Table 3.2 Influences on self-efficacy – implications for health promotion

Influences on self-efficacy	Examples of implications for health promotion
Direct experience	Provide experience through role play
Physiological state: 'people rely partly on information from their physiological state in judging their capabilities … Fear reactions generate further fear through anticipatory self-arousal. By conjuring up fear-provoking thoughts about their ineptitude, people can rouse themselves to elevated levels of distress that produce the very dysfunctions they fear'	Anticipatory guidance Stress management techniques
Verbal persuasion: 'to try to talk people into believing they possess capabilities that will enable them to achieve what they seek'	Various, well-recognized attitude change techniques, such as using credible sources, appropriate message style, right level of emotional arousal, minimizing reactance. Beware: changes may be short-lived and this strategy is not empowering and of dubious ethicality!
Vicarious efficacy information: 'information conveyed by modelled events … People judge their capabilities partly by comparing their performances with those of others'	Observation of credible/'homophilous' models achieving success

Source: Quotations from Bandura (1986: 399ff.)

Personality and behavioural intention

Personality is included in the portrayal of 'self' in the HAM. It is considered to be one of the factors contributing to behavioural intention. Personality differs from other psychological constructs in that it refers to the relatively fixed and enduring attributes of the individual. These attributes may be described in terms of 'traits', which may be further classified into 'types' and 'profiles'. Despite some earlier dalliance with attempts to link personality with health-related behaviour, traditional analyses of personality have not been considered to be particularly useful in health promotion.

We will make some reference to the use of 'depth psychology' in advertising in our discussion of mass media in Chapter 8, but for now we will limit ourselves to noting four instances where aspects of personality do seem to affect intentions and action to a greater or lesser extent.

Coherence, hardiness and resilience

The existence of a 'hardy personality' has been identified (for example, Kobasa, 1979) and it is of interest to our present discussion as its three major characteristics have special relevance to our discussion of empowerment and, in its reference to 'challenge', to radical health promotion. Hardiness has three main features:

- a sense of **personal control** – to all intents and purposes identical to locus of control
- **commitment** – a sense of purpose and involvement with community and life in general
- **challenge** – change is viewed as opportunity.

In addition to its similarity to Antonovsky's 'sense of coherence' (SOC, to which reference was made in Chapter 1), it is also virtually synonymous with the notion of 'resilience' that attracts increasing attention. Resilience 'refers to patterns of positive adjustment in the context of significant risk or adversity' (Luthar, 2003: 4) or, as Caltabiano and Caltabiano (2006: 1) put it, 'the ability of an individual to maintain competence and attain adaptation despite negative life circumstances'. Studies of resilient children have recorded, with some surprise, a tendency for them to recover rapidly from adversity, be well adjusted, have good social skills and, above all, a sense of personal control and relatively high self-esteem – all this, despite experiencing horrific circumstances, including being raised in dysfunctional families, being abused and even growing up in concentration camps (see, for instance, Werner, 1980, 1987). It is difficult to account for such phenomena when they are so inconsistent with the received wisdom of theories of learned helplessness. To the extent that such characteristics do reflect personality, it would seem necessary to have recourse to explanation in terms of inherited, 'temperamental' traits.

Resilience is strongly linked to mental health. Significantly, but perhaps not surprisingly, a positive correlation has been found between health-promoting behaviours and resilience (Ma et al., 2013). The notion of resilience receives increasing attention. There is also a focus in the literature on 'community resilience', which has been defined as a community's 'ability to withstand and recover from a disaster' (Chandra et al., 2013: 1181). More recently, the term 'collective resilience' has been used (Lyons et al., 2016). Collective resilience is related to community resilience but refers to all, or any, kinds of groups (for example, social groups, leisure groups, sports teams). Collective resilience is manifest by mutual support and connection as well as shared identity and purpose (Lyons and Heywood, 2016). A group's capacity to adapt, and higher levels of agency, results in the capacity for it to overcome challenges (Lyons et al., 2016). The concept of resilience has been criticized for being 'largely framed in Western understandings', 'unquestioningly accepted' and unchallengingly imposed on people (Usher et al., 2021: 1). Notwithstanding, resilience is clearly connected with concepts such as 'assets' and 'capacity'. The underpinning assumption of such concepts is that they can be built upon, strengthened or expanded, to improve health and health outcomes at an individual and community level. A decade ago, Whiting et al. (2012) argued that there was an increasing volume of literature exploring assets, which they define as those 'positive attributes of both people and communities' (p. 25). A recent example of this is research by Molina-Betancur (2021) in Colombia (see Abstract 3.2 for more details). These ideas are linked with notions of social capital and are discussed further in Chapter 9. The following study highlights the role of resilience in select health behaviours.

ABSTRACT 3.2

Community health assets mapping in a slum in Medellin (Colombia). Molina-Betancur, J.C., Agudelo-Suárez, A.A. and Martínez-Herrera, E. (2021)

Objectives: To describe how the community from El Faro neighbourhood identifies its community assets, uses them to face life's challenges through the capacity of collective agency; and by generating community development processes, applying the salutogenic theory that considers people as active subjects, with the capacity to conserve and generate health and well-being, through the use of their own resources called health assets.

Methods: A map of community assets was made in 2018 in El Faro neighbourhood, an informal settlement of Medellín, Colombia, following the phases recommended by other authors and from a qualitative, participatory approach that delves into the health situation of the community.

Results: In this process were identified 12 individual community assets, 12 collective, 13 institutional and 10 in the environment. The main community asset among the 47 described was community participation, from the agency capacity, mainly of its leaders who participating in their own organizations encourage development, identity construction and well-being.

Conclusion: Asset mapping served to identify intangible assets for the community and, in turn, this recognition was useful in strengthening the agency's capacity for community development. This is a territory transformed by community reflection processes allowing to understand situations of exclusion and poverty, seeking to create a more liveable place and developing a community capacity to solve their own problems, through solidarity and community support.

Type A and B personalities

The personality types that have received the greatest attention in relation to health are so-called Type A and Type B. The former has been characterized as 'an excess of free-floating hostility, competitiveness, and time urgency' (Bennett and Murphy, 1997: 20). In contrast, Type B is more relaxed and easygoing. Interest in the association with health derives from research (by Friedman and Rosenman, 1974) that demonstrated that Type As carried twice the risk of heart disease as Type Bs, after controlling for other risk factors such as smoking. A mixed profile has also been recognized, referred to as Type A/B or Type X. Clearly, from a health promotion perspective, it is not possible to change enduring traits such as personality. Nonetheless, the associated behaviours are amenable to modification.

The sensation-seeking personality

Another psychological construct having pretensions to a personality trait or type – and of relevance for health promotion – is the concept of 'sensation-seeking'. Individuals vary in the extent to which they actively seek sensations and Zuckerman (1990) developed a sensation-seeking scale (SSS). Bearing in mind earlier observations about risk-taking and phenomena such as edgework, the reality of this personality characteristic is of some importance to health promoters (and creates still more tension for the HBM's notion of susceptibility). Not surprisingly, a number of studies report a link between sensation-seeking and risk-taking (for example, Zuckerman and Kuhlman, 2000) and there appears to be some predictive value between sensation-seeking and risk-taking (Breakwell, 2007).

TRANSLATING INTENTION INTO PRACTICE: REMOVING BARRIERS AND EMPOWERING COMMUNITIES

The discussion so far has centred on self-empowerment and examined various psychological characteristics associated with those personal capabilities and characteristics that help an individual gain control over his or her life and health. However, bearing in mind the paramount importance of reciprocal determinism, it is not possible to seek to facilitate individuals' empowerment without paying due attention to the nature of the environment. Indeed, to do so is merely to engage in a more sophisticated form of victim-blaming. Accordingly, we will now consider what is involved in translating behavioural intentions into action.

Assuming that the complex of multiple influences between self, belief, motivation and normative systems have resulted in an intention to act, it is imperative to consider what more is needed to maximize the chances of individuals achieving the goals they have set for themselves. However, let us not forget – and taking into account the principles of self-efficacy – that an individual's beliefs about the nature and strength of environmental barriers and deficits may cause the intention to act to be aborted. Returning to the HAM (shown in Figure 3.2), it will be seen that three kinds of facilitating factors may be necessary before intention is translated into practice (or, conversely, three kinds of barriers may need to be removed). These will now be reviewed.

Facilitating health actions – knowledge and skills
The contribution of knowledge

In terms of the HAM, it is important to clarify the two different contributions made to health choices by knowledge. The first concerns the acquisition of information that may influence the formation of beliefs – ultimately, this may contribute to an intention to act. The second of these merely involves providing the information that people who are already committed to taking action need in order to help them translate their intention to act into practice.

With regard to the first of these two contributions made by knowledge, it is important to remember that knowledge alone, although necessary, will very rarely be *sufficient* to lead to behaviour. As we noted earlier, knowledge rarely leads to practice without, at the very least, a shift in attitude. We might also observe that, frequently, a positive attitude to making a particular health choice may lead to a search for knowledge to clarify and support the tentative intention to act. It is often said that knowledge is power, but this is true only up to a point. For example, while it is true that knowing about the existence of family planning clinics offering contraceptive advice might be essential to the routine adoption of condom use, social skills would also be necessary to interact confidently and assertively with professional staff – and, more importantly, to negotiate condom use with a partner. Knowledge thus has only a contributory role in empowering progress from intention to action. But, conversely, lack of knowledge can be completely disempowering.

The importance of skills

The development of personal skills is, of course, of central importance in health promotion and this is one of the five key areas outlined in the Ottawa Charter (WHO, 1986). There is no precise definition of skills in general – apart from an implication that they are goal-directed and would be applied to some practical purpose. However, a number of specific skills can be precisely identified, together with the conditions needed to acquire proficiency. The health action model includes consideration of **psychomotor, social interaction** and **self-regulatory** skills. Box 3.1 contains a summary of these three key sets of skills that are of concern to health promotion.

BOX 3.1   SKILLS FOR EMPOWERMENT

(May be referred to as 'health skills' if applied to specific health scenarios)

Cognitive skills

- **Literacy** – the ability to read and write is intrinsically empowering.
- **Decision-making skills** – competences associated with cognitive problem-solving, such as assessing the costs and benefits of particular courses of action.

Psychomotor skills

- Skills involving the integration of perception and movement, such as the hand–eye coordination involved in the correct use of a condom.

Social interaction skills

- **Life skills** – the use of skilled responses to a range of social situations. Although 'life skills' also incorporates applied knowledge and understanding, its emphasis is on the acquisition and practice of skills and particularly social interaction skills, such as how to deal with housing officials or how to work in groups and organize for radical social action.
- **Assertiveness** – a valuable package of the knowledge and skills needed to achieve desired goals while, at the same time, recognizing other people's needs and rights.

The vexed question of health literacy

Health literacy has been proposed as a set of skills that is critical to achieving a state of empowerment (Nutbeam, 1998a) enabling people to make decisions about their health (Pop et al., 2013). Health literacy is a key concept in health promotion and health communication (Thompson and Robinson, 2021). It has its origins in the USA in relation to the development of patient literacy and the ability

to comply with treatment regimens. While notions of compliance may seem at odds with empowerment, the converse position – not being able to understand what is needed – is totally de-powering.
The concept has now been applied to health more generally and there are several definitions of health
literacy in the wider literature (Quick et al., 2021). For example, Nutbeam (1998a: 10) defines it as:

> the cognitive and social skills which determine the motivation and ability of individuals to gain
> access to, understand, and use information in ways which promote and maintain good health.

Following a review of 13 different definitions, Berkman et al. (2010) proposed that health literacy is about the extent to which a person can obtain, process, understand and communicate about
health-related information necessary for making decisions about health. Abel (2007: 59) also makes
the point that 'adequate health literacy not only supports personal health management, but also
increases the chances of changing health-relevant living conditions'. Johnson et al. (2013: 949) assert
that health literacy includes a person's 'reading, writing and numeracy skills, as well as his or her cultural
experiences, understanding of health concepts and pathophysiology, and basic communication skills'.

Nutbeam (2000a) distinguishes three levels of health literacy:

- **functional health literacy** – concerned with knowledge about risks and health services and the
  adoption of prescribed actions
- **interactive health literacy** – additionally includes personal and social skills and the motivation
  and self-confidence required to take personal action
- **critical health literacy** – having the knowledge and skills that enhance individual resilience to
  adverse circumstances, and support effective social and political action as well as individual action.

It should be evident that health literacy incorporates the same constructs as empowerment. Indeed,
in a scathing critique, Tones (2002) argued that health literacy is merely a rebranding of empowerment. Nonetheless, it continues to gain currency. While its focus on the development of knowledge
and skills may offer some potential in enabling individuals to influence their environment, health
literacy – in contrast to comprehensive models of empowerment – pays scant attention to the reciprocal effect of the environment on their capacity to do so. Indeed, Meherali et al.'s (2020) systematic
review of health literacy interventions in low- and middle-income countries highlighting the links
between low levels of general literacy (education), poorly resourced/functioning health systems and
health literacy further emphasizes this point, whilst Quick et al. (2021) point to the limits of health
literacy as an individual-level variable in health outcomes. Health literacy, therefore, remains a contested concept in health promotion (see Chapter 7 in Cross, Davis and O'Neil, 2017b for a fuller
discussion). We now turn our attention to the role of the environment.

Empowerment – the role of the environment

The significance of environmental factors in determining health status has been emphasized
throughout this book and will, therefore, receive only brief attention here as a factor influencing the
translation of intention into action. Clearly, failure to address physical, social, economic and cultural

circumstances is to unwittingly blame the victim whose health suffers from those circumstances and whose scope for action is dramatically impeded by them.

The **physical environment** ranges from the drastic effects of natural and human-made disasters and the debilitating effect of squalor and preventable disease to access to clean water supplies and user-friendly health services, from smoke-free public places to wide availability of condoms. As we described earlier at some length, the **socioeconomic environment** is a key factor in health inequalities through the absolute effects of poverty, but also through the more subtle effects of having wide income differentials in society. The **sociocultural environment** includes those various normative practices that may either be intrinsically healthy or unhealthy and the social networks to which individuals may have recourse. Using a case study on youth empowerment in New Mexico, USA, Wallerstein (2002) highlights the links between powerlessness, poor material conditions and poorer health outcomes. These links are further exacerbated by the structural socioeconomic inequalities that are rooted within historical racism and sexism as illustrated by the experiences of powerlessness in African American women in the US (Thomas and González-Prendes, 2009).

The empowerment model of health promotion to which we subscribe in this book (described in Chapter 1) is premised on a need for action for self-empowerment, but, importantly for empowerment, directed at social and environmental change. One of the main strategies is the Ottawa Charter principle of the creation of 'active participating communities'. We now consider factors associated with the empowerment of communities and their relationships with the larger social system. First, we will consider the meaning of sick and healthy societies.

Healthy societies and communities

In our discussion of the determinants of health in Chapter 2, reference was made to the popular notion of social capital. As we noted, social capital is typically viewed as a feature of a healthy society, just as financial capital can be considered to contribute to *economic* 'health'. It will doubtless be apparent that, although some difference in emphasis may be discerned, the key features of social capital are virtually synonymous with what has alternatively been described in terms such as sense of community, trust and participation. We will not, therefore, repeat our earlier observations about social capital, but give some thought to the meaning of these parallel ideas and concerns.

At one level, it can be argued that a healthy society or community is an empowered one. Accordingly, it is important to look more closely at what are considered to be the key features of such a community. As it happens, some people might consider that a community is, by definition, healthy – or at least if the standard definition is used, which characterizes a 'genuine' community as a relatively small aggregate of people (probably in a relatively small geographical locality or neighbourhood) that has both a tightly knit network of relationships and a common sense of identity. The reference to a sense of identity is more commonly described as a 'sense of community' and this is frequently seen as highly desirable. However, while a sense of community might well be a feature of an empowered one, the converse is not necessarily true. Indeed, individuals may recognize that they are part of a social group and, for instance, take some comfort from their awareness of sharing a common predicament. This is not necessarily empowering, particularly if we accept the premises of social control by means of false consciousness!

Kindervatter (1979: 62) emphasizes the key elements of an empowered community as being: 'People gaining an understanding of and control over social, economic and/or political forces in order to improve their standing in society.' Laverack (2009), therefore, refers to community empowerment as a process. Rappaport (1987: 130) declared that empowerment was not just an individual attribute but also:

> an organizational, political, sociological, economic, and spiritual [construct]. Our interests in racial and economic justice, in legal rights as well as in human needs, in healthcare and educational justice, in competence as well as in a sense of community, are all captured by the idea of empowerment. The reason we care about fostering a society whose social policies appreciate cultural diversity … is that we recognize that it is only in such a society that empowerment can be widespread. We are as much concerned with empowered organizations, neighbourhoods, and communities as we are with empowered individuals.

Participation and empowerment

Reference was made earlier to the Ottawa Charter's emphasis on the virtues of empowered, participating communities. The question might legitimately be asked whether empowered communities generate participation or participation creates empowerment – and, ultimately, action. Kieffer (1984: 31) considered that the empowered state consisted of 'an abiding set of commitments and capabilities which can be referred to as participatory competence'. The effects of this were believed to be:

- the development of a positive self-concept
- a more critical understanding of the surrounding social and political environment
- the cultivation of individual and collective resources for social and political action.

Additional discussion of empowering communities features in our discussion of community development in Chapter 9.

Empowerment and the avoidance of relapse

It can be seen from the HAM that the single time choice of a specific health action is not the end of the story. Although there are instances where that is all that is required – for example, attendance at a clinic for a one-off vaccination – the more common requirement is that the health action should be sustained and become adopted as a 'routine'. Once this has happened, the results of that choice may be confirmed. 'Outcome efficacy' may be confirmed and individuals may continue to enjoy the benefits of the health action to which they have committed themselves. Not unusually, though, an individual may discover that the anticipated benefits fail to materialize or actual loss of gratification or discomfort may be experienced. In short, relapse may occur.

Relapse is traditionally associated with various kinds of addiction (a term that, we admit, is open to several interpretations) and, at this juncture, it is worth giving some thought to the applicability of a popular explanatory model – the 'transtheoretical model' (TTM). We will also consider its relationship to the conceptual schema used in the HAM.

A useful summary of the model is provided by Prochaska et al. (1997) and its origins are revealing. Prochaska and colleagues carried out detailed analyses of some 300 different theories of psychotherapeutic interventions and identified 10 processes of change. The model scanned these theories and processes (hence, 'trans'theoretical), then combined and reformulated them.

While the model can be applied to any behaviour, it has been most frequently applied to those health actions involving the sacrifice of gratification and the experience of discomfort, which create the consequent likelihood of relapse. So, smoking, alcohol and substance misuse, eating problems and obesity feature prominently in research using the model.

A key feature of TTM is its assumption that individuals move through a series of stages (see Box 3.2) but may relapse at almost any time. However, there is a high level of probability that many will move again from a stage of (temporary) 'precontemplation' and proceed through the various stages once more until, hopefully, they will be successful. The reason for the phrase 'revolving door model' being used as a synonym for TTM is thus, doubtless, apparent.

BOX 3.2 TRANSTHEORETICAL MODEL

Stage of change

1. Precontemplation – not even considering change
2. Contemplation – considering making a specific behaviour change
3. Preparation – serious commitment and preparation to change
4. Action – initiation of change
5. Maintenance – sustaining the change

OR

Relapse.

Source: Prochaska and DiClemente (1983, 1984)

For some behaviours, a sixth stage has been identified – 'termination' (Nutbeam et al., 2010). This would be applicable to addictive behaviours for example. Another point of considerable importance is that interventions designed to achieve behaviour change must be tailored to the individual and, therefore, take account of the particular stage that they have reached in their behaviour change career. As Upton and Thirlaway (2014) argue, it is important to understand where people are at in order to support them in changing. Initially designed by Miller for working with people with addiction, and later developed further by Miller and Rollnick, motivational interviewing is a technique that uses such an approach (Hillsdon, 2006).

Prochaska et al. (1997) provide an extensive list of approaches and techniques that have been used to maximize success and minimize the chance of relapse – including not only individual methods, such as 'consciousness-raising' and 'counter-conditioning', but also what they term 'social liberation' – broader, 'primary preventive' social measures to influence social norms that foster unhealthy behaviour.

How does the TTM relate to the HAM? Clearly, it relates well to the confirmation/relapse pathway that follows the period of 'trying out' the health action in question. The process of developing a routine – especially where the health action is problematic – may take some time. Following Prochaska's comment about the move from 'maintenance' to 'termination', it may take between six months and five years! However, as the precontemplation stage describes the state existing prior to the formation of an intention to adopt a healthy course of action, the HAM's analysis of the complex of beliefs, motivations, norms and factors associated with self and personality demonstrates that, at this point, the TTM analysis is somewhat superficial!

Returning to our focus on empowerment, one of the empowering approaches to minimize relapse involves attribution theory and, more specifically, reattributing individuals' perceptions of the nature of the barriers to maintaining their avoidance of negative behaviour, such as overeating or other 'addictions'.

Empowerment and self-control

The adoption of health practices is frequently dependent on having the requisite skills. The HAM incorporates one particular class of life or health skills that are similar to some of the intervention measures identified by Prochaska. These are skills derived from a long tradition of work in behaviour modification and are here termed self-regulatory skills.

Empowerment is ultimately concerned with self-determination and, as we have noted, environmental factors may limit the possibility of self-determination. Nevertheless, individuals can exercise a good deal of personal control. In short, freedom of will can be a reality. Central to the achievement of personal control are 'self-referent cognitions' – that is, beliefs about oneself – that also include 'meta cognitions' – the uniquely human capacity to think about thought and reflect on reflections.

The paramount importance of Bandura's application of the concept of self-efficacy in understanding how people can successfully interact with their environment is evident. Self-efficacy is of paramount importance in health behaviour change (Upton and Thirlaway, 2014). Not surprisingly, Bandura (1989: 1182) comments on the importance of self-efficacy beliefs in relation to self-regulation:

> Self-generated influences operate deterministically on behaviour the same way as external sources of influence do. Given the same environmental conditions, persons who have developed skills for accomplishing many options and are adept at regulating their own motivation and behaviour are more successful in their pursuits than those who have limited means of personal agency. It is because self-influence operates deterministically on action that some measure of self-directedness and freedom is possible … Self-regulatory functions are personally constructed from varied experiences not simply environmentally implanted … Through their capacity to manipulate symbols and to engage in reflective thought, people can generate novel ideas and innovative actions that transcend their past experiences. They bring influence to bear on their motivation and action in efforts to realize valued futures.

With respect to our current discussion, the 'valued futures' mentioned by Bandura above include freedom from addictions. Traditionally, behaviour modification has been employed to deal with these powerful drives. It has its roots in behaviourist attempts (typically in competition with counselling interventions derived from psychoanalysis) to deal with various kinds of mental illness, such as phobias and compulsive behaviour. Following, for example, Skinnerian 'operant conditioning theory', psychologists were concerned to shape unwanted and unhealthy behaviour into that which was acceptable to therapists, their clients (and society as a whole). Many of the methods used – such as counter-conditioning by means of electric shock – would seem to be diametrically opposed to the ethics and practice of empowerment. However, more recent developments have switched the emphasis away from 'therapist control' to 'client control'. In short, the DIY version of behaviour modification aimed to put clients in charge of their own 'therapy' and this approach has become integrated into various health promotion methods concerned with fostering behaviour change. See motivational interviewing for an example of this kind of approach.

Kanfer and Karoly (1972) were among the first to address the apparent paradox of employing behaviour modification techniques to achieve voluntaristic outcomes. They pointed out, for instance, how certain tactics that achieved desired behaviour change goals, at least in the short term, did not involve genuine self-control – that is, empowered decision-making. They noted, too, that genuine self-control occurs only when:

> an individual alters or maintains his [*sic*] behavioral chain in the absence of immediate external supports … Once an obese person has put a lock on the refrigerator or the alcoholic mixed an emetic in his drink [external factors] are sufficient to account for the resulting behaviour. (1972: 408)

Returning to observations made in Chapter 1 on voluntarism, it is interesting to note the parallel between these coercive measures at the micro level and the coercive potential of healthy public policy. This may go considerably further than making 'the healthy choice the easy choice' by seeking to make it the only choice!

Before considering the key skills needed to achieve self-regulation of behaviour, it is worth recalling that the kinds of behaviour currently under consideration are those where:

- a change in relatively recently adopted health actions occurs as a result of significant reduction in gratification or the experience of significant aversive consequences
- the emergence of a competing motivation of superior strength results in an undesirable behaviour.

An example of the first situation is provided by experience of negative effects after giving up smoking or when vigorous exercise proves painful. The second situation is illustrated by times when the sex drive overrides the motivating force of moral value and/or concern at the prospect of infection in the context of an unanticipated romantic encounter.

Self-regulatory skills – a model

Figure 3.9 seeks to describe key features of self-regulation in the particular context of combating relapse.

An essential feature of many, if not most, situations where people are seeking to change their behaviour is the provision of 'anticipatory guidance'. This term can be used to describe the whole package – including the provision of skills. It is used here to refer to providing 'cognitive control' – that is, a degree of empowerment by giving individuals a grasp of what will be involved in the aftermath of choice. More important is the use of methods to generate appropriate self-efficacy beliefs – for example, by using models, those who have successfully moved through the 'maintenance' stage and reached 'termination' (for instance, ex-smokers who have not smoked for more than one year).

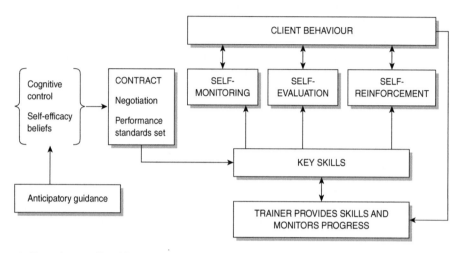

Figure 3.9   Self-regulation of health actions

A recommended and standard procedure for achieving self-control is the formulation of a contract between trainer and client. As with any contract, there is a process of negotiation and mutual agreement about the responsibilities and commitments of trainer and client, including what the client is prepared to do. The contract might actually be written or merely involve a verbal discussion. The procedure might involve contingency contracting. Examples of this include a cash deposit that will only be refunded once the target behaviour has been attained.

Three key processes are involved in the acquisition of a repertoire of self-regulatory skills:

- self-monitoring
- self-evaluation
- self-reinforcement.

It is generally accepted that, in order, ultimately, to handle motivational problems, clients should first of all be involved in conscious monitoring of behaviour and associated feelings. Monitoring involves paying attention to, and correctly interpreting, external environmental cues and internal, physiological events. For example, clients might ascribe the surge of excitement and gastronomic arousal to the display in the patisserie window prior to their succumbing to temptation!

'Proprioception' – the interpretation of internal states – is not only part of acquiring motor skills, it is also important in acquiring self-control skills. The individual learns to become aware of autonomic responses and associated thought processes. In self-monitoring, therefore, feedback is received from external stimuli, one's own behaviour and internal cognitive, affective and autonomic processes.

Self-evaluation consists of comparing self-monitored data with some standard of performance and judging the adequacy of the overall performance. This judgement then serves as a discriminating stimulus for either positive or negative reinforcement. In other words, the performance in the patisserie may serve as a cause of self-congratulation or harbinger of guilt!

Perhaps the most problematic of the three processes is that of 'self- reinforcement'. The key task is somehow to override the reinforcing qualities of the unwanted behaviour with some replacement reinforcer. The powerful gratifications delivered by the cream cake must somehow be reduced and/or replaced with a more powerful reinforcer. Unfortunately, it is often difficult to find a really enticing alternative. For instance, some of the suggestions offered in leaflets designed to help smokers quit their habit are distinctly uninspiring, such as, to take your mind off your need for a cigarette, fiddle with a paperclip, suck a mint or take a brisk walk! Interestingly, a systematic review on self-incentivizing and self-reward in behaviour change resulted in more questions than answers as to their effects, finding a weak effect size and a relative lack of studies. The authors argued that this 'raises the question of why self-incentivizing is such a widely employed component of behaviour change interventions' (Brown et al., 2018: 121).

Thoresen and Mahoney (1974: 22) identify four major categories of self- reinforcement:

- **Positive self-reward** – the self-administration or consumption of a freely available reinforcer only after performance of a specific, positive response, such as treating oneself to a special event after having lost weight
- **Negative self-reward** – the avoidance of, or escape from, a freely avoidable aversive stimulus only after performance of a specific, positive response, such as removing an uncomplimentary pig poster from one's dining room whenever a diet is adhered to for a full day
- **Positive self-punishment** – the removal of a freely available reinforcer after the performance of a specific, negative response, such as tearing up a dollar bill for every 100 calories in excess of one's daily limit
- **Negative self-punishment** – the presentation of a freely avoidable aversive stimulus after the performance of a specific, negative response, such as presenting oneself with a noxious odour after each occurrence of snacking.

Readers may experience doubts about the widespread applicability or acceptability of these tactics and favour less demanding reinforcement schedules such as public praise from peers or even self-satisfaction at meeting goals.

Self-reinforcement will frequently be supplemented by attempts to break the stimulus–response link between situation and gratification. Dieters might be advised not to shop when hungry and smokers might be advised to break habitual links.

One of the important issues in developing self-regulatory skills is the extent to which a skilled counsellor/trainer should be involved. For instance, as Kok et al. (1992) point out, it is important that attributions *after* failure should not lead to disillusionment. They cite Hospers et al. (1990), who demonstrate that people whose attributions of their failure are 'internal, stable and uncontrollable' are likely to feel that they lack the willpower to lose weight. The task of the trainer would be to change the attribution to 'unstable, internal and controllable' in order to reduce that expectation of failure and the associated guilt or anger that might be felt. Successful counselling would thus create higher persistence, hopefully leading to ultimate success. Attempts have been made to provide mediated help and guidance for individuals via booklets and computers, for example, that are based on targeting individuals and tailoring messages to their apparent needs, often in the context of a 'stages of change' analysis. Success in this endeavour would certainly be cost-effective, but the potential of such approaches must still be treated with a degree of scepticism.

CASE STUDY   THE HEALTH ACTION MODEL AND COVID-19

Individual-level responses to the COVID-19 pandemic required the uptake of several behaviours, some already familiar pre-pandemic, some less so. These include self-isolation, mask-wearing, handwashing, social distancing, testing and, later on, having a vaccine. These actions were designed primarily to prevent disease. Drawing on research, where appropriate, this case study applies the HAM to understanding behavioural intentions and outcomes in the COVID-19 context.

Systems contributing to behaviour intention

Self: Several factors concerned with self-concept appeared to play a part in behavioural intentions and outcomes. For example, Hammerman et al. (2021) found that higher self-efficacy was associated with greater levels of compliance with behaviours such as mask-wearing and social distancing whilst gender appeared to make a difference to risk perceptions. In a study by Rana et al. (2021), women were found to perceive themselves at higher risk than men. They were also more likely to comply better with government guidelines and to cope better generally in response to the pandemic.

Personality: Personality traits seem to have an effect. For example, Wang et al. (2021) found that during the pandemic Type A personality affected behavioural health in a number of ways including eating and sleep, whilst in Taha Can Tuman's (2022) study healthcare workers with Type D personality traits experienced more fear of contamination than those without Type D personality traits which is perhaps not surprising given that Type D personalities are characterized by social inhibition and negative emotional states.

Belief system: Beliefs played a big part in whether or not people complied with the prescribed behaviours and attitudes towards behavioural requirements and these tended to vary depending on perceptions of susceptibility, severity and risk. Trust in institutions was important for mandatory behavourial compliance (Hammerman et al., 2021).

Normative system: Interpersonal pressure played a part in people's behavioural responses. For example, the influence of family and friends on whether or not to have the vaccine was important. A study on Polish high school students showed that the majority were unwilling to vaccinate (Pasek et al., 2021), a pattern that was replicated in young people elsewhere. Social norms around certain behaviours changed very quickly during the course of the pandemic, for example, maintaining social distancing.

Motivation system: Many people were motivated to change their behaviour by not wanting to become ill or to infect others. Some felt a moral obligation to comply with government guidelines and policy. Attitudes towards certain behaviours varied with some people feeling negative towards mask-wearing for example. Other people experienced a compulsion to comply with the behaviour of the majority. Some people were motivated to comply by fear of getting ill (Rana et al., 2021).

Factors determining the likelihood that behavioural intention would become action

Knowledge: Knowledge about transmission and impact changed rapidly throughout the pandemic. Sources of knowledge were also important. In a study on knowledge about COVID-19 among student nurses in Australia and India a higher number of the students in India reported that they felt they had sufficient knowledge (Kochuvilayil et al., 2021). This was largely obtained from social media. There were large variations in preventative behaviours, however.

Skills (psychomotor, social interaction, self-regulatory): Compliance with several of the required behaviours required different skills. Doing a lateral flow test demanded specific psychomotor skills (hand–eye coordination) as well as a degree of literacy (reading and following through the instructions) and decision-making (when to test). Wearing a mask became part of social interaction as did the act of social distancing facilitated by many 2 metre markers in public spaces. Some people felt able to assert themselves in telling other people what they should (not) be doing.

Environment (physical, socioeconomic, sociocultural): The physical environment had a huge part to play: some people were not able to self-isolate due to living in crowded conditions, or couldn't wear personal, protective equipment in the workplace because it was not made available to them. Existing socioeconomic inequalities were exacerbated by the pandemic. For example, a study in China showed that overcrowding at a household had a detrimental effect on preventative behaviours whilst a higher household income had a positive effect (Ye et al., 2021).

Health action: Several preventative health actions were mandated or recommended as a result of the pandemic such as wearing a mask, regular testing and having a vaccine as well as the requirement to isolate when experiencing symptoms of infection. However, this was not unproblematic. For example, as Preusting et al. (2021) argue, having explored stigma and health-protective behaviours in the Netherlands, 'motivating adolescents to adhere to measures such as social distancing can be challenging, since adolescents are relatively more affected by them, while experiencing virtually no personal health benefit' (p. 1).

Routine: Wearing a mask, hitherto uncommon, became routine for most people, supported by mandatory requirements such as those imposed by the government of South Africa (Balkaran and Lukman, 2021) where the resultant public policy 'circumvented constitutional rights to individualism in the altruistic interests of the country' (p. 576). Likewise, routine testing was commonplace for many people.

Confirmation/Relapse: Confirmation of intention in this case study relates to the behaviour being carried out, whether that was wearing a mask or having a vaccine. It is not possible to relapse from having a vaccine; however, it is possible to be less vigilant about handwashing and mask-wearing. The latter more so when it ceases to be a mandatory requirement.

Nudge theory and choice architecture

This chapter on determinants of health actions would not be complete without a brief foray into the more recent ideas around choice architecture and nudge theory. Thaler and Sunstein published their book on the concept of 'nudging' in 2008 (Thaler and Sunstein, 2008). Their main argument is that people's behaviour can be changed by making small changes to their environment that encourage them to do things differently or make different ('healthier') choices, the focus being on changing the *environment of action* rather than changing the way in which people think. This is based on the premise that behaviour occurs as a result of two different processes – first, 'automatic' (behaviour resulting from uncontrolled, intuitive, emotional and unconscious processes) and second, 'reflective' (behaviour that results from conscious thinking and decision-making processes). The central thesis is that the majority of behaviour occurs as a result of automatic processes; therefore, the environment may be moulded to change behaviour. This links to one of the five action areas from the Ottawa Charter – creating supportive environments.

Choice architecture is directly related to the 'nudge' idea. It is concerned with designing environments and contexts in order to alter people's decision-making and behaviours (Cross and O'Neil, 2021). 'Choice architects' are, therefore, those who have influence over the design of space and available choices – they have 'responsibility for organizing the context in which people make decisions' (Thaler and Sunstein, 2008: 3). 'Nudges help redesign the choice environment by using deliberate and predictable methods of changing people's behaviour, modifying cues and activating unconscious processes of thought in decision-making that allow decision makers to make better choices' (Leal et al., 2022: npn). Although the question remains – *who* is deciding what the 'better' choices are?! Consequently, the links to marketing and advertising approaches to influencing behaviour are evident. There are, of course, some complex issues here to do with definitional, conceptual philosophical and ethical concerns, not least around the notion of empowerment. For example, influencing people on a subconscious level could be viewed as manipulating rather than facilitating choice, which is contrary to an empowerment approach. Changing the environment in which behaviour occurs may actually remove conscious choice rather than enabling healthier choices to be made. There are ethical implications to consider in adopting such approaches in an effort to promote health. Some of the dilemmas raised do not sit easily with a philosophy of empowerment. For a fuller discussion of nudge and choice architecture, see Marteau et al. (2011) and Cross, Davis and O'Neil (2017).

IMPLICATIONS FOR PROGRAMME PLANNING

Our discussion of communication of innovations theory examined in some detail major factors governing the adoption of new practices at the level of social systems. We then paid particular attention to the determinants of health actions at the individual level – especially from an empowerment perspective. It will doubtless be self-evident that any systematic and thoughtful attempt at devising effective interventions and programmes must categorically take account of these various influences on individuals and social systems. Indeed, understanding the determinants of health actions, and the complex interplay between determinants, is essential if we are to develop effective and efficient interventions to influence the factors that govern our health- and illness-related choices.

This principle does not apply only to individual behaviour change. Indeed, in accordance with our commitment to empowerment, we need to understand which characteristics of individuals and social systems can be influenced in order to enable them to gain control over their environmental and social circumstances.

Empowerment and the principle of reciprocal determinism are central to this endeavour. We are all influenced by our environments at macro and meso levels, and many of us are in a position to reciprocate and exercise power over our physical, social and economic circumstances. Regrettably, too many people have little influence in these areas and react passively to those circumstances. Understanding the determinants of powerlessness is, therefore, of special importance and using that understanding to develop empowering health promotion programmes must constitute our major *raison d'être*.

In the chapters that follow, we will be discussing models that might be used in planning efficient health promotion programmes. In Chapter 5, we seek to demonstrate that it is not only necessary to understand the determinants of health action but it is also important to use such 'evidence', together with other strategic information, for our programme planning.

KEY POINTS

- The adoption of new practices in social systems follows a consistent pattern.
- The rate of adoption is influenced by the characteristics of the innovation, channels of communication, the nature of the social system and time.
- Individual health intentions are the product of the interplay of beliefs (including beliefs about self), motivations (including self-esteem), normative influences and personality factors.
- Beliefs about control, both generalized (locus of control) and specific (self-efficacy beliefs), are central to both empowerment and health decisions.
- The translation of intention into practice is influenced by personal factors such as skills and knowledge, together with facilitating environmental factors.
- Maintenance of new behaviours is influenced by experience, and the development of self-regulatory skills can help to avoid relapse when this experience is perceived as negative.
- Individual empowerment is the product of self-esteem, beliefs about control, a sense of coherence, commitment and concern about others, and possession of a repertoire of appropriate life skills.
- There is reciprocal interplay between individuals and their environment, but environmental factors will significantly affect the amount of influence individuals have and their actual level of empowerment.

CHAPTER 3: INTERNATIONAL CASE STUDIES

The following case studies on the online resources website are relevant to the content of this chapter: 2, 3, 4, 5, 6 and 9.

CRITICAL REFLECTION AND APPLICATION TO PRACTICE

This chapter has critically considered the determinants of health actions at the community level and the major influences on individual health. Reflect on the people that you work with. What are the main factors influencing their health? How might they be tackled? At what level is action required? (For example, at individual, community or policy level? Or perhaps a combination?) What methods might be used to translate intention into positive behaviour? The chapter also considers the factors that contribute to control and empowerment. What are the implications of the concept of control for health promotion? What role does empowerment have to play in changing behaviour? How might health promotion interventions be designed to promote empowerment at an individual level? At the community level?

ONLINE RESOURCES

Please visit https://study.sagepub.com/greentones5e for all the online resources for the book, including recommended further reading on each chapter subject, useful weblinks (both introduced by the authors), as well as the abovementioned case study material.

4 HEALTH PROMOTION PLANNING – A SYSTEMATIC APPROACH

The world is divided into people who do things and people who get the credit. Try, if you can, to belong to the first class. There's far less competition.

Dwight Morrow (1873–1931), *Letter to his son*

OVERVIEW

The basic premise of this chapter is that well-planned interventions are more likely to be effective. The chapter will:

- establish the central importance of systematic planning
- introduce a number of planning models
- consider the factors associated with the quality of health promotion programmes
- recognize the need to develop partnerships and identify the characteristics of successful partnerships for health
- introduce social marketing as a planning model for health promotion.

INTRODUCTION

Over and above increasing effectiveness, a number of developments have emphasized the importance of a systematic approach to health promotion planning. These include the need for greater economic accountability, a target-driven climate and the general move towards evidence-based practice. By way of illustration, this chapter draws specifically at times on the UK context alongside other international examples. Within the UK, the adoption of market principles for commissioning services introduced by the health service reforms of the early 1990s led to a contract culture that required greater attention to the formal planning and costing of health promotion and quality assurance. As the fourth edition is updated, little has changed in this regard. It is also worth noting at the outset that relatively little has changed with regard to the core material within this chapter. For the larger part, it has yet to be replaced by better models and theories.

Speller et al. (1998) note the central importance of strategic planning to the quality of health promotion programmes, along with programme management and monitoring. Wills (2023) points out that systematic planning has had even greater emphasis due to an increasingly evidence-, economic- and target-driven focus. As argued by Ader et al. (2001: 187), 'methods for systematically following up and auditing health promotion have been in demand for a considerable period of time'. This is still the case over 20 years later. There is also an ethical imperative to make explicit the rationale for interventions and the assumptions, values and principles on which they are based.

It will be clear from the earlier chapters that health promotion can involve a wide range of different interventions to achieve health gain, used either on their own or in combination. Green and Kreuter (2005) summarize the purpose of health promotion as intervening to reduce, or prevent an increase in, the proportion of the population engaged in negative health behaviour or exposed to negative health conditions and, conversely, to increase the proportion that exhibits positive health behaviour or is exposed to positive health conditions. Sustainability is achieved by maximizing the conditions that enable individuals or groups to assume control over their health. Such support can range from putting policies in place to changing organizational practices and creating a supportive social and/or physical climate.

Bartholomew et al. (2001) note that health promotion programmes may be directed at a number of different levels – individual, interpersonal, organizations, community, society and supranation. Given the breadth of health promotion and the numerous options concerning possible interventions, the selection of an appropriate course of action can be perplexing and is often influenced either by ideological considerations or custom and practice. It is suggested that four core principles underpin the planning of health promotion interventions – firstly, the evidence base, secondly, strong evaluation, thirdly, ownership and, finally, relevance to the community or population of focus (Baldwin, 2020). A number of models exist that provide a guide through the complexity.

This chapter identifies the stages in the process of rational planning and provides examples of planning models. It also considers the issue of quality and health promotion. There is increasing recognition that tackling the complex factors that influence health status is not just the responsibility of the health sector, but requires the coordinated response of a number of different sectors. The participation of communities is also integral to effective health promotion. This chapter concludes by considering intersectoral collaboration and partnership working.

HORIZONTAL AND VERTICAL PROGRAMMES

Before providing an overview of selected planning models, we should note that practitioners are not always in a position to begin with a blank canvas. They may be appointed to a designated programme or required by managerial directives to address particular issues. Such programmes are often defined in terms of disease and are referred to as 'vertical programmes'.

Our earlier discussion of the determinants of health in Chapter 2 and the factors associated with changing behaviour in Chapter 3 would indicate that there are common issues across vertical programmes. Lifestyle factors, such as smoking, would be common to both cancers and cardiovascular disease. Similarly, at a more fundamental level, personal attributes, such as locus of control, self-esteem and life skills, will exert an influence on lifestyle. Furthermore, environmental factors will have an impact on lifestyle, as well as direct effects on health status. There is strong evidence linking poverty with a whole range of vertically defined problems. It is clear that not only are programmes more likely to be effective if they tackle these cross-cutting or *horizontal* issues, but also that reorientation towards a horizontal approach should lead to greater efficiency. Figure 4.1 illustrates how horizontal programmes can be applied to vertically defined problems. It also draws attention to the reciprocal relationship between environment and life skills. The exercise of democratic rights requires appropriate life skills and can be instrumental in achieving healthy (or healthier) public

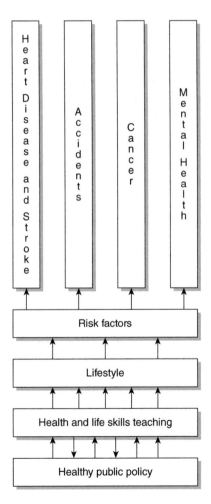

Figure 4.1   Horizontal and vertical programmes

policy. Conversely, public policy will limit individuals' freedom of choice and behaviour and may also determine what opportunities exist to develop life skills.

PLANNING MODELS

The overall purpose of systematic planning is to identify goals and the most effective means of achieving them. This involves making strategic decisions about the most appropriate courses of action together with operational decisions about the deployment of resources and ensuring that all the necessary elements are in place. Dignan and Carr (1992: 4) note that:

> Effective planning requires anticipation of what will be needed along the way towards achieving the goal. This statement implies that the goal is defined, as are the necessary steps involved in reaching the goal. Perhaps most importantly, it requires an understanding of the steps and how they interrelate.

We noted in Chapter 1 the wide range of activities that can be included under the health promotion umbrella. It follows that comprehensive health promotion programmes will need to include an appropriate combination of methods and involve a number of different sectors. Programmes are more likely to be successful if planning is approached in an inclusive way, involving all the major stakeholders. Not only does this create a bigger pool of experience to draw on, but it also establishes collective ownership of the programme. Furthermore, exclusivity runs counter to health promotion's commitment to participation. It is important at the outset, therefore, to identify the stakeholder community.

'Stakeholders' are all those individuals, groups or organizations with an interest in the initiative. They include those affected by the impact of an initiative and those who are in a position to influence its success. Stakeholder involvement is critical to the success of health promotion interventions (Morton et al., 2017). The different groups of stakeholders are outlined in Box 4.1.

BOX 4.1 STAKEHOLDERS

- Primary stakeholders are the potential beneficiaries – those who are directly affected, either positively or negatively, by the initiative.
- Secondary stakeholders are those involved in implementing the initiative.
- Key stakeholders are those whose support is essential to the continuation of the initiative – for example, fundholders.

The Ontario Agency for Health Protection and Promotion (2015) identified four levels of stakeholder:

- **Core** – on the planning team
- **Involved** – frequently consulted or part of the planning process
- **Supportive** – provide some form of assistance
- **Peripheral** – need to be informed.

The relative power and influence of the different stakeholders should be assessed together with their perceptions of, and willingness to support, the initiative. Such a stakeholder analysis can be instrumental in identifying potential alliances and partners and mobilizing the support required to get initiatives up and running. There are a number of tools available that are designed to enable a systematic stakeholder analysis. In health promotion, a key concern is who holds the power and what their level of interest in the programme might be. Those with high levels of power and high interest are therefore important. However, often the community itself, as the intended beneficiary or primary stakeholder, has relatively little power although high levels of interest. It is critical for success to involve all stakeholders and the process of developing a health promotion programme is also important. The Ontario Agency for Health Protection and Promotion (2015) highlight the following:

- working and planning *with* people, rather than for them
- consulting stakeholders at key points in the planning process
- involving the intended audience in programme design
- using a participatory approach.

More is written about these issues in Chapter 9.

The terminology associated with planning tends to be used somewhat loosely and interchangeably in health promotion literature. In the interests of clarity, we have defined the way in which we have used the terms here (see Box 4.2).

BOX 4.2 PLANNING TERMINOLOGY

- **Programme**: delineates the area that is being addressed. This is an umbrella term that includes all the activities involved in developing and running, for example, a coronary heart disease programme or a community development programme.
- **Strategy**: the preferred course of action for achieving immediate or longer-term goals. It is selected tactically on the basis of evidence, theory or experience. The term can be used at all levels – for example, an 'overall programme strategy' or an 'implementation strategy'.
- **Plan**: an outline of all the various components and how they relate to each other.
- **Aim**: a broad statement of what is intended to be achieved. Aims can be developed at different levels – for example, overall programme aims, educational aims, policy aims.
- **Objective**: precise and detailed statements of the intended outcomes that will contribute to the overall aim.
- **Intervention**: the activities or collection of activities that will contribute directly to the desired change.
- **Method**: specific approaches or techniques used.

Hubley (2004: 202) poses four questions to guide the planning process:

- Where are we now?
- Where do we want to go?
- How will we get there?
- How will we know when we get there?

While Scriven (2017) puts forward three key questions:

- What am I trying to achieve?
- What am I going to do?
- How will I know whether I have been successful?

These questions are integral to the planning model proposed by Dignan and Carr (1992), shown in Figure 4.2.

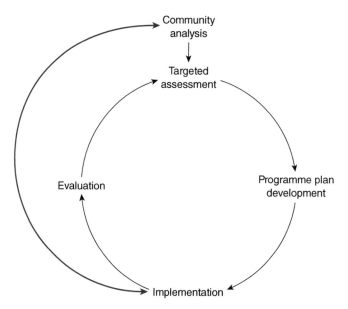

Figure 4.2 Dignan and Carr's planning model (Dignan and Carr, 1992)

In Dignan and Carr's model (as is the case with many other types of planning model), the process begins with a needs assessment. This involves a community analysis to identify the programme's focus and the characteristics of the community, followed by a more specific, targeted assessment to identify the determinants of any problems and the key issues that will need to be addressed to achieve change. The goals and objectives for the programme should then be identified, along with resource implications and any potential obstacles. The actual methods to be used in the intervention can then be selected. The logistics of implementation should be considered, and monitoring and evaluation systems put in place.

The apparent simplicity of this model belies the complexity of the decisions required at each stage. There is a fuller discussion of these issues at relevant points in this book – indeed, its structure reflects the various stages of the planning process. We have already discussed the determinants of health and health-related decisions in Chapters 2 and 3. Chapter 5 will consider needs assessment in more detail. Chapters 6, 7, 8, 9 and 10 will address different methods, Chapter 11 evaluation and Chapter 12, evidence. Our purpose in this chapter, however, is to focus on the planning process itself and the adoption of a systematic approach.

There are several different planning models. While conforming to the same broad outline as Figure 4.2, they vary in the level of detail and their relevance for particular purposes. We outline some examples below.

Precede–proceed

One of the best known planning models is the precede–proceed model (Green and Kreuter, 1991, 2005). As argued by Porter (2016), this planning model is one of the most comprehensive and widely used. A particular strength of this model is the attention given to identifying the numerous factors that affect health status as a basis for focusing on the subset of factors that need to be addressed by the proposed intervention. Indeed, the model is premised on the view that there are multiple determinants of health and that efforts to improve it require multidimensional and multisectoral action.

The starting point of the model is an assessment of the quality of life and any social problems experienced by the population. It then identifies any specific health problems that contribute to quality of life and establishes which of these should be prioritized. These are then analysed to establish both environmental and behavioural risk factors. The attention given to the environment acknowledges its importance in supporting health-related behaviour as well as its direct influence on health. Further analysis identifies the plethora of factors that influence health behaviour. These are grouped as follows:

- **predisposing factors** – personal factors that influence motivation to change, such as knowledge, beliefs, attitudes, values
- **enabling factors** – factors that support change in behaviour or environment, such as resources and skills, and also any barriers
- **reinforcing factors** – the feedback received from adopting the behaviour.

In essence, these various phases lead to a diagnosis of all contributory factors. Two key considerations influence the selection of factors to focus on in developing an intervention. The extent to which they contribute to the problem is clearly of fundamental importance. However, the resources available and the organization's capacity to deliver health promotion programmes will also be influential. In fact, an organizational assessment is one of the key components of this particular planning model (Issel, 2014).

An appropriate combination of methods can then be selected and the intervention implemented. Evaluation will include process, impact and outcome measures. Although presented as a linear sequence, the evaluation findings should feed back into the earlier stages, creating a more cyclical process.

The various phases of the model draw on a range of different disciplines. Phases 1, 2 and 3, for example, will draw on epidemiological methods and information; phases 3 and 4 on social and behavioural theory; designing interventions will require educational, political and administrative theory; and implementation will draw on political and administrative science and community organization theory. The precede–proceed planning model has been applied to a range of issues in a number of different contexts; more recent examples include oral health in Japan (Nomura et al., 2019), adherence to HIV treatment in Indonesia (Agustin and Murti, 2018) and health needs assessment in Australia (Handyside et al., 2021). A systematic review designed to summarize the research about the use of the precede-proceed model in the planning of health screenings concluded that it is very good for understanding the relationship between different variables such as knowledge and screening and that it provides an excellent framework for health intervention programmes (Sinopoli et al., 2018).

ABSTRACT 4.1

Engaging stakeholders and target groups in prioritising a public health intervention: the Creating Active School Environments (CASE) online Delphi study. Morton, K.L., Atkin, A.J., Corder, K., Suhrcke, M., Turner, D. and van Sluijs, E.M.F. (2017)

Objectives: Stakeholder engagement and public involvement are considered as integral to developing effective public health interventions and are encouraged across all phases of the research cycle. However, limited guidelines and appropriate tools exist to facilitate stakeholder engagement – especially during the intervention prioritization phase. The authors present the findings of an online 'Delphi' study that engaged stakeholders (including young people) in the process of prioritizing secondary school environment-focused interventions that aim to increase physical activity.

Setting: Web-based data collection using an online Delphi tool enabling participation of geographically diverse stakeholders.

Participants: 37 stakeholders participated, including young people (age 13–16 years), parents, teachers, public health practitioners, academics and commissioners; 33 participants completed both rounds.

Primary and secondary outcome measures: Participants were asked to prioritize a (short-listed) selection of school environment-focused interventions (e.g. standing desk, outdoor design changes) based on the criteria of 'teach', 'equality', 'acceptability', 'feasibility', 'effectiveness' and 'cost'. Participants were also asked to rank the criteria and the effectiveness outcomes (e.g. physical activity, academic achievement, school environment) from most to least important. Following feedback along with new information provided, participants completed round 2 four weeks later.

Results: The intervention prioritization process was feasible to conduct and comments from participants indicated satisfaction with the process. Consensus regarding intervention strategies was achieved among the varied groups of stakeholders, with 'active lessons' being the favoured approach. Participants ranked 'mental health and well-being' as the most important outcome followed by 'enjoyment of school'. The most important criterion was 'effectiveness', followed by 'feasibility'.

Conclusions: This novel approach to engaging a wide variety of stakeholders in the research process was feasible to conduct and acceptable to participants. It also provided insightful information relating to how stakeholders prioritize interventions. The approach could be extended beyond the specific project to be a useful tool for researchers and practitioners.

Table 4.1   A logical framework 4×4 matrix

	Narrative summary	Verifiable indicators	Means of verification	Assumption
Goal				
Purpose				
Outputs				
Activities				

Logical frameworks

Logical frameworks (or LogFrames) have their origin in military planning, but were adapted for use by the United States Agency for International Development (USAID) in 1969 and have subsequently been used by other aid programmes in response to demands for more effective planning (Nancholas, 1998). LogFrames provide a clear structure for planning health promotion interventions including the activities and methods of a programme, as well as the intended impacts and outcomes of it (Baldwin, 2020). Table 4.1 provides an overview of the logical framework matrix.

The vertical hierarchy corresponds to the stages in developing the LogFrame. It starts with the goal, which is usually expressed in very broad terms, such as reducing teenage pregnancy. The next level is the purpose, which is a statement of the desired achievement of the project. The purpose should make a direct contribution to the goal. Each LogFrame should contain only one goal and one purpose, which are often expressed in behavioural terms. Using the example of teenage pregnancy, the purpose of a programme might be to increase the proportion of sexually active teenagers who make use of the contraceptive services within a locality.

The outputs are then identified. These are the immediate results, or deliverables, of the programme and could include material factors, organizational change or behavioural change. A number of outputs may be necessary to achieve the purpose – for example, running young people's contraceptive clinics that are user-friendly and scheduled for a time that most suits their needs, along with raised awareness among young people of these services.

Finally, the activities that are required to bring about the outputs should be specified. These might include working with clinic managers to persuade them of the need to schedule sessions for young people, running focus groups with young people to establish how clinics could be made user-friendly and what times would be most appropriate for this age group, and providing training for clinic staff to make them aware of the views of young people. Similarly, activities to raise awareness might include developing and pre-testing posters, displaying posters in all schools in the locality and so on.

Bell (2001) summarizes the four vertical levels as:

- Why do the thing? (Goal)
- What is the thing for? (Purpose)
- What are the outcomes of the thing? (Outputs)
- How to do the thing? (Activities)

The vertical logic should then be verified by working backwards through these various stages and checking out, in principle, *if* one stage is in place, *then* the next will follow, as in Figure 4.3.

Such verification will reveal lapses in logic and identify both omissions and any redundancy. It will also make explicit any assumptions at each level. In our simple illustration, there are several major assumptions – for example, that the contraceptive service provider has both the capacity and resources to run designated young people's clinics, that young people are well motivated regarding using contraceptives, that schools will be willing to cooperate and display posters, that young people will read the posters and so on. Some consideration will need to be given to whether or not the assumptions are well founded or if they expose potentially fatal flaws in the vertical logic and overall design. 'LogFrames, when done well, can provide a clear and concise summary of the whole health promotion intervention' (Woodall and Cross, 2021: 258).

Returning to our example, if sufficient resources are not available, then, however supportive clinic managers and staff are of the proposed changes, they will be unable to put them into practice. Obtaining funding could be included as an additional output, along with an appropriate cluster of activities. Work may also need to be done to gain the support of those in the position of gatekeeper with regard to displaying posters in schools. If, however, schools have been actively involved with the development of the project, it may be reasonable to assume that their cooperation will be forthcoming. Nancholas (1998) notes that the process is 'reiterative' and each decision is reviewed and revised as necessary. The value of making explicit all assumptions is that it provides a check that all necessary conditions are in place to ensure the success of the project and that contingency plans exist for any problems that might be anticipated.

At this point, it is worth emphasizing that participatory processes are central to LogFrame planning and decisions should be arrived at by achieving consensus among the stakeholders. Relevant literature and research evidence should also be consulted (Nancholas, 1998). Furthermore, plans should be based on sound preliminary analysis, which would include:

- **stakeholder analysis** to identify the key players, their influence (positive or negative) and level of participation
- **problem analysis** to identify the nature of the problem and its determinants using a 'problem tree' that progressively homes in on the root causes needing to be addressed
- **risk analysis** to identify major obstacles and risks.

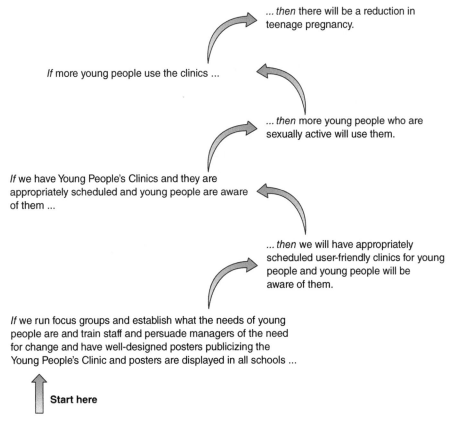

... then there will be a reduction in teenage pregnancy.

If more young people use the clinics ...

... then more young people who are sexually active will use them.

If we have Young People's Clinics and they are appropriately scheduled and young people are aware of them ...

... then we will have appropriately scheduled user-friendly clinics for young people and young people will be aware of them.

If we run focus groups and establish what the needs of young people are and train staff and persuade managers of the need for change and have well-designed posters publicizing the Young People's Clinic and posters are displayed in all schools ...

Start here

Figure 4.3   LogFrames – checking the vertical logical

Objectively verifiable indicators (OVIs) need to be specified for each level of the vertical hierarchy and would answer the question: 'How will you know that it has been achieved?' These are effectively the objectives of the programme and should be precise, including necessary detail, such as who, how much and when (for example, 80% of school pupils aged 15–16 will be able to recall the name, location and opening times of at least one young people's contraceptive clinic in the locality within a month of coming into service). The evidence required to provide objective verification – the means of verification (MOV) – should then be considered. Again, returning to our example, this could be a written questionnaire survey of 15- to 16-year-olds in all schools in the locality. Alternatively, in relation to the goal of reducing teenage pregnancy, an OVI might be a 10% reduction in births to teenage mothers within two years of the introduction of the young people's contraceptive service and the MOV would be routinely collecting data on births. The means of monitoring activities and evaluating outcomes are, therefore, embedded within the planning process.

The final stages involve operational, management and financial issues. The inputs required for each of the activities should be identified, overall costs estimated and a budget prepared. A time plan, covering implementation of all activities and milestones, will also need to be produced.

Clearly, the preparation of a LogFrame can be demanding in relation to the level of detailed decision-making required and the methodology is not without its critics. VSO Netherlands (undated) notes two major criticisms of LogFrames. First, predetermining objectives and indicators leaves no room for recording the often important, yet unanticipated, events that often arise. Second, the emphasis on consensus does not register differing views and diversity of opinion can be the source of innovation.

Broughton (2001) identifies the main weaknesses as being time-consuming, requiring sound understanding of the conventions used to complete LogFrames and, when completed, the danger of becoming 'frozen in time', hence limiting their applicability in rapidly evolving emergency situations. However, he also acknowledges their strength in bringing discipline to clarifying means, ends and assumptions and providing a framework for determining the way in which performance should be measured and for monitoring, evaluation and reporting. Furthermore, they contribute to collaborative working and consensus building.

Nancholas (1998) identifies similar advantages, along with some additional features. LogFrames have the capacity to combine the efficiency of rational planning models with flexibility. They also provide clear and concise summaries of whole programmes, which help to create overall visions of the programmes and communicate these to others.

Daniel and Dearden (2001: 2) note that LogFrames have been viewed as inflexible, restrictive and inappropriate for creative community projects and complex interventions. However, they argue that the approach embraces the key elements of successful projects, notably:

- short- and long-term objectives have to be clarified and coherent
- risks have to be identified and strategies developed to meet them
- indicators for successful intervention need to be agreed at the outset
- methods of collecting and recording evidence of change also have to be set in place.

Daniel and Dearden report on the experience in the UK of using LogFrames for planning Health Action Zone (HAZ) Innovation Fund projects – innovative projects set up to demonstrate new ways of working towards the HAZ inequality and modernization agenda. The advantages of using a LogFrame for planning were identified as being:

- a systematic, logical and thorough approach
- the discipline and structure that it imposes
- the identification of risks and assumptions
- the provision of a framework for monitoring and evaluation
- the encouragement of real partnerships
- flexibility and adaptability.

Conversely, disadvantages of the methodology included:

- conflict with other planning systems in place
- an emphasis on quantitative rather than qualitative indicators

- an assumption that partnerships exist
- its time-consuming nature
- its inflexible and controlling nature
- the use of a lot of jargon
- the requirement of appropriately timed training.

They conclude that 'the logical framework works' in this context and quote one of the trainers:

> LogFrames really do take the mystery out of project planning for local people, they are simple and clear. The problem for professionals is that [working with LogFrames] they have to be transparent – something we have all learnt not to be in order to survive in bureaucracies! Managing that change is the biggest issue, not necessarily managing the LogFrame process … (Daniel and Dearden, 2001: 6)

While we have shown how LogFrames can guide the whole planning process, others have used them more flexibly. See Freedman et al. (2014), who propose a framework for using logic models in training and education for the public health workforce in the USA. The Health Communication Unit (2001) suggests that they can be used at different stages – for initial 'visioning' and priority setting, for checking out draft goals and objectives to identify gaps and inconsistencies and during implementation in relation to presenting and evaluating the programme. The contribution of logic models to the planning process is summarized as:

- demonstrating how a programme's strategies contribute to the achievement of intended goals and objectives;
- identifying gaps and inconsistencies in a programme, such as objectives that are not being met, or activities that are not contributing to specific objectives;
- providing an effective communication tool that helps new stakeholders or potential sponsors to understand a programme;
- involving stakeholders in programme planning (through the collective development of a logic model); and
- building a common understanding of what a programme is all about and how the parts fit together. (Health Communication Unit, 2001: 1)

A final note reiterates the point that it is necessary to maintain a flexible approach in the use of LogFrames. Writing about the almost exclusive use of LogFrames in development evaluation in Japan, Fujita (2010: 4) notes the following:

> evaluations based on a LogFrame often face difficulties. One such difficulty arises from the futile attempt to develop an evaluation framework based on a LogFrame, which, in many cases, was prepared as part of the early-stage planning of the project and which then does not necessarily reflect a project's real situation at the time of evaluation. Although a LogFrame can be utilised initially as a tentative project plan, LogFrames are rarely revised even when the situation has changed. By the end of the project, the original LogFrame may not be an accurate embodiment of what the project is about.

In a comprehensive appraisal Hummelbrunner (2010) draws attention to the critique that the logical framework approach has encountered on both practical and theoretical grounds – concerns that are echoed by Bakewell and Garbutt (2005). Difficulties may occur, for example, around agreeing a clear set of objectives. Hummelbrunner (2010) argues that it is just as important to know when *not* to use LogFrames as well as being prepared to be flexible or make adaptations. In addition, Hummelbrunner points out that the LogFrame approach is often imposed externally as a rigid requirement attached to funding or donor support, asserting that the approach 'often fails to reflect the messy realities … thus producing confusion rather than clarity' (2010: 12). Despite its limitations, the logical framework approach has its merits and is still widely used; however, there are some who advocate using alternative approaches. Hummelbrunner (2010) details some alternatives that are being used in German development aid such as a variant called ZOPP (objectives-oriented project planning). For further details see Fujita (2010). Good examples of LogFrames can easily be found on the Internet in relation to a number of different issues.

A five-stage community organization model

Systematic planning is often aligned with top-down approaches and held to be inconsistent with community involvement. We would challenge this view and contend that strategies for involving communities are more likely to be effective if they are well planned. The key issue is that the planning process, in this instance, should explicitly address participation and draw on established principles of community development, together with relevant theory. Bracht et al. (1999), for example, describe a five-stage process for community organization, shown in Figure 4.4. Although the various stages are represented as discrete in the model, the authors note that there is some overlap between them.

Stage 1 is concerned with establishing the status quo and setting priorities. It involves:

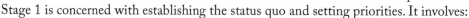

- defining the community
- constructing a community profile, which includes health and demographic data and information on the community
- assessing the community's capacity by identifying ongoing activities and those organizations, groups or individuals who could offer support – this will also include feasibility and identification of the financial resources required
- assessing any barriers within the community
- assessing readiness for change.

Stage 2 involves designing activities and setting up an organizational structure to mobilize and coordinate community support and involvement. The key components of this stage are:

- setting up a core planning group and identifying a local coordinator
- choosing an organizational structure
- identifying and recruiting members
- defining the goals
- clarifying roles and responsibilities of members
- providing training and recognition.

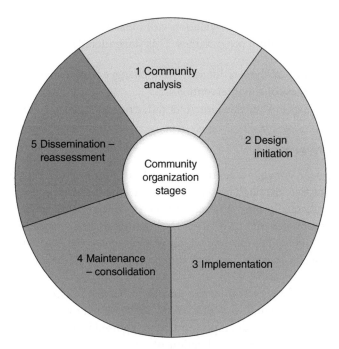

Figure 4.4   Bracht et al.'s community organization model (Bracht et al., 1999)

Stage 3 focuses on implementing activities to achieve goals and includes:

- selecting and prioritizing intervention activities – particularly, assessing whether or not activities are appropriate and sufficiently comprehensive to achieve the goals
- developing a time plan to sequence activities to achieve maximum gains
- generating broader community participation
- planning media coverage
- obtaining financial and other support
- setting up intervention evaluation monitoring and intervention systems.

Stage 4 takes place when the programme is well under way and appraises the current position and future directions. It is concerned with:

- sustainability by virtue of integrating activities into community structures
- establishing a positive organizational climate to encourage the retention of staff and volunteers
- having an ongoing recruitment plan for staff and volunteers
- acknowledging the contribution of volunteers.

Stage 5 involves dissemination and reassessment. Early dissemination of the evaluation findings in an appropriate manner will contribute to maintaining the visibility of the programme and provide a boost for those involved. Formative elements of evaluation will assist in shaping the development of the programme and a final summative evaluation will identify what has been achieved and lessons learned, which should inform future programmes. This stage includes:

- updating the community analysis to identify what changes have been achieved
- assessing the effectiveness of the interventions
- summarizing the findings in a suitable format for different constituencies and developing future plans.

Community empowerment

Empowerment, as we have noted, is a central tenet of health promotion. Yet, Laverack and Labonte (2000) assert that, in practice, although lip service is paid to the discourse of empowerment, top-down programmes maintain unequal power structures in society. Such programmes address issues defined by professionals and empowerment, in this context, becomes a means of achieving predefined goals. This contrasts with bottom-up approaches, which would involve the community in identifying and responding to its own needs. In such instances, empowerment would be a terminal goal – that is, an end in itself rather than a means.

Laverack and Labonte (2000) attribute the mismatch between discourse and practice to lack of clarity in how to operationalize empowerment within conventional top-down planning. They suggest that the two can be reconciled without empowerment being used instrumentally to achieve behaviour change goals, but that this requires consideration of empowerment at each stage of the planning process. They propose a model that pursues empowerment goals by means of a parallel track running alongside the conventional programme track, as illustrated in Figure 4.5, although it can also be used for bottom-up community development programmes.

At the design phase, sufficient time should be allowed for the often lengthy process of involving communities in an empowering way. Particular attention should be paid to the needs of marginalized populations who are least able to express their needs. Furthermore, programmes should begin with realistic aims and focus on relatively small-scale, achievable projects to generate early successes and build confidence. Programme planners need to question the ways in which planning processes and programme implementation will contribute to the nine domains of community capacity identified by Labonte and Laverack and listed in Box 4.3.

BOX 4.3 COMMUNITY CAPACITY DOMAINS

1. Community participation
2. Local leadership
3. Empowering organizational structures
4. Problem assessment capacities
5. Ability to ask 'Why?'
6. Resource mobilization
7. Links to others
8. Equitable relationships, outside agents
9. Community control over the programme.

Source: Labonte and Laverack (2001a, 2001b)

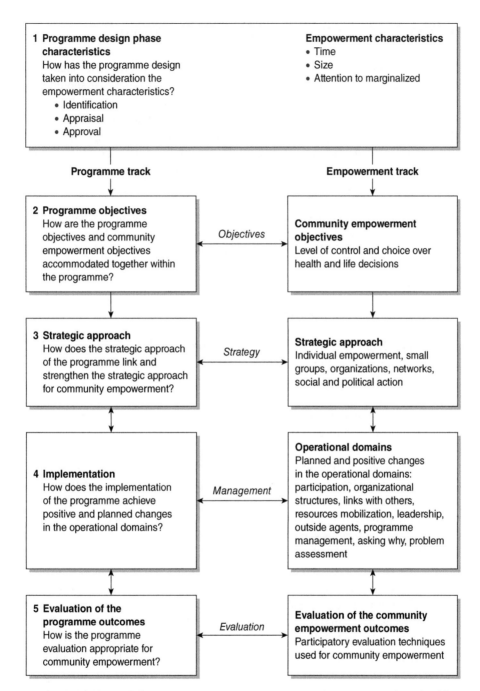

Figure 4.5 A planning framework for incorporating community empowerment into top-down health promotion programmes (Laverack and Labonte, 2000)

HEALTH PROMOTION PLANNING – REFLECTIONS

We have presented a number of planning models that differ from each other in relation to the levels of analysis that they include, the extent to which they specify the factors that should be considered at each level and the relative involvement of different stakeholders. Some models are more generic in orientation than others and, hence, applicable to almost any situation or problem, while others have been designed to suit more specific purposes. An interesting interchange between two groups of academics on the nature of planning models was sparked by an article by McLeroy et al. (1993), which suggested that planning models (such as PATCH, precede–proceed, coalitions/partnerships, lay health adviser approaches, social change models, organizational change models):

> are largely a-theoretical and a-contextual [and further] they are largely independent of the specific health problem being addressed, they ignore what we know about the social production of disease, they are not connected to the field's collective wisdom about what works, with whom, under what conditions and they may lead to inappropriate interventions for the communities in which they are to be used. (1993: 307)

They called for an ecological planning approach involving three stages:

1. **Theory of the problem** that involves analysis of problems and the intrapersonal, interpersonal, organizational, community, cultural and public policy factors that produce and maintain them
2. **Theory of intervention** that provides a state-of-the-art view of the relative effectiveness of different interventions
3. **Understanding the context of practice** that allows interventions to be matched to the local community or organizational context.

The riposte to this article by Green et al. (1994) highlights some key issues concerning planning models. They put forward a strong argument that they are, in fact, grounded in theory and are consistent with a multilevel, multisector analysis –that is, an ecological approach to health promotion. Furthermore, we noted above that a precede–proceed analysis should incorporate a range of theoretical perspectives into the various stages.

Green at al. (1994) acknowledge that no planning model is immune from misuse, but inappropriate interventions arise from lack of rigour in the detailed application of models rather than from the model itself. Models such as precede–proceed provide a guide through the causal logic underpinning the development of health or health problems and impose a framework for considering all pertinent variables – exposing any omissions and assumptions. Rigorous application of planning models should, therefore, reduce the probability of interventions being inappropriate. Moreover, some planning models specifically incorporate consideration of contextual factors by means of, for example, a community diagnosis or analysis. Green et al. (1994) also suggest that the step-by-step procedure of planning models such as precede–proceed leads to the selection of an appropriate theory to suit both the context and the emergent requirements rather than imposing a theoretical structure at the outset. A sequential approach to planning should, therefore, ensure both relevance and rigour.

MacDonald and Green's (2001) analysis of the process of using a planning model to develop alcohol and drug prevention programmes in schools raises some interesting issues. The project was premised on the view that drug education would be more effective if it were based on local needs and context. Prevention workers were expected to work with schools using the precede–proceed model to guide the planning process. One of the dilemmas facing the workers was achieving a balance between the proactive planning demanded by the project and the tendency of schools to respond to problems in a more reactive way. This raises questions about the suitability of rational planning models where there is a culture of reacting to problems and actions based on common sense and experience rather than analysis. A further issue was the variation in interpretation and application of the model by different workers. Training in the use of models and some assessment of the community's capacity to engage in the planning process will contribute to resolving these issues. However, the question still remains as to whether or not fidelity in implementing the planning model is realistic or possible. MacDonald and Green suggest that successful implementation requires some flexibility to allow adaptation to local circumstances. In reality, as Wills (2023) argues, 'planning health promotion is a more complex process than planning models suggest' (p. 326).

Consequently, an additional consideration is whether or not the complex interplay of factors and alliances associated with health can be addressed by essentially linear planning models. French and Milner (1993) are critical of a simplistic linear view of causality and emphasize the need to consider the many interrelated variables that impact on health behaviour and health status. They also call for realism in relation to what can be achieved and suggest that there can be a number of different starting points from which programmes of work can emerge. For example, the availability of funding for particular streams of work could be the starting point. They suggest that real planning, as illustrated in Figure 4.6, is a systematic, although non-linear, process. Wills (2023: 315) also notes that planning is often 'piecemeal or incremental. There is no grand design, but circumstances dictate many small reactive decisions.'

Notwithstanding this view, although we have presented the models in this chapter as a linear sequence, in practice it is not essential to start at the beginning – a point acknowledged by Green and Kreuter (2005). The planning process can, in principle, begin at some intermediate point, with the caveat that the preliminary stages should be worked through – retrospectively, as it were – in order to ensure logical and practical coherence. Furthermore, the possibility of including feedback loops between the various stages in the models provides opportunities for revisiting decisions in the light of emerging issues, thereby enhancing flexibility.

Writing from an evaluation perspective, Judge (2000) also highlights the problem of determining causality in complex social systems. We will provide a fuller discussion in Chapter 11, but this issue is also pertinent to a consideration of the inputs required to achieve change. Judge draws on the work of Pawson and Tilley (1997) to suggest that cause and effect are not 'discrete events', but mechanisms that interact with context to produce outcomes. It is not simply a question of whether or not something works, but more with whom and under what circumstances. The following formula provides a simple summary:

context + mechanism = outcome

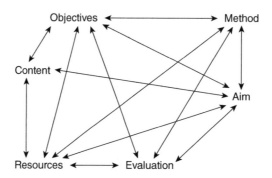

Figure 4.6   French and Milner's view of real planning (after French and Milner, 1993)

The mechanism for change is seen as 'modifying the capacities, resources, constraints and choices facing participants and practitioners' (Judge, 2000: 2). A programme will seek to manipulate these variables to achieve change, but the outcome is also contingent on the context. Therefore, planning appropriate interventions will require a thorough analysis of the context. Judge notes that a 'Theory of Change Approach' – originating from the work of Weiss et al. in the USA (Connell et al., 1995) – can help to clarify exactly how proposed actions are expected to achieve intended outcomes. Using this approach, those involved in planning and implementing initiatives are encouraged to make explicit the ways in which they envisage the links between the various programme components and outcomes – that is, to articulate their Theory of Change or the assumptive logic underpinning the change that they are trying to achieve. In this context, theory is defined as 'the professional logic that underlies a programme' (Bauld and Judge, 2000).

A systems checklist for health promotion planning

There are several concerns about health promotion programme planning being driven by rational processes and governed by formal planning frameworks rather than being allowed to evolve in a more organic way. This is particularly evident in relation to community participation. However, to set rationality and systematic processes against participation, flexibility and context specificity is to impose a false dichotomy. Planning models provide an ordered structure that ensures all relevant variables are considered. The way in which decision-making processes are handled and the information that is brought to bear on this can correspond to a number of different ideological positions. Similarly, goals can be framed in relation to disease prevention, behaviour change, empowerment or community development. The advantages of rational planning may be summarized as:

- making explicit the anticipated causal mechanisms underpinning desired change
- identifying all the necessary conditions for change
- scheduling the various components of an intervention appropriately
- ensuring that all conditions are in place to maximize effectiveness
- providing a forum for bringing together the various stakeholders.

Figure 4.7 provides a checklist of the key issues that need to be considered when developing health promotion programmes. The starting point involves establishing needs and stating the programme's aims or goals. Needs, as we will note in Chapter 5, may be defined in a number of different ways. The ideologies and values of those involved in planning and their conceptualization of health will not

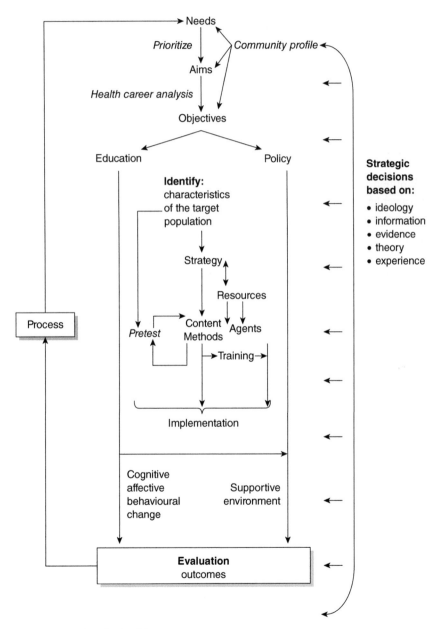

Figure 4.7   A systems checklist for health promotion

only inform the ways in which needs are defined and prioritized, but will also permeate each stage of the planning process. It is worth reiterating that the use of planning models does not in itself impose values on the planning process, but, rather, provides a vehicle for making explicit the values, rationale and assumptions underpinning any decisions. It also exposes those situations where rationality would dictate one course of action and political pressures another (classically demonstrated by the 'Heroin Screws You Up' campaign discussed later in this chapter).

Needs, then, could be professionally or lay defined and focus on positive health states or disease or their various determinants, either environmental or behavioural. Prioritization involves a number of considerations – not least the contextual factors revealed by community profiling. These include the:

- extent and severity of the problem – clearly, life-threatening problems will rate higher than those causing minor inconvenience
- urgency of the problem
- number of people affected
- power and influence of those affected
- possibility of achieving change/improvement
- level of concern, support and commitment among the major groups of stakeholders
- feasibility of taking action in the current context, based on an assessment of the capacity within the organization and/or community
- consistency with the ethics and values of those involved.

If the achievement of equity in health is, as we have argued earlier, a primary goal of health promotion, then some consideration should be given to this in prioritizing needs and the action to be

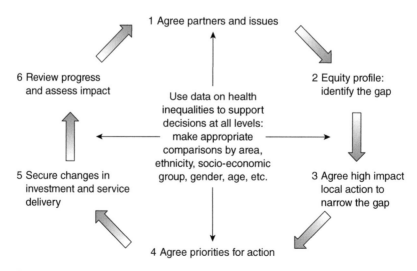

Figure 4.8 Health Equity Audit Cycle

Source: Derived from Office of the Deputy Prime Minister and Department of Health (2005: 94)

taken to address them. While the Health Equity Audit (Department of Health, 2003) was essentially introduced to enable services to be delivered more equitably, its principles are also applicable to the development of health promotion programmes. The Health Equity Audit uses 'evidence on inequalities to inform decisions on investment, service planning, commissioning and delivery and to review the impact of action on inequalities' (Office of the Deputy Prime Minister [ODPM] and Department of Health, 2005: 95). The stages of the Health Equity Audit Cycle are outlined in Figure 4.8. It allows gaps in health status to be identified. Priority can then be given to addressing those needs that would reduce the gap and targeting action appropriately.

Aims and objectives

Once priorities have been agreed, then a consensus should be achieved on the overall goal or aim of the programme. Not only does this provide a formal statement of intent as a point of reference to guide future action, but it also ensures that all those involved have a common understanding of what they are trying to achieve. Aims are general, global statements about what the programme intends to achieve (Dignan and Carr, 1992). Aims are sometimes also referred to as 'goals', defined as 'broad, encompassing statements about the impact to be achieved' (Issel, 2014: 215). However, vague, aspirational statements of intent, such as 'improving the quality of life', while perhaps serving a motivational purpose and acting as a rallying call, offer little in the way of establishing a common purpose. It therefore goes without saying that, although aims are expressed in broad terms, some precision is still required. Aims may be either long or short term and framed in a number of different ways, as shown in Table 4.2. Having clear aims and objectives is important in terms of knowing where you are going and what you are trying to achieve. They provide a common purpose and are often used as key performance indicators or outcomes, which become vital in a commissioning context.

Establishing the best way in which to achieve these aims demands a thorough analysis of the determinants of any problem or issue being addressed, along with the context. A health career analysis (referred to in Chapter 2) is a useful device for identifying the major influences on health status and locating possible intervention points. It also helps to identify appropriate target groups and agencies with which to develop collaborative working links. The characteristics of target groups will also need to be assessed.

Consideration of this information, along with relevant theory and empirical evidence of effectiveness, should enable a planning group to establish exactly what change needs to happen to achieve its goal. The broad vision encompassed within the stated aim can then be translated into more precise objectives. Whereas *aims* are, as we have noted, broad and relatively general statements of intent, *objectives* define goals in more specific terms. Thus, one aim may generate a number of subordinate objectives. As pointed out in a fact sheet for writing measurable objectives developed by the Department for Health in Australia (Women's Health West, 2010), objectives follow a general form: 'To do what, for whom, by when?'

Following our earlier discussion of health promotion as the synergistic interaction of policy and education, it should be possible to distinguish *policy* objectives from *educational* objectives. The former would be the specific goals to be attained in the development and implementation of policy, while the latter would be the specific learning outcomes that would result if the health education components of programmes were to be successful (see Box 4.4 for examples).

Table 4.2   Examples of aims

Focus	Example
Individual or groups	Increase levels of empowerment among teenage girls in a locality
	Build social capital within a community
Disease	Reduce the level of coronary heart disease in a community
	Reduce the injuries from falls in the over-60s in a locality
Health status	Increase the levels of cardiovascular fitness in senior citizens in a locality
	Reduce inequalities in health
Health behaviour	Reduce the level of smoking in a community
	Increase the uptake of physical activity in a community
Environment	Improve the safety of the community
Organizations	Introduce a health-promoting school initiative

The precise formulation of objectives is fundamental to the planning process for a number of different reasons. First, they indicate what strands of activity should be put in place and give structure to the programme. Second, the range of objectives should be sufficiently comprehensive to ensure that all the necessary conditions are achieved in pursuit of the overall aim. Third, as we will note in Chapter 11, they provide a means of evaluating the outcomes of the programme.

There is, at times, a tendency to use the looser term 'target' in policy documents. Notwithstanding the language used, the principle remains the same. It is essential to specify with precision exactly what is to be achieved. For the purpose of this text, we will use the term *objective*, bearing in mind that it is sometimes used synonymously with *target*.

BOX 4.4 EXAMPLES FROM THE WORKFORCE COUNCIL, AUSTRALIA

Sample aim (or goal):

Employees will have access to healthier food options within the workplace.

Sample objective:

All vending machines within the workplace will be modified to include at least 50% healthy food options by 1 September 2013.

Other sample objectives:

At least 90% of schools in the community will institute campus-wide no-smoking policies by 2015.

To reduce alcohol consumption by youth aged 14–16 years in Queensland by 5% by 30 December 2015.

To reduce the proportion of adults in Australia who smoke to 12% by 2015.

Source: Workforce Council of Australia (2013)

Objectives are highly specific and should be measurable. The acronym SMART is often used to describe the essentials of a clear objective (see Box 4.5).

BOX 4.5 SMART OBJECTIVES

Specific – target a specific issue for improvement

Measurable – specify a quantifiable indicator of success or progress

Achievable – should be attainable and acceptable

Realistic – what can realistically be done given the resources available?

Time limited – specify exactly when the results should be achieved by

Objectives should focus on outcomes rather than the process of achieving them. While objectives should be achievable, they should also be sufficiently challenging to attain worthwhile outcomes. The examples of objectives from the Workforce Council, Australia in Box 4.4 above specify the levels of outcomes expected in percentage terms. These should not, of course, be arbitrary, but derived from consideration of baseline data and existing time trends. One of the oldest political devices for guaranteeing success is to set objectives that will be achieved automatically if existing time trends continue, independently of any intervention. However, such subterfuge is clearly anathema to the achievement of *worthwhile* goals!

There is typically some variation in the specificity of objectives – the most rigorous objectives are held to be behavioural objectives. Wherever possible, therefore, objectives should be expressed as behavioural objectives that conform to the pattern:

who will be able to do *what* to *what extent* and *when*.

For example, 90% of four-year-olds in locality Z will have been immunized against measles, mumps and rubella within three years of beginning the programme.

Alternatively, if we are focusing on policy and environmental rather than behavioural change, an example would be: Y town council will have introduced traffic-calming measures in 10% of the residential streets in locality X within five years of beginning the programme.

Establishing such objectives presupposes that information is available on the levels of behaviour in question prior to beginning any intervention in order to set achievable, yet challenging, targets. For example, raising the uptake of immunization from 85 to 90% would offer a completely different challenge than from 30 to 90%. Moreover, it is not just a question of the magnitude of the change required. Reference to communication of innovations theory (Rogers and Shoemaker, 1971) in Chapter 3 would indicate that the early introduction of an innovation takes time (and *ipso facto* much health promotion effort) as the innovators and, subsequently, the early adopters accept the innovation. There follows a period of more rapid adoption and then the rate of uptake slows considerably as the laggards become involved. Increasing the uptake of behaviour from 5 to 10% is therefore likely to require more effort than from 50 to 55%, and the final 95 to 100% can be particularly problematic as laggards are notoriously difficult to change.

The most rigorous way of expressing behavioural objectives would (in addition to specifying what the learner should be able to do) also define the conditions and acceptable levels of performance. These three components are defined by Mager (1975: 21) as:

1. **Performance** – an objective always says what a learner is able to do.
2. **Conditions** – an objective always describes what the important conditions (if any) are, under which the performance is to occur.
3. **Criterion** – wherever possible, an objective describes the criterion of acceptable performance by describing how well the learner must perform in order to be considered acceptable.

While, at first sight, it could appear that behavioural objectives might be more appropriate and easier to formulate when the focus of an intervention explicitly addresses behaviour change, they are readily applied to educational goals. Indeed, their origins are within education and the pursuit of behavioural objectives became a major driving force in the USA in the 1960s and 1970s and the subject of fierce debate (see, for example, Popham, 1978; Stenhouse, 1975). Advocates of behavioural objectives claim that it is possible – and desirable – to develop appropriate behavioural objectives for all cognitive and affective learning outcomes.

One advantage of using behavioural objectives in an educational context is that this acknowledges the active role of the learner. It focuses attention on what we expect the *learner* to be able to do in the specification of outcomes rather than the teacher or health educator. The role of the 'educator' then becomes instrumental and involves putting the conditions in place to *enable* the learner to achieve the behavioural objectives. In that health promotion, by its very nature, is action-orientated, behavioural objectives are particularly relevant. Using behavioural objectives, therefore, specifies the target group and what we expect them to be able to do, along with how this would contribute to achieving the overall goal. However, we should emphasize that behaviour in this context is merely *indicative* of learning – it should not be taken to imply that the overall goal of the programme is necessarily concerned with behaviour change. For example, in pursuit of a safer environment, an appropriate objective might be: 'A majority of local councillors will vote in favour of the introduction of traffic-calming measures in locality X on date Y.' Achievement of this objective may require a series of subsidiary objectives, such as '90% of local councillors will respond accurately, when interviewed, that locality X has the highest rate of pedestrian injuries in the town within six months of starting the programme.'

Similarly, if participatory approaches are used, a behavioural objective could be phrased thus: 'Using participatory techniques, residents will produce a map identifying the high-risk areas within the locality within three months of starting the programme.'

Although we will return to this at greater length in Chapters 6 and 8, it is worth noting briefly at this point that programmes focusing on policy and environmental change require learning of some sort. This might include greater awareness of an issue, increased motivation to take action or the development of skills in advocacy and lobbying.

Clearly, the overall approach and the relative emphasis on environmental and behavioural factors will be fundamental to shaping objectives. A number of other key decisions will also influence the ways in which they are formulated – whether the programme is horizontal or vertical, the level of operation (individual, family, community, region and so on), the target groups and the timescale.

Listing the programme objectives provides an opportunity to check that consideration has been given to all the necessary elements required for the achievement of the programme's goal and identifies any omissions that may undermine the whole effort. Conversely, in the interests of economy, any overlap or redundancy can also be identified. Furthermore, it encourages articulation of the anticipated mechanism by means of which the change will be achieved – the so-called Theory of Change referred to above.

From objectives to action

Once programme objectives have been specified, the actual methods to be used – and combinations – can be considered. Clearly, these are many and various and so will be discussed more fully in Chapters 6, 7, 8, 9 and 10. The selection of methods will, again, be based on the intended purpose, local context and characteristics of any target group, theory and evidence of effectiveness – the art of health promotion practice lies in achieving the best fit in relation to all these. Attaching subsidiary objectives to the various activities clarifies their intended purpose. Any preconditions should also be identified. For example, effort may need to be directed towards building a sense of community before community action to improve safety can begin or, alternatively, school staff may need to be trained before a sex education programme can be provided for teenagers. Furthermore, materials and content should be pre-tested with the target group. Partnerships with other agencies may need to be consolidated and methods of achieving this will also need to be considered.

The so-called 'Penrith Paradox' (Adams and Armstrong, 1995) was born at a symposium to discuss the current state of health promotion theory and practice in the UK. It drew attention to the mismatch that often exists between the type of health promotion practice that might be expected, based on theoretical principles, and the dominant models seen in everyday practice, and it still has relevance today. Of particular concern was the emphasis on individualism in practice when evidence and theory point to the greater effectiveness of community development approaches. The paradox is summed up in Box 4.6.

BOX 4.6   THE PENRITH PARADOX

We talk of a theory–practice gap. Maybe it is more complex and pervasive than this. Some models of health promotion are well supported by theory, quality of theoretical debate and quantity of papers published (e.g. community development/social action). Others (e.g. individualism) are starkly unsupported; in fact greater volume of debate is focused upon criticizing than supporting them. The paradox arises when examining practice in the UK today. The theoretically weak models are dominant in practice whereas theoretically based models to which many practitioners subscribe struggle to be maintained or developed in practice in the UK today.

Source: Adams and Armstrong (1995: 3)

The solution to the paradox was held *not* to involve new models, nor was there a need to test current theories further. What was judged to be needed was a broad disciplinary alliance in both health promotion training and practice and more collaboration between academics and practitioners.

Political influences always shape the overall climate within which health promotion activity takes place and political factors can also be decisive in the selection of actual methods in health promotion. The 'Heroin Screws You Up' campaign in the UK was a classic example of flying in the face of expert opinion by allocating considerable resources to funding a high-profile mass media campaign (Tones, 1986). Conventional wisdom – and rationale planning – would dictate that drug education for young people should involve a comprehensive programme of personal, social and health education. What the programme did achieve was a demonstration to 'Middle England' that the government was taking action regarding the drug problem, albeit inappropriately.

Returning to the systems checklist (see Figure 4.7), at the implementation level, the 5WH formula (outlined in Box 4.7) is a well-known acronym for identifying which key issues to address.

BOX 4.7 5WH

- Who?
- What?
- Where?
- When?
- Why?
- How?

Clearly, with complex, multilevel interventions, all the activities need to be orchestrated so that everything is in the right place at the right time to maximize the effects of the programme and, indeed, minimize the risk of programme failure. Administrative issues such as funding, staffing and deployment need to be managed efficiently. Devices such as Gantt charts are helpful to this end and for detailed operational planning. Gantt charts are essentially bar charts that can be used to visualize the relationships between the various tasks required to achieve the programme's goal. By way of illustration, a brief extract from a Gantt chart is provided in Figure 4.9.

Each task should be specified. Durfee and Chase (1999) suggest that they should also be expressed as an action with a duration. Milestones are important points in the development of the project or programmes and can be marked. They serve as a check that everything is proceeding according to schedule. Beginning some tasks is dependent on the completion of others and this relationship can also be indicated.

The final stages are monitoring and evaluation, which will be discussed at some length in Chapter 11. However, we should note some key points here. First, evaluation should be an integral part of the planning process and considered at all stages. Second, precision in formulating plans and objectives provides a clear focus for monitoring what has been done and evaluating what has been achieved. Finally, plans are not set in stone. Formative evaluation, which would include the

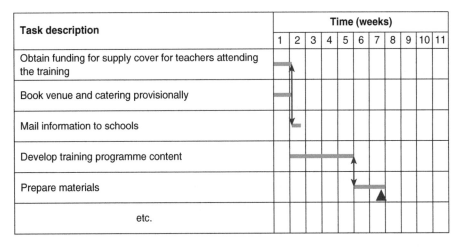

Task description	Time (weeks)										
	1	2	3	4	5	6	7	8	9	10	11
Obtain funding for supply cover for teachers attending the training											
Book venue and catering provisionally											
Mail information to schools											
Develop training programme content											
Prepare materials											
etc.											

▲ planned milestone

↕ relationship between different tasks

Figure 4.9 An extract from a Gantt chart for a sex education training programme for school staff

pre-testing of materials, aims to identify what is working well and what is working less well in order to make necessary modifications. Feedback loops in the planning cycle encourage such reflection and adaptation.

QUALITY HEALTH PROMOTION

Generally, the drive for greater efficiency within the health service has placed greater emphasis on value for money and cost improvements, yet the primary concern of the public – and, indeed, an overriding ethical imperative – is with the effectiveness and quality of the care they receive (Catford, 1993). The target-driven culture of the early twenty-first century has continued to focus on achievement of ends rather than the means of achieving them. Yet, to be consistent with its fundamental values, health promotion should also be concerned with quality and conforming to principles of good practice. As Wills (2023: 325) argues, quality not only implies excellence but also that something is 'fit for the purpose'. The principles of the Ottawa Charter have been a guiding force within the health promotion movement. As Jordan et al. (2011: 745) argue, 'monitoring and quality assurance are gaining in importance for the identification of needs and the effectiveness of prevention and health promotion activities'. Evans et al. (1994) suggest that the following core principles should be considered in relation to quality assurance:

- equity
- effectiveness
- efficiency

- accessibility
- appropriateness
- acceptability
- responsiveness.

Catford (1993) also proposes that there should be a common set of criteria to assess performance and quality organized around a number of themes – see Box 4.8.

BOX 4.8　THEMES FOR ASSESSING QUALITY

- Understanding and responding to people's needs fairly
- Building on sound theoretical principles and understanding
- Demonstrating a sense of direction and coherence
- Collecting, analysing and using information
- Reorientating key decision-makers upstream
- Connecting with all sectors and settings
- Using complementary approaches at both individual and environmental levels
- Encouraging participation and ownership
- Providing technical and managerial training and support
- Undertaking specific actions and programmes.

Source: After Catford (1993)

Quality assurance has been defined as:

> a systematic process through which achievable and desirable levels of quality are described, the extent to which these levels are achieved is assessed, and action is taken following assessment to enable them to be reached. (Wright and Whittington, in Evans et al., 1994: 20)

and

> the work that takes place within any work unit, so as to follow up and improve the unit's own activities and to prevent mistakes or defects from arising. (Berensson et al., 2001: 188)

Haglund et al. (1998) note the importance of establishing the purpose of quality assessment and whether it is concerned with checking if standards have been met (that is, providing a borderline between 'good enough' and 'not good enough') or a stimulus for continuous improvement. Speller et al. (1998) describe two main approaches to quality assurance that reflect this distinction: external standards inspection (ESI), where external standards are set in relation to a work process and monitored so that action can be taken if there is any failure to meet standards, and, in contrast, total quality management (TQM), which involves setting internal standards. TQM is also dynamic in approach and is concerned with continuous growth and improvement rather than just ensuring that minimum standards are met, which is typical of the more static approach of ESI. A survey of specialist health promotion services in England (Royle and Speller, 1996) revealed internal peer review as being the best way to monitor standards. Opinion was mixed about whether or not there should be a set of national standards and criteria for assuring quality. A 'standard' has been defined as 'a statement that defines an agreed level of excellence' and 'criteria' as 'descriptive statements which are measurable, that relate to a standard' (Evans et al., 1994: 103–4). Speller et al. (1998) also distinguish between 'quality assurance programmes', which aim to ensure the quality of all aspects of a service, and 'quality initiatives', in which standards for a particular project or intervention may be agreed.

Quality has been described (British Standards Institute, 1978: BS 4778) as:

the totality of the features and characteristics of a product or service that bear on its ability to satisfy stated or implied needs.

Speller notes that the assessment of the quality of interventions is often based, inappropriately, on outcomes rather than quality criteria. A consensus definition of quality assurance for health promotion was achieved by a European Commission-sponsored project in 1996:

Quality assurance in health promotion is the process of assessment of a programme or intervention in order to ensure performance against agreed standards, which are subject to continuous improvement and set within the framework and principles of the Ottawa Charter. (Speller et al., 1998: 79)

The principal concern of quality assurance, therefore, is with what is done and whether or not this conforms with agreed standards of practice rather than what is achieved – neatly encapsulated as: 'Doing things right is not enough if the right things are not done correctly' (Haglund et al., 1990: 100). The focus is therefore on *inputs* rather than *outcomes*. However, there is inevitably a reciprocal relationship between the two – quality health promotion should draw on evidence of effectiveness and be more effective. The argument that runs through this book is that health promotion should be planned well and that planning should draw on sound evidence at all stages and be informed by principles of good practice. The characteristics of good practice in health promotion are listed in Box 4.9.

BOX 4.9 CHARACTERISTICS OF GOOD PRACTICE

- An agreed philosophy
- A clear vision of health
- Decisions based on needs
- A planned approach
- Working in partnerships
- Strategic leadership

(Continued)

- Realistic aims and claims
- Use of effective methods
- Consumer involvement
- Disseminating results
- Reflection
- Motivated and skilled staff.

Source: After Evans et al. (1994)

Speller et al. (1998: 145) emphasize that quality assurance can ensure that interventions are 'acceptable, and applicable to the setting, and based on current best evidence'. They contend that only quality-assured programmes should be evaluated and, further, if they prove to be effective, clear guidance on what standards are expected in relation to implementation should be a necessary element of subsequent dissemination. As we will note in Chapter 11, such attention to quality would contribute to avoiding Type 3 errors in evaluation – that is, the inability to detect any effect when interventions were predestined to fail because of poor design and/or implementation.

Haglund et al. (1998) identify a number of tensions in applying models of quality assessment – largely deriving from the commercial and manufacturing sectors – to health promotion. First, quality production standards have generally been developed for routine and repetitive procedures, whereas health promotion interventions are usually unique. Second, quality standards are usually set by the consumer who, in the context of health promotion, may be difficult to define (is it the commissioning agency or the target group?) and also lack a clear voice. Third, health promotion is a multidisciplinary endeavour and views about quality may be influenced by the philosophies to which practitioners subscribe. Furthermore, quality assessment instruments are generally designed for analysing the activities of a single organization and do not adapt well to assessing the cooperation between them. As Wills (2023: 323) argues, quality in health promotion is 'less concerned with number crunching then with how the activity is perceived by the recipients'.

Audits are seen as the means of assessing the quality of service provision. Evans et al. (1994: 103) note that the term 'audit' is interpreted in a number of different ways, but that it can be defined as 'the systematic critical analysis of the quality of a health promotion programme' and taken to be synonymous with quality assurance. They propose a quality assurance cycle based on six stages:

- identifying/reviewing key areas for quality assurance
- setting standards
- selecting criteria with which to measure standards
- comparing practice with standards
- taking action
- reviewing the previous stages.

The outcome of the final review stage should feed back into stage one of a new cycle.

Health promotion, by its very nature, is wide-ranging and services are organized in a number of different ways. Speller et al. (1997a) argue that quality assurance should be applied to what might be considered the generic key functions of health promotion. Following a consultation exercise that reflected concern that quality assessment should be grounded in the reality of health promotion practice, they identified six key functions:

- strategic planning
- programme management
- monitoring and evaluation
- education and training
- resources and information
- advice and consultancy.

Strategic planning – particularly intersectoral planning – with a focus on health needs and healthy public policy was seen to be a core function of health promotion. Examples of standards that might be applied to some of these key functions are provided in Box 4.10. Alternatively, these could be developed by individual organizations, along with appropriate criteria.

BOX 4.10 EXAMPLES OF STANDARDS FOR SELECTED KEY FUNCTIONS

1. Strategic planning
    1.1   There is a group that addresses strategic planning issues in health promotion.
    1.2   The health promotion service makes an important contribution to this group.
    1.3   A health promotion strategy is produced and/or health promotion figures prominently within other strategy documents.
    1.4   The health promotion department's plan relates to the health strategies.
2. Programme management
    2.1   A group exists for the planning, implementation and review of each programme area.
    2.2   A range of health promotion methods and activities is considered for each programme area in order to determine action plans.

Source: Speller et al. (1997a: 220)

Haglund et al. (1990) contend that quality assurance can only be built into the planning phase of interventions. Rather than adopting the flexible TQM approach described above, they focus on the design and planning of interventions to ensure that all the necessary conditions for success are in place. The use of a standardized instrument enables the experiences of local projects to be collected and shared. The 20-item questionnaire used to systematize 'telling the story' of different projects at the Sundsvall Conference (Haglund et al., 1993) was subsequently found to have a role in improving planning. The key issues that were identified for reporting purposes were also the key issues that should inform the development of projects. This interconnectedness should not be altogether surprising. The questionnaire has been revised and now includes six dimensions that relate to the various stages of the supportive environments action model (SESAME) (Haglund et al., 1998), as shown in Figure 4.10.

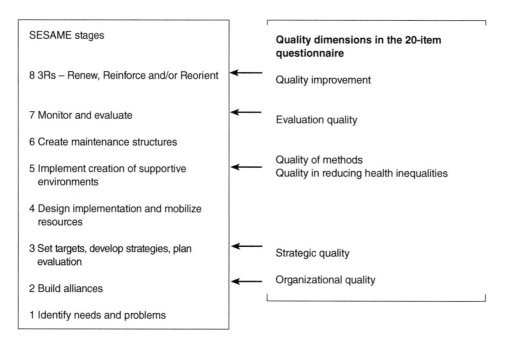

Figure 4.10   Quality dimensions associated with SESAME (after Haglund et al., 1998)

The approach to quality assurance adopted in the Netherlands is similar and aims to improve the effectiveness of programmes by encouraging 'systematic and critical reflection on programmes and projects' (Molleman et al., 2006: 10). A structured instrument is used – the PREFFI (Health Promotion Effectiveness Fostering Instrument), now revised as PREFFI2 (Health Promotion Effect Management Instrument). This includes contextual conditions (such as capacity and leadership), analysis of the problem and possible solutions, selection and development of interventions, implementation and evaluation. Quality criteria are specified for each condition with subsidiary questions about operationalization. In many ways, knowledge is central to the process and we will return to this issue in Chapter 11.

In essence, our discussion of quality has come full circle, returning to the assertion that the process of planning is fundamental to the quality of health promotion. Godin et al. (2007) propose that the degree of planning is an indicator of the potential success of programmes. They developed a tool to assess the planning process based on the 19 planning tasks in the 'intervention mapping' framework (Bartholomew et al., 2001). The tool was tested using data from 123 projects and the findings are summarized in Table 4.3.

Table 4.3 Proportion (%) of projects that completed tasks, stages and phases

Phase	Stage	Tasks	%
Preparatory		Identify problem	48
phase		Identify target population	89
(89%)		Identify determinants	12
		Analyse environment	97
Operational	**Stage 1**	Specify population	15
phases	Proximal	Overall objective	83
	objectives	Performance objectives	41
	matrices	Choice of determinants	7
	(15%)	Learning objectives	6
	Stage 2	Choose models	5
	Theory-practice	Translate into strategies	23
	(25%)		
	Stage 3	Organizational structure	79
	Producing the	Content of activities	59
	design	Producing material	66
	(68%)		
	Stage 4	Support of partners	80
	Adoption and		
	implementation		
	(80%)		
	Stage 5	Evaluation plan	48
	Evaluation	Process	78
	(39%)	Impact	8
		Communication	12

Source: After Godin et al. (2007)

Only 15% of projects properly completed the objective matrix stage and 25% the theory–practice stage. Of particular concern is the lack of attention to objectives and to the selection of theoretical models – identified as a major weakness in project development.

Haglund et al. (1998) suggest that improving the quality of health promotion rests on three cornerstones:

- user-friendly instruments for practitioners
- quality assessment instruments that reflect the reality of health promotion practice
- professional training for health promoters.

Clearly, quality is dependent on proper financing. Scriven and Speller's (2007) analysis of the global situation based on 10 regional field reports reveals 'a chronic shortage of resources, including difficulty associated with workforce capacity and capability for health promotion' (2007: 197). The effects of inadequate funding are summarized in Figure 4.11.

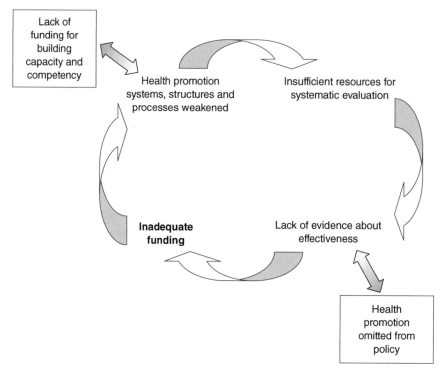

Figure 4.11　Consequences of inadequate funding

Source: Scriven and Speller (2007: 196)

ALLIANCES AND PARTNERSHIPS FOR HEALTH

 Recognition that health is determined by a wide range of factors automatically leads to the view that efforts to promote health demand the coordinated action of a number of different sectors and agencies. Hagard (2000: 2) contends that a successful strategy requires:

> concerted action by a number of different players, including government at all levels, many sectors of society, such as social services, education, environmental protection and healthcare, the media and nongovernmental organizations, and all public and private bodies that variously contribute to economic activity, social cohesion, justice and human rights.

This notion was recognized by the Ottawa Charter. It has been at the heart of the health promotion and 'Health for All' movements and is integral to settings approaches such as 'Healthy Cities' and the 'Health Promoting School' – indeed, Kickbusch has identified partnerships as the 'key to successfully promoting health' (WHO, 1998c). The Jakarta Declaration (WHO, 1997) identified the current challenge as that of releasing the potential for health promotion in different sectors and at all levels of society. Breaking down barriers between sectors and creating partnerships for health were seen as essential. In addition to reaffirming the importance of involving communities and families, the Jakarta Declaration also introduced the issue of investment and public/private partnerships. Overall, the priorities for the twenty-first century were listed as being to:

- promote social responsibility for health
- increase investment in health development
- consolidate and expand partnerships for health
- increase community capacity and empower the individual
- secure an infrastructure for health promotion.

Over the years, there have been changes in terminology concerning collaborative approaches to working – 'inter-agency working', 'intersectoral working', 'joint working', 'intersectoral collaboration', 'healthy alliances', 'coalitions' and, most recently, 'partnerships'. While it would be easy to dismiss these changes as merely rebadging a familiar concept, they do signal a subtle shift in emphasis – despite the lingering tendency to use them interchangeably.

The move towards using the term 'partnership' is perhaps indicative of a more explicit concern to involve members of the community, rather than assuming their implicit representation as a result of the involvement of organizations. Furthermore, the notion of 'partnership' draws attention to the issue of power and implies participation on an equal footing with the sharing of power. The term 'partnership' appears in the *Geneva Charter for Well-being* (WHO, 2021c: 4) which 'calls upon non-governmental and civic organizations, academia, business, governments, international organizations, and all concerned to engage in partnerships for decisive implementation of strategies for health and well-being'. Given the current emphasis on partnerships and alliances, we should consider the implications for planning health promotion before concluding this chapter. We will begin by looking briefly at alliances and intersectoral collaboration before moving on to partnerships.

Delaney (1994a) identifies four key features of organizations that contribute to effective collaboration. Similarity of structure and function is important, but there also needs to be agreement on respective remits and areas of responsibility, along with awareness of interdependence and the collaboration serving to meet needs (see Case study 4.1).

CASE STUDY 4.1 BOSTON PUBLIC HEALTH COMMISSION

An example of a collaborative initiative involving several services:

Homeless services
Infectious disease

(Continued)

Emergency medical services
Recovery services
Community initiatives
Child and family health

Tackling several issues including:

Children's health
Emergency services and preparedness
Health access
Health equity and social justice
Healthy eating and active living
Mental and emotional health
Sexual health
Violence prevention

Aiming to protect, preserve and promote the health and well-being of all Boston residents, particularly the most vulnerable.

Dependence on resources is a further stimulus for collaboration. Delaney (1994b: 475) notes Hudson's (1987) assertion that the 'absence of alternative sources of resources is a "prerequisite" for successful collaboration'. Resources are not necessarily financial – they can include human resources, services and information.

Collaboration is facilitated by formal commitments and structural arrangements for meetings and joint working. Formally ratified strategies and committee structures are a feature of some initiatives. However, networking and the informal working arrangements that develop among people who share the same broad goals are also important. Reticulist (networking) skills that support strategic thinking and crossing boundaries therefore contribute to effective collaboration. Please see Box 4.11 for some key features of successful collaboration. Delaney (1994b:9 cautions against seeing collaboration as 'a purely technical matter to be resolved by the right administrative arrangements' – it also involves negotiation and bargaining. Furthermore, drawing on the work of Lukes (see Chapter 1), she observes that the power relationships within alliances may be unequal and maintained in a variety of subtle ways so that particular organizations and values may come to dominate. At a very basic level, control may be exercised in the ways in which meetings are chaired and agendas constructed. Not only should the interactions within a collaboration be fair in themselves, but they must also be perceived to be fair. The optimal arrangement would appear to be formal structures coupled with informal networking within an overall climate of positive mutual awareness.

Delaney's (1994b) qualitative study of the factors perceived to influence intersectoral collaboration identified the following barriers to success:

- lack of vision and shared commitment
- lack of time
- competition:
  - between individuals and organizations
  - within and between professional networks and dominant or influential professional groups
- conflicting mechanisms and timescales
- different channels of accountability and communication.

BOX 4.11 KEY FEATURES OF SUCCESSFUL COLLABORATION

- Domain awareness and similarity of functions between agencies
- Shared vision
- Compromise and bargaining
- Needs of all parties should be met
- Resources exchange and commitment
- Formal recognition
- Organizational and communication structure, but also flexibility and opportunities to network
- Reticulist skills
- The interpersonal element
- 'Flat', less hierarchical structures rather than authoritarian organizational forms.

Identified by Tones and Delaney (1995: 22)

- Early vision and understanding
- Clarity of roles, rules, procedures and responsibilities
- Wide representation of stakeholders and a strong membership
- Leadership skills
- Communication between the diverse parties
- Human resource development
- Building on the identified strengths and assets of the partners
- Realistic timeframes and funding cycles.

Identified by Ansari (1998: 18)

(Continued)

Features of effective partnerships and coalitions

- Leadership
- Management
- Communication
- Conflict resolution
- Perception of fairness
- Shared decision-making
- Perceived benefits versus costs.

Identified by Bracht et al. (1999)

- Committed individuals
- Joint funding
- Pooling of resources
- Shared education and training opportunities
- Existing projects which span different agencies

Identified by Wills (2023: 133)

In relation to workplace health promotion interventions, Thesenvitz of the Health Communication Unit, Toronto, Canada, outlines nine conditions for success based on what was identified as being 'widespread agreement' in the literature (Thesenvitz, 2003: 4). Many of the nine conditions that were identified are transferable to other contexts. They are as follows:

- senior management involvement
- participatory planning
- primary focus on employees' needs
- optimal use of on-site resources
- integration
- recognition that a person's health is determined by an interdependent set of factors
- tailoring to the special features of each workplace environment
- evaluation
- long-term commitment.

Successful Partnerships: A Guide (Brandstetter et al., 2006) describes itself as 'a practical guide for practitioners and policy makers involved in partnership' (p. 3). It identifies the features of ineffective or 'unsuccessful' partnerships (see Box 4.12). The aim of working together effectively would be to avoid these types of pitfalls! In addition, Wills (2023: 133) points to some of the potential difficulties of partnership working which might occur due to 'differences in priorities, organizational ethos, funding arrangements, competition for contracts and geographical boundaries'.

Nelson et al. (2013) used a qualitative approach to establish features of successful partnership working in community-based interventions designed to promote physical activity in young people. Through a thematic analysis, they established that the following factors lead to stronger partnerships:

- continuity (history with partner, willingness to engage in future partnership)
- connectedness
- capacity (interest, enthusiasm and engagement, and clarity of roles and responsibilities).

BOX 4.12 UNSUCCESSFUL PARTNERSHIPS

A partnership is likely to be ineffective if...

- Partners do not share the same values and interests. This can make arrangements on partnership goals difficult.
- There is no sharing risk, responsibility, accountability or benefits.
- The inequalities in partners' resources and expertise determine their relative influence in the partnership's decision-making.
- One person or partner has all the power and/or drives the process.
- There is a hidden motivation which is not declared to all partners.
- The partnership was established just to 'keep up appearances'.
- Partnership members do not have the training to identify issues or resolve internal conflicts.
- Partners are not chosen carefully, particularly if it is difficult to 'de-partner'.

Source: Brandstetter et al. (2006: 11)

Gillies (1998: 101), commenting on a review of the literature on the effectiveness of partnerships, notes that those reported on fell into two broad groups:

- Micro level – alliances or partnerships that involve one or more collaborators among individuals or groups or organizations in the public, private or non-governmental sectors in the promotion of health, but that do not seek to affect the underlying systems or structures or architecture for health promotion.
- Macro level – alliances or partnerships that involve one or more collaborators among institutions, organizations or groups in the public, private or non-governmental sector that seek to affect the structural determinants of health.

While the published micro-level studies tended to focus on behavioural outcomes in assessing gains, Gillies notes that they could equally have focused on the wider environmental determinants. What clearly emerged from the review was that the stronger the representation from the community and the higher the level of involvement in practical activities, the greater and more sustainable were the gains. Mechanisms should, therefore, be put in place to involve local people in planning and practical health promotion activities. New Zealand's Ministry of Health (2003) published some general principles to guide health promotion practice that included working together with New Zealand's indigenous population and involving them at all levels in the decision-making, planning and delivery process. The document argues that 'working with communities and whanau groups to actively address health issues and structural factors impacting on health in an empowering way is the essence of health promotion' (p. 10). Furthermore, lay involvement should be based on power sharing and not mere tokenism. This view endorses that of Labonte (1993), who makes a clear distinction between consultation and participation. Central to participation is shared decision-making, negotiated relationships and openness to identifying problems and issues. Furthermore, he suggests that less powerful groups may need support so that they can participate on an equal footing. Strategies for engaging less powerful groups include providing staff training in cultural awareness, recognizing marginalized people as active participants, using various means of communication, and ensuring that physical spaces are accessible to everyone.

A review of the examples of best practice in alliances or partnerships for health collected from around the world (Gillies, 1998: 104) identified the key elements of good partnership to include:

> a relevant needs assessment combined with the setting up of committees crossing professional and lay boundaries to steer, guide and account for the activities and programmes implemented.

It was also noted that non-industrialized countries are leading the way in relation to partnerships and community-based health promotion. These examples of good practice placed less emphasis on behavioural outcomes than the published studies and were more concerned with their impact on the broad environmental conditions and process of change. Key outcomes in relation to process (Gillies, 1998: 112) were:

> getting agencies to work together; engaging local people; training and supporting volunteers and networks; creating committees; capturing politicians' interest and sustaining political visibility; resource allocation; reorientating organizations and services; promoting flexibility in working practices; and undertaking needs assessment as a way of identifying priorities and galvanizing interest …

Open communication and trust are essential ingredients of partnership working and are dependent on good networks for sharing information and establishing common values and goals. However, partners may be drawn from diverse professional, cultural and social backgrounds. The management of this diversity will also be integral to success. On the one hand, any conflict that would be a barrier to joint decision-making needs to be avoided – especially when it is associated with an imbalance of power.

Developing partnerships requires:

- leadership
- trust
- learning to continuously improve
- managing for performance.

An interactive tool is available to analyse how partnerships are working in relation to these dimensions (LGpartnerships – Smarter Partnerships, undated). Clearly, successful partnerships demand time and commitment, supportive organizational structures and appropriate skills among those involved. Individuals might need to develop their skills in order to engage constructively in partnerships, and organizations might need to change their internal ways of working. Capacity-building might be required in relation to individuals, communities and organizations before effective partnerships can be established.

It is possible to distinguish a number of stages in the development of a partnership (Educe Ltd and GFA Consulting, undated):

1. Forming
2. Frustration
3. Functioning
4. Flying
5. Failure.

Responding appropriately to the stage of development will help to ensure the success of the partnership: for example, at stage 1, developing a common vision will be important; at stage 2, demonstrating 'early wins'; and, at stage 4, paying attention to the future relevance of the partnership and sustainability. The characteristics of a 'healthy partnership' identified by LGpartnerships – Smarter Partnerships (undated) are:

- partners can demonstrate real results through collaboration
- common interest supersedes partner interest
- partners use 'we' when talking about partner matters
- partners are mutually accountable for tasks and outcomes
- partners share responsibility and rewards
- partners strive to develop and maintain trust
- partners are willing to change what they do and how they do it
- partners seek to improve how the partnership performs.

Notwithstanding the challenges, partnerships offer great potential for developing a coordinated response to the multiple factors that influence health status and achieving health gains. There are also potential gains for partner agencies that might be motivated to enter into such partnerships for reasons not necessarily related to health (see Box 4.13).

BOX 4.13 GENERAL BENEFITS OF PARTNERSHIP WORKING

- Achievement of organizational objectives and enhanced efficiency and effectiveness
- Improved coordination of policy, programmes and service delivery

(Continued)

- Broadening the scope of influence to include other services and activities
- Greater economy
- Less bureaucracy and regulation
- Business and commercial opportunities
- Access to data and information
- Access to a range of skills and competencies
- Opportunity for innovation and learning
- More involvement of local communities.

Source: After DETR (2001: Annex E)

ABSTRACT 4.2

Comparing the functioning of youth and adult partnerships for health promotion. Brown, L.D., Redelfs, A.H., Taylor, T.J. and Messer, R.L. (2015)

Youth partnerships are a promising but understudied strategy for prevention and health promotion. Specifically, little is known about how the functioning of youth partnerships differs from that of adult partnerships. Accordingly, this study compared the functioning of youth partnerships with that of adult partnerships. Several aspects of partnership functioning, including leadership, task focus, cohesion, participation costs and benefits, and community support, were examined. Standardized partnership functioning surveys were administered to participants in three smoke-free youth coalitions ($n = 44$; 45% female; 43% non-Hispanic white; mean age = 13) and in 53 Communities That Care adult coalitions ($n = 673$; 69% female; 88% non-Hispanic white; mean age = 49). Multilevel regression analyses showed that most aspects of partnership functioning did not differ significantly between youth and adult partnerships. These findings are encouraging given the success of the adult partnerships in reducing community-level rates of substance use and delinquency. Although youth partnership functioning appears to be strong enough to support effective prevention strategies, youth partnerships faced substantially more participation difficulties than adult partnerships. Strategies that youth partnerships can use to manage these challenges, such as creative scheduling and increasing opportunities for youth to help others directly, are discussed.

Investment for health

We noted in Chapter 2 that social and economic factors are the single major determinant of health status. Ziglio et al. (2000a) contend that health, as an essential personal and social resource, requires investment and, indeed, health promotion should be considered to be an investment strategy. Clearly, there is an inextricable link between health and social and economic development in that social and economic development leads to health improvement and, conversely, health supports social and economic development. Levin and Ziglio (1997: 363) note that, in many societies, the immediate priorities are 'economic competitiveness and fiscal soundness' rather than health priorities. The 'Investment for Health' (IFH) approach, which received considerable attention towards the turn of the twenty-first century, focused on integrating health promotion into mainstream social and economic development. This raises some questions about ends and means: is the emphasis on the promotion of health or is health merely instrumental to achieving wealth? However, the IFH approach acknowledges that priority social and economic policy areas, such as education, employment, transport and housing, have a major influence on health. Policy decisions and initiatives by governments – and the private sector – have the potential to improve or harm health. The major concern of IFH, therefore, is to ensure that efforts to improve social and economic standing also improve health status and are equitable, empowering and sustainable (Ziglio et al., 2000b). Kickbusch (1997) has identified three key questions that should inform the development of a sound health promotion strategy:

- Where is health promoted and maintained in a given population?
- Which investment strategies produce the largest population health gains?
- Which investment strategies help reduce health inequities and are in line with human rights?

Ziglio et al. (2000b: 4) add a fourth:

- Which investments contribute to economic and social development in an equitable and sustainable manner and result in high health returns for the overall population?

In the post-Ottawa era, there has been widespread acceptance of the importance of environmental influences on health, both directly and via their effect on behavioural choices. Latterly, there has been increased awareness of the complexity of environmental factors and the contribution of social networks, social capital and social inclusion to health. Ziglio et al. (2000a) suggest that, notwithstanding the widespread commitment to a socioecological model of health, the health promotion response has been oversimplified. Most change has been 'first-order change', achieving some minor adjustment but without affecting the major determinants of health. They call for a more radical approach in order to achieve 'second-order change' (2000a: 145), which involves new structures and processes – an approach whereby concern for health is interwoven into social systems and the focus is on the creation of health rather than disease prevention.

Organizational policies and activities tend to be sector-based, with little emphasis on intersectoral relationships. Watson et al. (2000: 17) refer to a 'silo model of governance', where different sectors, such as health, education and housing, traditionally have separate structures, funding, channels of accountability and professional 'domains' and there are few opportunities for links. In contrast, 'holistic governance' would be more flexible and involve 'shared objectives, a common understanding of what needs to be done and what others can contribute'. Similar arguments could also be put forward in relation to community involvement.

The issue of partnerships is, therefore, central to the IFH approach, along with accountability for health impact:

> The IFH approach therefore calls for a new form of partnership. In today's complex world, action for the promotion of health cannot come from the healthcare sector alone. It needs to be built on strong cross-sector alliances between health and healthcare, social development and equitable and sustainable economic development. (Ziglio et al., 2000b: 4)

It also involves policy at all levels, from national to local, and this will be considered more fully in Chapter 6. The core principles of IFH (Ziglio et al., 2000a) are:

1. A focus on health
2. Full public engagement
3. Genuine intersectoral work
4. Equity
5. Sustainability
6. A broad knowledge base.

Over and above the emphasis on partnerships and policy to address the structural determinants of health, the IFH approach draws attention to the capacity of systems to respond appropriately in order to foster health improvement. Ziglio et al. (2000a) refer to the importance of maximizing the health assets in a community as well as identifying and responding to the community's health needs. Indeed, the primary focus of IFH is on strengthening health assets. These assets, they found, include:

- policy investments
- regulatory changes
- the nurturing of non-governmental resources and programme initiatives
- the strengthening of health promotion infrastructures and decision-making
- a refocusing on education
- investment in research
- training in the requisite health promotion skills
- environmental improvement.

The principles of IFH offer a means of breaking down traditional barriers to partnership-working and spreading accountability for health beyond the narrow confines of the health sector. Hancock (1998) suggests that the involvement of the private sector offers particular challenges, given that the primary motivation is profit and this may well conflict with health interests. He does, however, recognize the potential benefits of working with the private sector, provided that partners and their subcontractors meet agreed ethical criteria. The proposed criteria are listed in Box 4.14.

BOX 4.14 ETHICAL PRINCIPLES FOR PARTNERSHIP WITH THE PRIVATE SECTOR

- The activities of the corporation are increasingly environmentally sustainable.
- Safe and healthy working conditions are provided for the workforce.
- Pay is fair with reasonable benefits, there is a right to collective bargaining and lay-offs are minimized.

- Taxes are paid fairly and economic activities do not increase poverty.
- Their activities do not pose a danger to consumers or the communities in which they operate and the public is fully informed about any potential hazards.
- There is respect for human rights.

Source: After Hancock (1998)

Social marketing as an approach to planning

As stated at the outset, this chapter unapologetically draws on classic material largely because there has not been a substantial amount of advance or change in this area. However, it is worth mentioning some more recent approaches to planning interventions designed to improve health outcomes and to promote health gains. Social marketing has become a popular choice in planning models in public health and health promotion efforts across the globe (Cross and O'Neil, 2021; Upton and Thirlaway, 2014). While not a theory of its own accord, social marketing does reflect a systematic way of planning an intervention and it involves several stages, similarly to the planning models discussed in this chapter. Social marketing uses a range of methods and approaches and may draw on a variety of different theories to underpin these. A basic social marketing strategy will contain the following elements:

1. Market analysis
2. Selecting channels and materials
3. Developing materials and pre-testing
4. Implementation
5. Assessing effectiveness
6. Feedback to refine the programme (cycle back to stage 1).

These stages are reflected in the social marketing wheel that was originally developed by Novelli in 1994 (cited in Nutbeam et al., 2010: 45). The similarities to generic health promotion planning stages we trust are clear. Social marketing is discussed in more detail in Chapter 8.

HEALTH PROMOTION PLANNING

We have argued in this chapter that effective health promotion is based on a systematic approach to planning. Indeed, planning is fundamental to the quality of health promotion. We have provided examples of a range of different planning models. While they differ to some extent in their orientation, there are several common features. They require the assessment and prioritization of needs and identification of objectives as a basis for appraising possible solutions and selecting the most appropriate courses of action. They also incorporate monitoring and evaluation elements. Perhaps the most important feature is that they provide a framework for integrating theory and empirical evidence into the various stages of the planning process. It is worth emphasizing that theory can be concerned with community participation and policy development as well as behaviour change.

Resistance to using planning models often derives from an association with reductionism and top-down styles of working. We would contend the reverse to be the case. When used appropriately, they can serve to open up the entire range of health promotion options and avoid any tendency towards being blinkered by custom and practice. Many health promotion programmes are destined to fail because they focus on too narrow a range of factors or are based on unsubstantiated assumptions. Rational planning processes will serve to expose such weaknesses and ensure that programmes address all relevant variables. Furthermore, the process of planning can be a vehicle for involving all stakeholders, ensuring wide ownership of plans.

The complex interplay of factors that influence health demands a coordinated response across a number of different sectors and at a number of different levels, from local to national and even supranational. The IFH approach is premised on the interrelationship between health and social and economic development, and seeks to strengthen the assets for health within communities by means of partnerships and policy.

Partnerships are seen to be the 'key mechanism for pulling together effective local planning and action' (Watson et al., 2000: 17). The involvement of communities and creating opportunities for participation on an equal footing are also instrumental to success. Building effective partnerships is undoubtedly challenging, but offers huge potential for developing whole systems approaches to promoting health, rather than reacting in a piecemeal fashion. However, this requires commitment from partners and new ways of working.

By way of conclusion, we would draw attention to Box 4.15, which contains a proverb about the elephant. This has been used as an analogy for taking a whole systems approach to tackling health issues (Newcastle Healthy City Project, 1997). It draws attention to the fact that there are a number of different perspectives on complex systems – all of which may be true but, equally, none represents a complete view. Understanding how the whole system operates depends on sharing knowledge. Members of the community concerned are more likely to interface with more components of the system and, hence, have a more complete picture than professionals, whose awareness may be confined to the remit of a particular agency.

BOX 4.15 WHOLE SYSTEMS AND ELEPHANTS

There is an old Indian proverb about three blind people describing an elephant. One holds the trunk and says, 'This is a snake.' One holds the tail and says, 'No, it's a rope.' The third grabs a leg and says, 'You're both wrong. It is a tree trunk.'

Each person has offered their perception of the truth, but they have failed to describe the elephant. Even putting all three descriptions together would not make a recognizable elephant.

Source: After Newcastle Healthy City Project (1997)

Furthermore, within complex systems, although all components could make a contribution to health and there are knock-on effects between the activities of different agencies, there is no single agency controlling and coordinating activity. Developing an intersectoral response to health issues and partnership working calls for a shift in emphasis away from the functioning of the 'parts' and towards their interrelationship and the functioning of the whole. The key to this is good communication, shared vision and clear strategic and operational objectives.

KEY POINTS

- The effectiveness and quality of health promotion programmes are dependent on good planning.
- The use of appropriate planning models ensures a systematic approach to planning.
- Consideration of equity at all stages of the planning process will prioritize action most likely to achieve narrowing of the gap in health status.
- The planning process can be a vehicle for involving all major stakeholders.
- Reference to theory and the development of clear objectives are essential, yet often neglected, components of the planning process.
- Partnerships between sectors and involving the community are essential for tackling the complex determinants of health and ill health.
- Successful partnerships require good leadership, a shared vision, clarity about roles and responsibilities, good communication, trust and respect.
- The development of partnerships is facilitated by having an appropriate infrastructure and the competencies required to work collaboratively.
- Investment for Health is an example of a partnership approach that recognizes the link between economic development and health.

CHAPTER 4: INTERNATIONAL CASE STUDIES

The following case studies on the online resources website are relevant to the content of this chapter: 2, 4, 8 and 9.

CRITICAL REFLECTION AND APPLICATION TO PRACTICE

This chapter outlines the planning process and argues for a systematic approach to planning for health promotion. Why is it so important to be systematic? How do the contents of this chapter apply to your work? Which planning model lends itself to the work that you do? What type of objectives (behavioural, policy, etc.) are most relevant in the context of the issues you deal with? How would you address the issue of quality in health promotion planning? Why is quality important? How would you ensure it? Reflect on your involvement in partnerships and collaborations in health promotion – what's worked well? What could have been improved?

ONLINE RESOURCES

Please visit https://study.sagepub.com/greentones5e for all the online resources for the book, including recommended further reading on each chapter subject, useful weblinks (both introduced by the authors), as well as the abovementioned case study material.

5 INFORMATION NEEDS

Certitude is not the test of certainty. We have been cocksure of many things that were not so.

Oliver Wendell Holmes, Jr (1841–1935), *Natural Law*

OVERVIEW

The purpose of this chapter is to consider the information required for programme planning. It will:

- consider the notion of need and different interpretations of health needs
- support the use of participatory approaches for identifying health needs
- note the importance of being aware of community profiles and wider contextual factors when responding to health needs
- emphasize the contribution of theory to understanding both the determinants of health and how to change them
- consider the nature of the evidence required to respond effectively to health needs.

INTRODUCTION

Planning for health promotion interventions and activities is an essential process that can be influenced by planning frameworks and theoretical concepts and tools. Importantly though, this application of frameworks and theories must be adapted to suit local needs (Fleming and Baldwin, 2020). The first stage of systematic programme planning involves establishing what the problem is and determining what the causes are, along with any other contributory factors. Some understanding of the nature of the community, its members and the context in which they live is also needed before appropriate courses of action can be identified. Not all health promotion interventions are planned well and the process can be *ad hoc* and lacking a systematic process (Woodall and Cross, 2021). Nutbeam's (1998b) linear approach to programme planning is some years old, but has been consistently use to aid decision-making and planning approaches. The first stage is 'problem definition', which highlights the necessity to utilize research processes, including epidemiological and demographic analysis, along with a community needs analysis to understand the 'problem' to hand. The next phase of 'solution generation', however, draws on theory and models, evidence of effectiveness and practitioner experience. Nutbeam (1998b: 33) provides a useful summary of the key questions that should be addressed at each stage of programme planning and implementation:

- **Problem definition**: What is the problem?
- **Solution generation**: How might it be solved?
- **Innovation testing**: Did the solution work?
- **Intervention demonstration**: Can the programme be repeated/refined?
- **Intervention dissemination**: Can the programme be widely reproduced?
- **Programme management**: Can the programme be sustained?

In Chapter 2, we examined issues associated with the measurement of health status and the broad determinants of health and, in Chapter 3, the factors influencing behaviour and action. The purpose of this chapter is to apply these ideas more specifically to identifying the information needed for making decisions about possible interventions. We will begin by considering definitions of health needs before looking at different approaches to assessing needs and profiling the community. We will then focus on the development of possible solutions and, particularly, the application of theory and evidence to the rational selection of intervention strategies.

Advances in information technology, together with the development of new information systems and sources of data, have done much to improve access to health information. Most data sources are now available publicly and can be used to great effect by health promotion and public health practitioners. The website 'Fingertips' is a large public health data collection resource managed by the Office for Health Improvements & Disparities (see: https://fingertips.phe.org.uk/). There can, however, be too much information and data that can be overwhelming to practitioners or indeed data collected that are relatively meaningless to inform planning and intervention development.

HEALTH NEEDS ASSESSMENT

Assessing health promotion needs is an important first step in planning health promotion activities (Hubley et al., 2021). An updated perspective on health needs assessment has recently been put forward:

> In health promotion, needs assessment incorporates consideration of the impact on health of a broad range of determinants of health, moderated by more locally defined needs and priorities. Community mobilization for needs assessment will better support the identification of priorities that are locally relevant and actionable. Needs assessment is not a one-off activity but a developmental process that is added to and amended over time. It is not an end in itself but a way of using information to plan health care and public health programmes in the future. (Nutbeam and Muscat, 2021: 1589)

A health needs assessment is a logical starting point in the design of a health promotion intervention (Laverack, 2014). In essence, a needs assessment allows health promotion planners to understand 'what is' and 'what should be' in a community (Bartholomew et al., 2011).

The nature of health needs

Given the debate about the nature of health and its determinants, the absence of a precise definition of health needs and the lack of a consensus about the means of assessing needs should come as no surprise. Given that the concept of 'health need' is somewhat loaded, several commentators have opted for the more neutral terminology of 'situation' analysis (Hubley et al., 2021). However, the interpretations of the term 'health needs' range from a narrow focus on heath service provision, through inclusion of a preventive element, to addressing social needs. There is an important distinction between health needs and healthcare needs. It will be clear from our earlier discussion that the broad remit of health promotion requires an analysis of needs that includes social and environmental concerns and also addresses well-being. However, in considering definitions of need, we will also draw briefly on interpretations of healthcare needs.

The traditional public health approach to assessing health needs has been to draw on epidemiological information to measure the disease burden or levels of ill health in communities, such as morbidity and mortality rates. This stems from a conceptualization of health as the absence of disease. More recently though, there has been more interest in focusing on salutogenesis as part of the situational analysis, or needs assessment, with growing interest in how well-being is incorporated alongside assessing moribidity or disease in communities (Mittelmark and Bull, 2013; Mittelmark et al., 2022).

An alternative conceptualization of need – one that addresses the issue of what can be done – is based on the capacity to benefit. Culyer (1977) considers a need for healthcare to exist when there is potential to improve health status or avoid reduction in it, but only if an intervention exists that can achieve positive outcomes. A person can be sick, for instance, but not in need of healthcare unless they can benefit from it (Morris et al., 2007). This resonates with the ideas of those who argue that health need is potentially infinite and resources limited and, therefore, decision-makers restrict themselves to what is known to be effective (Naidoo and Wills, 2016). A need is, therefore, determined not by the scale of the health problem, but by the ability to benefit. These two approaches should not necessarily be seen as incompatible.

An emphasis on the capacity to benefit acknowledges that some interventions offer greater potential for gain than others. A key issue for health economists is the notion of 'allocative efficiency', which is concerned with achieving maximum benefits from available resources. Comparison of the respective gains from spending on different interventions is viewed as essential if resources are to be deployed to achieve the greatest good. Needs identified in this way will clearly be relative and heavily influenced by judgements, not least in relation to how benefits are defined and measured. The measures frequently used in this context include QALYs and DALYs, which, as we noted in Chapter 2, have been the subject of controversy.

'Needs' can very considerably according to who is assessing the situation. There may be areas of overlap but there are also needs that differ between health services and communities. Hubley et al. (2021) differentiate between two elements of health promotion need – 'health service-determined needs' and 'community-determined needs or wants'.

A further interpretation of healthcare needs derives from an instrumental perspective. Rather than focusing on deficiency states, needs are identified in terms of what needs to be done or what conditions need to be in place to maintain or improve health. Within the broader context of health promotion, a useful example is provided by the list of prerequisites for health identified in the Ottawa Charter (WHO, 1986) – peace, shelter, education, food, income, a stable ecosystem, sustainable resources, social justice and equity. Liss's (1990) characterization of different views about healthcare needs provides a useful summary, one that could be applied more generally to health needs:

- **The ill-health notion** that equates a need for healthcare with a deficiency in health that requires healthcare.
- **The supply notion** that requires that acceptable treatment should also be available to respond to a deficiency.
- **The normative notion** that acknowledges that opinions about needs may vary and is based on an assessor believing that healthcare should be provided.
- **The instrumental notion**, based on the identification of care required to achieve certain states.

Bradshaw (1972) defined four types of social need, enshrined in his well-known taxonomy:

- **Normative need** is defined by experts or professionals often on the basis of a 'desirable standard' against which individuals or groups can be compared. However, normative needs may be defined differently by different professional groups and change over time. They cannot therefore be seen as absolute needs.
- **Felt need** is defined by lay people and equated with wants. It is limited as a measure of *real* need by people's perceptions, which may fail to recognize actual needs or else misrepresent wants as needs.
- **Expressed need** consists of felt need turned into action by seeking treatment or care.
- **Comparative need** is concerned with ensuring that people with similar characteristics receive equivalent levels of care and, if there is a shortfall, then individuals are in need.

Bradshaw (1994) acknowledges that there may be alternative views about normative needs and that comparative needs may themselves derive from normative judgements. Felt and expressed needs may differ widely, as illustrated in Figure 5.1.

As we noted in Chapter 2, even what purport to be objective assessments of needs based on disease burden remain essentially ideologically driven. A number of tensions exist in identifying health needs and derive both from the ways in which health and its determinants are conceptualized and where the focus of attention lies. These are summarized in Box 5.1.

BOX 5.1 TENSIONS IN HEALTH NEEDS ASSESSMENT

View of health

- positive or negative view of health
- holistic or atomistic view of health
- biomedical or social interpretation of determinants
- professional or lay perspective.

Focus of attention

- upstream (prevention) or downstream (treatment)
- individual or community.

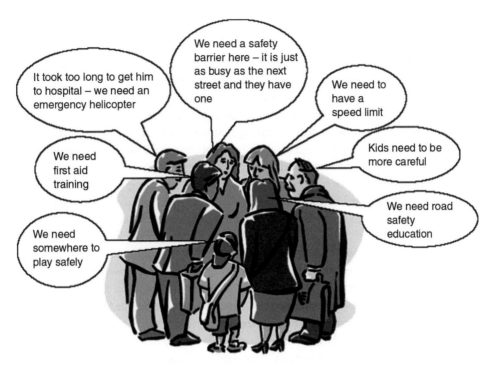

Figure 5.1   Alternative interpretations of need at the scene of an accident

Although Bradshaw's taxonomy provides a useful way to analyse different perspectives and, indeed, ensure that they are represented in any assessment of social needs, it offers little insight into the actual nature of need. Indeed, his assertion that 'real' need is likely to exist when all four types of need are present at the same time may be taken to imply that the individual 'types' are not sufficient in themselves as indicators of 'real' needs.

Two key issues remain unresolved – the distinction between needs and wants and whether needs are absolute or, ultimately, subjectively defined. Doyal and Gough's theory of human need sheds some light here.

Doyal and Gough's theory of human need

Doyal and Gough (1991: 9), in their meticulously constructed defence of the concept of objective and universal human need, recognize critics on both sides of the political spectrum:

> Many argue that it is morally safer and intellectually more coherent to equate needs with subjective preferences – that only individuals or selected groups of individuals can decide the goals to which they are going to attach enough priority to deem them needs.

Critics from the New Right are concerned about state collectivism and the intrusion of the 'nanny' state into matters of individual choice. In the absence of an agreed basis for identifying need, they advocate relying on individual preferences and market forces. Concerns on the Left and among minority and oppressed groups have their origins in the unequal power structure in society and the dominance of particular groups. The contention here is that needs are culturally determined and can only be fully understood by members of a group. They are, therefore, subjectively defined, but at the group collective level, rather than the individual. Doyal and Gough challenge both these positions, along with economic, sociological and postmodern interpretations of need, as relative and contend that objective need does indeed exist. Furthermore, demonstrating that there are objective universal needs creates a moral imperative to meet those needs and effectively establishes them as fundamental rights.

The term 'need' has been used to refer to drives or motivational forces that arise from some disequilibrium – for example, the need for sleep when tired or food when hungry. Maslow (1954) identifies a number of such needs that can be ordered into a hierarchy premised on the requirement to satisfy basic needs, such as hunger and warmth, before higher-order needs can be addressed. The identified needs are felt to be common in different cultures. The levels of the hierarchy are set out in Figure 5.2.

Each level is assumed to be necessary for the achievement of the next, although there is no requirement for 100% satisfaction before moving on to the next level. Maslow himself acknowledged that the hierarchy was not fixed. For example, for those who gain satisfaction from high-risk activities, such as mountaineering or hang-gliding, self-actualization needs may take precedence over safety needs.

Doyal and Gough reject the interpretation of needs as drives on the basis that needs and drives can exist independently of each other. For example, individuals may have a drive to consume alcohol that cannot be construed as a need and, conversely, they may have a need to take more exercise, although they may not feel driven to do so. While recognizing that choices are constrained by biological factors, Doyal and Gough are wary of placing too great an emphasis on biological determinism.

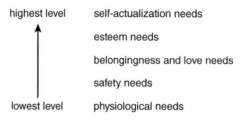

Figure 5.2   A representation of Maslow's hierarchy of needs (after Maslow, 1954)

An alternative way of looking at need is as a means of achieving a goal. Liss (1990) suggests that a goal therefore becomes a necessary precondition to there being a need. Hence, statements about need must conform to the pattern:

A needs X in order to G.

Wants would be distinguished from needs on the basis that wants can be expressed merely as preferences with no requirement to specify the relationship to goals. A further distinction between needs and wants can be made based on the nature of the goal. Doyal and Gough suggest that needs would only apply in relation to *universalizable* goals – that is, goals that are in everyone's interests to achieve.

Wants, in contrast, would vary from person to person, reflecting personal preferences. Such wants would be guided by individual perceptions, whereas needs draw on a shared understanding about the avoidance of harm. For example, an individual may say that they *need* a cigarette, but, from a *universalizable* goal perspective, they *want* a cigarette and *need* to give up smoking.

Doyal and Gough's analysis of universalizable goals identifies two key elements: the avoidance of serious harm and the ability to participate in a social form of life. They propose that the universal prerequisites for achieving these goals and participating fully in society constitute basic human needs, which are identified as:

- physical health
- autonomy.

Autonomy is seen to include mental health, cognitive skills and opportunities to participate in society. In order to meet these basic needs, 11 categories of intermediate needs are identified, as seen in the outline of Doyal and Gough's theory of need in Figure 5.3. While basic and intermediate needs are universalizable, the ways in which these needs can be met may well vary.

Needs assessment will be concerned with assessing how well these basic and intermediate needs are being met. This raises the issue of what standard should be set concerning the satisfaction of needs. In relation to basic needs satisfaction, Doyal and Gough reject both absolute minimum standards and relative standards. Instead, they advocate an optimum standard for basic needs and propose a 'minimum optimorum' level for intermediate needs – that is, the minimum level of input of intermediate need satisfaction to achieve optimal basic needs satisfaction.

The remaining question concerns how needs will be assessed. NHS Scotland (2019) suggest that there are some common steps to health needs assessment as follows:

1. Identify the issue – why are you doing the needs assessment and what do you want to understand?
2. Identify the population – is it everyone within a geographical area, or people with a particular characteristic or health condition?
3. Identify the sources of data you can use – these may include community profiles, local and national statistics, existing evidence about what works and stakeholder views.
4. Identify the gap between need and supply.

Doyal and Gough support the notion of informed participation by those whose needs are being assessed, although they caution that this can favour those already in privileged positions who may be more influential than others without such advantages. They suggest that the development of indicators of intermediate needs will be fed, in an iterative way, by the development of new codified and experiential knowledge. They recognize that both qualitative and quantitative indicators will be needed, but place considerable emphasis on the latter:

> To chart both basic and intermediate indicators we ideally require social indicators which are valid, distributive, quantitative and aggregated, but which are open to revision. These indicators should be open to disaggregation between groups. In this way profiles of the need-satisfaction of nations, cultural groups and other collectives can be compiled. (Doyal and Gough, 1991: 169)

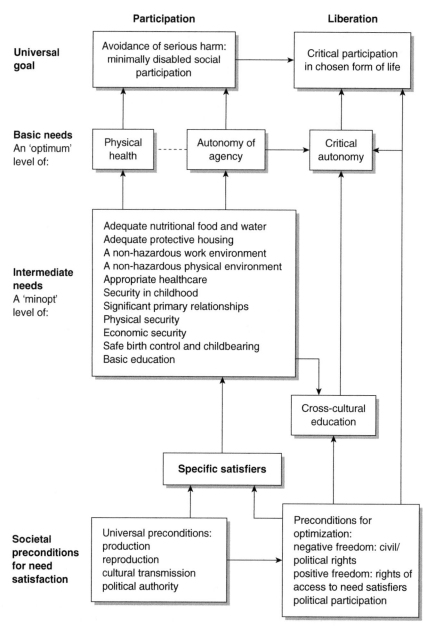

Figure 5.3 Doyal and Gough's theory of human need, in outline

When differences arise between the views of needs established by expert-led approaches, which draw on codified knowledge, and community-based approaches, which are grounded in experience, dialogue is proposed as a mechanism for resolving the situation.

Needs, wants and demands

Equity is recognized as one of the fundamental values of health promotion (Woodall and Cross, 2021).
Principles of social justice would presuppose that health resources should be distributed in relation to
needs. However, as is all too apparent, access to services and wider opportunities to promote health
are not necessarily governed by needs. Some time ago, Hart (1971) used the notion of the 'inverse
care law' to describe the generally poorer provision of services in those areas that are most deprived
and have the greatest burden of ill health. An emphasis on needs rather than wants or demands is,
therefore, integral to equity. More recently, tools have been developed to scrutinize health equity issues
in the needs assessment process. The Health Equity Assessment Tool (HEAT) developed by Public
Health England (2020) is one example of considering health inequalities related to programmes and
how these can be overcome by systematically examining factors leading to inequity.

The defining characteristic of need in Doyal and Gough's theory of need is its instrumentality in
achieving universal human goals. Wants, in contrast, are personal preferences and equate with what
Bradshaw might term felt need. These subjective, personal preferences may overlap with an objective
view of need or be completely different, as summarized in Figure 5.4.

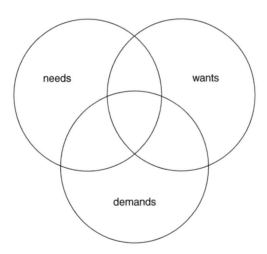

Figure 5.4   Needs, wants, demands

'Demand' is often linked to a broader principle of 'supply and demand' in economics (Woodall
and Cross, 2021). Mooney and Leeder (1997) describe demands as being based on wants, but
also involving action directed at fulfilling the wants. There is a clear parallel here with Bradshaw's
expressed need. Whether or not we accept that there are objective needs, decisions about the best
ways in which to achieve them will inevitably involve a degree of subjectivity. For some, the very
nature of needs remains subjectively determined. Therefore, the issue of values – both personal and
professional – cannot be ignored. At the most fundamental level, the distinction between needs,

wants and demands is value-laden. In short, there is rarely, if ever, enough resource to meet demands (Woodall and Cross, 2021) and this leads to the related question of who should arbitrate when there are conflicting views (Bartholomew et al., 2001).

A reductionist approach to needs assessment

The pursuit of the lowest-level causes of phenomena is referred to as 'reductionism'. Bringing a reductionist perspective to bear on the identification of needs would involve identifying the main health problems and constructing a causal chain that progressively homes in on factors that might be modified – that is, those factors that need to be changed to improve health status. Such a diagnostic approach would be very much in tune with the biomedical model of health promotion discussed in Chapter 1 and the public health approach to identifying needs referred to above. It could take either quality of life or disease as its starting point. This way of identifying needs would also equate with Bartholomew et al.'s view that a need is 'a difference between what currently exists and a more desirable state' (2001: 16). It typically draws heavily on epidemiological analyses and, by way of example, Figure 5.5 shows how it might apply to coronary heart disease.

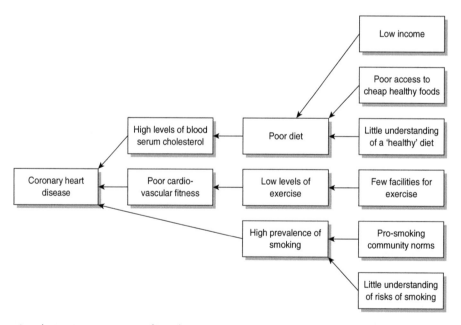

Figure 5.5   A reductionist assessment of need

The emphasis is on identifying modifiable risk factors. This approach has been criticized for attaching undue importance to behavioural risk factors. However, it could equally implicate social and environmental risk factors as the major determinants of problems. A further area of interest is the existence of any high-risk groups, defined as 'a group with a definable boundary and shared characteristics that have, or are at risk for, certain health and quality-of-life problems' (Bartholomew et al., 2001: 17).

As we will note below, reference can be made to major empirical studies and theoretical models to establish a framework for this type of enquiry. Such frameworks can be used to direct research at the local level towards identifying the key causative or contributory factors that should be considered when planning interventions. Analysis at the local level can then focus on identifying which of the generally recognized risk factors are the most pertinent in a specific context. As an example, a needs assessment of women in Al Ain, United Arab Emirates, identified using a cross-sectional survey that the prevalence of obesity in this group was very high and this in turn was used to focus health promotion interventions (Carter et al., 2011a). Green and Kreuter (1991) suggest that one advantage of this approach is that it allows workers to direct their efforts at achieving maximum gains. However, it does not formally acknowledge the value of community insights or gaining the active involvement of members of the community.

Participation in needs assessment

The importance of community participation was recognized in the Ottawa Charter (WHO, 1986) and reaffirmed since in global health promotion conferences and declarations.

The overall aim of involving lay, or community members, in the needs assessment process is to understand issues from the community, rather than professional, perspective. Perspectives can be ascertained using a myriad of approaches, including: informal discussion, focus groups, household surveys and interviews. Arguments supporting public participation in needs assessment can be based on the rights of individuals to have a voice and also, more pragmatically, on the premise that participation fosters higher levels of motivation and enhances the effectiveness of interventions (Watson, 2002). Participation can be a means to bridging the gap between planners and the community. As we noted in Chapter 3, when a community recognizes the existence of a problem and identifies its own solution, then adoption of an innovation is likely to be much more rapid than when an external agency prescribes a solution for a problem that the community was not aware of or does not consider to be a priority. Communities can also become a powerful voice for policy change when they are aware of unmet health needs.

Freire (1972) uses the term 'cultural invasion' for external agents bringing their own value systems to bear on the analysis of problems. The limitations of such top-down assessment of need are summed up by Gough (1992: 12):

Experts and professionals can put their own interest before the wellbeing of their clients or research subjects. Often too they will be so ignorant of the reality of life for ordinary people that their proposals can be counterproductive or just plain stupid.

BOX 5.2 HEALTH NEEDS AND PRIORITIES OF SYRIAN REFUGEES IN CAMPS AND URBAN SETTINGS IN JORDAN: PERSPECTIVES OF REFUGEES AND HEALTHCARE PROVIDERS

Research has shown some diametrically opposed perspectives between lay and professional perspectives. Syrian refugees in camps and urban areas reported their primary health concerns as poor living conditions; transportation challenges; cost of basic foods; insecurity; and mental ill-health, such as post-traumatic stress disorder and depression. In contrast, health professionals perceived that acute conditions (respiratory illness, fever, diarrhoea and injuries); high smoking rates; and a lack of necessary documentation such as marriage and birth certificates as the major concerns facing this population.

Source: Al-Rousan et al. (2018)

Knowledge held in the community must, therefore, become an integral part of any needs assessment. It offers a complementary insight that should be considered alongside epidemiological and economic approaches. For example, a health needs assessment of American Indians in Tulsa, Oklahoma, utilized a community advisory board to review and provide input on the assessment (purpose, design, methodology, instrument development and results); this board was made up of professionals alongside tribal elders and leaders, parents and young people (Johnson et al., 2010). A further example is provided in Box 5.2. Moreover, others have suggested that the use of 'citizens' juries' is a useful approach to ascertain local involvement in health assessments and decision-making (Laverack, 2014; Wells et al., 2021). The jury reaches a verdict on local issues and is often asked to consider questions such as, 'What would improve the health and well-being of residents in your community?' Studies have indicated that these are a practical and inexpensive way of gaining the lay voice (King et al., 2011; Ritter and McLauchlan, 2022). However, this clearly raises the issue of the weight attached to the views of the public in contrast to those of so-called professionals and how to deal with any differences. Comparison of the professionals' views of priorities in an area with the actual priorities of the community that emerged from a rapid assessment of women's psychosocial health needs (Lazenbatt and McMurray, 2004) demonstrates only too clearly how professional assessments can differ markedly from those of the communities concerned, as shown in Table 5.1.

Three decades ago, Stacey (1994) advanced the term 'people knowledge' to 'lay knowledge' as the term 'lay' often carries connotations of having less competence or worth. 'People knowledge' is often informal, experiential and mostly unwritten. It offers insights into the constellation of factors particular to specific situations from the perspective of those who are most familiar with them. The professional perspective, in contrast, draws on codified and systematized knowledge, often operating at a more general level.

Table 5.1   Mean ranks of women's psychosocial health needs in Northern Ireland (lowest score = highest priority)

	GP team view *n* = 6	PRA team view *n* = 6	Community view *n* = 25
Physical environment			
Political boundaries	1.9	1.5	1.8
Transport	2.0	1.8	1.6
Lack of facilities	3.0	2.9	2.2
Disease			
Breast cancer	2.1	2.0	1.7
Cervical cancer	2.4	2.9	2.4
Heart disease	1.5	2.1	2.3
Psychosocial health issues			
Depression	2.1	3.1	3.2
Stress	2.7	2.9	2.9
Anxiety and fear	3.1	2.8	2.7
Lifestyle			
Smoking	2.1	3.1	3.2
Alcohol problems	3.0	3.1	4.4
Access to services			
Baby clinic	3.4	2.7	2.4
Well-woman clinic	2.8	3.2	2.3
Asthma clinic	1.9	1.9	3.2
Socioeconomic			
Poverty	2.4	1.9	1.6
Unemployment	2.2	1.8	1.6
Low pay	3.0	2.8	2.7

PRA = Participatory rural appraisal

Source: Derived from Lazenbatt and McMurray (2004: 181)

Stacey is critical of the pressure to express lay understanding in official language and use acceptable research methods – that is, to operate within professionally defined parameters – and draws a number of lessons about participation:

- people's points of view should be understood in their own terms
- the distinction between people and professional is not rigid
- people knowledge is consistent and rational
- people are producers of health as well as consumers of healthcare
- lack of real influence in decisions alienates people from participation.

The Freirean notion of 'cultural synthesis' describes a situation in which professionals or external agents attempt to learn *with* the people about their experiences of the world.

Public participation in needs assessment can range from tokenistic consultation to having a controlling influence in arriving at what the needs are and how they should be prioritized. Arnstein's (1969) ladder of participation (see Figure 5.6) is a well-known device for distinguishing between genuine participation, mere tokenism and, indeed, attempts to manipulate. The degree of active participation increases progressively from none at the bottom to genuine control at the top.

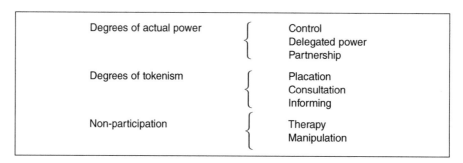

Figure 5.6   Arnstein's ladder of participation (after Arnstein, 1969)

Brager and Specht (1973) provide a similar analysis of the spectrum of participation. Their depiction of the various levels is particularly pertinent to health promotion planning and needs assessment.

A further consideration – over and above the actual level of participation – is the motivation underpinning attempts to involve communities. Clearly, the chief beneficiary of participation in needs assessment and planning processes should be the community itself. Participation should not be a covert means of furthering professional or organizational interests – a situation graphically encapsulated in a French student poster from the 1960s (see Box 5.3).

BOX 5.3 COMMUNITY PARTICIPATION: DECLINING THE VERB

Je participe

Tu participes

Il/elle participe

Nous participons

Vous participez

Ils profitent

A number of different vehicles have been used for consultation. These include postal panels, face-to-face panels, local involvement networks (LINks), local user and carer groups and surveys and opinion polls.

A further issue relates to the representativeness of the various groups. Clearly, surveys can explicitly attempt to obtain representative samples. In contrast, the selection of jury members, as discussed earlier, is usually more purposive and, despite membership generally rotating at intervals, cannot be regarded as being truly representative. There are several examples whereby the sample of people sharing their views may not be coherent or consistent with the demography or expressing the widely held views of the wider community (Kashefi and Mort, 2004; Ritter and McLauchlan, 2022). There are similar concerns about the composition of user and carer consultation groups and citizen panels.

Another pertinent issue is whether individuals are commenting on behalf of themselves or the group that they purport to represent – especially when there may be conflict between individual and community needs. Furthermore, within any community, the more articulate will inevitably be better placed to make their concerns known. Particular attention will, therefore, need to be paid to ensuring that the views of more marginalized groups are included. A variety of methods is likely to be needed to fully engage communities and the process itself can accordingly be resource intensive (Hubley et al., 2020).

The key aspects of the 'informed citizen process', which takes account of some of these concerns, are summarized by Blackwell and Kosky (2000):

- **information** – people must be presented with accurate, unbiased information
- **time** – sufficient time must be allowed to be informed and to be able to reflect
- **scrutiny** – opportunity must be provided to ask questions before making preferences
- **deliberation** – there must be a chance to reflect on information given
- **independence** – participants must have some control over how their findings are presented and to whom
- **authority** – participants must feel assured that their findings will be listened to.

In addition to improving understanding of health needs, participation can mobilize individuals and communities as agents for social change. Case study 5.1 provides an example of a project that has continued to inform sustainable change after its inception. It uses community-based participatory research, defined as:

A collaborative approach to research that equitably involves all partners in the research process and recognises the unique strength that each brings. [It] begins with a topic of importance to the community with the aim of combining knowledge and action for social change to improve community health and eliminate disparities. (Community Health Scholars Program, 2002, cited in Minkler et al., 2006: 294)

CASE STUDY 5.1 A COMMUNITY-BASED PARTICIPATORY RESEARCH PARTNERSHIP FOR HEALTH PROMOTION IN INDIANA

Initial partners:	University School of Nursing
	Healthy Cities Committee
Other key stakeholders:	included Members of City Council, newspaper editor, Fire Chief
Goal:	making the healthy choice the easy choice through changes in 'small p policies'
Methods used:	• data from census
	• door-to-door survey of 1000 households
	• mobilizing the community by raising awareness of health issues identified by the survey as compared with national health objectives (e.g. local smoking rate was double the national objective)
	• five health priorities established (smoking, exercise, alcohol use and abuse, mental health, dietary choices)
	• focus groups
	• statewide workshops, including sessions on data interpretation, priority setting, policy change
	• development of alliances between key stakeholders.
Achievements:	increased concern about health among the community – early: non-smoking areas in all city buildings; medium-term: building a playground on city owned land by 1200 community volunteers; longer-term: development of trails to encourage physical activity land use policy.

Source: Minkler et al. (2006)

Rapid assessment and appraisal

Rapid assessment techniques have their origin in the broad move towards community participation and recognition of the need for local knowledge. They emerged in lower-income countries as a response to inappropriate research by outside agencies – typified by overconfidence, lack of communication and consultation with the community or other professional groups, the use of theoretically rigorous but time-consuming methods and failure to translate research findings into action within a reasonable timescale (Vlassoff and Tanner, 1992).

Rapid assessment and appraisal attempts to overcome professional dominance and works towards developing a joint understanding of the needs of the community by bringing together the views of key stakeholders. It places emphasis on knowledge indigenous to a community and acknowledges the importance of qualitative research methods. However, it does not preclude the need for quantitative data (Kansiime et al., 2021).

A variety of terminology is used in relation to rapid assessment and appraisal, as summarized in Box 5.4. In the literature, a clear distinction has not always been made – indeed, some authors have used the terms interchangeably. Rifkin (1992), however, identifies two broad strands, which helps to resolve the semantic confusion. One emerged from epidemiology and is concerned with collecting information on ill health and disease – usually referred to as 'rapid assessment' or 'rapid epidemiological assessment'. It draws on all forms of local data, including routinely collected data and the views of the community, but the role of the community members is generally as informants only.

BOX 5.4 TERMINOLOGY FOR RAPID APPROACHES

REA Rapid epidemiological assessment

RA Rapid appraisal

RRA Rapid rural appraisal

PRA Participatory rural appraisal

PA Participatory appraisal

PNA Participatory needs assessment

RPA Rapid participatory appraisal

REA Rapid ethnographic assessment

PLA Participatory learning and action

The second strand originated in the 'rapid rural appraisal' techniques developed in the 1970s for use in agriculture and rural development and the move from extractive to participative methods of research. It gives greater attention to the *process* of gathering data and involving communities in data collection and analysis. This latter approach is referred to as 'rapid appraisal'. The terms 'participatory rural appraisal' and 'participatory appraisal' are also used and, as these names imply, they place particular emphasis on community participation.

The distinction between the two broad strands revolves around the level and nature of participation and the emphasis on particular methodologies. Is the assessment merely community-*based* or is it community-*led*, taking its direction from issues raised by the community?

Notwithstanding this difference, there is some overlap between the two schools. Both take a holistic view of health and aim to collect information quickly and at low cost to inform planning at the local level.

The use of the term 'rapid' should not be taken to imply any sacrifice of rigour or attention to quality. Speed is in some instances paramount and was highlighted during the response to COVID-19, where a range of rapid assessment and appraisal techniques were used in communities (Kansiime et al., 2021;

WHO, 2020). Other examples have shown the importance of speed – the Joint Rapid Assessment of Northern Syria was conducted during the conflict to ascertain the situation of conditions on the ground; the assessment found that more than 12.9 million people lack access to basic services of food, water and shelter (Coutts and Fouad, 2013). Speed is achieved by using a battery of research methods and involving a range of professionals and lay people. A rapid assessment of health needs in Aceh Jaya District, Indonesia, after the tsunami of 2004, for example, used a myriad of methods to collect quantitative and qualitative data in a timely manner. This included: observations obtained from the air and during a comprehensive walk around the community; interviews with key informants; a focus group discussion with local women; a review of medical records; and a questionnaire; indeed online methods and approaches have also been used to improve the rapid nature of this kind of assessment of health (Brennan and Rimba, 2005; Kansiime et al., 2021). There is, however, no emerging consensus on how long a 'rapid' assessment should take, with variability from 90 days to 6 months being reported in the literature (Vindrola-Padros et al., 2020).

Accuracy is also a major concern and triangulation is an important feature in relation to cross-checking the validity of findings (triangulation is considered more fully in Chapter 11). Rapid assessment and appraisal strategies usually incorporate opportunities, while still in the field, to reflect on findings and redefine data collection requirements in the light of any emergent conclusions or hunches. While there is considerable attention to validity, it should also be noted that this is counter-balanced with pragmatism and striking an equilibrium between rigour and resource (both time and financial resources) (Murphy et al., 2018). Heaver (1992: 14) sums this up as follows:

> The principles apply here of optimal ignorance – not trying to find out more than is needed; and of appropriate imprecision – not trying to measure what does not need to be measured, or not measuring more accurately than is needed for practical purposes.

Rapid appraisal techniques not only gather objective sources of information, but often also the perceptions and feelings of local communities or the health workforce itself (Mitchinson et al., 2021). For example, although the actual number of people using hard drugs within a community may be small, drug use may have consequences for a much wider group and, therefore, be perceived to be a major problem.

Heaver (1992) identifies a number of advantages of these approaches over and above speed and economy:

- the information generated is accurate and context-specific as it draws on people's in-depth understanding of the local situation and provides opportunities for cross-checking
- plans drawn up by insiders are more likely to work than ones created by those outside the community because they take account of the local context
- the process is empowering – it enhances people's understanding of problems and enables them to have a voice in decisions made about the most appropriate course of action.

Annett and Rifkin (1990) represent the key information needs of a community as a pyramid (see Figure 5.7). Data can be collected from a number of different sources and using a range of different methods for each of the levels.

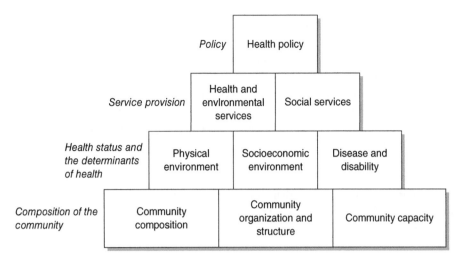

Figure 5.7   Information profile (derived from Annett and Rifkin, 1990)

The data collection methods used in rapid appraisal are many and varied. The use of visual and oral methods is particularly appropriate where there are low levels of literacy. The methods used in participatory appraisal are only limited by the creativity of individuals involved in the process, time and resources. Nevertheless, common techniques include:

- mapping
- transects
- social mapping
- body mapping
- timelines and trends, including seasonal trends
- historical transects
- photography
- ranking and scoring exercises
- sequence matrices
- causal and flow diagramming
- chapatti (Venn) diagramming
- case histories
- life histories
- diaries
- focus groups
- observations.

Professionals may well require training in the use of these methods. Moreover, if they are to operate within a true spirit of participation, they will also need to abandon their expert role and go into a community prepared to learn from the people – communication and listening skills are, therefore, particularly important. Similarly, if members of the community are to be more than just informants, they will also need to develop skills in data collection methods and interpretation. Online approaches to gathering information has also become commonplace and many rapid appraisal approaches have harnessed technology to optimize the data gathered.

An important practical issue is the selection of key informants and ensuring that they are representative of the community. How this should best be tackled will require consideration of local contextual factors. Chua et al.'s (2013) rapid rural appraisal in a village in Sabah, Malaysia, identified several groups of key informants:

- the head of the village
- the president and secretary of the village managing committee
- the assistant headmistresses of the local primary and secondary schools
- a random sample of villagers.

Moreover, in a rapid assessment of frontline healthcare workers' experiences with personal protective equipment during the COVID-19 pandemic in the UK, the following key personnel were identified to participate: doctor; nurse; medical associate professional; pharmacist; dietician; speech and language therapist; clinical support staff; management.

Chouinard and Cousins (2015) discuss the politics and power relations that are often inherent in participatory styles of evaluation. They highlight three key areas of power within the participatory evaluation context: relational, political and discursive. Relational power concerns the interpersonal relations between diverse stakeholder groups and how these play out in the participatory process. Political power refers to the potential barriers that may inhibit all members of the community from participation – those with power may deter marginalized or less powerful groups from participating in the process. Finally, discursive power is the least tangible but concerns the 'internalised norms and values that guide evaluation practice and that ultimately prevent some voices from being included in the process' (Chouinard and Cousins, 2015: 12).

The principles of participatory appraisal would require that the community should not merely be used as providers of information to slot into a conceptual framework already established by the researchers. True participation would involve the community members in developing the conceptual framework. It would also view them as equal partners in decision-making – especially if the tokenism referred to by Arnstein (1969) is to be avoided.

It will be clear from our earlier discussion of empowerment in Chapter 3 that community involvement in rapid appraisal and participatory appraisal can be empowering, with some arguing that the process of capacity-building and skill development in communities is the greatest strength of the approach (Chouinard and Cousins, 2015). The value of community members' knowledge and experience can be formally acknowledged and they can exercise power and control in decision-making and planning. However, there is always the risk of raising expectations that cannot be met, with consequent negative repercussions.

The key features of rapid and participatory appraisal can be summarized as:

- the community is involved in information collection and analysis – that is, they are done in/with/ and by the community

- action-orientated nature
- attempts to include all perspectives
- use of multidisciplinary teams and interactive methods
- emphasis on communication and listening skills
- use of a range of data collection methods and triangulation
- analysis is carried out while still 'in the field'
- iterative nature
- incorporates critical reflection and self-criticism
- flexibility – the direction of research may be reorientated as new information becomes available
- a holistic view of health and its determinants
- optimal ignorance and appropriate imprecision.

While developing countries have paved the way in the use of these methods, there has also been increasing interest in higher-income countries, certainly in response to the COVID-19 pandemic where information on a myriad of issues, for example personal protective equipment (Hoernke et al., 2021), was needed. Chouinard and Cousins (2015: 13) argue that the application of participatory techniques is different in lower- and higher-income countries – they suggest that 'the cultural, social, political and economic complexity across contexts, as well as the ongoing history of donor–recipient relationships in much of the developing world' create significant challenges. Participatory techniques have also been used in more diffuse communities, such as conflict-affected populations; sex workers; and prisoners (Chiyaka et al., 2018; Martin et al., 2009; Murphy et al., 2018). They have also been used with young people as a means to giving them a voice. Vaughan (2014), for example, describes a participatory health research project conducted with Papua New Guinean youth. The project focused on photovoice as a way to elicit the young people's views.

Critical reflections on participatory appraisal

Participatory appraisal has grown rapidly in popularity and has received huge financial support (Chouinard and Cousins, 2015). Cornwall and Pratt (2011) argue that participatory appraisal, particularly participatory rural appraisal (PRA), has been open to abuse since its origins in the late 1980s. They feel that the range of meanings of participatory appraisal, different conceptualizations of what it involves and the variety of practices carried out under its name, threaten its quality and create difficulties in establishing quality standards. A concern is that people may subscribe to the rhetoric without fully embracing the principles.

While recognizing the potential offered by rapid appraisal and the rewarding nature of working in this way, there are several valid criticisms of the approach (Murray, 1999; Vindrola-Padros et al., 2020). It tends to work best when there is a clearly defined, homogeneous community. Bias may occur if the informants selected have similar backgrounds and there is no conscious attempt to seek out any contradictory viewpoints. There may also be professional bias unless a multidisciplinary team is used and, in any event, there may be a degree of subjectivity in interpreting what people say. Any statistics generated may need to be interpreted with caution because of the rapid and highly focused nature of data collection.

Ethical review processes can be cumbersome and preclude rapid assessment from being undertaken. Where there are health emergencies, ethical review panels need to be swift and proportionate but there are several instances where this has not been the case (Vindrola-Padros et al., 2020). Further criticism centres on specific practical and methodological issues, including how lengthy or in some cases 'rushed' the process is and the quality of data produced. Moreover, some have highlighted the challenge of the timely sharing of findings so they could be used to inform decision-making and inform changes in practice – although this can be overcome by utilizing creative sources of dissemination, such as infographics (Vindrola-Padros et al., 2020). What is consistent in the literature is that the approach tends to work best when it conforms to a true spirit of participation and follows an agenda established by the community – a position that requires considerable skills in listening and facilitation on the part of those involved in the process. Problems tend to arise when the findings have to be slotted into a pre-existing agenda, which can lead to a mismatch between what the community is saying and what planners want to hear. As a method of working, it goes beyond merely providing a technical response to the issues of problem definition and solution generation to contributing to empowering communities by virtue of the value it places on individuals' contributions.

BOX 5.5 COMMON FINDINGS OF NEEDS ASSESSMENT EXERCISES

- Pollution and the environment
- Housing
- Employment
- Poor education and recreational facilities
- Vandalism and crime
- Transport
- Loneliness, stress and mental health
- Other diseases and disability
- Information on, and availability of, general practitioner and social services.

COMMUNITY PROFILES

Whichever way problems and needs are defined, additional information about the population or community is needed before decisions can be made about health promotion interventions and how they will be implemented. Hubley et al. (2020) emphasize the importance of getting to know the community as well as analysing its problems. A community profile will include information relevant to the assessment of needs, together with this wider contextual information. Some of the information may already be available in the form of records and published surveys; this information may need to be supplemented by gathering data directly from the community through surveys, interviews with key informants and community groups.

Nykiforuk and Flaman (2011: 69) define community health profiling as:

> the compilation and mapping of information regarding the health of a population in a community. Profiles can include data on health outcomes as well as direct and indirect factors that influence health. Sociodemographic characteristics, disease morbidity and mortality, health behaviors (e.g., physical activity, tobacco use, sexual practices), and policies (e.g., smoking bans, pesticide legislation) are just a few examples of variables that can be used. In profiling, these variables are linked with the spatial location of community infrastructure such as churches, restaurants, schools, grocery stores, hospitals and clinics, roads, and public utilities. This linkage, when done appropriately, permits examination of the general relationships between health and setting.

It provides a basis for setting priorities and planning. Community profiling should also take a strengths-based or asset-based approach to the population, identifying attributes and capabilities as well as the more traditional focus on weaknesses and inadequacies (see Box 5.6). The profile is the product of a process of community analysis. The term 'community diagnosis' has also been used, particularly in the North American context. Comparing community diagnosis with needs assessment, Stuart (in Quinn, 1999: 685) stated that:

> Diagnosis is much broader and aims to understand many facets of the community including culture, values and norms, leadership and power structure, means of communication, helping patterns, important community institutions and history. A good diagnosis suggests what it is like to live in a community, what the important health problems are, what interventions are likely to be most efficacious, and how the program would be best evaluated.

Although the two terms are synonymous, our preference here is to use 'community analysis', which we feel gives a better sense of the broad remit of the process and an emphasis on the positive aspects of a community. It reduces the risk of misinterpretation arising from associating the word 'diagnosis' with a narrow focus on the identification of problems.

As with the assessment of needs, a community analysis may be undertaken from a biomedical perspective or adopt community development principles and a more participative approach. It will include both quantitative and qualitative information derived from a variety of different sources, both primary and secondary.

There are several features of a community that would require consideration; some these include:

- specification of geographical boundaries
- assessment of social institutions – health, leisure, faith, education and so on
- identification of social interaction patterns
- examination of social control mechanisms and norms, both formal, via institutions such as the police, school and church, and informal, via values, norms and customs in the community. (Haglund et al., 1990; Hubley et al., 2020; Mulcahy and Downey, 2021)

BOX 5.6 DIFFERENT COMMUNITIES, DIFFERENT INTERVENTIONS

Community A:

- traditional
- homogeneous
- family ties and hierarchies within families important
- religious
- church leaders respected
- school curriculum controlled at national level – no provision for sex education
- general reluctance to talk about sex
- media are tightly controlled
- strong censorship laws
- strong sense of community.

Community B:

- progressive
- heterogeneous
- variety of different family structures and ties
- few members of the community belong to any religion
- schools are required to provide sex education, although the quality varies between schools
- young people laugh and joke among themselves about sex, but feel uncomfortable talking to their parents or teachers about it
- little control over the media
- censorship is very liberal and there is a considerable amount of sexually explicit material in the media
- no real sense of community.

Responding to the problem of HIV/AIDS would demand completely different intervention strategies in these two communities.

While establishing geographical boundaries is important in delimiting the area of enquiry, it should be noted that communities are not necessarily defined in geographical terms – they can be based on shared characteristics, such as ethnicity, gender, sexual orientation and disability. The concept of 'community' will be discussed further in Chapter 9.

Bartholomew et al. (2001) comment on the importance of assessing community competence, capacity and social capital because of their relevance as:

- **inputs** – factors that contribute directly to health promotion intervention
- **throughputs** – factors that will affect successful programme implementation
- **outputs** – the products of programmes.

'Community competence' focuses on how a community is currently functioning. The concept of 'community capacity' is closely related. It includes the notion of current competence, but also the potential within the community to respond to issues of common concern. There has been increasing emphasis on the concept of community capacity and some contemporary discussion about its role in health promotion (Nutbeam and Muscat, 2021); however, there has been relatively little attempt to define it, with some noting that the term covers 'almost any activity in the community health promotion domain, so it becomes somewhat academic to be too precise about terminological boundaries' (Raeburn et al., 2006: 85). Box 5.7 provides an overview of some of the definitions used.

BOX 5.7 SOME DEFINITIONS OF 'COMMUNITY CAPACITY'

Community capacity is defined as both a process and an outcome that requires collaborative action to promote healthy public policy and address systemic and structural inequities of community needs.

Source: Clark (2018: 246)

the characteristics of communities that affect their ability to identify, mobilize and address social and public health problems.

Source: McLeroy (1996), in Bartholomew et al. (2001: 26)

the degree to which a community can develop, implement and sustain actions for strengthening community health.

Source: Smith et al. (2001: 33)

Reference to our earlier discussion of social capital in Chapter 2 will confirm the considerable overlap with community capacity. However, social capital tends to focus on the networks, relationships and structural conditions rather than the resources that can be tapped into, material or otherwise (Warwick-Booth and Foster, 2020). Eight verifiable domains of social capital have been identified and are listed in Table 5.2. The notion of social cohesion is also closely related and refers to the bonds within communities based on shared social and cultural commitments.

The domains of community cohesion are listed in Table 5.2, along with the domains of social capital.

Table 5.2 The domains of social capital and community cohesion

Domain	Description
Social capital	
Empowerment	People feel that they have a voice that is listened to, are involved in processes that affect them, can themselves take action to initiate changes
Participation	People take part in social and community activities. Local events occur and are well attended
Associational activity and common purpose	People cooperate with one another by forming formal and informal groups to further their interests
Supporting networks and reciprocity	Individuals cooperate to support one another for either mutual or one-sided gain. An expectation that help would be given to, or received from, others when needed
Collective norms and values	People share common values and norms of behaviour
Trust	People feel that they can trust their co-residents and local organizations responsible for governing or serving their area
Safety	People feel safe in their neighbourhood and are not restricted in their use of public space by fear
Belonging	People feel connected to their co-residents, their home area, have a sense of belonging to the place and its people
Community cohesion	
Common values and a civic culture	Common aims and objectives, common moral principles and codes of behaviour, support for political institutions and participation in politics
Social order and social control	Absence of general conflict and threats to the existing order, absence of incivility, effective informal social control, tolerance, respect for differences, intergroup cooperation
Social solidarity and reductions in wealth disparities	Harmonious economic and social development and common standards, redistribution of public finances and opportunities, equal access to services and welfare benefits, ready acknowledgement of social obligations and willingness to assist others
Social networks and social capital	High degree of social interaction within communities and families, civic engagement and associational activity, easy resolution of collective action problems
Place attachment and identity	Strong attachment to place, intertwining of personal and place identity

Source: Forrest and Kearns (2000), in Home Office Community Cohesion Review Team (2001)

ABSTRACT 5.1

Perceptions of needs, assets, and priorities among black men who have sex with men with HIV: community-driven actions and impacts of a participatory photovoice process. Sun, C.J., Nall, J.L. and Rhodes, S.D. (2019)

Black men who have sex with men (MSM) with HIV experience significant health inequities and poorer health outcomes compared with other persons with HIV. The primary aims of this study were to describe the needs, assets and priorities of Black MSM with HIV who live in the Southern United States and identify actions to improve their health using photovoice. Photovoice, a participatory, collaborative research methodology that combines documentary photography with group discussion, was conducted with six Black MSM with HIV. From the photographs and discussions, primary themes of discrimination and rejection, lack of mental health services, coping strategies to reduce stress, sources of acceptance and support, and future aspirations emerged. After the photographs were taken and discussed, the participants hosted a photo exhibition and community forum for the public. Here, 37 community attendees and influential advocates collaborated with the participants to identify 12 actions to address the men's identified needs, assets and priorities. These included making structural changes in the legal and medical systems, encouraging dialogue to eliminate multiple forms of stigma and racism, and advocating for comprehensive care for persons with HIV. As a secondary aim, the impacts of photovoice were assessed. Participants reported enjoying photovoice and found it meaningful. Results suggest that in addition to cultivating rich community-based knowledge, photovoice may result in positive changes for Black MSM with HIV.

More recently, the identification of 'assets' within communities has been strongly supported by health promotion academics and practitioners (Woodall and Cross, 2021). Although this idea is not new, it places a focus on identifying positive aspects of individuals, organizations and communities. For example, assets of organizations may include: buildings, staff time, knowledge and expertise, leadership and so on (Warwick-Booth and Foster, 2020). Asset-based techniques stand in opposition to deficit-style assessments of need, but should not be conceptualized as being incompatible with more traditional techniques. Indeed, it should be regarded as a complementary approach (Brooks and Kendall, 2013).

It would be invidious even to attempt to draw up a generic checklist of all the issues that need to be considered before the detailed planning of interventions to improve the health status of a population can begin. However, they fall into five broad categories that are applicable, regardless of whether there is a professional or community-led approach to data collection and whichever ideological position underpins the endeavour:

- the health status of the population – identification of problems and any groups particularly 'at-risk'
- the key determinants of health status and disease – behavioural and environmental at micro, meso and macro levels
- motivation and capacity to respond – individually and collectively
- channels of communication and patterns of influence
- characteristics of the community and power structures within it and wider society.

Prioritization of health needs

Regardless of the approach taken, it is likely that a number of different health needs will emerge in view of the wide range of factors – both upstream and downstream – which impact on health status. Some prioritization will be necessary. Scriven (2017) argues that prioritization is not an exact science and that this ultimately comes down to normative judgements and resources available. Nonetheless, Cavanagh and Chadwick (2005) propose two initial selection criteria:

- impact – in terms of the severity or magnitude of the problem
- changeability – the feasibility of change.

Decisions can be based on the perceptions of the community, service providers and managers, health data and local, national and organizational priorities. The acceptability of change and the availability of resources are also important considerations. Clearly, the respective emphasis on these different criteria and the value attached to the views of different groups of stakeholders will be influenced by the approach taken to health needs assessment and its underpinning ideology.

SOLUTION GENERATION

The principal dilemma for those involved in health promotion planning is the selection of an appropriate intervention or combination of interventions. To an extent, the options considered will be constrained by ideological commitments. As we have noted in Chapter 1, those who subscribe to the ideology of empowerment will opt to work in participative ways. In contrast, more authoritarian, top-down approaches would be consistent with a preventive model. The range of options can be represented using models – either iconic or analogic (see Box 5.8). There are many models of health promotion that demonstrate a wide range of ideological views and indeed strategies for promoting health (Woodall and Freeman, 2020). Beattie (1991) provides a useful analogic taxonomy of the range of different health promotion approaches.

BOX 5.8 ICONIC AND ANALOGIC MODELS

- Iconic models are descriptors or characterizations that offer a simplified view of a recognized aspect of reality.
- Analogic models provide a framework to assist understanding of reality and use analogies or metaphors that need not necessarily currently exist.

Source: Rawson (1992)

Beattie's model, as represented in Figure 5.8, incorporates two fundamental dimensions – the mode of intervention, which ranges from authoritative to negotiated, and the focus of intervention, which is either on the individual or the collective. An individual's personal and professional values will have a bearing on the preferred mode of operation, but critics have noted how the model reinforces the extremes of agency and structure and overlooks nuance and more sophisticated ecological approaches (Woodall and Freeman, 2020).

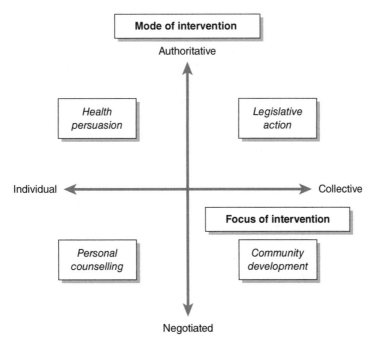

Figure 5.8   Beattie's model of health promotion (Beattie, 1991)

Rawson notes that the advantage of analogic models over iconic models is that they have a theoretical structure, which can assimilate new forms of practice. However, the disadvantage is that 'they may seem remote from the detail of reality' (1992: 211). Clearly, the demarcation between authoritative and negotiated approaches is not absolute (Woodall and Freeman, 2020). Rather, they represent polar extremes, with some possible gradation between the two. For example, we have already observed that community participation can range from a minimal, tokenistic consultation to the community having genuine control and a recognized decision-making role. Similarly, there is the possibility of differing levels of authoritarian control. Indeed, we might postulate that this could even include the instrumental use of participative methods – not because of any commitment to negotiated styles of working, but because it is the best way to achieve predefined goals. The focus of intervention will also be subject to parallel variation. A collective approach could involve change at the group, setting, community or population level.

Notwithstanding an ideological commitment to broad styles of working, the rational selection of specific methods will be based on a combination of:

- theory
- evidence about effective practice
- context
- professional judgement based on experience.

The role of theory

Recourse to theory will be useful both in pursuing the cause of health problems and in identifying what should be done to tackle them. Indeed, good theory is exceptionally useful to aid practice (Lynch et al., 2018), but most health promotion practitioners and commissioners are unsure what, if any, underlying frameworks or theories they are utilizing. One significant challenge in health promotion practice is applying the right theory to the appropriate practice context. Moreover, the diversity of issues, target groups, settings and contexts often necessitates the use of a plethora of theoretical ideas (Laverack, 2014).

In short, theory supports the identification of key relevant variables and helps practitioners and academics in their thinking and intervention development (Lynch et al., 2018). Explanatory theory will guide the search for modifiable risk factors. For example, if the proportion of young people taking up smoking has been implicated as the problem, a health action model (HAM) analysis would direct attention towards exploring the principal determinants of young people's behavioural intention concerning smoking – that is, their belief, motivation and normative systems and self-concept. Furthermore, investigation of any factors that facilitate or act as a barrier to their translating intentions into practice would also be required.

In contrast, change theory will inform decisions about the most appropriate strategy. It will make clear any assumptions underpinning the chosen strategy and also check that all the necessary elements of the intervention are in place (see Box 5.9).

BOX 5.9 A VIEW OF THEORY AND PROFESSIONAL PRACTICE

Like an expert chef, a theoretically grounded health education professional does not blindly follow a cookbook recipe, but constantly creates it anew, depending on the circumstances. Without a theory, she or he has only the skills of a cafeteria line worker.

Source: National Cancer Institute (1997)

Unless a full, rational appraisal of the problem and possible solutions is undertaken, interventions might easily:

- address wrong or inappropriate variables – that is, miss the target completely
- tackle only a proportion of the variables required to have the desired effect – that is, hit only a few of the total possible targets and not enough to achieve any meaningful change. (Green, 2000)

The potential for theory to guide the development of interventions and programmes is substantial (Nutbeam et al., 2010):

> Interventions without a clear theoretical rationale almost always fail or achieve only a semblance of success that disappears when submitted to critical examination. (Eiser and Eiser, 1996: 43)

However, this type of theoretical analysis of problems and possible solutions is not without its critics. It has been aligned with authoritarian, individualistic approaches and the preventive model discussed in Chapter 1. A particular concern is that it objectifies human experience and is, therefore, inconsistent with the central tenets of health promotion – holism and empowerment. Buchanan (1994) attributes scepticism about the relevance of theory to health promotion practice to a narrow view of theory equated with the natural sciences and positivism. This interpretation of theory would see it as establishing the relationships between factors (independent variables) and some outcome (dependent variable). It should also be possible to predict the changes in outcome that would be caused by manipulation of the independent variable/s and, indeed, verify this by testing. The role of the health promoter would, therefore, simply be to identify and change the relevant independent variables to achieve the desired outcome. Failure to achieve success would demand a more thorough and detailed analysis of the variables and ever more precise targeting and tailoring of interventions. 'Targeting' involves designing interventions to suit the characteristics of particular subgroups (such as age, gender, ethnicity, social class, occupational group), whereas 'tailoring' adapts interventions to meet the specific requirements of individuals.

Noar and Zimmerman (2005) argue that, although there are numerous health behaviour theories, there is no consensus about which offers most precision in explaining health behaviour. One important thing to consider in theory selection is the appropriateness-of-fit, which is determined by each study's needs and aims, rather than there being a 'wrong' choice *per se* (Lynch et al., 2018). Further, despite the similarity between the constructs of different theories, the use of different terminology gives the illusion that they are different. They call for more empirical testing and comparison of theories in order to refine them as a means of understanding health behaviour.

Buchanan, in contrast, contends that human action is not governed in the same law-like way as natural processes and, hence, the methods used to study natural phenomena cannot be applied to human behaviour. The role of human agency in constructing reality is well recognized in this regard (see Box 5.10).

BOX 5.10 HUMAN AGENCY AND REALITY

Human beings are not 'things' to be studied in the way one studies ants, plants or rocks, but are valuing, meaning attributing beings to be understood as subjects and known as subjects ... To impose positivistic meanings upon the realm of social phenomena is to distort the fundamental nature of human existence.

Source: Hughes (1976: 25)

Buchanan (1994: 274) does not reject the need for theory *per se*, but calls for a broader conceptualization of theory that recognizes that 'knowledge is contingent and contextual rather than universal, determinate and invariable'. The purpose of theory, then, is not to offer universal explanations or predictions, but to clarify understanding of complex situations (Lynch et al., 2018). It therefore needs to interplay with a range of contextual factors. This is further reiterated by Nutbeam et al. (2010: 7):

Ultimately, theories and models are simplified representations of reality; they can never include or explain all of the complexities of individual, social or organizational behaviours. However, while the use of theory alone does not guarantee effective programs, the use of theory in the planning, execution and evaluation of programs will enhance the chance of success.

Buchanan proposes Aristotle's notion of *phronesis* or 'practical reason' as a means of understanding the unique features of each situation. This contrasts with *episteme* or 'theoretical knowledge' based on universal laws that Aristotle himself recognized could not capture the complexity of the social world. Practical reason (Buchanan, 1994: 279) is the:

> ability to recognize, acknowledge, pick out and respond to the singular salient features of a complex and unique situation. It is not deduction from abstract generalizations ... Practical reason is the thinking process involved in deciding what to say or how to do that which best suits the particular situation at hand. Practical reason is involved in weighing which of the available courses of action is more appropriate given the specific circumstances.

Theory, then, can provide important insights into the nature of problems and the strategies that could be adopted. As Kurt Lewin is famously noted to have said, 'there is nothing so practical as a good theory' (Marrow, 1969). However, as we have noted above, an abstract analysis alone is insufficient. A complementary understanding of specific contextual factors is also required before a decision can be made about the most appropriate course of action.

CASE STUDY 5.2 THE USE OF THE HEALTH BELIEF MODEL TO UNDERSTAND FACTORS ASSOCIATED WITH THE ACCEPTABILITY OF SOLAR DISINFECTION OF DRINKING WATER IN NEPAL

Uptake of solar disinfection (SODIS) 9%

Beliefs

Beliefs about susceptibility and seriousness:

Don't know what causes diarrhoea
Diarrhoea is a normal situation
Headache, not diarrhoea, was the main reported health problem

Barriers:

Heavy workload
No bottles available

No place to expose bottles all day

Temperature/taste of water different

Solar disinfected water was seen as a 'leftover' and not culturally acceptable

Effectiveness of preventive measures:

Don't know if SODIS works or not

Self-efficacy:

Solar disinfection is easy to understand

Cues to action

Ill family members

Turbidity of water

Presence of researcher during data collection

Efforts to increase uptake would need to address the beliefs of the community.

Source: Derived from Rainey and Harding (2005)

Health promotion has a plethora of theories to draw on (Nutbeam et al., 2010). A key issue concerns the selection of appropriate theory for the task in hand – see Case study 5.2 for an example of the use of the health belief model. The factors that influence health status range from micro-level individual factors to macro-level policy and environmental issues. The various levels of an ecological approach identified by the National Cancer Institute (2005) are:

- intrapersonal level
- interpersonal level
- community level

  o institutional or organizational factors
  o community factors
  o public policy.

Clearly, each level will have its own repertoire of theory to draw on. Lynch et al. (2018) suggest practical ways to select theory and how to implement theoretical considerations before, during and after an intervention. Relevant theory at the intrapersonal level might, for example, include the health belief model (HBM), and theory of planned behaviour (TPB); at the interpersonal level, social cognitive theory; and, at the community level, diffusion of innovations. Some theories will bridge different levels – for example, the health action model (HAM). Comprehensive multilevel approaches will, therefore, need to combine different theories from the different levels of analysis. McLeroy et al. (1993: 305) contend that '*no single theory*, certainly no psychological theory, is adequate for developing truly effective and comprehensive health education programmes'. They also note that there are no guidelines for selecting individual theories, let alone combinations of theories. Box 5.11 lists some key questions to consider when assessing how well a theory is suited to the task.

BOX 5.11   WHICH THEORY?

- Does it include all relevant variables?
- Is it parsimonious (does not include any redundant variables)?
- Does its use make logical sense in the particular situation?
- Has it been used by others for similar purposes?
- Are there any published studies that use the theory for similar purposes?
- Is it consistent with the values integral to the work?

Nutbeam et al. (2010) and Laverack (2014) would suggest the addition of:

- Is it consistent with everyday observations?

The application of theory

The choice of theory will clearly be influenced by ideological perspectives. By way of illustration, let us pursue the example of high levels of heart disease in a socially disadvantaged community, where it is recognized to be a problem by both professionals and the community itself.

A major risk factor is the diet of many members of the community, which is known to be high in saturated fats and refined carbohydrates. An authoritarian or preventive approach would search for the key variables to address by means of the application of cognitive behavioural or psychosocial theory – for example, the HAM would identify the main factors associated with dietary practice and the stages of change model would assess the readiness of the community to change. A two-pronged strategy might be adopted. One strand would focus on attempting to change behavioural intention concerning a healthy diet and develop skills in preparing healthy meals at low cost. The selection of actual methods should also be informed by a range of relevant theories – learning theory, diffusion of innovations theory and communication theory. The other strand would be concerned with making healthy foods available at lower cost – for example, by working with local shops to gain their cooperation. The selection of methods to achieve this would be enhanced by reference to diffusion of innovations theory and organizational change theories. Should the remit of the programme be more ambitious and attempt to influence food policy more generally, then recourse to policy theory would be needed.

In contrast, a negotiated approach would draw on community development theory to identify ways of working with the community to enable it to identify the main causes of the problems it is experiencing and the most feasible solutions. These might include the need to empower people to achieve a healthy diet on a low income, either individually or by working collectively to reduce food costs by setting up food cooperatives. Both may require some form of learning and, again, communication and learning theory will be important as will community organization theory. Should any environmental change and political action be needed – for example, getting the council to set aside

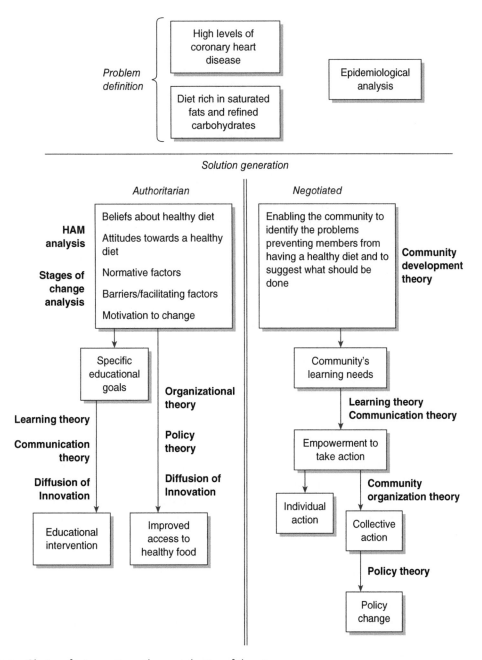

Figure 5.9 Choice of intervention – the contribution of theories

land for allotments so that people can grow their own food – then additional lobbying and advocacy skills will be needed, together with an understanding of how to influence political processes derived from policy theory. An overview of both these approaches is presented in Figure 5.9.

Evidence-based practice

The latter part of the twentieth century witnessed a move towards evidence-based practice in health and social care generally, but also in health promotion. Indeed, the 51st World Health Assembly (WHO, 1998a) urged all member states to 'adopt an evidence-based approach to health promotion policy and practice, using the full range of quantitative and qualitative methodologies'. Further exploration of this is given in Chapter 12.

While evaluation has been recognized as being integral to good practice in health promotion, there is now even greater emphasis on the *utilization* of evaluation evidence in practice. The need for such evidence of effectiveness has been a major driver for the production of systematic reviews, and groups such as the Cochrane Collaboration have played a leading role. Much of the discussion about evidence-based practice in the past has focused on ways of measuring effectiveness. A particular concern has been the emphasis on positivist methodology and the use of randomized controlled trials (RCTs). Indeed, calls for more evidence in the public health community are often synonymous with conducting more RCTs as opposed to other non-experimental study designs (Petticrew et al., 2012). We will focus on the issue of evaluation and the generation of evidence in Chapter 11. However, we should note, in passing, that there is a developing consensus – endorsed by the WHO (1998a) – on the value of methodological pluralism for health promotion evaluation and, as highlighted by Juneau et al. (2011) and Woodall et al. (2018), the need for a broader view of evidence.

Notwithstanding these concerns and the ongoing debate, it is still the case that greater weight is attached to evidence from experimental or quasi-experimental studies – see, for example, the hierarchy of evidence for assessing interventions given in Table 5.3.

 Furthermore, some of the central concerns of health promotion – participation, empowerment, policy development and environmental change – present a greater challenge for robust evaluation than individually orientated behaviour change. It is perhaps not surprising, therefore, that there is less evidence to draw on in relation to these areas than is the case for others. Tilford (2000) notes that, as health promotion has evolved from health education, there has been a time-lag in evaluations focusing on the social rather than the individual determinants of health. Indeed, many interventions that are evaluated may not actually be conceptualized as 'health-promoting' interventions in their broadest sense, given that they are often focused on discrete individual behaviour change (Juneau et al., 2011).

At present, there is a lack of understanding about how evidence is used by health promotion practitioners (Juneau et al., 2011). Ideological commitments will, again, influence views about the credibility and utility of different types of evidence and its appeal to practitioners. However, over and above the issues associated with evaluation methodology, systematic reviews (and, indeed, published evaluations more generally) are recognized as having a number of limitations for the end-users. These issues are summarized in a paper identifying the barriers to the uptake of evidence from systematic

Table 5.3 Levels of evidence for studies on the efficacy of public health interventions

Level of evidence	Type of evidence
1++	High-quality meta-analyses, systematic reviews of RCTs or RCTs (including cluster RCTs) with a very low risk of bias
1+	Well-conducted meta-analyses, systematic reviews of RCTs or RCTs (including cluster RCTs) with a low risk of bias
1−	Meta-analyses, systematic reviews of RCTs or RCTs (including cluster RCTs) with a high risk of bias*
2++	High-quality systematic reviews of, or individual, non-randomized controlled trials, case-control studies, cohort studies, controlled before-and-after (CBA), interrupted time series (ITS), correlation studies with a very low risk of confounding, bias or chance and a high probability that the relationship is causal
2+	Well-conducted non-randomized controlled trials, case-control studies, cohort studies, controlled before-and-after (CBA), interrupted time series (ITS), correlation studies with a low risk of confounding, bias or chance and a moderate probability that the relationship is causal
2−	Non-randomized controlled trials, case-control studies, cohort studies, controlled before-and-after (CBA), interrupted time series (ITS), correlation studies with a high risk of confounding bias, or chance and a significant risk that the relationship is not causal*
3	Non-analytic studies (for example, case reports, case series)
4	Expert opinion, formal consensus

* Studies with a '−' level of evidence should not be used as a basis for making a recommendation.

Source: National Institute for Health and Care Excellence (NICE) (2005: 31), reproduced with permission under the NICE UK Open Content Licence.

reviews, which included: lack of access to systematic reviews, lack of awareness, lack of familiarity with systematic reviews, lack of perceived usefulness and the limited use and applicability of reviews in practice (Wallace et al., 2012). More specifically, in relation to health promotion, Tilford (2000) cites the main issues as being:

- insufficient attention to the quality of interventions
- the theoretical basis of interventions is not always made clear
- insufficient information on the process of implementation of interventions
- the tendency for reviews to focus on health education rather than the broader sphere of health promotion
- the short-term follow-up time of many studies
- the dominance of studies from the USA.

She notes that the mismatch between the types of interventions that have been rigorously evaluated and those commonly used in practice further limits the relevance of the evidence base for practitioners. It is self-evident that innovative approaches will have little, if any, evidence to draw on.

South and Tilford's (2000) study of the use of research by health promotion specialists in England found two different interpretations of evidence-based practice among practitioners. On the one hand, it was associated with using sound empirical research and, on the other hand, it was conceptualized more broadly as additionally drawing on theory, principles of good practice, the academic literature and national policy. Some practitioners used a systematic approach to retrieve and appraise evidence, whereas for others this was done on a rather more *ad hoc* basis or, alternatively, seen as falling within the general context of keeping up to date. Practitioners also used their professional judgement to make decisions about the appropriate level of evidence required. The valuable contribution of research to planning interventions was recognized, but only as one element alongside theory and professional expertise. Other studies have suggested that many health promotion practitioners do not consistently use research evidence to inform their practice, relying instead on tacit knowledge and professional wisdom (Woodall and Cross, 2021).

Nutbeam (1996) identifies three levels of practice that differ in the extent to which they are based on research evidence – planned, responsive and reactive. *Planned* health promotion is based on a rational and systematic review of evidence concerning health needs, effectiveness of interventions and contextual factors. *Responsive* health promotion involves addressing the expressed needs of the community in ways it sees as most appropriate – the use of research evidence is only one factor in the decision-making process. Although this style of working is consistent with the rhetoric of the Ottawa Charter, Nutbeam (1996: 321) cautions that:

> the interventions chosen may not be effective or efficient, and not tackle fundamental problems even though they are strongly supported by the community.

Reactive health promotion takes the form of a rapid and often high-profile response to a problem or crisis. Political imperatives may drive both the pace and type of response – for example, the early public awareness campaigns about HIV. The short timescale of this knee-jerk type of response does not allow sufficient time for rigorous evidence-based planning.

Although evidence-based practice had been narrowly equated with evaluation research, a broader interpretation will provide a more secure base for practice. This view, as we have noted, is reflected in the field, where there is some concern that other forms of evidence may be omitted from decisions about interventions (South and Tilford, 2000). Green (2000) has argued for a greater emphasis on the contribution of theory to evidence-based practice. Furthermore, empirical evidence and theory are not alternatives, but should be inextricably linked. In short, research evidence about the effectiveness of interventions should contribute to the development of intervention theory, which will itself shape subsequent interventions and the ways in which they are evaluated. Sackett et al. (1996: 71) also draw attention to the importance of professional expertise in their definition of evidence-based medical practice as 'integrating individual clinical expertise with the best available external clinical evidence from systematic research'.

A combination of these elements should allow state-of-the-art solutions or interventions to be identified and an appropriate selection made. McLeroy et al. (1993) refer to this as the 'theory of intervention' – statements or summaries of what we know about the relative effectiveness of different intervention strategies with particular populations.

Professional judgement and context

We have already noted the importance of the professional perspective in our discussion of the contribution of both theory and evidence-based practice to solution generation. At grassroots level, this derives from experience and is grounded in familiarity with particular contexts and specific groups, which enables the most appropriate course of action to be identified. Adherence to the professional values of health promotion will also make some approaches more acceptable and preclude others. These values have been discussed at length in Chapter 1.

Realist approaches to evaluation are attracting considerable attention and will be discussed more fully in Chapter 11. Unlike other approaches, they focus particularly on attempting to understand the contexts and mechanisms underpinning observed outcomes (Pawson and Tilley, 1997). However, much of the research evidence about effectiveness and theoretical analyses remains largely context-free. Health promotion, though, does not operate within a vacuum. Effective health promotion interventions must be designed to have a good fit with contextual factors and local circumstances. For example, any attempt to bring about organizational change will need to give due regard to the culture and norms within the organization. Similar attention should be given to the range of relevant contextual factors, regardless of the level of the proposed intervention – be it individual, group, community, organization, environmental or policy change.

We noted above the broad range of factors included within a community profile that are relevant both to understanding needs and the contextual factors that will influence the response. McLeroy et al. (1993) emphasize that this understanding should include the capacity of families, social networks, communities and organizations to address the needs of their members and that health promotion interventions should take a form that strengthens this. Otherwise, health promotion interventions risk becoming a substitute for these local mechanisms, reducing the community's capacity to cope independently – effectively becoming a de-powering, rather than an empowering, influence.

Over and above contributing to strategic decisions, contextual information also informs operational planning. It identifies who the most appropriate target groups are and what channels are most appropriate for reaching them. It also identifies any gatekeepers. Indeed, it may be more appropriate to target gatekeepers than those it is hoped will ultimately benefit. For example, attempts to improve the nutrition of young children will need to target families, particularly mothers. In patriarchal societies, improving women's access to contraception may require working with men to gain their support. Similarly, if access to interventions is controlled by gatekeepers, their cooperation will be needed. For example, schoolteachers have an important gatekeeper function in relation to young people's access to health education materials. If there are important opinion leaders or referent groups, then it is also wise to work with them.

Understanding what channels of communication exist will increase the potential for success. This might be something as obvious as access to radio or television and details of listening audiences at particular times of day, if a mass media campaign is being planned, or details of social interaction networks, if a peer education programme is being developed. Larkey et al. (1999), for example, used systematic network measurement techniques to identify individuals who were most centrally and socially connected before offering them the opportunity to train as peer health educators for their

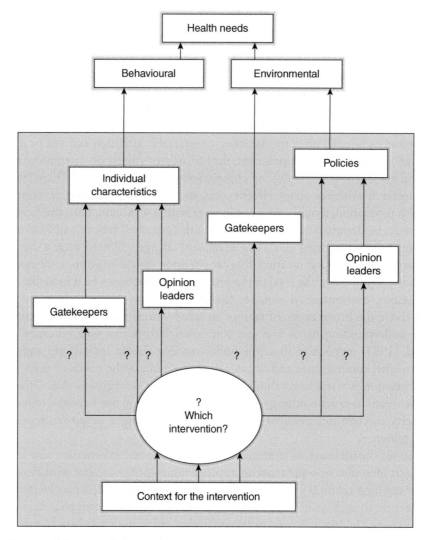

Figure 5.10 Contextual factors and choice of intervention

worksite dietary change intervention. Similarly, effective lobbying and advocacy is dependent on being able to identify and target those with most political power and influence. An overview of how these various strands fit together is provided in Figure 5.10.

INFORMATION AND HEALTH PROMOTION PLANNING

This chapter has focused on identifying the information needed to plan interventions. A theme running through the chapter has been the tension between different approaches to defining needs and proposing solutions – particularly between:

- participative, bottom-up and professionally led top-down approaches
- subjective and objective interpretations
- reductionist and interpretive perspectives.

This will inevitably influence the ways in which health needs are defined and prioritized and the types of solution proposed.

Health promotion, by its very nature, is action-orientated towards improving health status – whether this is viewed as addressing specific problems or creating conditions that are supportive of health. Health promotion interventions are more likely to be successful if they respond to the needs recognized by individuals or a community and are based on an analysis of environmental, social and behavioural determinants. Identifying appropriate solutions requires recourse to theory, research evidence of effectiveness, analysis of contextual factors and professional judgement. Furthermore, the use of participative approaches at all stages will draw on the practical knowledge and experience of the community.

Whichever approach is adopted, information is needed to answer the following key questions:

- What is the nature of the problem?
- Who is affected?
- What are the causes?
- What are the contextual factors?
- What do we need to do to tackle it?
- How should we do it?

KEY POINTS

- Assessing health needs is the first stage of systematic programme planning.
- Understanding of contextual factors and community profiles should also inform the planning process.
- The approach to health needs assessment will be influenced by ideology.
- Participatory approaches place people at the centre of the process and are consistent with the principles of health promotion.
- Developing effective responses to health needs requires reference to relevant theory, existing empirical evidence and the insight of practitioners and the community.

CHAPTER 5: INTERNATIONAL CASE STUDIES

The following case studies on the online resources website are relevant to the content of this chapter: 1 and 5.

CRITICAL REFLECTION AND APPLICATION TO PRACTICE

This chapter has reviewed the notion of health needs and explored a myriad of techniques for appraising needs. How are individual and community health needs identified in your professional context? Which techniques outlined in the chapter best resonate with your own experiences? To what extent are deficiencies in individuals and communities still examined in assessment techniques? A– are 'asset-based' approaches common, or perhaps stronger in rhetoric than reality? How do you deploy theory in your choice of interventions and to what extent does professional judgement override empirical evidence in decision-making?

ONLINE RESOURCES

Please visit https://study.sagepub.com/greentones5e for all the online resources for the book, including recommended further reading on each chapter subject, useful weblinks (both introduced by the authors), as well as the abovementioned case study material.

6 HEALTHY PUBLIC POLICY

He has sat on the fence so long that the iron has entered his soul.

David Lloyd George (1863–1945)

OVERVIEW

This chapter will look at the role of policy in influencing health and establishing supportive environments for health. It will:

- define healthy public policy
- consider the process of policy-making and implementation
- identify the contribution of health education to policy development through awareness-raising and development of political skills
- outline the contribution of advocacy to policy-making and consider advocacy strategies
- consider the role of power in the policy process and how to bring pressure to bear
- examine the contribution of health impact assessment to building healthy public policy.

INTRODUCTION

Effective engagement with the policy process is an increasingly important role for those involved in health promotion and recognized as a core competency for professional practice (Woodall and Cross, 2021). Within England, for example, responsibility for public health and health promotion has shifted into local government, having formerly been located in the National Health Service. This transition has meant that senior health promotion practitioners have a need to be increasingly more engaged with politicians and elected officials to influence and shape local policy decision-making and budgeting (Homer et al., 2021). Nonetheless, policy-making has become more difficult and complex in the twenty-first century as Kickbusch and Gleicher (2012: 27) note:

> the nature of policy-making has changed. It has become more complex as it attempts to address wicked problems and systemic risks, confront multiple possible futures, include many players and stakeholders and reach agreement on courses of action based on the understanding that the amount of evidence is always increasing and is rarely final.

The defining feature of health promotion has been its emphasis on the environmental determinants of health rather than individual behaviour, and healthy public policy has been seen as the vehicle for 'creating supportive environments to enable people to lead healthy lives' (WHO, 1988: 1). The use of public policy measures to protect health is not new. Many of the health improvements in the UK in the nineteenth century were achieved by public policy, such as the Public Health Acts of 1848 and 1875, which attempted to control aspects of the environment – water supply, sewage disposal, slaughtering of animals, parks and open spaces, isolation hospitals and the beginnings of housing control (Jones and Sidell, 1997; McKeown and Lowe, 1974).

The emphasis of the importance of environmental influences on health underpinned the emergence of health promotion and 'The New Public Health' movements in the latter part of the twentieth century. However, contemporary conceptualizations of the environment have broadened to include social and economic as well as physical aspects, such as housing, economic and environmental regeneration, strategic planning, education, children and young people's services, fire and road safety. Today, in the twenty-first century, 'wicked' health problems and other contemporary challenges to health (e.g. climate change) create unique situations that require policy responses to mitigate their effects. Contemporary society has been described as VUCA – an acronym that suggests we live in times characterized by: volatility, uncertainty, complexity and ambiguity (Worley and Jules, 2020). This chapter considers the role of policy in two broad ways. First, it looks at the development of policy explicitly to tackle health issues – policy as the solution to health concerns. There are clear links with the sections on media advocacy and persuasive communication in Chapters 7 and 8 and community activism in Chapter 9. Second, the chapter considers the effects on health of policy designed for other purposes and the use of health impact assessment to identify these potential effects. However, we will begin by examining the WHO position on healthy public policy.

HEALTHY PUBLIC POLICY – THE WHO POSITION

The central role of healthy public policy has been a consistent theme running through major WHO documents on health promotion, as discussed in Chapter 1. The Ottawa Charter (WHO, 1986) – which has been a constant source of reference in the development of health promotion and 'The New Public Health' – identified building healthy public policy and the creation of supportive environments as two of its five priority action areas. This commitment has been reaffirmed in subsequent statements.

 The Jakarta Declaration (WHO, 1997) noted the importance of multisectoral and partnership working along with a commitment to healthy public policy. The pursuit of social responsibility for health involves decision-makers in the public and private sectors adopting polices and practices that:

- avoid harming the health of individuals
- protect the environment and ensure the use of sustainable resources
- restrict the production of, and trade in, inherently harmful goods and substances, such as tobacco and armaments, as well as discourage unhealthy marketing practices
- safeguard both the citizen in the marketplace and the individual in the workplace
- include equity-focused health impact assessments as an integral part of policy development. (WHO, 1997: 3)

Healthy public policy was the specific focus of the 2nd International Conference on Health Promotion held in Adelaide, which defined it as 'characterized by an explicit concern for health and equity in all areas of policy and accountability for health impact' (WHO, 1988: 1).

The recommendations of the Adelaide Conference formally recognized that the activities of a number of different government sectors influence health status and that there should be accountability for health impacts. This would include effects on the social and physical environments, which may influence the possibility and ease of making healthy choices or, alternatively, effects that are directly health enhancing or damaging. Health was also seen as a fundamental right and sound social investment.

A central concern was equity and narrowing the health gap in society by means of policies that attach high priority to disadvantaged and vulnerable groups. Furthermore, developed countries were considered to have an obligation to ensure that their own health policies impacted positively on developing nations.

Healthy public policy was seen to be important at all levels of government, from national to local, and 'public accountability for health ... an essential nutrient for the growth of healthy public policy' (WHO, 1988: 2). Community action can, therefore, provide the motivational force for policy development. The other side of the coin is that governments should assess and report the impact of policies in a way that can be understood by all groups in society.

Although government was seen to have a key role, other groups – such as the private and business sectors, non-governmental and community organizations – were also identified as important influences that could be harnessed for health promotion.

The 5th Global Conference on Health Promotion held in Mexico City identified the central responsibility of governments for health and social development. It acknowledged that in order to achieve equity and health for all, 'health promotion must be a fundamental component of public policies and programmes in all countries' (WHO, 2000a). A strong theme to emerge from the Mexico City conference was the need to 'work with and through existing political systems and structures to ensure healthy public policy, adequate investment in health and facilitation of an infrastructure for health promotion' (WHO, 2000b: 21). This was held to require:

- democratic processes
- social and political activism
- a system of equity-orientated health impact assessment
- reorientation of health services
- improved interaction between politicians, policy-makers, researchers and practitioners
- strengthening existing capacity for implementing health promotion strategies and supporting synergy between different levels – local, national and international.

The responsibility of governments in relation to health promotion was reiterated in the Bangkok Charter (WHO, 2005), along with the need to 'make the health consequences of policies and legislation explicit, using tools such as equity-focused health impact assessment'. Further, the charter also emphasized the importance of establishing mechanisms for global governance to address the harmful effects on health of trade, products, services and marketing strategies. In 2009, the Nairobi Global Conference on Health Promotion (WHO, 2009) raised the importance of health in all policies and this was reasserted both in the Rio Declaration on Social Determinants of Health (WHO, 2012) and in Helsinki at the 8th Global Conference on Health Promotion (WHO, 2013e).

Health in All Policies, vehemently espoused in recent WHO charters and declarations (WHO, 2009, 2012, 2013e) – although somewhat de-emphasized in the 9th WHO Conference on Health Promotion (WHO, 2016a) – has as a central basis the recognition of health impacts of policy across all sectors (e.g. transport, education, agriculture, and so on). Indeed, decisions influencing people's health not only concern 'health service' policy, but also decisions in many different policy areas:

> the core of 'Health in All Policies' is to examine health determinants that are mainly controlled by policies of sectors other than health. (Puska, 2007: 328)

Health in All Policies (HiAP) is not a new concept, but momentum for this has gathered pace in recent years. Health in All Policies is an approach to public policies across sectors that systematically takes into account the health implications of decisions – it is consistently cited as a way to tackle the intersectoral requirements of the Sustainable Development Goals (SDGs), and as an important strategy for achieving Universal Health Coverage (UHC) and Health for All (Nutbeam and Muscat, 2021). It remains though that in health, much policy analysis has tended to be dominated by health service policy activity (Coveney, 2010). That said, the move to policy-making through highly networked, multilevel, multistakeholder governance is now seen as the way forward to tackle complex health issues (Kickbusch and Gleicher, 2012: 30). To provide some examples, in Barcelona concerted efforts to modify transportation policies in relation to cycling, better public transportation and traffic calming led to impacts on population health. Research which measured key health outcomes prior to and subsequent of the transport policy modifications showed impressive increases in walking and cycling trips registered on working days in Barcelona and decreases in the number of pedestrian or cycling injuries or deaths (Pérez et al., 2017). Health in All Policies has more recently been used as a framework to consider the prevention of non-communicable diseases in low- and middle-income countries (Ndubuisi, 2021) and moreover the notion of 'mental' Health in All Policies in the context of war and conflict has been suggested (Kienzler, 2019). At the 9th Global Health Promotion Conference in Shanghai (WHO, 2016a), WHO had a less explicit focus on 'Health in All Policies' albeit a strong commitment to achieving health and sustainable development through policy was asserted. Supporting legislation, regulation and taxation of unhealthy commodities was provided as a commitment, as was the implementation of fiscal policies to generate added revenue for investments in health and well-being.

HEALTHY PUBLIC POLICY – MEANINGS AND SCOPE

Health, as we noted in Chapter 1, is both a relative and contested concept. The notion of policy is equally nebulous, as encapsulated in the metaphor, 'Policy is rather like the elephant – you recognize it when you see it, but cannot easily define it' (Cunningham, 1963: 229).

While the term 'policy' is one that enters the dialogue of most public health and health promotion professionals (Porter and Coles, 2011), it is subject to variation in meaning and usage in different contexts. Stoneham and Edmunds (2020) describe policy as a map which provides strategic guidance. Milio (2001: 622) offers an alternative definition:

Policy is a guide to action to change what would otherwise occur, a decision about amounts and allocations of resources: the overall amount is a statement of commitment to certain areas of concern; the distribution of the amount shows the priorities of decision makers. Policy sets priorities and guides resource allocation.

While policy is often associated with government activity, it also exists outside of government circles and is developed at the national as well as local and regional levels.

Colebatch (1998) identifies three key elements of policy:

- **authority**: the implication that there is official endorsement
- **expertise**: applied to a problem area and identifying what should be done about it
- **order**: decisions are not arbitrary but consistent and structured.

Jenkins (1978: 15) provides a useful definition that focuses on the instrumentality of policy and emphasizes that it should not merely be aspirational, but also within the control of those responsible for making policy:

A set of interrelated decisions taken by a political actor or group of actors concerning the selection of goals and the means of achieving them within a specified situation where these decisions should, in principle, be within the power of these actors to achieve.

While the implication of this definition is that policy is concerned with action, it can equally involve inaction – deciding what *not* to do. Ignatieff (1992, in Walt, 1994: 40) draws attention to the longer-term view of policy in his acerbic commentary on short-term economic policy:

A policy ought to be something more than a galvanic twitch. It ought to have legs for distances longer than those implied in a 'dash for growth'. It ought to have some end in view larger than seeing an addled government through the next month … policy is not about surviving till Friday. Nor is policy to be confused with strategy, which is about getting through to Christmas. Policy is the selection of non-contradictory means to achieve non-contradictory ends over the medium to long term.

What, then, is healthy public policy? There is a clear distinction between 'public health policy', which can be viewed either as public sector (government) policy for population health or any policy concerned with the public's health (de Leeuw et al., 2015). Healthy public policy is concerned with the role of government and the public sector in creating the conditions that support health. Milio (2001: 622), who played an influential role in shifting the emphasis from health policy to healthy public policy and raising its profile within WHO, offers the following definition of public policy:

Public policy is policy at any level of government. Some levels may have formal or legal precedence over others. Policy may be set by heads of government, legislatures, and regulatory agencies empowered by other constituted authorities. Supranational institutions' policies, as those of the World Trade Organization or United Nations Conventions, may overrule government policies.

The key characteristics of healthy public policy are listed in Box 6.1.

BOX 6.1   CHARACTERISTICS OF HEALTHY PUBLIC POLICY

- Commitment to social equity
- Recognition of the important influence of economic, social and physical environments on health
- Facilitation of public participation
- Cooperation between health and other sectors of government.

Source: After Draper (1988)

Given the plethora of factors that influence health status (discussed in Chapter 2), the scope of healthy public policy is necessarily wide-ranging. Recent health emergencies, for instance, have shown that policy-making focusing on animals and ecosystems is critical to avoid unanticipated consequences (Stephen, 2020). Some indication of the breadth of healthy public policy is provided by Terris (in Tesh et al., 1988) in an editorial submitted to the Yale Symposium on Healthy Public Policy:

> The logic of our discipline makes it necessary to support a healthful standard of living through full employment and adequate family income; improved working conditions; decent housing …; effective protection from environmental discomforts …; good nutrition that will foster optimal physical and mental development; increased financial support to public education and elimination of financial barriers to higher education; improved opportunities for rest, recreation, and cultural development; greater participation in community activities and decision-making; an end to discrimination against minority groups based on race, gender, age, social class, religious belief, national background or sexual preference; and freedom from the pervasive fear of violence, war and nuclear annihilation.

Policy can support health in a number of different ways:

- fiscal/monetary – incomes and incentives
- regulation – economic and environmental
- provision of goods and services
- supporting participation
- research, development, information, education.

The notion that policy implementation can be upstream and downstream is relatively well understood. The former would include, for example, the development of preschool education to meet the needs of disadvantaged families or reducing the fear of crime and violence and creating a safe environment. In contrast, the latter would focus on policies intended to prevent disease, such as fluoridation of drinking water or ensuring equitable access to healthcare.

Within the health promotion field there is an acceptance that health has little to do with healthcare policy, together with a shared understanding to move away from monocausal models and reductionist analyses and towards recognition of the complex interplay of factors that impact on health (Tremblay and Richard, 2014). In relation to alcohol consumption as a public health risk, for example, Kelly and Barker (2016: 113) note:

> Habitually policy makers and politicians refer to the misuse of alcohol as if the consumption of alcohol was a single behaviour and as if it was possible to find a single solution to the problem of alcohol misuse.

Tesh et al. (1988), however, have a number of concerns about the adoption of multifactorial models of causality. First, they offer little insight into exactly how to prevent disease. Because everything is interlinked, any one action may appear insignificant, yet it is unlikely that sufficient resources will be available to tackle everything. The enormity of the task can become a reason (excuse) for not taking action and thus lead to inertia.

Second, because all elements of a multicausal web appear equally weighted, policy-makers are provided with an opportunity to seem to be responding to a problem while at the same time opting for interventions that are less socially disruptive or costly and may well be less effective than some other course of action – for example, providing smoking-cessation clinics rather than tackling poverty, or encouraging people to improve their diet rather than addressing the issue of whether or not those on low incomes or receiving state benefits can afford a healthy diet.

This also provides the opportunity effectively to opt out of responsibility for a health issue by attributing major responsibility elsewhere. For example, there would be no need to address the activities of the food industry if the major influences on a healthy diet were perceived to be acceptable minimum levels of income and awareness of what constitutes a healthy diet.

The third point is that an emphasis on cause overlooks those who are more likely to experience ill health – notably those of lower socioeconomic status. Recognition of the 'primacy of poverty' (Tesh et al., 1988: 258) presupposes that all elements of the web are not equal, but that some have more fundamental significance. Therefore, constructing a hierarchy of causes may be necessary to target those that are likely to have the greatest impact on health.

Clearly, when considering policy options, there will be a need to make tradeoffs in choosing one course of action rather than another and between those groups that benefit and those that bear the costs. Proposals for airport expansions and growth projects are good examples of the driver for increasing economic productivity through policy-making, but at the expense of environmental impact and potential noise pollution (Griggs and Howarth, 2018).

Christoffel (in Tesh et al., 1988: 259) asserts that 'Knowing how to solve a public health problem is not enough when powerful interests are threatened by the solution, which seems to be the case most of the time.' He sees the major problem for health as not being an overall shortage of resources, but an uneven distribution of them. The redistribution of resources would require that some (albeit a minority) lose and these are, in general, those who hold 'critical political power' (in Tesh et al., 1988: 260). Christoffel concludes that the main barrier to healthy public policy is the concentration of wealth and power among those who stand to lose.

Delaney (1994c) makes the distinction between policy as *problematic* for health promotion and policy as the *solution*. The former focuses on identifying the negative impacts of policies on health status. The growing field of health impact assessment is concerned with analysing the potential health impact of policies (we will return to this below). The latter is concerned with the use of policy to tackle the problems and create conditions that are supportive of health, with a recognition that well-conceived and effective policy can be critical to tackling and addressing significant health inequalities in society (Woodall and Cross, 2021).

Choice and control

Recognition of the duty of governments to create conditions that support health and enable community participation is a core principle of health promotion. Individuals are also seen as having a responsibility – individually and collectively – to contribute to health. A fundamental question is: what should the respective roles and responsibilities be of the individual and the state in controlling the determinants of health?

As we observed in Chapter 1, one of the core ethical principles of health education has been a commitment to voluntarism, or free choice. This was aptly summarized in the North American Society of Public Health Educators' Code of Ethics: 'change by choice not coercion' (Society of Health Education and Health Promotion Specialists, 1997). Milio (1981: 277) contends that: 'There is no "free choice" but only "choice" within a limited number of options.' The key issue is what options will be made available and how health-promoting or damaging those options are. For example, 'hard paternalism' may be needed to tackle inequalities. The best examples here have been seen in relation to tobacco products, alcohol and some junk-food and how this is addressed through policy imperatives. Evidence shows that price rises in unhealthy products, for example, leads to restrictions in people's purchasing and consumption (Hawkins and McCambridge, 2020) (see Box 6.2).

BOX 6.2 ROLES OF GOVERNMENT IN OBESITY PREVENTION

Leadership

- Providing a visible lead
- Reinforcing the seriousness of the problem
- Demonstrating a readiness to take serious action

Examples

- Being visible in the media
- Role modelling healthy behaviours (at an individual level)
- Role modelling healthy environments (at a government agency level)
- Creating mechanisms for a whole-of-government response to obesity
- Lifting the priority for health (versus commercial) outcomes

Advocacy

- Advocating for a multisector response across all societal sectors (governments, the private sector, civil society and the public)

Examples

- Advocating to the private sector for corporate responsibility around marketing to children
- Creating a high-level taskforce to oversee and monitor multisector actions
- Encouraging healthy lifestyles for individuals and families

Funding

- Securing increased and continuing funding to create healthy environments and encourage healthy eating and physical activity

Examples

- Establishing a health promotion foundation (e.g. using a hypothecated tobacco tax) to fund programmes and research
- Moving from project funding to programme and service funding for obesity prevention
- Creating centres of excellence for research, evaluation and monitoring

Policy

- Developing, implementing and monitoring a set of policies, regulations, taxes and subsidies that make environments less obesogenic and more health-promoting

Examples

- Banning the marketing of unhealthy foods to children
- Subsidizing public transport and active transport more than car transport
- Requiring 'traffic light' front-of-pack labelling of food nutrient profiles
- Restricting the sale of unhealthy foods in schools

Source: Derived from Swinburn (2008), reproduced with permission under the Creative Commons Attribution Licence.

The concern of healthy public policy should be to ensure that the environment does not damage health and that there is an equitable distribution of 'health-important resources'. Policy is often utilized as a way of protecting citizens and efforts to improve their health. Most recently, the power of the state has been seen in relation to managing and controlling COVID-19 in almost every global nation. History has shown how effective state intervention has saved lives and improved the health of communities, but this has always come against a backdrop of heavy debate and disagreement as not everyone believes that state intervention is proportionate or even justifiable (Woodall and Cross, 2021).

Healthy public policy is generally seen as a vehicle for tackling structural and environmental threats to health – as both protective and opening up healthy choices by removing constraints to action. However, we should also note that, over and above making the healthy choice the easy choice, policies can make it the *only* choice (Tones and Tilford, 1994). Beattie (1991) sees legislation and policy as an authoritarian approach directed at the collective (see Figure 6.1).

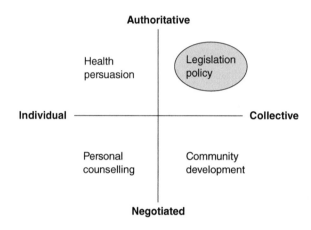

Figure 6.1   Health promotion – alternative approaches (after Beattie, 1991)

Curtailing individual choice can clearly be defended when exercising that choice may put others at risk. The most recent examples were in relation to managing the spread of COVID-19, but there are other examples: it would be difficult to uphold the rights of individuals to choose to drive through residential areas at excessive speed or while intoxicated or subject others to inhaling tobacco smoke.

However, control takes on a more coercive complexion when applied to behaviour that only places the individual concerned at risk. Such an approach equates with a narrow, preventive model of health education and leaves health promoters open to accusations of health fascism. The anti-health lobby has been quick to pick up on this element of coercion and frequently uses arguments about liberty and civil rights in its activities. For example, the Freedom Organisation for the Right to Enjoy Smoking Tobacco (FOREST, 2008) describes its purpose as 'to protect the interests of adults who choose to smoke or consume tobacco in its many forms'. The pro-gun lobby in the USA and the opponents of pool-fencing in Australia take a similar stance.

The soda tax, a piece of public policy originating in the USA, was an illustration of the possible overreach of authorities into people's lives (Wiley et al., 2013). Despite soda companies opposing the policy to raise taxes on sugary drinks to reduce consumption, many jurisdictions across the USA implemented this tax increase to prevent the consumption of sugary drinks and, indeed, saw reductions in consumption (Gostin, 2017). More recently, guidance and policy mandating mask-wearing during the COVID-19 pandemic caused polarization in relation to the state's control and influence on people's lives and choices (Fischer et al., 2021).

So, to what extent should government and authorities intervene through policy measures and to what extent should adults have the right to make their own free choices? The debate is complex, although politicians and those in positions of authority are known to be hesitant to use policy to intervene in such health matters as it can jeopardize their own popularity (Zalmanovitch and Cohen, 2015). Nonetheless, it seems that trust in some governments was unwavering during policy decisions to mandate mask-wearing during the COVID-19 pandemic, suggesting that a more paternal approach was welcomed by communities (Sheluchin et al., 2020).

Sparks (2011) urges the health promotion community not to be distracted by critics of healthy public policy and those who suggest that it is a form of intrusion into people's lives through restricting freedom of choice. Nonetheless, the ideological debate on the role of healthy public policy within health promotion is influenced by right or left leaning views on the way health promotion is broadly conceptualized and indeed practised (Brown et al., 2018).

The restriction on people's choices by governments is often labelled 'nanny statism' by critics of paternalism. Wiley et al. (2013) suggest that the term 'nanny state' in itself is a loaded and evocative word that conjures negative images and is, therefore, frequently used by proponents of free choice in health matters. Jochelson (2005) points out that: 'Almost every government intervention in the public health arena has been criticized ... as a sign of tyranny, nanny statism, or the end of individual freedom' (2005: 29), despite the capacity to bring about changes that individuals are unable to do on their own. Other contemporary commentators note the importance of state regulation and protection to limit potential public health harms arising from private companies and industry (Steele et al., 2021).

In relation to the views of the public, a survey by the King's Fund revealed strong support 'across the social spectrum for government action to prevent illness and improve health' (2004: 4), reiterated by research conducted during the COVID-19 pandemic in Canada (Sheluchin et al., 2020). Three types of measures that a government can take were identified:

- encouraging measures that inform and advise, warn about health risks and encourage employers to promote health
- enabling measures that help to create favourable social, economic and environmental conditions
- restrictive measures that prevent actions that put others' health at risk or actively discourage people from putting their own health at risk. (King's Fund, 2004: 4)

Research often shows a more nuanced picture in relation to the public's views on government legislation and intervention for public health improvement. Stronger support, for instance, was seen in relation to some matters than others – clear food labelling on packaging (i.e. using a traffic light system indicating high, medium and low levels of fat, sugar and salt) garnered more endorsement than the use of graphic images on tobacco packaging to deter smoking behaviour. Interestingly, the study, based on a sample of respondents from Sweden and the USA, found differences in views between these two countries, with the Swedish sample being more likely to endorse policy and government interventions to promote and improve population health than those from the USA (Hagman et al., 2015).

Health education and health promotion – lifestyle and structure

Healthy public policy is generally associated with attempts to influence the structural determinants of health. Health education, in contrast, is seen as a means of influencing lifestyle. However, this representation is overly simplistic and ignores the complexity of the interplay between these various elements.

As we have noted earlier, structural factors can have a major influence on lifestyle and behaviour – and vice versa. Similarly, a major goal of policy can be to widen access to education, as evidenced by, for example, efforts to secure universal primary education. Education policy will influence the content of education generally and, more specifically, the opportunities afforded for health education.

Critical consciousness-raising, as we note in Chapter 7, is at the heart of Freirean approaches to education. Furthermore, health education can develop the skills required for political activism, including lobbying and advocacy skills.

Thus, it can be seen that representing health education and healthy public policy as competing options for promoting health is to create a false dichotomy. As Figure 6.2 illustrates, health education is a major driver in the process of policy development.

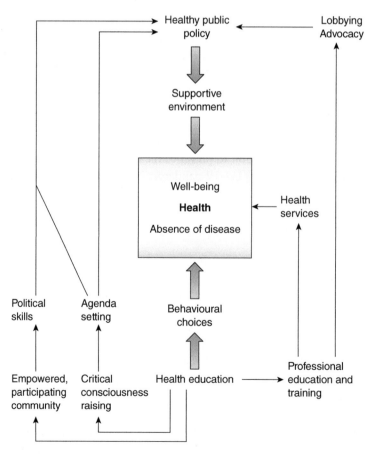

Figure 6.2 Health education and health promotion (after Tones and Tilford, 1994)

DEVELOPING POLICY – FROM RHETORIC TO REALITY

The potential for organizations and communities to influence public policy will inevitably be dependent on the structure of the state. Walt (1994) notes that, in contrast to more authoritarian regimes, liberal democracies will, at least in theory, encourage participation, and that participation can be both direct and indirect.

Direct participation involves explicit attempts to shape the development of policy by means of involvement in the policy-making process or through lobbying and advocacy. Clarke et al. (2016), for example, highlight how advocacy or lobbying processes can be useful techniques in influencing local and national obesity prevention policies. Alternatively, indirect participation consists of exercising influence via electoral processes. Walt also notes that opportunities for participation may be limited in relation to 'high politics' where consideration of major issues may be dominated by small 'elites'. High politics has been defined as 'the maintenance of core values – including national self-preservation – and the long-term objectives of the state' (Evans and Newnham, 1992, in Walt, 1994: 42). High politics, more often than not, is determined by 'policy-makers'; this is a broad term deployed in the literature that implies that 'policy-makers' are a clearly identifiable, internally homogeneous group (Smith and Katikireddi, 2013). Clearly, 'policy-makers' are not homogeneous and have varying attributes and characteristics.

In contrast, there may be a greater opportunity for participation in more run-of-the-mill issues of policy – that is, 'low politics'. Generally, individuals have little direct influence on the role of policy-making and their voice is more likely to be heard as part of a collective or via organizations. Nabyonga-Orem et al. (2016) suggest that policy-dialogue works best when there are diverse stakeholders in the policy-making discussion and where an open, inclusive and informed discussion among stakeholders takes place. Where such conditions are facilitated, there is a greater likelihood that policy is tailored to the specific needs of groups and individuals.

Walt (1994) identifies other contextual factors that influence policy development and, following Leichter (1979), categorizes these as being:

- **situational factors**: temporary conditions or situations
- **structural factors**: relatively stable elements of society polity
- **cultural factors**: the values within communities and society
- **environmental factors**: factors external to the political system, or international factors such as international trade agreements, international aid and the activities of transnational corporations.

Understanding the machinery of government and the relative roles of local, national and supranational organizations is clearly a necessary precondition for those seeking to influence policy. However, Delaney (1994c) contends that this is insufficient in itself. Healthy public policy is essentially a political undertaking (Draper, 1988; Signal, 1998; Tesh et al., 1988) and analysis of the location of political power and influence is of critical importance to the process of policy development. Yet, Signal (1998) comments that the politics of health promotion receive comparatively little attention.

There are several different perspectives on the politics of policy-making. Buse et al. (2012) distinguish between pluralist and elitist views. Pluralism presupposes that power is dispersed throughout society and that no single group dominates. The alternative position is that the political arena is dominated by 'ruling elites' whereby policy is dominated by a privileged few. In this view, policy is said to reflect the 'ruling elites' rather than the people (Buse et al., 2012). The former is consistent with neo-Marxist interpretations and the latter with the new institutionalism.

Hogwood and Gunn (1984: 71) note that the concentration of power in elite groups is seen as deriving from 'office-holding, political power, or the way the state is structured to favour the interests of the dominant class'. Norsigian (Tesh et al., 1988), writing from a feminist perspective, contends that women have a major role in supporting health by their childrearing, caregiving, homemaking and food production and preparation roles, yet have a very limited role in policy-making. The former administration in the USA led by President Donald Trump, for example, had only four women in a cabinet of 24 members (Mosendz and Randall, 2017). Moreover, in particular parts of sub-Saharan Africa, women have consistently been excluded from leadership roles, with men dominating political spaces (Coffe and Bolzendahl, 2011).

'Pluralist interest group theory' is seen as offering a micro-level analysis of the interest groups within the policy arena and their influences on public policy. Identifying the key players and the location of support and opposition is necessary for building alliances to achieve desired policy changes and tackling any opposition.

Signal (1998) uses 'the new institutionalism' as a meso-level theory to explore the effects of institutional characteristics in shaping the process of policy-making – focusing on the effects of organizational structure, together with the ways in which organizations operate, the rules that guide their operation and the ideas integral to their functioning. Clearly, there will be a stronger impetus to address issues of healthy public policy among those organizations that have a 'health promotion mandate' or those that perceive health issues as falling within their legitimate sphere of activity. Furthermore, wider recognition of health being part of an organization's accepted remit will lend authority to its voice within the policy arena. Key issues to consider in assessing the potential of different interest groups are summarized in Box 6.3.

BOX 6.3 ASSESSING THE POTENTIAL OF DIFFERENT INTEREST GROUPS

- How well organized is the group?
- What resources are available – financial, time, skills, experience?
- What strategies are used to influence the political process?

Source: After Signal (1998)

We noted in Chapter 4 that institutions vary considerably in their degree of openness and the extent to which they interlink with other institutions and involve communities. This will inevitably impact on alliance-building and responsiveness to the community's needs.

Finally, Signal draws on neo-Marxist theory to analyse macro-level political and economic factors that set the broad context for policy. She refers to two traditions within neo-Marxist analysis – the functional perspective and the political class perspective. The former is concerned with the organization of the state in relation to capital accumulation and emphasizes the importance of locating health promotion policy development within the broader economic and social policy context. The political class perspective focuses on power and the capacity to take collective action among the three main political class groupings – organized capital, organized labour and political parties. In particular, it draws attention to the need to harness the forces of business, labour (and the trade unions) and political parties in the interests of healthy public policy.

We might summarize the key points as follows:

- Know your potential allies and adversaries.
- Know the structures with which you are working.
- Know the context within which you are working.

Rational and incremental approaches

There are two broad schools of thought about the process of policy-making – the 'rational' and the 'incremental'. The former conforms with the principles of rational decision-making to be discussed in Chapter 7 and assumes that policy-making is a linear, sequence-based process in which a problem is identified and then solved (Warwick-Booth and Rowlands, 2021).

The view that policy is the product of such rational processes is considered to be overly idealized and has consistently faced criticism (de Leuuw and Breton, 2013). A more realistic interpretation is offered by incrementalism, which describes policy as evolving gradually rather than representing radical and fundamental change (Porter and Coles, 2011). An example of policy incrementalism is climate and energy change policy development in Europe whereby there is an incremental transition to a low-carbon society rather than radical transformation which is being called for from some sectors (Kulovesi and Oberthür, 2020).

Climate change is an example where the enormity of the task at hand and its complexity arguably fit well with an incrementalist approach, although it could be argued that more radical proposals would be more impactful. The choice is, therefore, between inaction in the face of the magnitude of the problem or working incrementally to ensure that the right course of action is being taken or at least that some headway is being made. The notion of 'bounded rationality' accepts that rational decision-making will inevitably be constrained by factors such as cost and practicability. A further factor limiting the practical feasibility of purely rational approaches is that policy-makers are not value-free (Walt, 1994). Indeed, we have identified the core values of health promotion in Chapter 1 and, clearly, health promotion policy should be consistent with these core values.

Incrementalism is characterized by:

- lack of a clear distinction between goals and the means of achieving them
- consideration of a restricted number of alternatives
- identification of the major consequences rather than all consequences

- no ideal policy option – the best option is the one that policy-makers agree is the most appropriate
- achieving small changes to existing policy rather than major change. (After Walt, 1994)

Incrementalism is also typical of pluralist, democratic approaches. Decisions about policy are arrived at by means of bargaining and compromise between different interest groups – referred to as 'partisan interaction' and 'mutual adjustment' (Lindblom, 1979; Lindblom and Woodhouse, 1993). Each attempts to pursue its own interests but, in order to accommodate the interests of other groups, may be prepared to fall back to a compromise position (Janis and Mann, 1977: 34):

> Whenever power is distributed among a variety of influential executive leaders, political parties, legislative factions, and other interest groups, one centre of power can rarely impose its preferences on another and policies are likely to be the outcome of give and take among numerous partisans. The constraints of bureaucratic politics, with their shifting compromises and coalitions, constitute a major reason for the disjointed and incremental nature of the policies that gradually evolve.

Small changes are held to be more feasible than radical ones. Incrementalism, therefore, tends to maintain the status quo (Ike, 2020). The incrementalist view is that small changes can be made quickly and a series of small changes can, when judged as a whole, achieve major change. It is, therefore, associated with serial policy-making – that is, revisiting and readjusting policy (Benson and Russel, 2015).

The notion of mixed scanning (Etzioni, 1967) adopts a middle-ground position and attempts to capitalize on the strengths of both rational and incremental approaches. It involves developing a broad overview of the policy field as a basis for distinguishing between those areas that can be approached incrementally and those requiring a more thorough analysis of options before making major strategic decisions.

Conflict and consensus models

'Conflict models' see groups as having their own interests and competing to ensure that they achieve their own goals. For example, the potential role of the food industry in shaping the UK childhood obesity strategies (Gregg et al., 2017) and the role of manufacturers with commercial interests influencing policy developments in relation to the use of insecticide-treated bed nets in Southern African countries (Woelk et al., 2009).

Bunton (1992) sees the state as having an important role when major corporations bring power to bear to thwart public health interests. Equally, the state must balance economic and other interests with public health concerns. A recent example was described by Thompson et al. (2021), who cite Transport for London (TfL) – the local government body responsible for the transport system in Greater London – who took the decision to restrict advertisements of high fat, salt and sugar foods across its network (colloquially defined as a 'junk-food ad ban'). This example perhaps illustrates the balance between protecting public health and income generation through advertisements.

International agreements may also be necessary to meet the challenge to health posed by multinational companies or, indeed, when the activity of one country has negative effects on the health of others. Taking tobacco control as an historical example, the Framework Convention on Tobacco

Control – the first treaty negotiated by WHO – came into force in 2005 to address the global problem of tobacco consumption. It includes measures to reduce both the demand for and supply of tobacco products (see Box 6.4).

BOX 6.4 WHO FRAMEWORK CONVENTION ON TOBACCO CONTROL

Core demand reduction provisions – Articles 6–14

- Price and tax measures to reduce the demand for tobacco, and
- Non-price measures to reduce the demand for tobacco, namely:

  o Protection from exposure to tobacco smoke;
  o Regulation of the contents of tobacco products;
  o Regulation of tobacco product disclosures;
  o Packaging and labelling of tobacco products;
  o Education, communication, training and public awareness;
  o Tobacco advertising, promotion and sponsorship; and,
  o Demand reduction measures concerning tobacco dependence and cessation.

Core supply reduction provisions – Articles 15–17

- Illicit trade in tobacco products;
- Sales to and by minors; and,
- Provision of support for economically viable alternative activities.

Source: WHO (2008a)

Tobacco and the control of tobacco seems to be a policy area where there is continual conflict globally (Peruga et al., 2021). Indeed, in 2012, this policy issue came back into the spotlight when the ban on the display of tobacco products at the point of sale in England entered into force on 6 April in large stores and supermarkets (with a floor area exceeding 280 m^2) (ASH, 2013). A report by the Centre for Tobacco Control Research (2008) stated that retailers were concerned about the policy move, arguing that it would result in practical and logistical problems: namely economic damage to the retailer (through reduced sales or increased shop-fitting costs); burdens for staff; and increases in shoplifting and illicit sourcing. Moreover, retailers claimed that the ban on the display of tobacco products at the point of sale would compromise legitimate commercial freedoms. Internationally, there remains more to be done in the tobacco control field. Commentators suggest that smoke-free environments should be extended further and that plain tobacco packaging with large pictorial health warnings should be further promoted in some parts of the world. It is argued that bold political decisions are further required, including a ban on added ingredients that are currently used to increase the attractiveness of tobacco products; and curbing the tobacco industry's corporate social responsibility initiatives (Peruga et al., 2021). There have been some demonstrable successes in bold policy-making though – in several prison systems (England and Wales in 2016, for instance) smoking has been banned for all people (staff and people in prison) in all areas of the institution (including outdoor smoking and smoking within prison cells). The results of the ban have shown in some studies markedly improved health outcomes for people in prison, with one study suggesting particular improvements for people in prison aged 50 years and older and who had been heavy smokers. Quitting smoking on admission to prison led to a reduced heart age of between two and seven years for all participants (Perrett et al., 2022).

Since the rise in popularity of electronic cigarettes (e-cigarettes), policy discussions have recently shifted to this issue rather than discussions on tobacco and the control of tobacco. However, there is a spectrum of policies and strategies around e-cigarettes across the world with no consistent picture emerging (Campus et al., 2021). In the UK, legislators have chosen not to ban e-cigarette use in all public places and workplaces. This decision has been based on a myriad of factors, including the risk of harm to others (Bauld et al., 2016). It seems that the evidence is not yet there to support a policy to prohibit e-cigarette use in enclosed public places, but it is likely that lobby groups and other influencing stakeholders may challenge this moving forward.

ABSTRACT 6.1

E-cigarette use in public places: striking the right balance. Bauld, L., McNeill, A., Hajek, P., Britton, J. and Dockrell, M. (2016)

Countries have adopted different approaches to the regulation of electronic cigarettes (e-cigarettes) and other alternative nicotine delivery devices. Some jurisdictions have decided to prohibit use in all indoor workplaces and public places where smoking is not permitted. However, is this the right approach? The United Kingdom has not adopted comprehensive public places bans, for at least three reasons. The first is that the scientific evidence of harm to bystanders from exposure to e-cigarette vapour is very limited and all the existing evidence suggests that the risks are far lower than that for second hand smoke. With this in mind, applying smoke-free laws to e-cigarettes is not currently warranted on health grounds. Secondly, there is growing evidence that e-cigarettes help smokers to stop, and concern that banning them indoors sends the message to smokers that these are harmful products and may deter switching. This is particularly important as surveys show that smokers increasingly believe e-cigarettes are as dangerous as tobacco, a misperception that could undermine efforts to reduce smoking rates. Thirdly, in England, the national public health agency has conducted an extensive consultation with employers and other key stakeholders. This has produced a framework to assist decision-making about which premises choose to introduce restrictions on vaping indoors. Our view is that this type of dialogue is helpful to reach consensus and to balance the public health benefits of e-cigarettes while also acknowledging concerns about their use.

Clearly, conflict models are marked by a power struggle that results in some groups 'winning' or an impasse. The power strategies that are used in groups and organizations to exert control are summarized in Box 6.5. Variations between different groups in their access to resources will influence the pressure that they can bring to bear. The structure of the policy environment may be such that some groups are excluded and, where there are steep social gradients, the most disadvantaged will have greatest difficulty in making their voices heard (Bunton, 1992).

BOX 6.5 POWER STRATEGIES

- Physical power: coercive power, either real or threatened
- Resource power: (also referred to as reward power) deriving from possession of valued resources that may or may not be material
- Position power: (also referred to as legitimate power) associated with position or status
- Expert power: attributed to individuals on account of acknowledged expertise
- Personal power: emanates from the personality and is associated with charisma
- Negative power: the inappropriate use of power outside the recognized domain of interaction. Its intention is subversive, for example not passing on information.

Source: After Handy (1993)

The power strategies that are used in groups and organizations to exert control are summarized in the box above. These strategies include: physical coercion (either real or threatened); the use of expertise or knowledge (expert power); or position or status (position power).

Lindblom and Woodhouse (1993: 128) identify three methods for conflict resolution:

- non-rational and irrational persuasion, as via propaganda campaigns or symbolic rhetoric
- logrolling – that is, steamrollering – vetoes, bribery or other interpersonal means for inducing acquiescence without actually persuading on the merits
- informed and reasoned persuasion.

Profound differences in ideological commitments between different groups make it unlikely that reasoned persuasion will be effective and it may, therefore, be necessary to resort to less rational and more persuasive – or, indeed, coercive – strategies. A 'consensus model' is premised on the view that it is possible to reach agreement and is consistent with pluralism and the 'muddling through' notion of incrementalism.

Bunton (1992) contends that the development of healthy public policy can be built on cooperation and collaboration. Agreements are reached by means of negotiation and bargaining – partisan mutual adjustment. The role of health promotion is to influence the process to maximize health gain via persuasion techniques, such as 'information dissemination, incentives and sanctions' (Bunton, 1992: 146).

Lindblom and Woodhouse (1993: 120) contend that, overall, the level of fundamental disagreement in society is surprisingly small:

Instead, politics normally proceed on the basis of what some call the 'underlying consensus' in a society. Is this agreement brought about by reasoned persuasion, or does much of it evolve through social indoctrination processes … ? Who has the capacity and incentive to use schooling and other socializing institutions to bring about widespread agreements?

Their views draw attention to the narrowness of contemporary debates and raise the question: why has there not been a greater challenge to issues such as inequality? That said, it is apparent that contemporary politics and debate have become more polarized with far greater competing views, perhaps stimulated in the UK by issues such as Brexit. However, inequalities in health have remained a relatively under-discussed issue in society and clear strategies for tackling root causes of inequality have not been forthcoming from policy-makers.

The players – terminology

'Policy actors' are those individuals, groups or organizations involved in policy-making. Their level of involvement may well vary at different stages of the policy development process. For example, groups that are at the forefront of lobbying activity may have a less prominent role in the formulation of policy but might be critical in policy-making 'issue attention' (Brandenberger et al., 2022); politicians, however, are essential players in policy design (Zalmanovitch and Cohen, 2015). An important consideration at each stage is not only who is included but, equally, who is left out. 'Stakeholders' are all those who stand to be affected, in whatever way, by the introduction of a policy and who may be, but are not necessarily, involved in policy-making.

The 'policy keeper' is the agency that, either by mandate or its own initiative, holds a policy and moves the policy forwards during any phase of policy-making (Milio, 1988). The identity of the policy keeper may change during these different phases.

There are various different groups that seek to influence policy. The term 'interest or pressure group' is generally used for groups that exist outside government. Interets groups tend to be concerned with maintaining or increasing their share of resources from governments. Evidence demonstrates that interest groups can influence policy decisions; however, what is less clear are findings that systematically relate interest groups to policy outputs (Breunig and Koski, 2018).

Lindblom and Woodhouse (1993) note the lack of precision in the term 'interest group'. They suggest that business interest, for example, cannot be seen as a 'group' in the conventional sense, but that businesses are organized bureaucracies dominated by a small number of executives. Some of the so-called interest groups may, in fact, be highly influential individuals who take on interest group activity to influence the direction of policy. Somewhat unusually, Lindblom and Woodhouse also suggest that government departments and officials may seek to shape the development of policy by lobbying on behalf of their own interests – operating in substantially the same way as private interest groups – for example, the ministry of health trying to influence fiscal policy on tobacco or transport policy.

Interest groups fall into two broad divisions – those concerned with protecting the interests of their members, such as trades unions, disability rights groups and gay rights groups, and those coming together around a specific issue, such as abortion, pollution or opposition groups to local planning developments. It follows that membership of the former will be restricted to particular groups, whereas in the latter it will be open to anyone with an interest in the issue.

The terminology for these groups varies – Buse et al. (2012) suggest 'sectional' and 'cause' groups. Walt (1994) also notes a further distinction between 'insider' and 'outsider' groups. Insider groups are respected by policy-makers, there are often close working relationships and, because of their recognized legitimacy, these groups tend to be consulted on policy issues and invited to participate in policy-making. Outsider groups, in contrast, have greater difficulty in gaining access to the policy process and may resort to direct action to make their voices heard. Walt cites the activities of Greenpeace, drawing attention to the pollution generated by industry, or anti-abortion groups demonstrating outside clinics. Other activity would involve advocacy and lobbying on behalf of a cause.

An alternative strategy would be to move from outsider to insider status. Walt notes that groups such as the Family Planning Association in the UK and HIV activist groups in a number of countries have achieved insider status by providing services and building up acknowledged expertise in particular areas. Walt also draws attention to the important role of non-governmental organizations (NGOs) in developing countries and Constantino-David's witty categorization (see Box 6.6). While not formally recognized as interest groups, NGOs may consciously seek to influence policy or ensure the public accountability of the state.

BOX 6.6 NON-GOVERNMENTAL ORGANIZATIONS (NGOS)

BINGOS big NGOs

GRINGOS government-run or inspired NGOs

BONGOS business-orientated NGOs

COME'NGOs   NGOs set up opportunistically and that do not last long

Source: Constantino-David (1992) in Walt (1994: 116)

Generally members of the public do not, as individuals, engage directly in the policy-making process. Their influence is more usually via action groups or contributing to creating a collective opinion, such that adoption of a particular policy becomes the most prudent course of action for politicians seeking to maintain their popularity with the electorate. As an example, Mumsnet, the online support community for mothers, has been influential in shaping policy decisions on various issues, including the support available for miscarried parents and preventing the premature sexualization of children. There are, however, notable exceptions where committed individuals have managed to secure policy change. A well-known example is the case of Victoria Gillick, who challenged a Department of Health circular stating that young people under the legal age of consent could receive confidential contraceptive advice and treatment. She succeeded in 1984 in winning a Court of Appeal ruling that girls under 16 should not be given contraceptives without their parents' consent, although this was subsequently overturned by a House of Lords decision in *Gillick* v.

West Norfolk and Wisbech Area Health Authority and Another [1986] 1 AC 112. More recently, Laura Ahearn is known for her work in attempting to change policy on the prevention of child sexual abuse and the introduction of 'Megan's Law' in the USA.

A 'policy network' is the 'collection of actors and organizations that influences decision making in a policy sector' (John, 1998: 205). A network is made up of a number of 'policy communities'. John (1998: 83) suggests that this term implies that 'the participants know each other well and … share the same values and policy goals' and defines it (1998: 204) as 'a restricted set of actors and organizations which influence decisions on a policy sector'. A good example is in relation to climate change where policy communities from sectors such as defence, development and environmental protection form collaborations based on shared interests (Abrahams, 2021). From this perspective, policy decisions are viewed as the outcome of discussions within policy networks and this approach emphasizes the possibility of influencing policy through diverse routes (for example, via journalists or NGOs) (Smith and Katikireddi, 2013). Think tanks (for instance, the Global Warming Policy Foundation, Policy Exchange and Copenhagen Institute) are also regarded as policy networks able to influence policy decisions; these organizations exist independently of government and can offer fresh perspectives on policy solutions (Bennett et al., 2012). Think tanks traditionally develop ideas, make policy proposals to political stakeholders, develop and try to influence public opinion (Allern and Pollack, 2020). However, commenting on the power of think tanks in Bangladesh, Rashid (2013) states that their direct impact on policy outcomes remains limited. That said, in other parts of the world, such as the UK, think tanks can exert substantial influence over the policy-making process (Arshed, 2017).

Coalitions

In that networks include different public, private and commercial organizations, it is likely that a range of different viewpoints will be represented. 'Coalitions' may, therefore, develop between groupings sharing similar values. They can become a major force within the policy arena and, indeed, 'The more people you have on your side the greater your influence' (Hubley et al., 2021: 190). Coalitions, community partnerships and collaboratives are increasingly being seen as a viable vehicle to create population-wide, macro-level changes, and communities with strong coalitions tend to access more resources, cultivate greater power and are able to mobilize change (Lardier Jr et al., 2019). Coalitions have been defined (Feighery and Rogers, 1989, in Butterfoss et al., 1993: 316) as:

> an organization of individuals representing diverse organizations, factions or constituencies who agree to work together to achieve a common goal.

Box 6.7 describes the importance of coalitions, but the key elements can be summarized as:

- unity in working towards a common goal
- pooling of resources
- increased capacity to achieve the goal.

Butterfoss et al.'s (1993) review of the literature on coalitions identifies three types of coalition, based on Feighery and Rogers (1989):

- **grassroots coalitions**: generally set up by volunteers to respond to a crisis, such as closure of a local hospital
- **professional coalitions**: formed by professional organizations
- **community-based coalitions**: usually initiated by an agency, but involving professionals and grassroots leaders.

Hubley et al. (2021) note difficulties and barriers with forming coalitions, including: differing concepts of health promotion, values, visions and aims; concerns that smaller organizations may get swamped by larger ones; concerns over loss of identity; and concerns that the coalition might be slow to respond to political events.

BOX 6.7 THE IMPORTANCE OF COALITIONS

- Coalitions spread responsibility across a number of organizations and enable them to become involved in a broader range of issues.
- Coalitions both demonstrate and mobilize public support for an issue.
- Coalitions can maximize the power brought to bear on an issue and achieve a 'critical mass' to mobilize system change.
- Coalitions can minimize duplication of effort.
- Coalitions provide access to a wider range of talent and resources – human and material – and can 'enhance the leverage' of groups.
- Coalitions are a vehicle for recruiting additional groups to enhance knowledge, understanding, skills and resources – across a range of constituencies – to a cause.
- The flexibility of coalitions enables them to draw on new resources as situations change.

Source: Butterfoss et al. (1993); Hubley et al. (2021); Lardier Jr et al., 2019

Clark et al. (2010) reported on the policy and system changes produced by a community coalition – the Allies Against Asthma programme – to address childhood asthma in low-income communities of colour across the USA. This coalition established policies related to improved clinical practices and system coordination for children with asthma. As an example, a policy was established that permitted children with asthma to carry and self-administer life-saving medication in school settings; moreover, legislation was passed in Puerto Rico that protects a child's right to take asthma medication in school.

We have already considered the issue of intersectoral working and healthy alliances in Chapter 4. However, we should note here some of the factors associated with the success of coalitions (see Box 6.8).

BOX 6.8 FACTORS ASSOCIATED WITH COALITION FUNCTIONING

Member characteristics and perceptions

- Member benefits
- Member participation
- Member satisfaction and commitment
- Members' skills and training
- Representativeness of members
- Member recruitment
- Member expectations
- Ownership.

Organizational or group processes

- Conflict resolution
- Decision-making
- Clear mission
- Quality of action plan
- Formalized roles and procedures
- Technical assistance
- Resources available.

Organizational or group characteristics and climate

- Community context and readiness
- Group relationships/collaboration
- Communication
- Strong leadership.

Impacts and outcomes

- Linkages to other groups/community
- Policy advocacy/change
- Empowerment/social capital
- Community capacity
- Institutionalization.

Source: Granner and Sharpe (2004)

One of the key elements in coalition formation is the development of a clear goal to which all members can subscribe (Lardier Jr et al., 2019). Indeed, research by McCartan and Palermo (2017) on a rural food policy coalition in Australia demonstrated the importance of a shared vision and direction. While a whole range of factors related to structure, leadership and interpersonal factors will affect the maintenance of the coalition, member satisfaction is important – members need to perceive the coalition as beneficial. Achieving some short-term success will increase motivation and the credibility of the coalition. However, this should not detract from a focus on the overall goal. Clearly, evaluation of outcomes is essential in demonstrating progress and sustaining momentum. Feighery and Rogers (1989) found that the following influenced members' satisfaction with the coalition:

- it is managed effectively
- it has good communication among membership
- it has low costs of, and barriers to, participation.

Gottlieb et al. (1993) recommend:

- formalization of agreements, mission statements, and goals and objectives
- attention to the process of group formation
- clarification of expectations.

Health social movements

Since the industrial revolution, health movements have been an important feature in advocating and agreeing occupational health and safety measures for employees (Daykin, 2019). According to Laverack (2013: 24), health social movements:

> challenge state, institutional and other forms of authority to give the public more of a voice in health policy and regulation.

Health social movements deploy a broad range of tactics, including: engaging in the legal realm; shaping public health research; employing creative media tactics to highlight the need for structural social change; and engaging in the policy arena (Brown and Zavestoski, 2004). They can be progressive, reformist or conservative in their outlook and view of the world (Daykin, 2019). Both Brown and Zavestoski (2004) and Laverack (2013) suggest that people have become more accepting of challenging health policy because of the growing level of awareness about health through the Internet. This has been coupled by the negative publicity received about, for example, experimentation with contraceptives, radiation and immunization, that has created a heightened level of cynicism in the public. People have realized that as a collective they can apply significant pressure to influence policy that affects their health at both an individual and a collective level. An example of a health social movement is the Scottish Dementia Working Group (SDWG), who are a campaign group set up and run by people with dementia and whose aim is for people with the condition to unite and influence policy (Weaks et al., 2012). Bartlett's (2013) research on dementia activism suggests a number of reasons motivating individuals to participate in social movements. One finding, worthy of further investigation, suggested that activism prevented individuals from further decline in their health from the condition. Barlett's participants perceived their actions to have an 'energizing quality' that gave individuals 'a terrific buzz from [activism]'. That said, academic critiques of activism in the field of dementia has offered a different perspective, suggesting that such approaches can exacerbate stigma (Fletcher, 2021).

POLICY-MAKING

According to Milio (2001: 622), policy-making is 'driven by organisations and groups that have an interest in the outcomes'. The main stages in policy-making are problem identification, policy formulation, implementation and evaluation. While this may be taken to imply a chronological sequence, in reality, the process may be more iterative and complex.

Delaney (1994c: 7) cites the questions posed by Anderson (1975) as a means of identifying key issues at each stage and proposes adding 'Why?' and 'Why not?' to expose more fundamental concerns – particularly the location and operation of political power:

1. **Problem formation.** What is a policy problem? How does it get on the agenda of government?
2. **Formulation**. How are the alternatives for dealing with the problem developed? Who participates?
3. **Adoption**. How is a policy alternative adopted or enacted? Who adopts?
4. **Implementation**. What is done, if anything, to carry a policy into effect? What impact does this have on policy content?
5. **Evaluation**. How is effectiveness measured? Who evaluates? What are the consequences?

Milio (1988) also offers a series of generic issues to consider in relation to policy-making and these are set out in Box 6.9.

BOX 6.9 POLICY-MAKING – ISSUES TO CONSIDER

- Agenda setting – whether or not a given public issue is an appropriate problem for public policy
- Problem framing – determining the definition and scope of the problem
- Priority setting
- Option setting – finding possible optional solutions, including goals and strategies
- Criteria selection – by what criteria options should be chosen
- Policy selection – who bears the responsibility to decide
- Means choice – how, and by whom, the policy should be implemented
- Success indicators – determining the criteria and sources of evaluation
- Changing goals or means – how the policy should be reformulated.

Source: After Milio (1988: 266)

There is clearly a need for those wishing to influence policy to form alliances and identify 'points of entry' into the policy-making process. In the same way that healthy public policy should make the healthy choice the easy choice, efforts to influence policy should make the healthy policy option the most attractive option. Clearly, both insiders and outsiders will need political skills and acumen to exert influence effectively in the policy arena.

Ideally, policy should be based on sound evidence and there is clearly a need to produce relevant information to inform the policy-making process. A recent study by Homer et al. (2022) showed how elected politicians often found making research-led policy decisions challenging due the culture and environment in local government. Research was not prioritized organizationally and research active staff members within local government were the exception, rather than the rule. Some studies have suggested how elected politicians working in local authorities rely on rudimentary Internet searches to find information to inform their practice – often due to the inaccessibility of peer-reviewed research publications (Le Gouais et al., 2019). In addition, barriers to accessing research that is contextually specific to the local area is a common problem that elected politicians face when utilizing evidence to inform decision-making (Ige-Elegbede et al., 2021).

The reality is that policy-making is heavily influenced by assumptions, vested interests and power positions. Clarke et al. (2016), for instance, showed how, in policy formulation in relation to obesity prevention, professional judgement and political ideology were stronger drivers than research evidence. In a reflective paper written by public health professionals, the challenges of influencing electronic cigarette policy using research evidence were highlighted:

> We learned that our position could be challenged even though we were sharing evidence-based and evidence-informed policy options, and we needed to be prepared to respectfully but convincingly counter arguments from the electronic cigarette industry and 'vaping' advocates. (Garcia et al., 2015: 165)

Bearing in mind our various earlier discussions, it will be apparent that the relative power of the key groups of players is of paramount importance. At a government level, conflict between ministers is a well-known phenomenon.

Key assumptions in the policy-making process concern 'cause and effect' and 'intervention effect' – that is, if we do X then Y will follow. While data can be collected to establish the nature of a problem and predictions can be made about the effects of policy change, the challenge is to convert research findings into a form that conveys a powerful message that appeals to dominant values. It is also important to understand the power structures in the policy arena and how to manipulate them. As Milio (1988: 265) suggests, the development of 'policy relevant' information requires consideration of the following issues:

- how to extrapolate the policy implications of data
- how to propose feasible policy options
- how to judge the social and political responses to issues and proposals
- who to contact, when and how.

The notion of 'creative epidemiology' is concerned with making research findings and epidemiological data more accessible. It is a way of restating data that makes the information more compelling and visual – it is not about embellishing or exaggerating as this can undermine the message (Anderson and Miller, 2016). For example, expressing death rates from smoking-related diseases in conventional epidemiological terms as rates per 100,000 or as relative risk – while undoubtedly essential in establishing evidence of the effects of smoking on health – has little impact outside professional circles. Expressing the data though in relation to, for example, 'the number of smokers that die each day' is easier for audiences to conceptualize.

Infographics are becoming increasingly recognized as a way to communicate 'creative epidemiology' information and were seen consistently throughout the COVID-19 pandemic to communicate health risks to communities. Recent research by Egan et al. (2021) has shown that infographics have aided people's understanding of correct mask-wearing techniques and compliance. Infographics aided the recall of correct mask techniques by highlighting salient steps and reducing cognitive burden. Infographics were also identified as providing individuals with greater levels of trustworthiness in the message than text-only guidance. Infographics often translate complex evidence into meaningful ways for lay audiences and for policy-makers. Historically, WHO (2018c) has invested heavily in the production of infographics, producing these on a variety of issues from smoking to malaria to mental health. As an illustration of the use of 'creative epidemiology', WHO's (2018c) infographic on suicide states that 800,000 suicides happen each year or one suicide every 40 seconds across the world.

Agenda setting

The 'policy agenda' has been defined as the:

> list of issues to which an organization, usually the government, is giving serious attention at any one time with a view to taking some sort of action. (Buse et al., 2012: 65)

A key question concerns how issues get on to – or fail to get on to – the policy agenda. Jones and Sidell (1997) refer to the well-known UK example of the effective 'burying' of Sir Douglas Black's report, *Inequalities in Health* (Department of Health and Social Security [DHSS], 1980), by tactics such as producing a limited number of copies and its publication on an August bank holiday, which ensured minimum publicity. Whitehead's update on inequality, *The Health Divide* (1987), suffered a similar fate and there was only tacit reference to inequality in the first national health strategy, *Health of the Nation* (Department of Health, 1992).

Notwithstanding the lack of national political attention, sound research evidence demonstrating inequality to be a major public health issue generated a groundswell of opinion at local and national levels, including public health professionals, academics, pressure groups and the public. Against this backdrop, inequality has received progressively increasing government attention, although the type of policy instrument to tackle inequalities, for example obesity, is often ideologically driven with neoliberal viewpoints often protecting economic development 'at all costs' (Clarke et al., 2016).

Timing is a critical factor when attempting to get an issue on the policy agenda (Korenik and Węgrzyn, 2020), evidenced in the development of Arkansas's childhood obesity policy where the timeliness of several factors opened up a 'policy window' that enabled childhood obesity to be on the political agenda (Craig et al., 2010). Hogwood and Gunn (1984) suggest that an issue is most likely to get on the policy agenda if any of the following apply:

- It has reached crisis proportions.
- It has achieved particularity – that is, it exemplifies a larger issue.
- It has an emotive aspect.
- It is likely to have wide impact.
- It raises questions about power and legitimacy in society.
- It is currently 'fashionable'.

Other factors, such as the role of influential personalities, or an event of some kind that triggers widespread media interest can influence the agenda. For example, the 2018 inquest verdict that the death of child asthma sufferer Ella Roberta Kissi-Debrah was directly linked to air pollution on busy London roads, the announcement that actress Barbara Windsor had dementia in 2018, and rugby international Gareth Jones sharing his story of being HIV positive in 2019 all led to increased public interest in the particular policy issues (Hubley et al., 2021). However, the influence of 'agenda setters' (see Box 6.10) can also be pivotal (Hubley et al., 2021). As we have already noted, the elitist viewpoint (Hogwood and Gunn would also include anything other than the most naive pluralist interpretation) acknowledges that there may be unequal access to the policy agenda. John (1998: 147) suggests that:

> the distribution of power is the underlying factor, but it is more normal in radical accounts to stress the salience of ideas and political language which marginalizes certain interests and ideas. Power is expressed through the hegemony of certain ideas. Created by the middle or upper classes and by economic interests, ruling ideologies ensure that certain issues are off the agenda and others are on it.

BOX 6.10 AGENDA SETTERS

- Organized interests
- Protest groups
- Political party leaders
- Senior government officials and advisers
- Informed opinion
- Mass media and social media

The notion of 'bounded pluralism' has been applied to gaining access to the policy agenda. Elite groups may have dominant influence over major issues, of high politics, whereas there may be much more open debate on more minor and less politically sensitive issues. In addition to what gets on to the policy agenda, an important consideration is what is kept off. Elite groups may take on a gatekeeper function in relation to major – potentially politically damaging – issues (Hubley et al., 2021). Efforts to confine the agenda to safe issues can simply involve filtering out more contentious ones, but also, and perhaps rather more sinisterly, implicitly or explicitly shaping people's perceptions of what they want and need (Lukes, 2021). Reich (2002) maintains that policy change is dependent on the political will of leaders. The role of policy advocates, therefore, is to create that political will. This requires political analysis to identify the key stakeholders and their intentions, potential losers and winners, and where support and opposition will lie. It also requires the adoption of appropriate political strategies.

ADVOCACY

Healthy public policy depends on political vision and leadership and Draper (1988: 218) contends that leadership 'must begin with the people who have a strong professional responsibility for public health'. Despite advocacy being regarded as a core competency for health promotion practice, both in some national (Public Health England, 2016) and international frameworks (Barry et al., 2009), advocacy tends to be an underdeveloped element of health promotion and public health practice, arguably being seen as a lower priority than programme planning and implementation. Garcia et al. (2015) suggest that health promoters lack experience in policy advocacy and perhaps because of this, Radius et al. (2009) propose improving the professional preparation of health educators to take on an advocacy role.

Defining advocacy

Advocacy was identified as a key strategy by the Ottawa Charter (WHO, 1986) and is one of the three major strategies for health promotion (Nutbeam and Muscat, 2021). The term 'advocacy' has traditionally been used to describe activity on behalf of those in a less powerful position. Laverack (2013) also notes that advocacy concerns influencing the outcome of decisions. It is about protecting vulnerable individuals in society, empowering people and tackling inequalities – with contemporary examples including how health promoters are advocating political institutions to consider their policies on climate change and health (Patrick et al., 2019).

The International Union for Health Education (1992) identified three main areas in which advocates can operate:

- influencing government to develop healthy policies and legislation
- influencing commercial and other organizations to consider the health impact of their activities and exert pressure on governments and citizens
- influencing individuals and groups to make healthy choices and support initiatives to promote health.

Advocacy for health has been defined as:

> A combination of individual and social actions designed to gain political commitment, policy support, social acceptance and systems support for a particular health goal or programme. (Nutbeam and Muscat, 2021: 1588)

Wallack et al. (1993: 27) suggest that:

> Advocacy is a catch-all word for the set of skills used to create a shift in public opinion and mobilize the necessary resources and forces to support an issue, policy, or constituency. Advocacy involves much more than lobbying in support of a certain piece of legislation. Health professionals routinely engage in a wide array of advocacy activities, including patient advocacy, client advocacy, and policy advocacy, all designed to make the system function better to meet health and safety goals ...

They draw on Amidei (1991, in Wallack et al., 1993: 28) to identify several characteristics of advocacy:

- Advocacy assumes that people have rights, and those rights are enforceable.
- Advocacy works best when focused on something specific.
- Advocacy is primarily concerned with rights and benefits to which someone or some community is already entitled.

Policy advocacy is concerned with ensuring that institutions work the way they should. Patient and client advocacy are concerned with ensuring that individuals obtain their rights. Our concern here is with the broader area of policy advocacy – specifically, healthy public policy advocacy and issues affecting collective rights. The related activity of lobbying is taken to apply narrowly to attempts to persuade members of government to take up a cause.

Walt (1994) distinguishes between 'commercial lobbyists', who will take on any cause, and 'cause lobbyists', who are seeking to further the specific cause to which they subscribe. Both may adopt similar tactics and seek close relationships with civil servants as well as elected representatives.

In contrast, the target of advocacy may range wider than government circles to generate support among interest groups, the media and the general public. Based on the premise that democratic governments tend to act in line with major public opinion – or at least not risk alienating it – the overall intention of public health advocacy is to create a climate of support for healthy policy options.

As Milio (1981: 304) argues:

> The development of organized advocacy for the public's health may well be necessary to demand that government use its resources for health-making purposes. If so, advocacy must go far beyond the usual voicing of discontent, or of admonitions to individuals to change their ways. The message must be conveyed in ways that create widespread and informed public debate. Usable translations of the message are necessary. Explanations are needed of the complexities of the health problem, of alternate health strategies, and of their costs and gains. The true costs of not preventing illness must be addressed, as well as the protections that are possible for those whose livelihoods might be harmed during transitions. Workable formats for presenting the message and convenient forums for discussion are needed for the general public and for its subgroups, for the mass media and specialized professional media, for policymakers, and for scientists and methodologists. Such groundwork seems essential to effective policy-influencing action. Its ultimate strategic purpose is to make health-promoting policy decisions easier for policymakers to choose.

Wise (2001) contends that, although the overall aim may be to change the legislative, fiscal, physical and social environment, advocacy is fundamentally a political process that aims to influence political decisions. She draws on Wallack (1998) to distinguish between advocacy and public education or social marketing. Although they may use the same media to communicate their messages, the latter are predicated on the assumption that problems are due to a lack of information and focus on filling the information gap. Advocacy, on the other hand, focuses on the *power* gap and problems are seen to be due to a lack of sufficient power to achieve social change. Advocacy, therefore, attempts to mobilize support and political involvement. McCubbin et al. (2001) note two interrelated facets of advocacy as a health promotion strategy:

- prescriptive or campaign-style advocacy
- empowering or community development-style advocacy.

Strategies

Effective advocacy involves identifying and assessing the power of opposition groups and supporters as a basis for targeting action to build support and develop coalitions, along with undermining the opposition.

Advocacy relies on the tactical use of persuasive communication. Presenting the evidence is not enough. Effective advocacy must, in Klein's words, be 'logically persuasive, morally authoritative, and capable of evoking passion. Furthermore, effective advocacy campaigns often use a 'simplifying concept' – catchy phrases that communicate more complex ideas such as 'global warming' and 'second-hand tobacco smoke'. Symbolic representations can also be useful; for example, the red ribbon for HIV awareness or white wrist band as the symbol of the Make Poverty History campaign.

Advocacy involves framing issues to convey their fundamental essence and constructing arguments to appeal to potential supporters. The various players present what is in the best interests of their group by filtering information from factual reality.

Given that there is no objective reality, public health policy initiatives are open to a range of interpretations (Chapman and Lupton, 1994). These will inevitably be influenced by values and ideological commitments. Milio suggests that we need to understand how a policy will affect major stakeholders and how they frame their support or opposition.

Effective advocacy requires careful framing of arguments and, conversely, understanding of the way the opposition is framing its own arguments so that an appropriate response can be mounted. In planning advocacy programmes the following questions need to be considered (see Box 6.11).

BOX 6.11 PLANNING ADVOCACY PROGRAMMES: KEY QUESTIONS

- What is the ultimate objective you wish to achieve?
- What are the intermediate objectives you need to achieve on the way to the ultimate objective?
- Who are the people you need to reach – the decision-makers and gatekeepers?
- At what level do they operate – community, organizational, district, regional, national or international?

Source: Hubley et al. (2021)

Efforts to sway public and political opinion will need to draw on a whole repertoire of proactive and reactive, creative, dramatic and news-grabbing tactics. An example is provided in Box 6.12.

BOX 6.12 ADVOCACY IN ACTION

Surfers against Sewage (SAS) launched the Return to Offender campaign in April 2006 at the opening of the O'Neill Highland Open Surfing international competition in Thurso, Scotland. Companies identified from litter collected on local beaches were contacted by competitors to persuade them to:

- improve 'the anti-littering' message on their products
- look at using less harmful packaging to ensure products can break down naturally without putting wildlife at risk
- promote recycling and/or reuse wherever appropriate, including more involvement with community 'anti-litter' initiatives.

Source: SAS (2008)

The media can be particularly effective in bringing issues to the public's attention and in influencing opinion (Laverack, 2013). Chapman and Lupton (1994: 19) note that relatively few key decision-makers need to be convinced before action is taken and that highly placed individuals – politicians, senior bureaucrats and heads of non-governmental organizations – are 'often highly sensitive to the ways in which the media are framing issues and setting public expectations about the roles they should perform'. Furthermore, where there is dispute, the media can become the 'battlegrounds on which each side seeks to secure the most powerful connotations for its cause, and to attribute to its adversaries the most negative associations' (Chapman and Lupton, 1994: 99). They contend that the success of an advocacy campaign can hinge on the way in which issues are framed in the media and how they are reframed to respond strategically to the efforts of the opposition.

BOX 6.13 ALTERNATIVE FRAMES FOR CHARITABLE ACTION

Archbishop Helder Camara of Brazil said, 'When I feed the hungry, they call me a saint. When I ask why they have no food, they call me a Communist.'

Source: Cited by Wallack et al. (1993)

Given that many – if not most – public health pressure groups have insufficient funds to buy advertising space in the media to publicize their causes, maximizing free media coverage becomes essential.

Like the well-known acronym for giving information to politicians – KISS (keep it short and simple) – gaining access to the media demands brevity rather than protracted rational argument. In this regard, the Internet and other social media (for instance, Twitter) has increasingly been seen as a tool for publicizing causes and to bring about social and political change (Laverack, 2013). E-petitions, as an example, have been used to advocate for improved services or to generate public support for a cause (Baringhorst et al., 2009). Hubley et al. (2021) offer the following advice on using the Internet for advocacy activity:

1. Provide information on your issue, including a calendar of events, details of meetings, critical dates when policy decisions are being made by authorities, suggestions for letter-writing to decision-makers.
2. Set up an online petition to which people can add their name.
3. Invite visitors to your website to send emails describing their own advocacy activities and views about the topic.
4. Compile a page of Frequently Asked Questions (FAQs) on your issue.
5. Include a web forum on which people can post and exchange messages.

As noted previously, the association of a celebrity with an issue or cause can attract considerable publicity. Well-known individuals, such as Arthur Ashe, Rock Hudson, Earvin (Magic) Johnson and Freddie Mercury, brought the issue of HIV and AIDS to the forefront of public attention by generating substantial media coverage. Bono, the lead singer of the rock group U2, drew attention to health and social issues in Africa and Angelina Jolie has raised political consciousness of the plight of displaced people in Sierra Leone and beyond (Thrall et al., 2008). Celebrities endorsing or highlighting issues via social media has become an increasingly prominent part of contemporary life with research showing that by celebrities simply retweeting health campaign measures, this can significantly increase awareness and exposure in populations (Chung, 2017; Macnab and Mukisa, 2018).

We will consider the issue of media advocacy more fully in Chapter 8. Box 6.14 provides a set of tips for gaining media coverage.

BOX 6.14 TIPS FOR GETTING ITEMS INTO THE MEDIA

- Get to know the media – know what types of stories they publish.
- Develop good relationships with local journalists and local radio and television.
- Build up a list of contacts of people who handle your sort of story.
- Be realistic about the amount of interest your story will attract.
- Find a local angle.
- Use concrete examples rather than abstract ideas.
- Find a human interest angle.
- Think visual and use a good picture.
- Involve celebrities.

While the media may be very effective in raising awareness of issues, Walt (1994) notes that policy-makers are unlikely to be influenced by a single media account and poses the question of how long media coverage has to be sustained before an issue is put on to the policy agenda.

Campaign groups will, therefore, need to consider strategies for maintaining the visibility of issues over a protracted period. In some parts of the world, state control of the media casts doubt on its impartial reporting. Similarly, economic interests may dictate what gains coverage. Newspaper editors and radio and television producers occupy a key gatekeeping role. Over and above dominant ideological frameworks shaping the content of the media, there may also be more conscious filtering of information. Walt refers to the 'propaganda model' of Herman and Chomsky, which is based on the view that the media are controlled to further the interests of the state and powerful groups. Factors that may affect the filtering of news coverage include ownership, profit orientation, advertising and sources of information.

Returning to the more general issues of advocacy, Baum (2001: 107) suggests that successful advocacy strategies should:

- set an agenda
- frame the issue for public consumption
- advocate specific solutions.

The 'A' Frame for Advocacy developed by the Johns Hopkins Center for Communication Programs (undated) identifies six stages in the advocacy process:

1. **Analysis** of the problem, the need for policy change, stakeholders and, specifically, supporters, opponents, decision-makers and vote swingers, policy-making structures and processes and means of influencing decision-makers
2. **Strategy** based on clear objectives suited to the context
3. **Mobilization** of potential partners and coalition building to maximize collective resources and power
4. **Action** achieving maximum visibility for the cause using credible messages and appropriate channels, including the media
5. **Evaluation** to identify what has been achieved and what still needs to be done
6. **Continuity** planning for the longer term, keeping coalitions together, keeping arguments fresh and adapting them to current circumstances.

Having clear objectives is a key factor in coordinating activity during the various stages. Furthermore, advocacy efforts are more likely to be successful if decisions about the most appropriate courses of action are based on an analysis of contextual factors and the location of power and influence. Chapman and Lupton (1994: 130) also caution that those involved in advocacy should be clear about their goals and not lose sight of 'the big picture'. Moreover, advocacy should not become an end in itself, but a means of achieving public health goals.

Key questions to guide an advocacy strategy are therefore:

- What are the public health objectives?
- Who are the main stakeholder groups?

- What alliances/coalitions can usefully be formed?
- Who is the target? Who has the power to bring about change?
- What is the message?
- How can the message be framed to appeal to the target group/s?
- Which channel/s will be most effective for reaching the target?
- What other action will achieve visibility for the cause and a supportive climate of public opinion?
- What opposition is there?
- How can opposition be countered?
- How will you know you have been successful and what milestones are there en route to success?

ADOPTION AND IMPLEMENTATION

Whether polices are adopted or not will depend on a range of factors. There is often an 'implementa-tion gap', defined as the 'difference between what the policy architect intended and the end-result of a policy' (Buse et al., 2012: 129). As an example, Amuyunzu-Nyamongo et al. (2009: 185) have argued that in the African Continent there has been a 'worrying disconnect' between policy formulation and implementation, which remains one of the fundamental challenges to the development of health pro-motion. Warwick-Booth et al. (2021) suggest that barriers to implementation include:

- practitioners and their level of commitment, experience, attitudes and time available
- lack of resources (financial and human resources)
- policy overload and contradictions
- poor communication
- partners who are not on-board or who undermine implementation.

Furthermore, Bunton (1992) notes that policies may be modified and considerably watered down during the process of development and implementation. This may be the product of powerful inter-ests bringing their weight to bear or, alternatively, the decisions and routines established by what Lipsky (1997) terms 'street-level bureaucrats' – workers in public services, such as welfare departments, schools, health services and so on. As an example, Woodall and Tattersfield (2018) showed how some prison officers were likely to ignore the complete smoking ban in all areas of the prison estate as they themselves were smokers or believed that their time was too constrained to 'police' or enforce this policy.

Walt (1994: 165) also sees that the implementation of policy requires the cooperation of many different groups and that 'policy formulation, even in the form of a legal statute, is not a sufficient condition for implementation'. Hogwood and Gunn (1997) contend that the perfect implementation of policy is extremely unlikely and specify the conditions that would need to exist for this to happen:

- circumstances external to the implementing agency not imposing crippling constraints
- adequate time and sufficient resources being made available
- the required combination of resources being available
- the policy being based on a valid theory of cause and effect

- the relationship between cause and effect being direct and few, if any, intervening links
- dependency relationships being minimal
- understanding of, and agreement on, objectives
- tasks being fully specified, in the right sequence
- perfect communication and coordination
- those in authority being able to demand and obtain perfect compliance.

Springett (1998) notes that intersectoral policy is notorious for failure during implementation. Clearly, ensuring that the conditions specified are met is particularly problematic when a number of different agencies and sectors are involved. Colebatch (1998: 56) states that there is held to be a problem in implementation when 'the outcome was likely to be quite different to the originally stated intentions'. By way of illustration, he quotes the title of the seminal work by Pressman and Wildavsky (1973): *Implementation: How Great Expectations in Washington Are Dashed in Oakland: or, Why it's Amazing that Federal Programs Work at All, This Being a Saga of the Economic Development Administration as Told by Two Sympathetic Observers Who Seek to Build Morals on a Foundation of Ruined Hopes.* The problems identified by Pressman and Wildavsky include having a large number of participants and diversity of goals, such that approval is needed to be obtained at a number of different points.

Colebatch provides a useful overview of the ways in which implementation problems are perceived. The vertical perspective assumes a top-down approach and sees implementation as requiring compliance with the directives of those in authority. In contrast, a horizontal perspective recognizes that participants have their own agendas and interpretations of policy. It also acknowledges that the flow of influence is not only vertically within organizations, but that there is negotiation with people external to them.

The horizontal perspective views the implementation of policy rather more flexibly than the vertical. It would see implementation as a collective action that evolves to be compatible with the policy goals and the perspectives of participants rather than a strict adherence to top-down directives.

A further distinction is between normative frameworks, which are concerned with what 'ought to be', and empirical frameworks, which are concerned with 'what is'.

Colebatch equates the vertical perspective on implementation with normative frameworks and the horizontal with empirical frameworks. He notes, too, that there can be two coexisting accounts of the implementation process – the *sacred*, which presents the ideal, and the *profane*, which is a more realistic account of what actually happened.

The means of securing policy implementation will inevitably vary according to the perspective. The vertical perspective will focus on policy goals and compliance, whereas the horizontal will pay greater attention to processes and the people involved.

HEALTH IMPACT ASSESSMENT

We turn our attention now to the wider issue of health impact assessment (HIA). As we noted earlier, the notion of healthy public policy is not just concerned with the development of policies to tackle health issues, but also requires an appraisal of the health impact of all policies. While the practice of

HIA can vary according to different international contexts and approaches (Khomenko et al., 2021; Winkler et al., 2013), HIA is defined by Green et al. (2021: 2) as:

> a decision-informing tool which can support the development and implementation of policy decisions by identifying a broad and holistic health impact across the determinants of physical, social, environmental and mental health and well-being

Over the last 10 to 20 years, HIA has been particularly high on the public health agenda in Europe as its capacity to assess differential impact on various groups within the population makes it an important tool in efforts to achieve equity in health (Hubley et al., 2021). As mentioned, HIA can apply to policy, programmes, projects and industrial and commercial activity. For example, a comprehensive HIA was conducted prior to the Glasgow Commonwealth Games in 2014 and outlined the potential positive or negative health impacts of the Games on individuals and communities (Glasgow City Council, undated) and, more recently, an HIA was undertaken to assess air pollution in European cities (Khomenko et al., 2021) and also the impact of 'staying at home and social distancing' during COVID-19 (Green et al., 2021). Our focus in the remainder of the chapter, however, is principally with the use of HIA in policy development.

Kemm (2001) suggests that healthy public policy is dependent on predicting the health consequences of different policy options and ensuring that the policy process gives consideration to these potential consequences at all stages. Winkler et al. (2013: 298) also suggest that:

> HIA is used to assess the likely effect of a policy, programme or project in a specific situation by drawing on the available evidence.

HIA, therefore, leads to informed policy-making and provides the opportunity to adapt decisions in order to avoid potential harm. It is considered to add value to policy and decision-making processes (Green et al., 2021) and in some countries, for example Thailand, HIA is a legislative requirement. Indeed, in Thailand HIA is used to settle conflicts between government and civil society in that citizens have the right to request an assessment when they have concerns about government policy decisions (Leppo et al., 2013). Other benefits of HIA are listed in Box 6.15.

BOX 6.15 THE BENEFITS OF HEALTH IMPACT ASSESSMENT

Health impact assessment can:

- promote equity, sustainability and healthy public policy in an unequal and frequently unhealthy world
- improve the quality of decision-making in health and partner organizations by incorporating the need to address health issues into planning and policy-making

- emphasize social and environmental justice (it is usually those who are already disadvantaged who suffer most from negative health impacts)
- encourage public participation in debates about public policy issues
- give equal status to both qualitative and quantitative assessment methods
- make values and politics explicit, and open issues to public scrutiny
- demonstrate that health-relevant policy is far broader than health-care issues.

Source: Scott-Samuel and O'Keefe (2007: 212)

Despite the benefits of HIA for policy development, it is apparent that such an approach is not always fully utilized. In some parts of the world, for instance, the development of HIA has been less thorough, as shown in Caussy et al.'s (2003) article on the use of HIA in South East Asian countries and Winkler et al.'s (2013) discussion of HIA in developing countries. To respond to this, advocates have lobbied the WHO to develop and promote HIA, especially in Africa. They argue that the WHO's website has very few examples of HIA deriving from low and medium human development index countries (Winkler et al., 2013).

Identifying the potential health impact of policy is necessarily complex – given the plethora of factors that interact to influence health status, both directly and indirectly. Moreover, policy development in one sector may have a knock-on effect in another. The key questions to consider in planning to undertake an HIA are summarized in Box 6.16.

BOX 6.16 KEY QUESTIONS CONCERNING HIA

- What

  - o ... policies will be screened and what are the criteria for deciding?
  - o ... impacts will be assessed? Will these include health outcomes, determinants, risks and equity?

- How

  - o ... will HIA happen? Will it be integrated or conducted separately? Will it be a voluntary or legal requirement?
  - o ... can we infer causality between policy and outcome?

- When

  - o ... will HIA be introduced into the policy process?

(Continued)

- Who

  - ... does the assessment? Will this be the policy proponent or an external agency?
  - ... pays?

- Where

  - ... at international, national or local levels?

Source: After European Centre for Health Policy (1999: 8)

To have maximum influence, HIA will need to be integrated into the various stages of policy-making. Kemm (2012a) notes the importance of HIAs fitting into the 'windows of opportunity' that arise during the policy-making process. There is general agreement that HIA should be carried out early enough for there to be sufficient fluidity in the decision-making process to respond to the findings. Although, optimally, HIA will be predictive in order to enable remedial action to be taken, the National Assembly for Wales (1999) identifies three types of assessment:

- **prospective:** predicts the effects of policy before it is implemented
- **retrospective:** identifies the consequences of a policy already implemented (such evidence may inform future prospective assessments)
- **concurrent:** undertaken during policy implementation.

Banken (2001) identifies two conceptual streams that have informed the development of HIA – namely, environmental impact assessment, which focused on the environmental consequences of projects, and the public health emphasis on the social and environmental determinants of health. Lerer (1999) notes that the current focus tends to be on identifying health hazards and health-risk management, but there is clearly scope to broaden this. Although HIA is usually concerned with policies in the non-health sector, Kemm (2001) suggests that it also has a role in identifying the indirect and unanticipated consequences of health-sector policy. Latterly, there have been links with the inequality and human rights agendas.

The potential remit, then, is enormous and this raises questions about the feasibility of assessing the health impact of all policies. There are two responses to this. The first is to filter out for scrutiny only those policy areas that are likely to have health consequences. The second, more radical approach, is to make HIA an integral part of all public policy development and part of the mindset of those involved (Barnes and Scott-Samuel, 2000: 2):

> In the longer term it [HIA] has the potential to make concern for improving public health the norm and a routine part of all public policy development.

This latter approach undoubtedly has the advantage of institutionalizing concern for health. Kemm (2001) sees ownership of HIA by the policy proponent as the ideal state – one that supports shared understanding of values and, at a more practical level, allows HIA to be embedded in all stages of policy development. This is in marked contrast to the situation in environmental impact assessment, where there is usually an external regulatory authority.

Banken (2001) is also supportive of institutionalization of HIA, but cautions that raising health to superordinate status may be perceived by other players in the policy arena as health imperialism, resulting in some resistance. She emphasizes that the aim should not be to increase the power of public health actors, but to 'add health awareness to policy making' by enabling those in non-health sectors to 'produce public health knowledge for use by decision makers' (Banken, 2001: 30). Clearly, this may require the development of skill and awareness among those involved. She also suggests that enabling non-health actors to produce this kind of information needs to be followed through with quality control to ensure rigour and avoid tokenism. As Bartlett (1989, in Banken, 2001: 31) notes:

> the politics of bureaucracy provide an environment in which the effectiveness of impact assessment can be tempered, subverted, and broken in the absence of adequate provisions for external accountability.

It has been suggested that the use of an alternative term to HIA might advance the cause more effectively. Kemm (2001) suggests 'overall policy appraisal' and Banken (2001) 'human impact assessment'.

The main stages in the process of HIA identified by the technical briefing for the WHO Regional Office for Europe (2002b) are:

1. **Screening** to quickly establish whether a particular policy, programme or project is relevant to health. This assessment may involve the use of checklists or other tools (see, for example, Department of Health, 2007b). It will flag up if there is a need for a more detailed assessment.
2. **Scoping** to identify the relevant health issues and public concerns that need to be addressed during appraisal. It generates questions, maps out possible connections, and sets the boundaries and terms of reference for the appraisal.
3. **Appraisal** to identify, and when possible quantify, the potential impacts on health and well-being in the context of available evidence and the knowledge, experience and opinions of stakeholders. It can be a *rapid* or an *in-depth appraisal*, depending on the level of detail and quantification needed to inform the policy decision, and may include mitigation and health-promoting measures.
4. **Reporting**, that is, communicating with stakeholders about the expected impacts on health and about how the policy, programme or other development could be modified to minimize negative and maximize positive impacts.
5. **Monitoring** of compliance with recommendations and of expected health impacts following the implementation of the policy or programme. This allows the existing evidence base to be expanded.

The final stage often includes evaluation of the quality of the HIA process to inform future assessments. Although the stages are presented sequentially, the process is essentially iterative and should conform with the key principles of HIA (see Box 6.17).

BOX 6.17 KEY PRINCIPLES OF HIA

- A social model of health and well-being
- An explicit focus on equity and social justice
- A multidisciplinary, participatory approach
- The use of qualitative as well as quantitative evidence
- Explicit values and openness to public scrutiny.

Source: Barnes and Scott-Samuel (2000: 2)

During the appraisal stage all significant health impacts should be identified and the implications of each should be considered in relation to quantity and quality of life. Resource costs in the healthcare and other sectors can also be considered. However, it is unlikely that sufficient information will be available to allow this to be done in monetary terms. The various impacts identified may well have contradictory effects on health or, indeed, on different groups and, in principle, this could be reduced to an overall net effect. However, it is more useful to maintain an overview of the various pathways that might improve or harm health. See the example in Table 6.1.

Kemm (2001) also emphasizes the importance of differentiating between winners and losers by including consideration of which groups are affected as well as the nature and magnitude of health impacts. For example, in the development context, the construction of a dam may secure a supply of potable water, support irrigation schemes to increase agricultural yields and increase health and prosperity for some, but may require others to relocate, losing homes and farmland, and shift the distribution of diseases such as schistosomiasis. Douglas et al.'s (2001) case study of three possible scenarios for developing transport policy in Edinburgh differentiated the effects on various subgroups of the population, as shown in Table 6.2.

It is axiomatic that HIA should be based on sound evidence. Kemm (2001) distinguishes two main approaches to assessment. One is characterized by a 'tight focus', based on an epidemiological model of exposure and dose–response relationships. Outcomes are usually defined in terms of death and disability, but could potentially be extended to include additional dimensions. The other 'broad focus' adopts a more wide-ranging approach and draws on informed opinion and local knowledge. A combination of the two is held to be most likely to generate a complete picture. HIA, therefore, relies on both qualitative and quantitative information and a multidisciplinary input. Kemm (2001: 82) suggests that this multidisciplinary input is particularly relevant to:

- **situational validation** – will the policy objectives be relevant to the problem?
- **societal vindication** – will the policy have instrumental value for the health of society as a whole?
- **social choice** – will the fundamental ideology of the policy be compatible with health?

Table 6.1 Health impact assessment

Extract from the assessment of the impact of the operational phase of the Merseytram Scheme on lifestyle		
Lifestyle	Direction/scale	Likelihood
Travel behaviour		
Increase in sustainable, healthier transport modes	+	probable
Modal shift from bus to tram	–	probable
Modal shift from car to tram	+	possible
Physical activity		
Some increase in cycling, walking, reduced risk of developing heart disease, diabetes (2), obesity, fall in hypertension, etc.	++	probable
Reduction in health inequalities between Merseytram zone and elsewhere	+	possible
Mobility		
Increase in mobility, increased access to job, education opportunities, social networks	++	probable
Reduction in health inequalities between Merseytram zone and elsewhere	+	probable
Safety		
Low, but increased risk of accidental injury involving the tram and pedestrians, cyclists	–	possible
Reductions in fear of crime associated with public transport increased use of tram	+	probable
Electromagnetic effects – the National Radiological Protection Board has concluded that there is no clear evidence that electromagnetic fields emanating from alternative or direct currents to which people are exposed to in everyday activities can give rise to adverse health effects	negligible	probable

Source: Derived from Prashar et al. (2004: 13)

While acknowledging the persuasiveness of quantitative data and providing guidance on the production of robust quantitative HIA, Mindell et al. (2001) express a number of reservations:

- not everything that can be quantified is important
- not everything that is being quantified at the moment should be
- not everything that is important can be quantified.

Communities may well have different perceptions of risks and benefits than professionals – telecommunication masts for mobile phones is one area where often lay individuals and experts disagree on their potential impact on health (Kemm, 2012b). Nonetheless, there is general consensus on the importance of the role of community involvement in the HIA process.

Table 6.2 Health impacts on different population groups under transport scenario 1 (low spend) and scenario 3 (high spend)

	Accidents		Pollution		Physical activity		Access to goods and services		Community network	
	1	3	1	3	1	3	1	3	1	3
Young children										
Affluent	+	+	+	+	+	−	−	+	−	++
Deprived	+	+	−	+	+	+	+	+	−	++
Adolescents										
Affluent	−	++	+	+	−	+	+	++	+	++
Deprived	+	+	−	+	−	++	+	++	+	++
Elderly										
Affluent	−	++	−	+	−	++	−	+	−	++
Deprived	−	+	−	+	−	++	−	++	−	++
Working people										
Affluent	O	+	+	+	−	+	−	++	−	+
Deprived	−	+	−	+	−	++	+	++	−	++
Unemployed										
Deprived	−	+	−	+	−	+	+	++	+	++

Key:

++ very positive impact   O no impact   – very negative impact

+ positive impact   – negative impact

Source: After Douglas et al. (2001)

 Careful consideration will need to be given to ways in which to involve the public. Mittelmark (2001) notes that the trend towards more technical and complex methods of assessment, along with the use of inaccessible jargon, makes it difficult for the average citizen to participate. He calls for an approach to HIA that is user-friendly and inclusive and cites the example of the People Assessing Their Health (PATH) project in Eastern Nova Scotia. This involved members of the community in developing local HIA tools suited to the needs of the community. Indeed, an often-cited critique of involving communities in the HIA process is the representativeness of those involved and whether these individuals *truly* reflect the community viewpoint (Kemm, 2012b). As we have noted, commitment to participation is a central concern of health promotion and is supported by the Gothenburg statement's list of values governing HIA (see Box 6.18). Furthermore, there are clear links with health advocacy and ensuring that there are opportunities for individuals who stand to be affected by policy to have a say in shaping its development.

BOX 6.18   THE GOTHENBURG STATEMENT'S VALUES GOVERNING HIA

- Democracy
- Equity
- Sustainable development
- Ethical use of evidence.

Source: European Centre for Health Policy (1999)

Notwithstanding the rhetoric about the importance of participation, Mathers et al. note some tension between the participatory and knowledge-gathering dimensions of HIA. They note the tendency to give 'pre-eminence to expert and research generated evidence' (2005: 58).

While decision-makers need to be confident that the conclusions of HIA are robust (Mindell et al., 2001), predicting the consequences of policy will inevitably be associated with some uncertainty. In some instances, there will be evidence on which to draw, whereas in others, predictions may need to be based on informed opinion, experience of similar situations and theory. Examples of evidence and data collection methods (from Taylor and Blair-Stevens, 2002) include:

- depth/key informant interviews
- focus group discussions
- equity audits
- surveys/questionnaires
- secondary analysis of existing data
- community profiling
- health needs assessment
- expert opinion
- documentary sources.

Identifying indirect effects may be particularly problematic, especially if they operate via complex systems. It may be possible to extrapolate precise figures and attach confidence intervals to these, but, equally, predictions are often expressed as crude ordinal scales from very certain to very uncertain (Kemm, 2001) or very positive impact to very negative impact, as shown in Table 6.2. The National Assembly for Wales (1999: 6) recognizes this and suggests that those involved:

> should make the best assessment they can using the information and skills available to them and by accepting that some degree of uncertainty may be unavoidable.

The Gothenburg Consensus (European Centre for Health Policy, 1999) emphasizes the importance of taking into account the values and goals within a given society and suggests that the process of HIA should be informed by the core values identified in its statement (see Box 6.18 above). Furthermore, it identifies three categories of HIA that can be instigated following the scoping exercise:

- **rapid health impact appraisal**: based on existing knowledge and the exchange of information between experts, decision-makers and representatives of those affected by the proposed policy
- **health impact analysis**: involving a more in-depth analysis based on existing evidence and, if necessary, the generation of new data
- **health impact review**: used when policies are very broad, it aims to produce a convincing estimation of the major impacts of a policy on health without disentangling the detailed impacts of the various policy components and is more concerned with broad relationships than precise cause-and-effect ones.

While it is not possible here to pursue in detail the actual process of conducting risk assessment, numerous guides and checklists are available – see, for example, European Centre for Health Policy (1999), Barnes and Scott-Samuel (2000), Kemm (2007), Department of Health (2007b) and Birley (2011). However, we will conclude with this the list of recommendations developed by Douglas et al. (2001: 152):

- screen to select policies for HIA
- negotiate
- share ownership
- be timely
- define and analyse the policy
- define and profile the population
- use an explicit model of health
- be aware of underlying values
- be systematic
- think broadly
- use appropriate evidence
- involve the community
- take into account local factors
- recognize differences within communities
- monitor impacts continuously following an initial prospective HIA
- make practical recommendations.

HEALTHY PUBLIC POLICY, HEALTH PROMOTION AND HEALTH EDUCATION

We have established that healthy public policy is a central concern of health promotion. It is a means of upholding the rights of individuals to health by creating a supportive environment – one that:

- does not threaten health
- provides the conditions to:
  - make the healthy choice the easy choice
  - encourage the participation of citizens.

While policy can be explicitly developed to further health goals, the contention is that all policy should consider potential impacts on health – direct and indirect.

A key theme running through this discussion has been the location and exercise of power. Advocacy and participation in HIA have been identified as ways of influencing policy development.

Health education and healthy public policy have been seen by some as competing options – the former associated with individual behaviour change and victim-blaming, and the latter with an emphasis on structural factors and enabling. However, making healthy public policy a reality is dependent on the skills and awareness of those involved. Health education, viewed more broadly, can therefore be a major driver in developing healthy public policy by virtue of its contribution on a number of different levels – from consciousness-raising and the development of the skills needed for advocacy and community activism through to professional training and lobbying.

KEY POINTS

- The development of healthy public policy is central to health promotion practice.
- Public health professionals can be important advocates for policy to improve public health and need to understand policy processes.
- Health education has a key role in the development of healthy public policy by raising awareness of health issues among 'policy actors' and also by developing political skills among those seeking to influence policy.
- Health impact assessment is a means of assessing the potential effect on health and health equity of any policy in order to recommend ways of minimizing negative and maximizing positive effects.

CHAPTER 6: INTERNATIONAL CASE STUDIES

The following case studies on the online resources website are relevant to the content of this chapter: 1, 2, 4, 8 and 9.

CRITICAL REFLECTION AND APPLICATION TO PRACTICE

This chapter has outlined the role of healthy public policy and the policy-making process. To what extent should healthy public policy be used to shape people's health behaviours? In what circumstances would using policy be inappropriate? How does the use of policy align with core values in health promotion, such as choice and empowerment? Thinking about your own professional practice and role, how are local policies devised, upheld and evaluated?

ONLINE RESOURCES

Please visit https://study.sagepub.com/greentones5e for all the online resources for the book, including recommended further reading on each chapter subject, useful weblinks (both introduced by the authors), as well as the abovementioned case study material.

7 EDUCATION FOR HEALTH

Those that know, do. Those that understand, teach.

Aristotle (384–322 BC)

OVERVIEW

The purpose of this chapter is to consider the contribution of education to health promotion. It will:

- establish the central importance of health education as the major driver within health promotion
- consider the ethical implications of alternative approaches to health education
- present an understanding of the factors involved in communication and their relevance to health education
- distinguish different types of learning
- identify key source, message and audience factors of relevance to communication, health education and efforts to persuade
- consider the appropriateness of different learning methods for achieving particular learning outcomes
- explore the potential of health education as a strategy for social and political change.

INTRODUCTION

In Chapter 1, we provided a technical definition of 'health education' as a planned process designed to achieve health- and illness-related learning. Discussion focused on its philosophical and ideological dimensions – attempting to answer the question of what education ought to be about. Its role was seen to involve more than traditional attempts to persuade individuals to comply with received wisdom about health behaviour and include empowerment and social and political change. The term 'New Health Education' is used to distinguish this broader conceptualization. We now turn our attention to the technical aspects of what is involved in achieving educational goals, together with the nature and dynamics of the learning process.

In Chapter 1, a number of different kinds of influences on learning were identified. These were arranged on a spectrum of coercion. At one end of this spectrum was empowerment, which fulfils the requirement of voluntarism that characterizes true education and the model of health promotion that is espoused in this book. Other activities, indicative of a much wider range of potential interventions, were also represented on the spectrum. Some may be ideologically neutral; others, such as brainwashing, are unacceptable in the context of our empowerment imperative.

BOX 7.1   PROCEDURES TO PROMOTE LEARNING

Education	Social marketing	Facilitating
Indoctrination	Instruction	Brainwashing
Advising	Conditioning	Persuasion
Teaching	Lobbying	Counselling
Propaganda	Training	Advocating

The negative connotations of at least some of the activities listed in Box 7.1 will doubtless be obvious through their association with coercion. For others, there may be more debate. It is interesting, for instance, to consider the use of 'propaganda', which currently has negative associations, but this was not always so. For instance, in the early days of health education, 'health propaganda' was considered perfectly acceptable. The use of propaganda by politicians and dictators – particularly in wartime – has resulted in a more tarnished image.

Notwithstanding ethical and ideological considerations, all the various activities listed in Box 7.1 have in common a capacity to influence learning to a greater or lesser extent and potentially contribute in some way to health education. However, in line with the emphasis we are placing on empowerment, we will give particular attention to health education's radical imperative and its concern to create social change. We will, however, start by examining a process that is a prerequisite for *all* kinds of learning. That process is communication.

THE COMMUNICATION PROCESS

The word 'communication' is sometimes used to refer to the whole educational process. For instance, Fletcher (1973: 2) viewed communication as synonymous with learning, as the first of his principles of communication demonstrates:

> The purpose of communication is not just to deliver a message but to effect a change in the recipient in respect of his [*sic*] knowledge, his attitude or, eventually, in his behaviour.

However, there is an important distinction. Whereas communication is a necessary prerequisite for learning, it is learning *per se* that is responsible for change. The communication process itself is essentially concerned with the transmission and reception of messages. While in many instances some learning will also take place, it is also possible to envisage situations in which it does not; for example, telling someone that it is raining when they already know this to be the case. Furthermore, mere transmission of information is not the same as the relatively permanent change in knowledge, disposition or capability that is central to our earlier definition of learning. Nonetheless, the form and effectiveness of communication will have some bearing on the achievement of learning goals.

The model shown in Figure 7.1 developed out of work in telecommunications. An information source sends a message via a transmitter and this, hopefully, reaches its destination and is decoded by a receiver. Inevitably, the process is afflicted to a greater or lesser extent by noise. This is not just technical interference, but may refer to psychological as well as physical 'noise'. It would thus include any distortions resulting from the beliefs and attitudes of individuals, as well as defects or limitations in their sensory systems.

Key features of the communication process

The communication process involves three components:

- a sender
- a message
- a receiver.

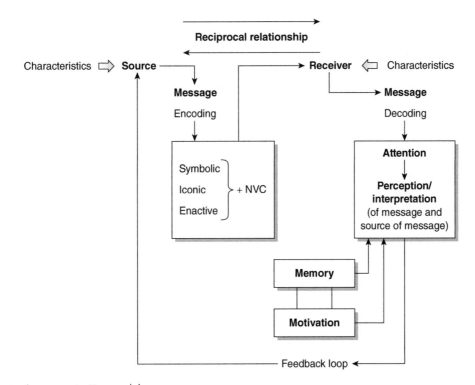

Figure 7.1 A communication model

Terminology may differ. For instance, the sender may merely be described as the 'communicator'. More commonly, the originator of the message may be called the 'source' – in which case, the receiver is likely to be defined as the 'audience' (even if it is an audience of one). The source may be personal or 'mediated' – that is, it may be in the form of a poster or leaflet or any other variety of mass media. Whenever the source is present in person, non-verbal communication (NVC) will accompany the message. The source constructs or, more accurately, *encodes* the message and it is the task of the receiver to decode it.

The coded message may be 'symbolic', using spoken or written language (or, of course, mathematical and scientific symbols). Alternatively, it may be 'iconic', using pictorial or diagrammatic presentations, or 'enactive'.

As stated, it is the task of the receiver to decode the message. First of all, the message must reach the receiver's senses (if this does not happen, communication and learning fail at this initial stage). It is obviously the responsibility of the communicator to avoid such failure. Second, the receiver must pay attention to the message for as long as it takes to achieve the goals of the communication. Third, the processes of perception are brought into play – the message must be correctly interpreted. Attention and accurate perception will be determined by past experience (stored in the memory) and current motivation (also partly determined by past experience).

The nature and success of the communication process will be influenced by the characteristics of both the source and the receiver. The source (and his or her non-verbal communication – NVC) is an integral component of coding and transmitting messages. For instance, the receiver's perception of the source may influence whether or not he or she pays attention or interprets the message appropriately. As we will note later, the credibility of the source will also have a major effect – not only on communication, but on learning. Indeed, identification and manipulation of source characteristics are two of the main concerns in devising 'persuasive communication'. Clearly, receiver characteristics are all-important in the decoding process – cultural beliefs, language skills, intellectual capabilities and personality traits will influence attention and, in particular, perception and interpretation of messages.

Figure 7.1 includes an 'immediate feedback loop', which shows the reciprocal relationship between communicator and receiver, between source and audience. (Note also the 'long-term' feedback system in Figure 7.2.) As has frequently been remarked, communication is (or should be) a two-way process. A critically important part of this reciprocity is the (immediate) feedback loop, which forms an integral part of the interaction. The only way in which communication can be maximized is when the source of the message constantly checks the reactions of the receiver (often by accurately perceiving his or her NVC). Successful communication occurs when the receiver's interpretation of the message exactly matches the communicator's intended message.

Readability

Written communications constitute one of the most common forms of symbolic coding used by health educators. The use of such materials assumes that the target audience is literate. Clearly, it is incumbent on communicators to ensure that their written materials match the audience's level of competence. In a study of sexual health education leaflets, Corcoran and Ahmad (2016) concluded that the readability was too high for the intended recipients and argued that this could contribute to

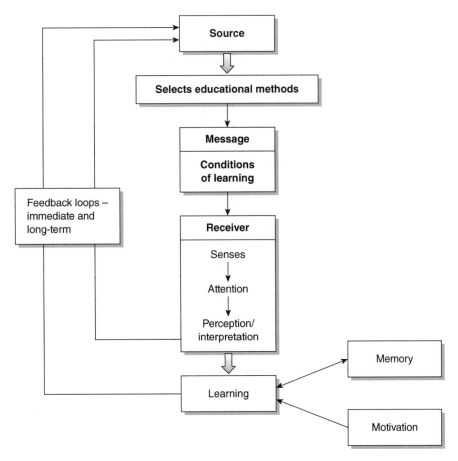

Figure 7.2   The communication to learning process

inequalities in sexual health. Key issues influencing the ease of reading appear to be sentence length, the number of words, word length, the inclusion of 'difficult' words and writing in the passive voice. A plethora of tests of readability – or 'reading ease' – have been developed to assess the degree of difficulty of written communications: for example, Flesch, FOG (frequency of gobbledygook) and SMOG (simple measures of gobbledygook). Some express the results as a score associated with the level of difficulty, whereas others use a school grade or number of years of education equivalent. In an era when many people use the Internet as their first source of health information, issues of readability are even more salient. Laplante-Lévesque et al. (2012) carried out a study assessing the readability of English-language websites providing information about hearing impairment from Australia, Canada, India, the UK and the USA. Readability was measured using the Flesch Reading Ease Score, Flesch–Kincaid Grade Level Formula and SMOG. The results indicated that, on average, people needed at least 11 to 12 years of education in order to read and understand the contents of the websites, whereas the recommended number of years is 9 (Walsh and Volsko, 2008, cited in Laplante-Lévesque et al.,

2012: 619) or at/below Grade 6 reading level (Kehl and McCarty, 2012). Other more recent studies have also found that the readability of online health information tends to be much higher than the recommended level (e.g. Burns et al., 2021; Marsh et al., 2020).

While readability tests offer some insight into the intelligibility of written material, none of these tests measures the *actual* level of understanding of the target audience. Only a direct test of people's ability both to read and to understand a particular communication will do that. In addition, Begeny and Greene (2014: 198) argue that: 'there is limited direction … regarding which readability formulas (if any) are appropriate indicators of actual text difficulty'. Importantly, communicators need to be aware of the cultural interpretations and emotional reactions of their audience to written communications. It is essential, therefore, to undertake a comprehensive pre-test of communications to ensure that the information is received as intended/appropriate and so that amendments can be made (Centers for Disease Control and Prevention [CDC], 2009). As de Silva et al. (2017: 815) argue in relation to the promotion of oral health literacy in Australia, 'where possible, market-testing [resources] with target client groups will provide the best indicator of what is an appropriate resource for them'. Corcoran and Ahmad (2016) make some specific suggestions for improving the design of print materials, particularly for lower literacy audiences (see Box 7.2). Health inequalities are linked to health literacy. There is evidence that the most disadvantaged in society are the most likely to have lower levels of health literacy (National Institute for Health and Care Research, 2022). It is therefore vital that those charged with the responsibility for producing health information, in whatever form, do so in an accessible way. This is particularly the case for online health information. As Skierkowski et al. (2021) argue, there is a risk of exacerbating existing inequalities if the recommended guidelines about readability and accessibility are not adhered to.

BOX 7.2 DESIGNING PRINT MATERIALS

- Change complex words to words with fewer syllables.
- Include techniques that encourage engagement and reader interaction, such as true/false quizzes.
- Use graphics and images to support the written text.
- Review the cultural suitability of written materials and tailor to specific cultural groups where appropriate.

The National Cancer Institute (2007) has provided very detailed guidance for designing printed materials for breast cancer screening:

- Write simply and clearly.
- Write with the audience in mind.
- Make headings work.
- Keep paragraphs short.
- Consider using a Question & Answer format.

- Emphasize important points without distracting from the readability.
- Write about one concept at a time.
- Consider incorporating informed decision-making concepts.
- Frame the information in culturally appropriate ways.

While printed materials have been a popular form of disseminating health information, the growth of web-based health promotion resources has been seen in recent times. An American survey in 2010, for example, showed that 50% of those surveyed said that they looked online for health information (Deloitte, 2010) and it is estimated that almost 80% of Australians who are active online have sought out health information this way (Cheng and Dunn, 2015). This could include accessing information from:

- websites
- blogs – online journals where authors can write about a topic of interest
- message boards – online platforms where users can post questions and receive responses from other users
- social networking sites – an opportunity to create online communities through sites such as Facebook
- wikis – allow content on a topic to be created by multiple users
- YouTube.

One of the drawbacks to the Internet is that anyone can set up a webpage and website content is not often regulated. This unregulated nature of the Internet and lack of quality control of information provided does mean that issues such as readability are not always considered (Hubley et al., 2021). Indeed, the use of jargon, acronyms and abbreviations are integral to the popularity and way in which social networking sites and message boards operate. However, many of the principles outlined in the lists above should apply to 'reputable' websites of organizations involved in health promotion (for instance, the WHO).

Reflections on empowerment

People have a right to information and communication can serve to meet that need. Communication may, therefore, be seen as essentially empowering – provided due consideration is given to accessibility to the target audience. However, the source–audience relationship frequently involves an imbalance of power. The selection and manipulation of symbols may reflect cultural assumptions or more conscious efforts on the part of the communicator to persuade.

A goal of an empowerment model of health promotion, and indeed health literacy, would be to enhance the ability of the audience to obtain information and, moreover, to question the content and challenge the sources of messages directed at them. More generally, empowerment seeks to shift the power balance between communicators and audiences.

As Kehl and McCarty (2012: 242) argue, 'many health care materials are not written at levels that can be understood by most lay people'. The same can be argued for health information generally. This can lead to frustration for the user, disparities in experience and, ultimately, increased health inequality

(Rutten et al., 2019). The US National Cancer Institute (1998) advocates involving lay people (the 'audience') at an early stage in order to develop culturally relevant material. Doing so can help to establish the following:

- Understanding of relevant physical, behavioural, demographic and psychographic characteristics.
- What your audience already knows; what rumours, myths and misinformation may exist.
- How your audience feels about the topic; what questions and information gaps there are.
- What specific ethnic, cultural and lifestyle preferences might exist.

Daghio et al. (2006) advocate involving lay people in the production of written materials to redress any imbalance, through the following process:

1. Priority setting to identify the topic
2. Critical appraisal of evidence
3. Collective writing of the key messages
4. Calculation of readability scores
5. Assessment of readability by an independent reading panel
6. Assessment of comprehensibility by an independent panel.

A case study in the USA by LePrevost et al. (2013) involved the participation of farm-workers at risk of pesticide exposure in the development of health and safety materials. Farm-workers were involved in developing and selecting specific symbols and illustrations to communicate hazards to the workforce. The authors emphasize 'the need to engage low-literacy end-users [of health information] in the production of health education materials' (LePrevost et al., 2013: 975) and such approaches as a way to recognize and incorporate lay expertise. Emphasis on involving lay people in the design of health communication has increased over recent years and we are seeing a much-needed move away from a deficit model of public communication (where experts hold the knowledge and power) towards a recognition of the importance of dialogue, participation and co-production (Campbell, 2021).

HEALTH EDUCATION AND LEARNING

Clearly, learning is linked to communication, as shown in Figure 7.2, which also indicates the centrality of selection of methods and development of the message.

In Chapter 1, we distinguished between two often-conflicting approaches to health promotion – the preventive medical model and the empowerment model. The contribution of health education to each was characterized as:

- Health education as persuasion – associated with 'coercing' people into adopting 'approved' behaviours to prevent disease and improve health.
- Health education as empowerment – concerned to strengthen individuals' capacity to control their own health (self-empowerment) and work collectively to achieve supportive environments for health (community empowerment).

It is also useful to note a radical variation on the empowerment model of health education that is primarily concerned with developing the capacity to achieve social and political change in the interests of promoting public health. While this is integral to the empowerment model described in this book, efforts that focus on developing this capacity may be distinguished as 'critical health education'.

Patient education can also be legitimately located under the health education umbrella. However, perhaps because of its association with the medical model, it has become marginalized by mainstream health promotion. This is unfortunate. Not only is the education of patients a task of major importance, it can be comfortably accommodated within the general empowerment model of health promotion. Indeed, empowering strategies typically result in more effective preventive outcomes than so-called victim-blaming approaches. In fact, the only real logical distinction between patient education and other varieties of health education is the fact that it is, by definition, concerned to promote the health of people who have been defined as patients!

The role of health education is to create the conditions necessary for achieving the required learning. The key questions that will inform the selection of methods are:

- What learning is required?
- Who is the target (group)?
- How large is the group?
- What are the contextual factors?

A theme running through this book is that, regardless of whether the focus is on policy, behaviour or empowerment, achieving change is ultimately dependent on learning. Clearly, the actors will differ and the type of learning required will vary. The adoption of a systematic approach to planning and the application of theory should produce a clear specification of what type of learning is required and by whom. For example, this could involve attempts to shift the attitudes of those holding the balance of power in policy development or consciousness-raising and the development of community activist skills with a community group or assertiveness skills with young women. The framework developed by McLeroy (1992) (see Table 7.1) provides a useful overview. Green (2000) contends that, without a full theoretical analysis, interventions risk addressing inappropriate variables or failing to tackle the whole combination of variables required to bring about the desired effect.

A taxonomy of health learning

It is worth reiterating here our earlier definition of learning as a 'relatively permanent change in capability or disposition'. This might involve change in:

- knowledge and understanding
- ways of thinking
- beliefs
- values
- attitudes

and

- the acquisition or development of skills.

Table 7.1　Targets of change and strategies for different ecological levels

Ecological level	Targets of change	Strategies and skills
Intrapersonal	Developmental processes	Tests and measurements
	Knowledge attitudes	Educational approaches
	Values	Mass media
	Skills	Social marketing
	Behaviour	Skills development
	Self-concept, self-efficacy, self-esteem	Resistance to peer pressure
Interpersonal	Social networks	Enhancing social networks
	Social support	Changing group norms
	Families	Enhancing families
	Workgroups	Social support groups
	Peers	Increasing access to normative groups
	Neighbours	Peer influence
Organizational	Norms	Organizational development
	Incentives	Incentive programmes
	Organizational culture	Process consultation
	Management styles	Coalition development
	Organizational structure	Linking agents
	Communication networks	
Community	Area economics	Change agents
	Community resources	Community development
	Neighbourhood organizations	Community coalitions
	Community competences	Empowerment
	Social and health services	Conflict strategies
	Organizational relationships	Mass media
	Folk practices	
	Governmental structures	
	Formal leadership	
	Informal leadership	
Public policy	Legislation	Mass media
	Policy	Policy analysis
	Taxes	Political change
	Regulatory agencies	Lobbying
		Political organizing
		Conflict strategies

Source: Derived from McLeroy (1992), reproduced with permission

In terms of designing effective interventions for influencing learning, four key principles emerge from the seminal work of Gagne (1985):

1. There are various different and separately identified types of learning and learning outcome.
2. Learning is hierarchical – typically 'lower-order' learning outcomes must be fulfilled before higher levels of learning can be attained.
3. Successful learning requires that learning-specific internal and external conditions be supplied – where internal conditions relate to previously acquired capabilities and dispositions and external conditions are provided by the deliberate organization of external events to facilitate learning.
4. Those who seek to influence learning – via persuasion, training, education and so on – must check that the necessary internal conditions have been met and then provide the appropriate external conditions by using the right educational methods for the situation.

The simplest classification of learning has been mentioned in Chapter 3, which categorizes it as cognitive (concerned with knowledge and beliefs), affective (concerned with values and feelings) and conative (concerned with purposeful action and change).

Learning also includes the development of skills. The term 'skill' is often used in a general sense merely to indicate a high level of competence. Three kinds of skill are of particular relevance to health promotion. These are: psychomotor, social interaction and problem-solving or decision-making skills.

The cognitive domain

A detailed technical analysis of cognitive learning is beyond the scope of this chapter. At a common-sense level, it is clear that a distinction may be made between the rote learning of facts and acquiring deeper levels of understanding. While factual data may be useful, understanding is necessary for the transfer of learning and its application to problem-solving. As we noted in Chapter 3, beliefs are best conceptualized as cognitive constructs and, as indicated in our discussion of the health action model (HAM), perhaps the most important goal of health education is to create or modify health-related beliefs.

Cognitive skills – problem-solving and decision-making

Problem-solving is usually categorized as a cognitive skill. For instance, Gagne (1985) defines it primarily as a 'cognitive strategy' that 'enables the learner to select appropriate information and skills and to decide when and how to apply them in attempting to solve the problem'.

Problem-solving ability can be enhanced through two main types of learning – first, the acquisition of new principles and associated concepts and, second, the development of generalizable problem-solving skills. For instance, consider the case of diabetic labourers working on building sites. Two problems that they face are finding ways to inject themselves at work and eat regularly and appropriately. Forward planning might allow them to come up with a workable solution. Furthermore, a thorough understanding of the need to balance dietary intake, exercise and insulin will enable them to have greater control over their lifestyle. This learning can be generalized so that they can successfully apply problem-solving skills in a variety of different situations. However, such transfer of learning is only likely to occur where there is a good deal of similarity and common ground between the different types of problems to be solved.

As mentioned above, it is difficult in practice to distinguish between problem-solving skills, social interaction skills and decision-making skills. They all tend to be viewed as part and parcel of 'life skills' (or 'action competences') that form an integral part of education for empowerment. They will be discussed more fully in the context of critical health education later in this chapter.

Decision-making is closely related to problem-solving and the terms are often used synonymously. Decision-making is frequently conceptualized as rational, but as we noted in the discussion of the HAM, may also be influenced by emotional and social pressures. Janis and Mann (1977) distinguish between 'cold' decisions taken in a calm, detached state and 'hot' decisions that involve issues that matter more to the individual and are hence more emotionally charged. These include issues of immediate safety as well as longer-term issues such as the choice of a lifetime partner. The Conflict Model of Decision Making (Janis and Mann, 1977; Newman and Brown, 1996) focuses on these decisions that matter. The model is based on the tension between maintaining and changing current behaviour. Three main groups of influence have a bearing on the quality of decision-making: awareness of the risk associated with current activity (and indeed change); recognition that there may be a better alternative; and the amount of time to assess alternatives. Depending on the mix between these variables, five different patterns emerge that influence the way in which information is processed and decisions are taken, as outlined below:

- Unconflicted inertia – no serious risk is recognized with current behaviour, therefore there is little stress associated with continuing.
- Unconflicted change – serious risk is recognized with continuing current behaviour and none with change, therefore little stress is associated with change.
- Defensive avoidance – serious risk is associated both with current activity and change, with no hope of a better solution, therefore stress is high. Decision-making may be cut short or postponed.
- Hypervigilance – the risks of changing and not changing are both recognized, but there is insufficient time to pursue all options. Stress is high (akin to panic) and decisions may be taken on partial information, or responsibility delegated to others.
- Vigilance – the ideal when there is recognition of the risk of continuing current behaviour and ample time to appraise the alternatives.

High-quality, vigilant decision-making involves:

- seeking out a wide range of alternatives
- carefully assessing the known risks and costs associated with each, as well as any benefits
- searching for additional information
- reassessing the alternatives in the light of new information
- planning implementation including contingency plans to deal with anticipated risks.

Before moving on to affective learning, we will briefly consider other types of skill development.

Psychomotor skills

The relevance of psychomotor (or motor) skills to health education is doubtless self-evident. They range from simple to complex and the following examples will serve to illustrate this particular kind of learning:

- use of a toothbrush for the efficient removal of plaque
- using a condom
- competence in cardio-pulmonary resuscitation.

Social interaction skills

The skills involved in interacting with other people are fundamental to social health. Furthermore, capabilities such as assertiveness are of importance in empowering individuals and groups and increasing the likelihood of their gaining control over their lives and the political systems that govern them. Health literacy, as we noted in Chapter 3, involves the acquisition of cognitive and social skills to obtain, understand and use health information along with the motivation to do so.

There is an important parallel with psychomotor skills learning – as Michael Argyle, one of the key authorities in researching social interaction, has amply demonstrated. Indeed, in the 1960s, he made particular reference to a 'motor skills model' of social interaction (Argyle, 1978), shown in Figure 7.3. Social interaction skills, like psychomotor skills, involve accurate perception of and response to both external environmental cues and internal proprioceptive cues. In learning to drive a car, the learner must respond appropriately to visual information about the road situation and to those muscular sensations involved in controlling the steering wheel. Similarly, socially skilled communicators will accurately

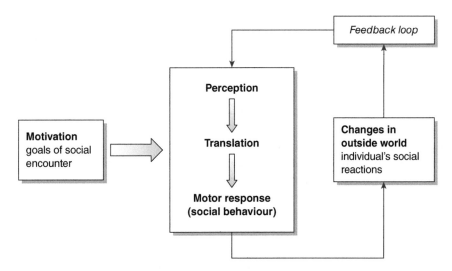

Figure 7.3 Motor skills model of social interaction (after Argyle and Kendon, 1967)

interpret the non-verbal cues provided by other people – such as facial expressions – and, at the same time, will be in control of their own non-verbal responses, such as gesture and tone of voice. A socially skilled person makes an appropriate choice from a wide repertoire of potential responses on the basis of incoming interpersonal information, then he or she reacts in the most appropriate way.

It will be apparent that the ability to interpret and use non-verbal communication (NVC) is also of central importance to the acquisition of social interaction skills. For instance, respect, empathy and genuineness have been described as the 'holy trinity' of counselling. It is relatively easy to *say* the right things, but a lack of genuineness or empathy is readily revealed by what has been called 'non-verbal leakage'. NVC is of paramount importance in communicating feeling and attitudes. Numerous studies have demonstrated, for example, that when there is a contradiction between verbal and non-verbal messages, the non-verbal is more powerful. A verbal expression of interest can so easily be undermined by tone of voice and facial expression. Table 7.2 sets out some of the key features of NVC.

Table 7.2   Key features of non-verbal communication (NVC)

Channel	Examples
Proxemics	Personal space, territory, body orientation, seating arrangement, body angle
Haptics (touch)	Playful, ritualistic, aggressive, affection
Chronemics (time)	Waiting time, punctuality, duration, urgency
Kinesics	Direction of gaze, facial expression, smiling, gestures, head movements, posture, gait
Physical appearance	Body shape, weight, height, hair and skin colour, clothing, cosmetics, adornments
Vocalics	Tempo, pitch, loudness, dialect, fluency, pauses, articulation, breathiness
Artefacts	Volume of space, size, ventilation, furniture arrangement, decor, lighting, temperature

The affective domain

We now turn our attention to affective learning. The different aspects of affective learning are encapsulated in the motivation system of the health action model (HAM), discussed in Chapter 3. These include values and attitudes along with emotional states and associated drives such as fear. The model identifies two sets of influences on motivation. The first operates via the mediation of the belief system, while the second provides a direct input into the motivation system itself – for instance, by using emotive imagery to generate anxiety or other feelings directly.

We have consistently challenged the use of coercive methods to achieve the goals of health promotion on the grounds that it conflicts with empowerment. Yet the use of 'persuasion' and 'attitude change' techniques has traditionally been associated with coercion. Clearly, any attempt to change attitudes should be subject to ethical scrutiny.

It is important to distinguish between *deliberate* attempts to persuade and coerce by generating emotional responses and, on the other hand, those situations in which emotional responses occur as an almost *incidental* effect of learning. For instance, to the extent that people come to understand and accept the reality of personal risk or realize the ways in which social injustice is associated with ill health, it is quite probable that emotions will be roused. In the first instance, it may involve anxiety or concern over personal vulnerability. In the second instance, it may result in feelings of indignation and commitment to take political action. Moreover, while the deliberate use of attitude-change techniques are most closely associated with attempts to manipulate rather than empower – and, thus, are ethically dubious – there is, paradoxically perhaps, a situation where persuasion rather than empowerment is justified. As we noted in Chapter 6, the use of persuasion is standard practice for lobbyists and other political activists seeking to bring about changes in health-related policy. It is presumably acceptable, therefore, for health promotion activists to become skilled in the use of attitude-change techniques. There is, of course, a difference in degree between, say, a community health worker utilizing persuasive techniques with a local politician and advertisers' use of persuasive messages to persuade young children to pester their parents to buy them unhealthy products.

The conative domain

Conative learning is associated with proactive behaviour and is central to self-direction and autonomy. Conation influences whether cognition (knowing) and affect (feeling) result in behaviour. It is an essential, yet often overlooked, aspect of learning in general and health-related learning. It clearly has particular relevance to empowerment. Huitt (1999) attributes this lack of attention to the fact that it is so closely enmeshed with the cognitive and affective domains. However, some key aspects derived from Huitt's review are summarized in Table 7.3 and the implications for health education are identified.

Huitt draws on Bandura's social cognitive theory to identify past experience of achieving mastery as an important influence on self-efficacy and a predictor of future success. Enabling learners to be successful and experience success can, therefore, help individuals to be successful in other areas of their lives.

Table 7.3   Aspects of conative ability

Aspects of conation	Sub-components	Implications for health education
Direction	Awareness of human needs	Exercises to enable individuals to identify their own needs
	Visions and dreams – awareness of what is possible	Raise awareness of possibilities
	Making choices	Develop decision-making capability
	Setting goals:	Encourage setting difficult but attainable goals
	Mastery goals – concerned with developing competence	Develop self-efficacy beliefs
	Performance goals – concerned with achieving outcomes	

(Continued)

Table 7.3   (Continued)

Aspects of conation	Sub-components	Implications for health education
	Social goals – concerned with the individual fitting into a group or group performance	
	Develop plans	Enable individuals to develop a clear view of their desired specific outcome and to identify the steps to take to achieve this
		Encourage commitment – ideally writing plans down or at least telling others of intentions
Energizing	Potential for positive returns from the effort must outweigh any negative aspects of change and fear of failure	Attention to early gains
		Attention to self-efficacy beliefs
Persistence	Linked to the level of motivation, expectation of success, high self-esteem, previous experience of success or failure, praise for effort and public display of achievement of outcomes	Praise
		Reinforcement
		Public acknowledgement of success

Source: Based on Huitt (1999)

FACILITATING LEARNING

The purpose of health education is to achieve health- or illness-related learning and the task of the health educator is to marshal those methods that provide the conditions needed to ensure efficient learning. There is a considerable repertoire of methods on which to draw, backed up by numerous manuals on their detailed application. Educational methods range from formal, top-down, didactic ones to participatory methods and the target from a single individual (as in the one-to-one encounter) to whole populations. Figure 7.4 attempts to order selected educational methods with respect to the size of the target group and the level of participation. Our purpose here is not to review the utility of specific methods, but, rather, to draw out key principles that will inform approaches to promoting learning. Clearly, ideology will have some influence but, over and above such concerns, the selection of an appropriate mix of activities will be governed by:

- the type of learning required
- the characteristics of the learner
- the characteristics of the teacher
- other factors – context, availability of resources, time, feasibility.

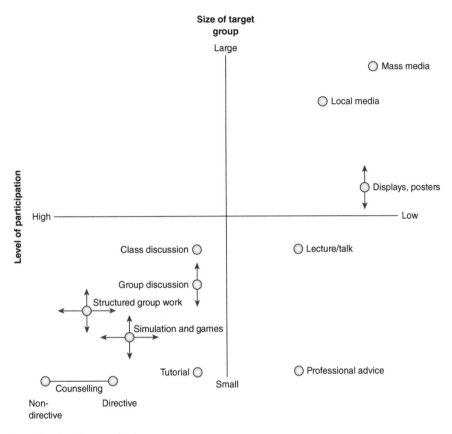

Figure 7.4   Health education methods

The need for participation

A fundamental principle of Carl Rogers's approach to education is that we cannot teach, but can only facilitate learning (Barrett-Lennard, 1998). Work undertaken some time ago at the Industrial Training Research Unit at the University of Wales Institute of Science and Technology (Belbin et al., 1981) found that poor learners were characterized by a passive attitude towards learning, used a narrow range of learning methods and frequently inappropriate methods. The active involvement of the learner is, therefore, essential – encapsulated in the maxim:

- I hear and I forget
- I see and I remember
- I do and I understand.

Not only does active involvement maximize learning, it also contributes to empowerment. Please see Box 7.3 for some techniques that encourage active learning. It underpins life and health skills teaching and the development of action competences and, as we will see, is central to Freirean approaches.

> # BOX 7.3 TECHNIQUES FOR ACTIVE LEARNING
>
> - Ice-breakers
> - Educational games
> - Tours and field trips
> - Presentations
> - Outside speakers
> - Role playing
> - Record keeping
> - Exchanges
> - Contests.
>
> *Source: Active Teaching – Active Learning: Teaching Techniques and Tools* (Van Winkle, 2002)

Tones (1993) attributes the shift from formal to more participatory methods of health education over the last 50 years to ideological considerations – notably a commitment to participation and empowerment. A further influence has been the development of theory that has supported their use and evidence of greater effectiveness of these approaches. This shift has been accompanied by an increasing awareness of the importance of process as well as content. Furthermore, there has been a gradual move away from seeing learners as empty vessels to be filled with knowledge towards acknowledging and building on their prior learning and experience. The role of the health educator has correspondingly changed from expert to facilitator and the role of the learner from passive acceptance to active involvement.

A number of different terms refer to methods for achieving active learning – 'experiential learning', 'participatory learning', 'active methods', 'student-centred learning', 'confluent education'.

The notion of the 'experiential learning cycle' derives from the work of Kolb et al. (1971), shown in Figure 7.5. The cycle begins with a new experience or some device for drawing on the learner's past experience, followed by reflection and sharing of learning. This is followed by processing, which involves an analysis of the learning in cognitive, affective and conative domains and its relevance. The learner may appreciate the need for additional skills or knowledge. Anderson (undated) suggests that the role of the 'teacher' or the trainer at this point can be to provide input that is outside the experience of the group. Provided the input is linked to the learner's needs and experiences, this is not seen as compromising commitment to active learning. Finally, if it is to be meaningful, learning should be applied to the real world, with opportunities for subsequent reflection and review.

Ryder and Campbell (1988) draw on the work of Settle and Wise (1986) and Brandes and Ginnis (1986) to contrast experiential methods with more traditional approaches, as shown in Table 7.4.

The mainstay of experiential learning is structured groupwork. The effective functioning of groups as a means of promoting learning is dependent on good facilitation and attention to two broad areas of functioning, although there may be some overlap, namely:

- task-orientated functions – designed to achieve specific learning
- group-orientated functions – designed to build and maintain the cohesiveness of the group.

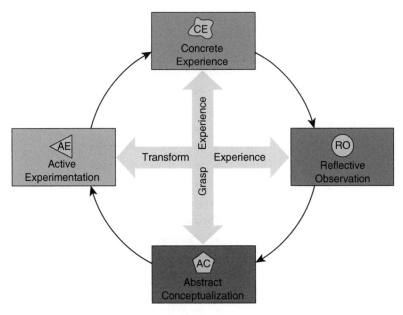

Figure 7.5   The experiential learning cycle

The selection of appropriate methods is made easier if learning objectives are formulated precisely – and optimally if framed as behavioural objectives (that is, they specify what the learner will be expected to be able to *do*, under what conditions and over what timescale – see Hubley et al., 2021). For example, following the groupwork session, participants will:

- when asked, list the main routes of transmission of HIV (knowledge)
- demonstrate to the group, using a condom and banana as visual aids, the correct way to put on a condom (skills)
- in a role-play situation, use three different strategies to refuse pressure to have unprotected sex (skills).

Clearly, the development of knowledge will require different methods from those used in the development of skills. Belbin et al. (1981) produced a simple taxonomy using the acronym MUD to distinguish between appropriate methods for memorizing, understanding and doing (see Figure 7.6). The development of skills requires the opportunity to learn from the practical experience of trying out the skill. Complex skills may need to be broken down into components and, once each of these has been mastered, grouped together to achieve competence in relation to the whole.

Ryder and Campbell observe that, in experiential learning, the affective and cognitive domains tend to flow together to achieve confluent learning. They cite Rogers's (1983) view that the personal involvement in learning central to experiential approaches necessarily touches feelings, even when it has a cognitive orientation or the impetus comes from outside.

In some instances, it will be possible to identify detailed and specific learning objectives, leading to sharply focused interventions. Furthermore, as we will note below, messages can be tailored with

Table 7.4　Contrasting teaching styles

Experiential	Traditional
Role of learner – active:	Role of learner – passive:
• negotiating content	• teacher determines content
• negotiating ground rules	• teacher sets rules
• communicating with other learners	• talk between learners discouraged
• displaying work	• teacher controls display of work
• management of resources	• teacher manages resources
• maintaining behaviour as agreed	• teacher maintains standards of discipline
Teacher as facilitator or guide	Teacher as expert – transmits knowledge
Uses active methods:	Focuses on memory, practice and rote learning:
• collaboration	• individual and competitive
• groupwork	• concerned with academic standards
• starts from what the learner knows or is concerned about	• confined to the classroom
• not confined to the classroom	
• regular review and evaluation (of self and group performance)	• emphasis on tests and grades
Subject matter integrated	Traditional boundaries between subjects
Uses the intrinsic motivation of students	Motivation external and based on rewards and punishments
Focuses equally on cognitive and affective domains	The affective domain is neglected
Students encouraged to reflect on, and talk about, their learning	Little attention to learning behaviour
Process is valued as well as content	Little attention is paid to process

Source: After Ryder and Campbell (1988)

increasing sophistication to match the characteristics and precise learning needs of individuals. This effectively demands greater precision – and potentially control – on the part of those responsible for designing interventions. This approach may be more relevant in the context of vertical rather than horizontal programmes and is certainly less applicable when the objectives are couched in broader terms, such as the development of empowerment or social capital. While it would, in principle, be possible to conduct a detailed analysis of the constructs of empowerment and put together an appropriate collection of methods to address each of these, an alternative approach would be to use methods that are more wide-ranging and have a multidimensional impact. These allow the learner to take from the learning experience whatever meets his or her own learning needs and achieve confluence between the different learning domains rather than compartmentalization of knowledge. The potential of the creative arts for contributing to community health has begun to receive attention and, as Clift (2012) argues, creative arts are receiving increasing worldwide attention in terms of the benefits to health and well-being. We will conclude this section with a brief consideration of their role in health promotion.

M Memorizing	U Understanding	D Doing
Facts	Concepts	Skills
Methods of learning		
Association: • visual • verbal Repetition: • written • verbal • aura • visual Self-testing	Listening Questioning: • ourselves • others Discussing Comparing Solving problems Acting out Experiencing Imagining	Practice Demonstration Teaching others Trial and error Doing and reviewing

Figure 7.6   Appropriate learning strategies (after Belbin et al., 1981, in Anderson, undated)

The creative arts and health promotion

The capacity of the arts in general to enhance well-being is well recognized, as is their capacity to improve communication by increasing aesthetic appeal and arousing emotions and, indeed, to raise awareness of oppression and social inequality. However, in contrast to the visual and performing arts, the explicit use of the arts to promote health is characterized by participation and active involvement in the creative process – hence, the term creative arts projects (see Box 7.4 for an example).

BOX 7.4 HEALTH BENEFITS FOR CHILDREN OF CREATIVE ACTIVITIES

A rapid review of evidence was undertaken to ascertain the effects of participating in creative activities on health and well-being outcomes of children and young people. Twenty studies were included in the review with the majority of these deriving from UK sources. The majority of the studies (12) reported in the review used drama, performance art or forum theatre as the main activity, but studies on visual arts, dance and music were also included. While there were methodological limitations in many of the studies due to the complexity of the interventions and the challenges in measuring outcomes, the authors concluded that participating in creative activities can have a positive effect on behavioural changes, self-confidence, self-esteem, levels of knowledge and physical activity levels of young people.

Source: Bungay and Vella-Burrows (2013)

The materials produced may take a number of forms – from posters and leaflets to banners, artworks, music and drama performances – and may or may not have an additional educational purpose. For example, a giant mobile developed by pupils on the importance of clean air and the polluting effects of smoking displayed in a school entrance hall communicated the message to the whole school community without a word being said. However, it is important to distinguish the effects that it had on two major constituencies. Those who developed the mobile benefited from having participated in the creative process. However, for those who had not taken part, it was simply a means of communicating a message – comparable to professionally developed materials, albeit benefiting from local relevance and a certain homophily between the designers and the audience (Green and Tones, 2000).

Participating in creative arts projects will contribute to the learning of those taking part in a number of ways. Learning may be concerned with substantive content and developing knowledge, raising awareness and changing attitudes. Additionally, the process itself may be empowering as a result of its developing skills, which, together with the concrete evidence provided by the successful production of materials, will contribute to self-efficacy beliefs, confidence and a sense of control. Clearly, if others recognize the value of the 'products' or artefacts, then there will be further enhancement of self-esteem. In short, it will influence the basic constructs of empowerment (and indeed health literacy). The development of these attributes will apply outside the boundaries of the arts projects to more general areas of people's lives. If those involved feel that they are achieving worthwhile goals, then the meaningfulness of their involvement will lead to an enhanced sense of coherence (Antonovsky, 1984) and the achievement of salutogenic goals. Furthermore, contact with other individuals may generate a sense of social connectedness, contributing to a sense of community and the development of social capital.

Community-based art for health involves 'the use of art to address health and well-being' (Angus, 2002: 2). An earlier review of the literature on the impact of community-based arts projects indicated that changes occur in different areas that include: personal change such as making new friends and feeling happier; social change such as bringing people together; economic change such as enabling people to find work; and educational change such as improved performance at school (Newman et al., 2001). There are many projects and they can be varied, ranging from using participatory theatre in mental (ill)health recovery (Torrissen and Stickley, 2018), to the use of dance for older people in acute hospital settings to promote physical activity, social interaction and well-being (Bungay et al., 2022) to using collaborative community arts projects to address issues of social justice and equity (Epstein et al., 2021).

A review of good practice in community-based 'arts for health' projects (Health Education Authority [HEA], 1999a) noted that the quality of the artefacts was of central importance in generating a sense of pride and influencing the extent to which the participants took the activity seriously. It also saw no conflict between an emphasis on the rigorous teaching of basic skills (and, if necessary, correcting them) and commitment to participation. Rather, it found that this contributed to the quality of the artefacts. Similarly, Angus (2002) argues that many practitioners advocate for the importance of quality in the art that is produced but notes that this can create a tension between the intended health and social outcomes of a project and the quality of art that results. The participatory models that were found to work best were 'well-structured, well-organized and specifically related to the acquisition of skills or of resources for self-expression' (HEA, 1999b: 5).

Creative arts projects have also been used to explore health needs. Their capacity to put people in touch with their feelings and engage their imagination to envisage how things *might* be is particularly valuable in this regard. The materials produced can themselves have a powerful advocacy function. For example, one community arts project involved different generations in depicting their views about the health of their community through the medium of art. A display of their work was described by one observer as 'chilling' (Tones and Green, 1999). It communicated to policy-makers the fear of crime and going out at night, the problem of traffic and the issue of loneliness more powerfully than perhaps any other medium could. Creative arts projects also have the potential for positive impacts at an individual level. A community art programme in South Africa for children affected by HIV and AIDS found that attendance at the programme was a predictor of significantly higher self-efficacy and the authors advocate for the use of similar programmes for vulnerable children (Mueller et al., 2011).

The creative arts can also have a role in developing awareness of issues and the motivation to take action about them. This critical consciousness-raising is a central concern of Freirean approaches and liberatory education that will be discussed more fully later. In particular, creative arts can contribute to critical reflection on reality and the belief that change is possible. The use of theatre has been popular in this regard and notably forum theatre, which is attributed to Freire's fellow Brazilian, Augusto Boal.

In forum theatre, members of the audience with ideas for change go on stage and act out their ideas, becoming transformed from spectators into 'spectactors'. This enables the audience to envisage change, act it out and reflect collectively on outcomes and potentially empowers the audience to take social action. As an example, Sriranganathan et al. (2012) report on the work of 'YouthCo', who train and deploy peer youth facilitators to act out scenes and encourage participants to intervene and participate. Their focus is often on issues such as sex, sexualities, drug use and self-esteem.

Theatre is becoming more widely used in health education – for example, in HIV, AIDS and drugs education. However, theatre can only be included under the umbrella of 'creative arts' if the audience actually participates. There is a well-recognized repertoire of theatre in education (TIE) activities to encourage such participation – role-play, simulation and problem-solving. The use of theatre can be particularly relevant to developing empathy, clarifying values and exploring moral dilemmas.

Day (2002) provides an example of the use of forum theatre in schools to enable young people to put themselves in other people's shoes and try out moral behaviour with regard to the homeless and refugees. Taking a slightly different approach, Stevens et al. (2008) report on a project that involves children and young people in interactive performances encouraging them to think about a range of health issues including bullying, obesity, drug use and so on. At points during the production, the audience is asked: 'What would you do?'

In summary, creative arts offer the potential for enhancing learning in relation to both cognitive and affective issues and have a particular capacity for developing individual empowerment, a sense of community and social capital.

The HEA (1999b: 2) review of arts for health projects proposes a broad range of possible outcomes, which would include:

- enhanced motivation – within the project and in the participants' lives generally
- greater social connectedness
- people perceiving that they have a more positive outlook on life

- reduced sense of fear, isolation and anxiety
- increased confidence, sociability and self-esteem.

Participation was identified as a key element linking the arts activity with health outcomes, and the principal contributions of projects (HEA, 1999b) were seen as:

- development of interpersonal skills
- opportunities to make new friends
- increased involvement.

The study by Comedia (Matarasso, 2001) identified some 50 social impacts deriving from participation in arts projects. While they might all influence empowerment and health in a general way – for example, in terms of enhanced educational opportunity and increased employability – a selection of immediate relevance to health is provided in Box 7.5.

BOX 7.5 SELECTED SOCIAL IMPACTS OF ARTS PROJECTS

- Increase people's confidence and sense of self-worth
- Provide a forum to explore personal rights and responsibilities
- Reduce isolation by helping people to make friends
- Develop community networks and sociability
- Build community organizational capacity
- Encourage local self-reliance and project management
- Help people extend control over their own lives
- Be a means of gaining insight into political and social ideas
- Facilitate effective public consultation and participation
- Strengthen community cooperation and networking
- Help feel a sense of belonging and involvement
- Create community tradition in new towns or neighbourhoods
- Help community groups to raise their vision beyond the immediate.

Source: After Matarasso (2001: 159–60)

Characteristics of the learner

Using educational approaches and content suited to the age and stage of development of the learner is fundamental to good educational practice. The notion of 'cognitive matching' (Bruner, 1971) underpins the concept of the spiral curriculum, which introduces ideas in a simple form and revisits them with increasing sophistication and levels of abstraction as the learner matures.

The work of Piaget has been influential in relation to understanding the cognitive development of young people. While a full discussion of developmental psychology is beyond the scope of this chapter, a summary of Piaget's developmental stages is provided in Box 7.6. Ryder and Campbell (1988: 101) characterize the development in reasoning through these stages as:

- taking things at face value
- exploring relationships between tangible entities
- recognizing relationships involving unseen events
- abstract conceptualization.

Approximately 20% of adults do not reach the stage of having developed full formal operational thought and the capacity for hypothetico-deductive reasoning.

BOX 7.6 PIAGET'S DEVELOPMENTAL STAGES

Sensory-motor	0 – 1½/2 years
Pre-operational	1½/2 – 7/8 years
Concrete operations	7/8 – 11/12 years
Formal operations	11/12 – 15 years/adolescence

Source: Piaget and Inhelder (1969)

As well as consideration of the stage of development, the need to 'start where children are' has informed the development of school-based health education projects.

While the relevance of didactic methods for teaching young people is questionable, the use of these methods is particularly inappropriate to the needs of adult learners. The idea that adult learners have different learning needs to those of children and the use of the term 'andragogy' to refer to adult learning has been associated particularly with the work of Knowles, who built on the earlier work of Lindeman dating back to the 1920s. Knowles's seminal text, *The Adult Learner: A Neglected Species*, was published in 1973 and is now in its ninth edition (Knowles et al., 2020).

The core principles of adult learning that can usefully inform the development of health education interventions for adults are as follows:

- Adulthood is associated with a self-concept of being self-directed and in control – adults therefore need to feel responsible for their own learning.
- Adults have large reserves of experience on which to draw, so learning should utilize this experience.
- The willingness to learn is associated with its contribution to carrying out roles and coping with life situations.

- The relevance of the learning needs to be clear and immediate rather than deferred.
- The motivation to learn is internal and linked to coping with real-life situations.

Over and above the stage of development, within any group there will be differences in preferred learning style, linked to personality.

There are several different instruments for assessing learning styles. Perhaps the best known of these is the Myers–Briggs Type Indicator (MBTI), developed from Jungian theory and first published in 1962 (see Box 7.7). The 'Health Skills Project' used a simpler version, based on two dimensions – 'doer-intuiter' and 'feeler-thinker' – to identify four basic personality types as shown in Figure 7.7.

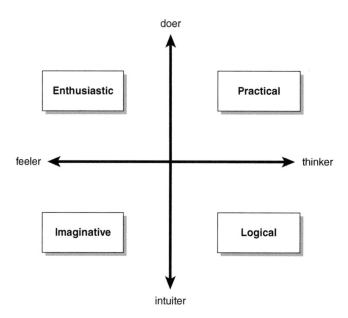

Figure 7.7 Personality types (based on Anderson, undated)

BOX 7.7 THE MYERS–BRIGGS TYPE INDICATOR (MBTI)

On the basis of the four dimensions below, there are 16 possible combinations:

extraversion (E) vs introversion (I)

seeing (S) vs intuition (N)

thinking (T) vs feeling (F)

judging (J) vs perceptive (P).

Teaching methods will vary in their appeal according to an individual's learning style. For example, extraverts (spelt as in Myers–Briggs) often learn by explaining to others, whereas this may not appeal to introverts who prefer to have a logical framework to order their learning. The tendency is also to teach in one's own preferred learning style but, given that in any group there is likely to be a mix of styles, variety is essential to ensure that the needs of all learners are met at some point.

In addition to developmental and personality factors, the effective facilitation of learning also requires sensitivity to issues such as gender, ethnicity and culture. Such sensitivity is central to the core values of health promotion, as well as being instrumental to success. Clearly, educational interventions are more likely to be effective if they are perceived to be personally relevant. A key consideration is the extent to which interventions are designed to suit the specific requirements of individuals – that is, the extent to which they are targeted or individually tailored.

Targeting and tailoring

Reference to social marketing theory would indicate that health education is more likely to be effective if there is a good fit between the message and the characteristics of the target group.

The notion of 'targeting' applies the principle of market segmentation to the design of materials for specific subgroups in relation to particular characteristics, such as age, gender, ethnicity, social class, occupation. In contrast, 'tailoring' refers to adapting the educational approach to meet the needs of the individual (Kreuter and Skinner, 2000):

> any combination of information or change strategies intended to reach one specific person, based on characteristics that are unique to that person, related to the outcome of interest, and have been derived from an individual assessment.

Kreuter and Skinner provide a useful analogy, comparing off-the-peg clothing (targeted) and bespoke tailored clothing (tailored).

Holt et al. (2000) identify a number of empirical studies that have demonstrated the superior effectiveness of tailored materials, but also note that factors such as personality and locus of control play a part. They suggest that developments in information technology offer considerable potential for tailoring health education materials to suit individual psychosocial and behavioural profiles. However, their effectiveness will ultimately be dependent upon being able to identify, with some precision, all relevant variables.

The most commonly used approach to tailoring is 'behavioural construct' tailoring, which draws on theories of behaviour. Constructs such as stages of readiness to change, identification of barriers to change and self-efficacy for changing behaviour are frequently used. As yet, however, there is little advantage over well-designed non-tailor-made materials that address these constructs. This could, perhaps, be expected, given that little attention is paid to cultural and personality factors. Kreuter et al. (2000) suggested that the inclusion of a wider range of variables, including non-behavioural factors such as preferred learning styles, would increase the relative advantage over non-tailored material. A meta-analysis of tailored print health behaviour change interventions concluded that there was evidence of effectiveness and that numerous factors appear to influence the effects of tailoring (such as length of material, what behaviour was being focused on, and whether or not the intervention drew on theoretical concepts of behaviour change) (Noar et al., 2007). A subsequent meta-analysis specific to tailored web-delivery health behaviour change interventions concluded that tailoring resulted in significantly better health outcomes across a variety of medical conditions and populations (Lustria et al., 2013). A study by Shirazi et al. (2015) highlighted the importance of using participatory approaches to targeting and tailoring practice in relation to breast screening interventions and found that tailoring to match a specific community's needs was vital in order to tackle inequalities in breast cancer (see Abstract 7.1 for details).

ABSTRACT 7.1

Targeting and tailoring health communications in breast screening interventions. Shirazi, M., Engelman, K.K., Mbah, O., Shirazi, A., Robbins, I., Bowie, J., Popal, R., Wahwasuck, A., Whalen-White, D., Greiner, A., Dobs, A. and Bloom, J. (2015)

Background: Members of underrepresented minority (URM) groups are at higher risk of disproportionately experiencing greater breast cancer-related morbidity and mortality and thus require effective interventions that both appropriately target and tailor to their unique characteristics.

Objectives: The study sought to describe the targeting and tailoring practices used in the development and dissemination of three breast cancer screening interventions among URM groups.

Methods: Three national Community Network Programs (CNPs) funded by the National Cancer Institute were focused on breast cancer screening interventions as their major research intervention. Each targeted different populations and used participatory research methods to design their intervention tailored to the needs of their respective audience. The Alameda County Network Program to Reduce Cancer Disparities partnered with community members to design and conduct two-hour 'Tea Party' education sessions for Afghan women. The Kansas Community Cancer Disparities Network co-developed and deployed with community members a computerized Healthy Living Kansas Breast Health Program for rural Latina and American Indian women. The Johns Hopkins Center to Reduce Cancer Disparities employed a train-the-trainer COACH approach to educate urban African American women about breast cancer.

Conclusions: Each CNP targeted diverse URM women and, using participatory approaches, tailored a range of interventions to promote breast cancer screening. Although all projects shared the same goal outcome, each programme tailored their varying interventions to match the target community needs, demonstrating the importance and value of these strategies in reducing breast cancer disparities.

The stages of change model (Prochaska and DiClemente, 1983) offers the possibility of designing interventions that are appropriate to the various stages, and can be applied to both targeting and tailoring. Miilunpalo et al. (2000) describe the basic elements of the model as being:

- **motivational** – concerned with attitudinal readiness, intention building and decision-making
- **behavioural** – tentative performance up to regular practice.

Progression through the stages of change from precontemplation to contemplation, preparation, action and maintenance is marked by a shift in emphasis from motivation to behaviour. Figure 7.8, developed from Cabanero-Verzosa (1996), indicates how learning needs will vary depending on the stage an individual or group is at.

A study by Cornacchione and Smith (2012) examined the stages of change model and message framing. The purpose of the study was to establish whether gain- or loss-framed messages were more or less effective at motivating smokers towards intention to quit at different stages. The authors concluded that gain-framed messages were more likely to make individuals move from contemplation to preparation but there did not appear to be difference at other stages. However, a key concern is whether or not the individuals at a particular stage are, in fact, a homogeneous group. Miilunpalo et al. (2000), for example, suggest that, in relation to physical activity, the precontemplation stage may be subdivided into two groups: 'negative precontemplation', in which individuals may be consciously resistant to change; and 'neutral precontemplation', in which little consideration, if any, has been given

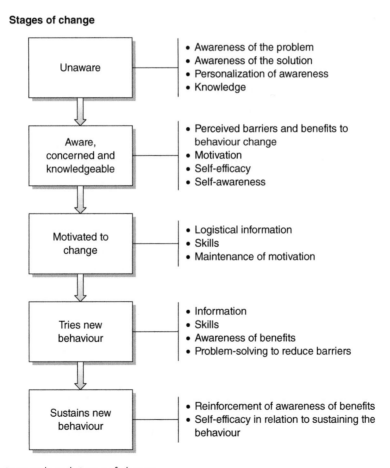

Figure 7.8   Learning needs and stages of change

to the possibility of change. The findings of Dijkstra and de Vries (2000) also confirm that the precise tailoring of smoking interventions would need to recognize that there are subgroups within the precontemplation stage.

The principles of targeting and tailoring support the development of interventions to suit particular needs. Clearly, tailoring is more challenging in that messages are designed for individuals and depend on an analysis of pertinent individual-level factors. However, we should also note that the process of checking out individual characteristics is integral to the interchange that takes place in one-to-one counselling. For example, 'motivational interviewing' (Rollnick et al., 1992) was developed as a means of helping people to work through ambivalence about behaviour change and is structured to respond to different needs at the various stages of change. Furthermore, well-designed experiential groupwork has the capacity to achieve highly individualized learning outcomes. However, one-to-one counselling or small groupwork may only be feasible in relatively small-scale projects. Targeting and tailoring offer the potential for improving the effectiveness of larger-scale programmes by means of the individualization of messages.

Characteristics of the teacher

Social learning theory – which has been a major influence on the development of health education interventions – recognizes the contribution of the characteristics of the teacher to the learning process through 'modelling'. Ryder and Campbell (1988) cite McPhail et al.'s (1972) research for the 'Lifeline Project' on moral education, which found that young people were critical of being told how to behave when this was not reflected in the behaviour of their teachers. This applies to a whole range of 'teacher' behaviour, but is particularly pertinent to fundamental principles such as integrity and respect.

These principles are also integral to Rogerian and Freirean approaches. Rogers refers to 'realness' or 'genuineness' as a key attribute of a facilitator, along with acceptance, trust and valuing of the learner. He also notes the importance of being able to empathize with the learner (Rogers, 1967). The 'Health Skills Project' (Anderson, undated) used the acronym REG to summarize these requirements – respect, empathy and genuineness. To avoid any gender bias, it also offered RUBY – respect, understanding and be yourself. Reference to Freire's message to the coordinator of a 'cultural circle' in Box 7.8 reveals similar views about what makes a good coordinator. More information about cultural (or culture) circles is provided later on in this chapter and in Chapter 9.

BOX 7.8 TO THE COORDINATOR OF A CULTURAL CIRCLE

In order to be able to be a good coordinator for a 'cultural circle', you need, above all, to have faith in man [sic], to believe in his possibility to create, to change things. You need to love. You must be convinced that the fundamental effort of education is the liberation of man, and never his 'domestication'. You must be convinced that this liberation takes place to the

> extent that man reflects upon himself in relationship to the world in which, and with which, he lives ... A cultural circle is a live and creative dialogue, in which everyone knows some things and does not know others, in which all seek, together, to know more. This is why you, as the coordinator of a cultural circle, must be humble, so that you can grow with the group, instead of losing your humility and claiming to direct the group, once it is animated.
>
> *Source*: Freire (1972: 61)

Over and above the content of any message, the style of interaction adopted by the health educator can contribute to empowerment to a greater or lesser extent, as shown in Figure 7.9.

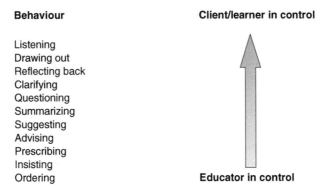

Figure 7.9   Empowering or de-powering

Our discussion of communication of innovations theory in Chapter 3 also highlighted the importance of the change agent's characteristics, particularly the principle of homophily (Rogers and Shoemaker, 1971). The growth in popularity of peer education in recent years is premised on the notion that peer educators will automatically have more credibility than other teachers and that people learn best from those who share similar characteristics. A systematic review by Harden (2001) concluded that the evidence for effectiveness for peer-delivered health promotion with young people was not yet clear; nevertheless, peer education has grown in popularity in recent years. Given the development of what Frankham (1998) refers to as the 'dogma' of peer education, we will briefly consider its relevance for enhancing learning.

Peer education

According to South at al. (2015), peer education is conceptualized as the teaching and communication of health information, values and behaviours between individuals who are of equal social status or share similar characteristics or have common experiences. There is some variation in the terminology associated with peer education (see Box 7.9), which Milburn (1995) suggests signals subtle differences in roles and styles of working – particularly regarding the level of control and authority.

BOX 7.9 PEER EDUCATION – THE TERMINOLOGY

- Peer education
- Peer training
- Peer tutoring
- Peer counselling
- Peer facilitation
- Peer leader
- Peer helper.

A number of claims have been put forward to support the use of peer education. Turner and Shepherd (1999) identify the following. Peers are:

- a credible source of information
- acceptable sources
- more successful than professionals
- able to reinforce learning through ongoing contact
- positive role models.

Peer education:

- is empowering for those involved
- is beneficial to those involved
- utilizes established channels of communication
- provides access to those who are hard to reach through conventional methods
- is more cost-effective.

Furthermore, the use of peers as educators may enable groups to be reached who may ordinarily be difficult to access or engage, a point reiterated by Cross et al. (2021). For example, peer-based approaches have been consistently implemented in prisons across the world, particularly Europe, North America and Canada, and are regarded as a way to expand the range of services on offer in the criminal justice system and also increase access to health information and education. While the evidence of peer education in this context is 'patchy', as noted by a systematic review by Wright et al. (2011), many studies demonstrate positive outcomes as a result of peer education, including, for example, uptake of HIV-testing (Zack et al., 2013), efficacy in increasing knowledge and awareness of potentially sensitive issues such as sexual health (Kannappan and Shanmugam, 2019), and knowledge, skills improvement and increased self-efficacy in breast self-examination (Yurt et al., 2019). In a systematic review on peer education and support in prisons, Bagnall et al. (2015) concluded peer interventions in this setting have a positive effect on the peer educators/supporters as well as on the recipients, maintaining and improving health and well-being. Like others, Fisher and Fisher (2018) argue that peer education has benefits for the peer educators themselves and can be an empowering and transformative process. However, Moore (2021) introduces a cautionary note, contending that peer education does not always empower or engage the peer educator and is an outdated mode of health promotion – albeit in the context of college students promoting health with their peers.

More traditionally, peer education has been consistently used in relation to young people's health (Cross et al., 2021). For example, research by Denison et al. published in 2012 demonstrated how a Zambian 'youth-led' volunteer peer-education intervention to teach HIV prevention and reproductive health in schools showed positive outcomes for young people in relation to improved knowledge and self-efficacy and lowered levels of sexual risk-taking behaviours. Peer education is an approach that is commonly used in schools, colleges and universities to educate and reach out to students in order to promote health (Moore, 2021). Clearly, peer education is more than a device for educating 'others'. Those who take on the role of peer educator stand to benefit from improved knowledge, skills, self-confidence, self-esteem and standing within their social group. This may derive from the training that they receive, but may also stem from their role as 'educators', as summed up in the aphorism *qui docet discit* – who teaches, learns!

Fundamental questions in the development of peer education projects concern who is a peer and who defines this, together with the related issue of how peer leaders/educators are selected. Age has often been seen as a key determining factor – many projects have focused on young people and there has been an interest in peer education programmes for senior citizens. However, other commonalities may also be relevant, such as common status (being a pupil in a school, for example, or a member of the workforce of a company) or experience that is relevant to the programme (such as breastfeeding or quitting smoking). Turner and Shepherd (1999) note that the principles of social learning theory (Bandura, 1986) would suggest that the effectiveness of peers as educators will be influenced by their standing within the group. Typically peer educators will self-select or be selected as 'suitable' by project coordinators.

Peer education projects fall into two broad groups: those that tap into existing social and friendship groups and those in which groups are more artificially constructed for the purpose of 'receiving' peer education (Milburn, 1995). Furthermore, the method of delivery can be through 'formal', planned sessions or informal social contacts. There is no rigid boundary between the two approaches and, whichever is used, the involvement of peer leaders in the selection and development of methods helps to ensure relevance. Backett-Milburn and Wilson (2000) noted that young peer leaders were aware of the advantages of informal approaches in that they could choose the right moment and adapt what they said to suit the needs and experience of the person they were speaking to.

Turner and Shepherd (1999) assert that many peer education projects lack a sound theoretical base and that, given its diversity, peer education will need to draw on a number of theories. Box 7.10 provides a list of the theories that they identify as being relevant to peer education.

BOX 7.10   THEORIES RELEVANT TO PEER EDUCATION

- Social learning theory (Bandura, 1986)
- Social inoculation theory (Duryea, 1991)
- Role theory (Sarbin and Allen, 1968)
- Communication of innovations theory (Rogers and Shoemaker, 1971)
- Differential association theory (Sutherland and Cressy, 1960)
- Subculture theories (for example, Cohen, 1955).

A review of the effectiveness of peer-led approaches in adolescent sexual health education found positive results in some trials (for example, a reduction in chlamydia incidence), but the authors concluded that the findings 'did not provide convincing evidence that peer-led education improves sexual outcomes among adolescents' (Kim and Free, 2008: 144). Similarly, Frankham (1998) expresses concern about the way in which claims made for the relevance of peer education for young people are repeated as dogma without being substantiated by research evidence. She takes the 'key tenets of the faith' and subjects them to critical scrutiny in relation to peer sex education.

- The claim that young people talk openly to each other about sensitive issues, such as sex and drugs:
  - o little factual learning takes place between friends and the content of conversations in groups is limited by the need for girls to protect their reputation and boys to be seen as 'one of the lads'
  - o young people are more likely to turn to friends for advice than parents, but friends are not necessarily seen as credible sources
  - o giving advice to friends can be seen as 'breaking the unwritten rules of friendship'.

- The claim that peer pressure is a powerful influence on young people's behaviour:
  - o young people appear to choose peer groups that suit their preferences, rather than their preferences being dictated by the group (a view endorsed by Michell, 1997) and allegiance to such groups is concerned more with identity formation than being pressured to fit in
  - o the portrayal of young people as a homogeneous group or, alternatively, as members of stable subgroups, appears to be erroneous – there are several subgroups and the boundaries between them are relatively fluid.

- The claim that peer education is participatory and empowering:
  - o peer educators facilitating sessions with groups may feel the need to set themselves up as experts and model the behaviour of those who trained them
  - o peer educators often see maintaining control of the group as part of their purpose – it may, therefore, be difficult for young people to use participatory forms of education
  - o peer leaders may not be representative of young people generally and the agenda that they set may reflect their own needs rather than responding to others' needs.

Frankham (1998: 190) concludes that peer education 'seems to sit (often uneasily) at the intersection of two cultural domains – the professional cultures of health education and the peer cultures of young people who are the intended recipients'. Young peer educators are confronted with the challenge of bridging both worlds. She also sees an inherent contradiction in submitting to peer influence in the context of peer education, but resisting it in other areas of life. Milburn (1995) also notes the ethical dilemma of placing peer educators in a position in which they feel responsible for influencing behaviour when the principal determinants of that behaviour are social and environmental factors beyond their control.

The EPPI-Centre review (1999) called for a clearer understanding of the processes involved in peer education and the ways in which they impact on outcomes. Backett-Milburn and Wilson (2000) concur with this view. Their process evaluation of a young people's peer education project noted the reluctance of adults to relinquish control to young people and that this was attributed to concerns about passing on inaccurate information. They emphasize the importance of distinguishing between concerns that can be addressed by means of the quality of the training given to peer educators and the more general concerns about handing over power to young people, such as fear that they might talk about sensitive subjects, such as sex, in ways that might not be approved of by adults.

The insight into the peer education process provided by Backett-Milburn and Wilson (2000) allows us to identify a number of key factors that impinge on it:

- **the recruitment process** – the extent to which peer educators are recognized as natural leaders within the group
- **setting** – the formality of the setting and consistency with the informality of peer education, the opportunity to maintain protected time for peer education, enthusiasm and commitment of staff, good liaison and evidence of success as a motivational factor
- **organizational context** – role of various stakeholders in decision-making and the extent to which power rests with the peer educators themselves
- **personal development of participants** – the development of the skills and acquisition of information needed to be peer educators
- **ongoing support for peer educators** – whether or not this is in place as they carry out their role.

Peer education offers the opportunity to capitalize on the shared characteristics of 'the teacher' and 'the learner' to enhance learning. However, it needs to be based on a full understanding of the social context in which it takes place (Frankham, 1998; Milburn, 1995). Furthermore, to maximize its potential, the peer educators need to be fully involved in developing the agenda and making decisions about process and content rather than merely acting as agents delivering a professionally defined programme.

ABSTRACT 7.2

Developing a typology for peer education and peer support delivered by prisoners. South, J., Bagnall, A. and Woodall, J. (2015)

(Continued)

Peer interventions delivered for prisoners by prisoners offer a means to improve health and reduce risk factors for this population. The variety of peer programmes poses challenges for synthesizing evidence. This article presents a typology developed as part of a systematic review of peer interventions in prison settings. Peer interventions are grouped into four modes: peer education, peer support, peer mentoring and bridging roles, with the addition of a number of specific interventions identified through the review process. The article discusses the different modes of peer delivery with reference to a wider health promotion literature on the value of social influence and support. In conclusion, the typology offers a framework for developing the evidence base across a diverse field of practice in correctional care.

Other factors

Educational interventions will necessarily be influenced by contextual factors. These can be thought of as falling into two broad groups. First, there is a set of factors that will determine the practical feasibility and acceptability of different methods and this is largely outside the control of those responsible for implementing interventions. This would include the availability of resources (financial and other), size of the target group, experience of the staff and so on. Cultural and professional norms will also influence the acceptability of programmes – to both recipients and key gatekeepers.

Second, there are several contextual factors that health educators might consciously seek to control to enhance the quality of the learning environment. Ryder and Campbell (1988) see part of the educator's role as that of providing an appropriate learning climate. This can include psychosocial as well as physical factors. Some of the key factors identified by the 'Health Skills Projects' are listed in Box 7.11.

BOX 7.11　KEY FACTORS IN THE LEARNING ENVIRONMENT

Physical factors

- Space – appropriate for comfort and closeness
- Seating – to allow eye contact with all participants
- Bright, stimulating environment
- Protected from outside distractions
- Convenient timing for participants – and sufficient for the task.

Psychosocial factors

- Appropriate style of leadership
- Negotiated ground rules
- Appropriate size of group

- 'Unfinished business' or members' mental baggage cleared away
- Any conflict is brought into the open and dealt with
- Clear expectations and purpose
- Reactions of the group are checked out regularly
- High levels of trust and cooperation
- Constructive feedback
- Appropriate use of humour
- Interactions between all members of the group – and leader's attention shared evenly
- Good group management skills.

Source: Adapted from Anderson (undated)

We have considered the various elements that impact on learning. We now turn our attention to consider attitude change in more detail and then go on to conclude the chapter by considering critical health education and strategies for social and political change.

PERSUASION AND ATTITUDE CHANGE

Attitude change has occupied a prominent part in traditional health education as health educators have searched for ways to persuade individuals to adopt healthy practices. We have already noted the potential conflict with empowerment.

We identified earlier four interrelated motivational constructs featured in the HAM – drives, emotional states, values and attitudes. Attitudes were conceptualized as specific rather than general and deriving from 'higher-order' motives. Emotional states can result from basic drives, such as fear, while attitudes emerge from values. Both values and emotional states may influence attitudes – that is, determine the importance attached to certain objects, people or courses of action.

The significance of the hierarchical dimension for health education is doubtless obvious. Given the enduring power of values, attempts to change attitudes may be ineffectual or counterproductive *unless* these underlying values are acknowledged. From the plethora of theories, we will use the Yale–Hovland model as a framework for this relatively brief analysis of attitude change. It was explicitly designed to develop efficient ways to influence public attitudes. An early concern, for example, was with finding the best way to convince American servicemen – in the middle of a general euphoria over victory in Europe in the Second World War – about the (erroneously) anticipated long and difficult struggle with Japan.

The general framework of the approach derived from Lasswell's (1948) recommendation to examine: 'who says what to whom via what medium and with what effect?' Hovland et al., therefore, researched the relative contributions of the message, the source of the message, the characteristics of the audience for whom the message was intended and the nature of the action resulting from the process of attitude change (for a more complete review of the early work, see Hovland et al., 1953).

Figure 7.10 has been adapted from McGuire and colleagues (McGuire, 1989), who have made a major contribution to the development of the Yale–Hovland model and its evaluation. Our adaptation aims to accommodate the model to the analysis of communication and learning presented at the beginning of this chapter and to our subsequent discussions of mass media and methods in Chapter 8. The figure provides a matrix relating source, message and audience factors to the various key stages in the communication and learning processes. The idea of a 'channel' has also been included and allows us to consider and contrast the relative roles of mass media and interpersonal methods.

Level of difficulty in achieving each stage **LOW** ↑	Communication characteristics				
	Communication and learning outcomes	Source	Message	Channel	Audience
	Exposure to message				
	Attention: • attract • sustain				
	Perception/interpretation				
	Recall of essential information				
	Understanding of message				
	Beliefs: Accept truth of message				
	Positive attitude to recommended action				
	Acquisition of skills				
	Adopt approved action				
↓ **HIGH**	Sustain approved action				

Figure 7.10   Relationship of major communication variables to the communication to learning process (adapted from McGuire, 1989)

Figure 7.10 not only shows the various stages in the communication to learning process, but gives an indication of the relative ease or difficulty in achieving the necessary change. Certain stages are of greater relevance to typical attitude-change initiatives. For instance, although it would be essential to understand and remember information associated with attitude change and the actions ensuing from that, the learning of principles and concepts would not normally be of concern – indeed, genuine understanding might militate against persuasive pressure! The cells in the matrix (following McGuire's formulation) can be used as a convenient evaluation device in the form of a checklist to assess to what extent various intermediate, process and outcome objectives have been achieved.

Before proceeding further, a cautionary note should be introduced. Psychology is replete with studies that have demonstrated statistically significant effects of particular approaches to attitude change. These are most commonly achieved in the laboratory. The effect is real, but their applicability to real life may be limited, insignificant or completely irrelevant. This is typically due to the fact that minor effects revealed in the laboratory are completely submerged by much more powerful real-life influences – often in combination with other equally powerful influences. As a full discussion of the complicated field of attitude theory is beyond the scope of this book, a selection of factors that do seem to be relevant to real concerns for health promoters will be outlined below.

Source factors

Reference was made earlier in this chapter to the role of the communicator or 'source' in both the communication and learning process. The real and perceived characteristics of the source are considered to be pivotal in the attitude-change endeavour and have been extensively researched. We must content ourselves here with merely listing the most important features identified by research:

- power and leadership
- source credibility:
  - o legitimate and expert authority
  - o perceived trustworthiness
  - o source attractiveness

- homophily and referent authority
- group pressure.

Message factors

Considerable research effort has also been devoted to the relative effectiveness of different ways of presenting persuasive messages in producing changes in attitudes and behaviour. Five key aspects emerge:

- repetition, primacy and recency
- sidedness
- the use of positive affect
- fear appeal
- arousal.

Repetition, primacy and recency

One of the most common assumptions is that, generally speaking, the more frequently a message is repeated, the more effective it will be. By contrast, a good deal of laboratory evidence has been accumulated to demonstrate that a message delivered first or last in a sequence of different persuasive attempts is more likely to be influential.

Sidedness

An important consideration in the construction of the message is whether greater attitude change would be produced by a one-sided persuasive argument or if both sides were presented. This is referred to as 'sidedness'. The outcome would seem to depend on the audience. If it is well educated, intelligent or both, a two-sided approach should be adopted. If the audience is uneducated/unintelligent or it could be guaranteed that it would never be exposed to the counter-arguments, the one-sided approach might be used.

One of the findings to emerge from the work on sidedness was that people exposed to two-sided messages who already favoured the advocated measure (such as fluoridation) maintained their support, even when exposed to attempts to change their commitment. This phenomenon provoked not only further research, but also, ultimately, resulted in deliberate measures designed to 'inoculate' individuals against attempts to persuade them to adopt unhealthy practices, such as smoking. McGuire (1970: 37, cited in Pfau, 1995: 100) played a substantial role in this research and his position is clear:

> We can develop belief resistance in people as we develop disease resistance in biologically overprotected man [*sic*] or animal, by exposing the person to a weak dose of the attacking material strong enough to stimulate his defences but not strong enough to overwhelm him.

Pfau distinguishes inoculation 'proper' from '*social inoculation*'. He defines this latter as an approach that uses a combination of strategies designed to anticipate future anti-health arguments and pressures. The essence of the technique involves 'threat and *refutational preemption*'. The threat might be an anticipated challenge to existing attitudes, such as a threat to existing negative feelings about smoking. Pfau (1995: 103–4) summarizes the situation as follows:

> adolescents commence the transition from the primary to middle grades with strong attitudes opposing smoking. 'They have *already been persuaded* that smoking is bad' (Pfau and Van Bockern, 1994: 420) … these attitudes often do not persist during the two years following the transition from elementary school to junior high school. The large majority of adolescents began this transition with negative attitudes towards smoking, but those attitudes deteriorated during the next two years. Adolescents grew more positive towards smoking, more positive towards peer smoking, and less likely to overtly resist smoking (Pfau and Van Bockern, 1994) … at the point of transition from the primary to middle school grades, adolescents possess reasonably established attitudes opposing smoking. What is needed at this point is a strategy to protect these antismoking attitudes from deterioration during the turbulent middle school years.

'Refutational preemption' is the proposed strategy. Individuals are made aware that at some future point there may be an 'attack' on their attitude that is vulnerable to change: that is to say, there is a threat. They are exposed to weak negative messages. The process of countering these messages prepares them to deal with any subsequent exposure 'in real life' to potentially stronger messages. Typically, the approach has involved peer leadership as discussed earlier in this chapter, peer modelling and videos.

Interestingly, the analogy of immunization can be further extended to include the use of 'booster' doses of education to maintain immunity. Botvin (1984) added these to his successful 'life skills training model', which demonstrated a reduction of 50% or more in school students' recruitment to smoking.

A further consideration is whether or not greater attitude change would result when conclusions are explicitly drawn for the audience or when the audience is allowed to reach its own conclusions on the basis of the information included in the message. Again, it seems to depend on the audience. A more informed or intelligent audience would demonstrate a greater shift in opinion and attitude by drawing its own conclusions, whereas less experienced or less intelligent people might need to be told much more directly what they should believe!

Positive affect

The majority of communications will produce an affective reaction of some kind in the audience, whether revulsion, humour or just interest. However, we are concerned here with *deliberate* attempts to design a message to produce affective responses that will lead to attitude and behaviour change.

Two important situations merit discussion. These relate to generating *positive* affect – that is, creating positive emotional responses in the audience; and, by contrast, the use of negative affect – an approach more usually described as 'fear appeal'. Positive affect is generally underutilized (Guan and Monahan, 2017) despite some evidence of some success for such approaches (see, for instance, Monahan, 1995; Murphy and Zajonc, 1993; Zajonc, 1980). Most research has concentrated on the creation of negative affect in the form of fear appeal. However, Guan and Monahan (2017) reviewed research from a range of disciplines including health communication, which showed that a focus on positive incentives, feelings and outcomes can promote risk-reducing behaviours. They argue that 'people who feel good during and after exposure to a health message tend to have favourable attitudes toward the message, which in turn, establishes more open, rather than resistant, attitudes toward the issue or risk-reduction behaviour promoted in the message' (Guan and Monahan, 2017). Two key strategies appear to influence this – using gain-framed appeals (emphasizing reward) and inducing positive feelings such as happiness (by attaining goals, for example). Guan and Monahan (2017) point out that the challenge is to understand how and when to use positive affect.

In all events, there can be no real objection to using positive messages as, at the very least, they attract attention and are likely to be more memorable than dry, factual data. Provided, of course, that messages fulfil the ethical requirement of not being economical with the truth. In contrast, there may be fundamental objections to the use of negative affect in changing attitudes and behaviour, irrespective of the question of effectiveness.

Fear appeal – creating negative affect

The use of fear appeal in general – and for health promotion in particular – is still highly controversial, both regarding the ethics of its use and its relative effectiveness. Fear appeals are 'in vogue', once again, especially in deterring individuals from health behaviours such as smoking, unsafe sexual practices, drug use, alcohol abuse and impaired driving (Gagnon et al., 2010). Attitudes have shifted back towards the benefits of using fear appeals for health, although some researchers have recommended that these techniques should be used sparingly (Brown and Richardson, 2012). Research into the use of fear to bring about an attitude change was famously triggered by the work of Janis and Feshbach (1953). Their influential study into the use of different levels of fear appeal in persuading individuals to brush their teeth regularly seemed to demonstrate that there was actually an inverse relationship between the level of fear and (reported) tooth-brushing behaviour. Those experiencing a very high level of fear were least likely of all to change their dental practices, while those experiencing a relatively neutral presentation were most likely to report an increase in dental hygiene. The results of those receiving the mid-level of arousal were, naturally, located somewhere in the middle!

Innumerable studies into the use of fear followed this counter-intuitive result, but generally these studies lacked methodological rigour. This was noted by Ruiter et al. (2014: 67), who reviewed the current state of empirical evidence on the effectiveness of fear appeals. One of their conclusions was that:

> after more than 60 years of experimental research into the persuasive effects of fear appeals, only six studies could be identified that provide high quality experimental tests.

Current evidence on the effectiveness of fear appeals then is inconclusive and suggests that more research evidence is required. Nonetheless, there is perhaps a broader moral and ethical question: 'Is the arousal of fear, guilt, anxiety and panic a price worth paying to get messages across' (Hubley et al., 2021: 147)? Some have argued that fear and distressing advertising can be ethically defensible if 'conditions of effectiveness, proportionality necessity, least infringement, and public accountability are satisfied' (Brown and Whiting, 2014: 89). Lupton (2015: 6), however, takes a slightly different angle and suggests that:

> If there is a convincing argument that a public health campaign fails to meet ethical principles, unless a simple utilitarian ethical stance is taken (whereby the ends always justify the means), whether or not it is effective is beside the point.

Arousal

Some insight into the effect of arousal on learning is provided by the so-called 'Yerkes–Dodson law' (Yerkes and Dodson, 1908). It has also been applied in the attitude change field, although some workers have questioned the generalizability of this phenomenon (for example, Winton, 1987). In short, the Yerkes–Dodson law demonstrated that both a very low level of arousal and a very high level of arousal resulted in poor learning. This is entirely consistent with common sense – an individual who is totally disinterested will neither be motivated to learn nor to perform. An individual whose state of arousal has resulted in an attack of panic and is paralysed with terror will also not be in a position to learn or act. Moreover, complicated and intricate learning tasks are disrupted at lower levels of arousal (that is to say, more easily) than simple tasks.

The Yerkes–Dodson law is often described in terms of an inverted 'U' curve where some optimal level of arousal figures at the top of the 'U'. While the effect of extreme levels of arousal is unchallengeable, it is more problematic finding evidence of a smooth curve – although a nicely constructed piece of research by Krisher et al. (1973) into the uptake of mumps vaccination did produce results consistent with the curvilinear predictions of Yerkes–Dodson.

It also seems clear that the shape of the curve or the level of 'threshold arousal' will depend on the nature of the proposed actions. For example, presenting immediate action opportunities that are perceived to be attainable would increase the likelihood that a relatively high level of arousal might lead to action. Without such opportunities, high levels of arousal can backfire and be associated with denial and avoidance.

Again, as noted above by Leventhal (1980), audience characteristics would also be important. High self-esteem and self-efficacy certainly tend to result in vigilance and people having such characteristics would be able to cope with relatively high levels of arousal without resorting to defensive behaviour or succumbing to paralysis! However, Witte and Allen (2000) note that personality factors and demographic characteristics such as gender appear to have little influence on the way fear appeal messages are processed.

Audience factors

The final aspect of attitude change under consideration here is the contribution of the audience itself. As emphasized in Chapter 4, detailed information about the target group of a health promotion intervention should be an essential part of effective planning. Attitude change theory, too, urges persuaders to know their audience. It is, self-evidently, important to know people's existing attitudes and the values from which they are derived.

At a macro level, there is evidence that there may be social class differences in reactions to persuasive messages (see our discussion of social marketing in Chapter 8). At the micro level, there also seems to be some variation in individuals' suggestibility, which can render them more amenable to persuasive influences. Moreover, reference has already been made to the importance of self-esteem in several contexts. It is generally accepted that individuals having high self-esteem (and belief in their capacity to control their lives) are better able to make vigilant decisions following exposure to health education messages – whether or not they use fear appeal. Yet high self-esteem may confer some protection against persuasive attempts to change attitudes. To pursue this further, we will consider the notions of cognitive dissonance and reactance.

Dissonance and reactance

Cognitive dissonance theory (Festinger, 1957) is one of a group of so-called 'balance theories' that contend that a state of imbalance between psychological components, such as belief, attitude and behaviour, results in an uncomfortable state of dissonance and creates pressure for change. Accordingly, an imbalance between one's beliefs and attitudes and behaviour should result in a change of one or more of these in order to restore 'consistency' or 'congruence'. In Chapter 3, we located 'dissonance' in the motivation system of the HAM, equating it with such emotional states as guilt and anxiety in terms of its capacity to influence intentions to act. For instance, a smoker who is health-conscious and concerned about her or his family's welfare is likely to experience a high degree of dissonance about exposing the family to passive smoking. Clearly, this dissonance could readily be resolved by quitting or only smoking outdoors. However, smokers who feel unable to do this often resort instead to denying the risk.

Festinger and colleagues performed an ingenious series of experiments demonstrating the effects of dissonance and attempts to reduce it (for a comprehensive account, see Aronson, 1976). One example will suffice to indicate the lengths to which people will go to achieve dissonance reduction. Aronson was concerned with the way dissonance reduction was related to the justification of cruelty in the context of significant US policy decisions. He described a notorious situation at Kent State University when four students were shot and killed by the Ohio National Guard during a demonstration against the Vietnam War. According to Aronson (1976: 121, citing Michener, 1971), the guilt and dissonance experienced by the community in relation to respectable students could only be assuaged by modifying beliefs and attitudes so that the killing could be justified:

> several rumors quickly spread to the effect that: (1) both of the slain women were pregnant (and therefore, by implication, were oversexed and wanton); (2) the bodies of all four students were crawling with lice; and (3) the victims were so ridden with syphilis that they would have been dead in two weeks anyway.

Two of the more important generalizations from research are, first of all, that dissonance is proportional to the seriousness of the issue that creates the dissonance. Second, it seems clear that the level of dissonance is also proportional to the level of self-esteem. Someone having high self-esteem who 'acts out of character' or in contradiction to moral values that he or she has espoused is likely to experience such discomfort that the mere contemplation of the act is likely to result in its rejection.

The second audience characteristic of relevance to attitude change is 'reactance'. One of the important facts of life is that most people do not like to be bludgeoned into taking action, even if they believe it is for their own good. Brehm (1966: 9), who studied this characteristic extensively, provides a key definition:

> Reactance is the motivational state experienced whenever any behaviour that the audience might have freely engaged in is either eliminated or threatened; its aim is to re-establish freedom of choice. Freedom will be re-established by changing attitude in a direction away from the advocated position.

Sutherland's commentary on the negative reaction to the historic establishment of the (English) General Board of Health in 1850 provides a common-sense example of reactance in the field of public health. In his words:

> Many local 'interests', however, resented the central power of the Board, and particularly Chadwick's thrustful, tactless methods, and these probably led *The Times* to comment: 'We prefer to take the chance of cholera and the rest than to be bullied into health.' (Sutherland, 1979: 7)

The objections to healthy public policy illustrated above clearly involved a clash of political and economic interests. However, this is not the same as the psychological phenomenon of reactance. The 'law of reactance' developed by Brehm and colleagues (Brehm, 1966; Brehm and Brehm, 1981) makes the simple, but highly relevant, point that, whenever individuals feel that their freedom of action will be curtailed, they tend to react against the message and its source. Dowd (2002) distinguishes reactance and resistance. Resistance always involves some sort of obstructive or oppositional behaviour. In contrast, reactance is characterized as a motivational psychological attribute that may be expressed through developing a negative attitude to the message (even if the individual was initially favourably disposed towards it) or through behaviour. Crossley (2002) cites as an example the tendency among gay men to reject safer sex messages despite being made aware – through years of intensive health education – of the risks they might incur.

Resistance to health promotion messages is held to involve:

- a challenge to the idea that 'unhealthy' or 'risky behaviours' are 'irrational'
- a recharacterization of 'unhealthy' or 'risky' behaviours as an intelligible response and assessment of 'risks' in a risk-laden society
- an argument for the need to understand such activities rather than simply explain them away
- a characterization of the 'dominant' health promotion perspective as dominant or 'hegemonic' – a perspective which imposes and/or prioritizes a medical/scientific 'worldview' over the 'lay' perspective. (Crossley, 2002: 108)

Some individuals appear to have a greater tendency to be oppositional than others. For instance, Dowd (2002) identifies an association between reactance and Type A behaviour linked to the individual's need to have a sense of control. This is somewhat paradoxical given the emphasis of health promotion on enabling individuals to have control over their health.

Even the best-intentioned health education can, therefore, backfire, resulting in reactance and oppositional behaviour – either at an individual or a group level. What, then, is the best strategy to adopt? Crossley argues that greater exposure to 'accurate' information fails to engage with alternative 'worldviews' about risk. Rather than repeating simple messages, she advocates critical discussion and debate that allow concerns to be brought out into the open.

Channels and methods for attitude change

Reference was made earlier to the importance of taking into account both the channel used to deliver persuasive messages and the particular methods used. Mass media are often deliberately employed to change attitudes by utilizing influential sources and messages that are deliberately tailored to specific audiences and take account of their characteristics. We will consider the role of mass media more fully in Chapter 8. However, we should note the limited capacity of mass media to bring about attitude change. Participatory and interpersonal methods, as discussed earlier, offer much more potential in this regard.

In contrast to the persuasive role of health education, we will now turn our attention to its more radical and emancipatory role – arguably, its most important function for health promotion. We use 'critical health education' as a generic term to describe this function.

CRITICAL HEALTH EDUCATION – STRATEGIES FOR SOCIAL AND POLITICAL CHANGE

Although critical education incorporates all of the categories of learning described in this chapter, its major concerns are essentially affective. It aims to motivate people to take action to achieve the various goals that characterize health promotion's ideological commitments. The key difference between critical education and the kinds of attitude change that we have discussed above is that the attitudes to be changed relate to achieving social and political outcomes that, in turn, address issues of equity and social justice. It is, therefore, closely linked to empowerment and informed by critical theory. It is essentially political (see Box 7.12).

BOX 7.12 HEALTH PROMOTION AS A POLITICAL ENTERPRISE

Health promotion is an inherently political enterprise. Not only is it largely funded by government, but the very nature of its activity suggests shifts in power. Its recognition that peace, shelter, food, income, a stable ecosystem, sustainable resources, social justice and equity are basic prerequisites for health implies major redistribution in power and wealth.

Source: Signal (1998: 257)

In discussing the application of critical theory to research, Tones and Tilford (2001: 164) cite Harvey (1990: 2), as follows:

> At the heart of critical social research is the idea that knowledge is structured by existing sets of social relations. The aim of a critical methodology is to provide knowledge which engages the prevailing social structures. These social structures are seen by critical social researchers as *oppressive* structures.

Again, discussing implications of critical theory for health promotion research, Connelly (2001: 118) leaves no doubt about the social activist goals of health promotion:

> Reality is produced and reproduced by the causal powers of generative mechanisms whether these are our activities and attitudes or our encounters with social structures. Why we should want to strengthen some or undermine other generative mechanisms emerges from the inescapable reality of making ethical and political decisions in the light of our human interest in emancipation and enlightenment.

We have emphasized the relationship between health education and healthy public policy. We have also asserted the primacy of education in achieving health promotion outcomes. Accordingly, critical health education is viewed here as potentially the most powerful means of achieving the supportive environments needed to empower choice. Although, as noted earlier in this chapter, health education can achieve individual empowerment, at this point, our focus is primarily on those empowering strategies that influence the physical, socioeconomic and cultural environment. In other words, to build environments that facilitate healthy choices and remove the barriers that militate against these. There are five separately identifiable (but frequently overlapping) approaches to achieving this end:

- activism and social action
- critical consciousness-raising
- providing 'life skills' and 'action competences'
- community organization
- media advocacy.

We will consider activism, social action and community organization more fully in Chapter 9 and media advocacy in Chapter 8. For the purpose of this chapter, we will focus more specifically on the contribution of education and learning.

As we explained earlier, health education is concerned with health- (or illness-) related learning. Moreover, we argued that education and policy development and implementation were mutually interdependent; it is rare to find examples where healthy public policy does not in fact involve – and, indeed, depend on – health-related learning. However, social action has not infrequently been contrasted with 'traditional' health education and its focus on individuals. Our view is that *critical* health education is the major means for achieving social action.

Persuasion and other forms of education are central to achieving change through 'non-violent disruption', exemplified by Ross and Mico (1980) as Gandhi's civil disobedience and Martin Luther King's civil rights movement. Ross and Mico also included the work of Saul Alinsky, whose radical approach is relevant to current conceptions of the social determinants of health. Alinsky's (1969, 1972) main concerns were with alienation and social disadvantage. His approach included the recruitment and training of a cadre of leaders and, in the words of Minkler and Wallerstein (1997: 243):

> This *social action organizing* emphasized redressing power imbalances by creating dissatisfaction with the status quo among the disenfranchised, building communitywide identification, and helping community members devise winnable goals and non-violent conflict strategies as means to bring about change.

For further discussion of Alinksy's approach, see Pruger and Specht (1972).

Freudenberg (1978, 1981, 1984) has been consistently associated with a radical approach. He reminded us that radical action for health is not a recent phenomenon and described how, between 1910 and 1920, Dr Alice Hamilton investigated health conditions in the lead and mercury industries (1984: 40):

> When employers refused to allow her on their premises, she set up clinics in the back rooms of bars and social clubs ... she also instructed them on how to protect themselves against toxic exposure and she lobbied forcefully for stricter regulations of these metals.

A flavour of activism in the field of health and safety is provided by a case study of the work of the Delaware Valley Toxics Coalition (DVTC). As Freudenberg (1984: 41) reports:

> Among their educational methods were demonstrations at polluting companies, testimony of victims of poisoning at public hearings, and written reports by scientists, physicians and epidemiologists. They developed a flair for using the media creatively. [See Chapters 6 and 8 on media advocacy.] At one city council hearing, a union member who was appearing in support of the bill sprayed an unmarked canister into the chamber. 'Stop that', the legislators shouted, 'you're poisoning us.' The unionist replied, 'This can has only air, but everyday we have to work with chemicals we know nothing about.' His testimony made headlines in the local paper.

Critical consciousness-raising – the Freirean perspective

Paulo Freire, who died in 1997, is probably the best-known advocate of a radical, libertarian approach to education for social change. His work originated with literacy programmes for impoverished cane-cutters in plantations near Recife in Brazil in 1958. He rapidly realized that de-powered individuals viewed reading and writing as alien to them. The way in which to achieve literacy was, therefore, by developing a radical challenge to poverty and the social systems that created it. Only in this way could illiterate workers be empowered. Freire's emancipatory approach has inspired not only those concerned with promoting social justice, but also those who seek to promote the health of the disadvantaged. His approach mirrors the empowerment model we propose in this book in that it not only seeks to liberate people from environmental barriers derived from oppressive power structures, but also to free them from their perceptions of an 'external locus of control' revealed in 'magical thinking'.

Following our earlier discussions of the meaning of education, we can say that Freire is committed to 'true education' – that is, to voluntarism and depth of understanding rather than persuasion and propaganda. Indeed, Freire criticizes the 'activism' of revolutionary leaders who fail to genuinely educate the populace (1972: 43):

> [Unless] one intends to carry out the transformation *for* the oppressed rather than *with* them … the oppressed … must intervene critically in the situation which surrounds them and marks them: propaganda cannot achieve this … It is my belief that only this latter type of transformation is valid. The object in presenting these considerations is to defend the eminently pedagogical character of the revolution.

In justifying his educational approach, Freire (1972: 67) cites Mao Tse-tung:

> We should not make the change until, through our work, most of the masses have become conscious of the need and are willing and determined to carry it out … There are two principles here: one is the actual needs of the masses rather than what we fancy they need, and the other is the wishes of the masses, who must make up their own minds instead of our making up their minds for them. (Mao Tse-tung, 1967)

Over and above any radical concerns, Freire's humanistic approach to education frequently includes references to the intrinsic value of people. These are essentially similar to Rogerian notions of 'unconditional positive regard' – a mainstay of non-directive counselling, which affirms that, although individuals' behaviour may be a cause for condemnation, their essential humanity must be respected. Freirean observations are also often reminiscent of the transactional analysis notion of healthy 'life positions' (Berne, 1964; Harris and Harris, 1986). It is argued that, as a result of early socialization and life experiences, individuals adopt basic attitudes to the self. There are four such positions, deriving from the extent to which people accept that they and other people are 'OK'. Turner (1978) adopted the term 'OK Corral' to describe the matrix shown in Figure 7.11.

I'm OK You're not OK **A**	I'm OK You're OK **B**
I'm not OK You're not OK **C**	I'm not OK You're OK **D**

Figure 7.11   The OK Corral

Source: Turner (1978: 72)

As will probably be apparent, the 'healthy' state is depicted in the top right cell, indicating an individual belief that the people in question feel content with themselves and have good self-esteem, but also trust others and feel concern for them. In other words, we have a remarkably concise definition of mental and social health, having links to such concepts as a 'sense of coherence'.

The pedagogy – educational methods

An emancipatory curriculum such as Freire's includes both cognitive and affective factors and the pedagogical methods employed take this into account. They are concerned with creating a level of critical awareness and translating that awareness into action.

A core feature is *'conscientizacao'*, or 'conscientization' that, in the words of the translator of *Pedagogy of the Oppressed* (Freire, 1972: 16, footnote), 'refers to learning to perceive social, political, and economic contradictions, and to take action against the oppressive elements of reality' and is most readily translated as 'critical consciousness-raising'.

The link between consciousness-raising and action is defined in terms of 'praxis'. Praxis is the interactive process of reflection and action. Action without reflection is mere 'activism'; reflection without action can involve mere detached intellectualism. The method is primarily 'dialogical' and involves problem-solving approaches.

Freire compared traditional educational approaches that treat learners as empty vessels to be filled by a teacher, referred to as 'banking', with a problem-posing approach that seeks to engage learners and put them in control of their learning. The distinction between 'banking' and 'problem posing' is not new, as we noted earlier in our analysis of rote learning, problem-solving and decision-making. The novelty here lies in the purpose of education – that is, it is radical, political and essentially affective.

The banking approach is not viewed merely as a technical method of teaching, but has deep ideological connotations – namely, in respect of the emphasis on the inequality of the teacher–learner relationship and the consonance between 'banking' and political domination. It is characterized as follows:

- The teacher teaches and the students are taught.
- The teacher knows everything and the students know nothing.
- The teacher thinks and the students are thought about.
- The teacher talks and the students listen – meekly.
- The teacher disciplines and the students are disciplined.
- The teacher acts and the students have the illusion of acting through the action of the teacher.
- The teacher chooses the programme content and the students (who were not consulted) adapt to it.
- The teacher confuses the authority of knowledge with his or her own professional authority, which he or she sets in opposition to the freedom of the students.
- The teacher is the subject of the learning process, while the pupils are mere objects.

The specific techniques employed by Freire in problem posing include the use of 'culture circles' – that is, informal groupwork. The culture circles explore their thematic universe, which is composed of a complex of generative themes that refer to key social and cultural issues. The culture circle (or 'thematic investigation circle') is presented with 'codifications of reality' – in other words, pictures or other triggers to discussion that incorporate major social issues, of which the participants are not yet conscious. The 'decoding' process works through dialogue and group members typically:

- reflect on aspects of their reality, such as poor housing
- search for a root cause of the problem
- consider implications and consequences
- devise a plan of action.

Because of its relevance to community development, we will revisit Freirean methodology in Chapter 9. It has also been adapted for a variety of health promotion purposes. For instance, Macdonald and Warren (1991) amalgamated the Freirean approach with Frankena's (1970) model for analysing the philosophical basis of educational programmes and applied this to primary healthcare (as prescribed by the WHO). Figure 7.12 outlines this amalgamation.

The Freirean perspective – problems and prospects

The ideological approach intrinsic to Freire's pedagogy is entirely consistent with the commitments and concerns of empowering health promotion. However, there are problems to be addressed by those health promoters seeking to utilize Freirean enlightenment. For example, it has been argued that Freire's focus on overtly oppressive state control and class is not relevant to all societies and cultures. However, Freire himself argued that his approach could be adapted to fit all those situations in which there was oppression and a lack of empowerment. The techniques can, and have, been applied to different contexts – for example, as a feminist challenge to male hegemony.

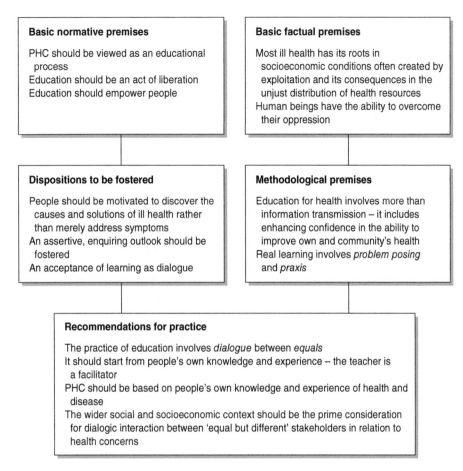

Basic normative premises

PHC should be viewed as an educational
  process
Education should be an act of liberation
Education should empower people

Basic factual premises

Most ill health has its roots in
  socioeconomic conditions often created by
  exploitation and its consequences in the
  unjust distribution of health resources
Human beings have the ability to overcome
  their oppression

Dispositions to be fostered

People should be motivated to discover the
  causes and solutions of ill health rather
  than merely address symptoms
An assertive, enquiring outlook should be
  fostered
An acceptance of learning as dialogue

Methodological premises

Education for health involves more than
  information transmission – it includes
  enhancing confidence in the ability to
  improve own and community's health
Real learning involves *problem posing*
  and *praxis*

Recommendations for practice

The practice of education involves *dialogue* between *equals*
It should start from people's own knowledge and experience – the teacher is
  a facilitator
PHC should be based on people's own knowledge and experience of health and
  disease
The wider social and socioeconomic context should be the prime consideration
  for dialogic interaction between 'equal but different' stakeholders in relation to
  health concerns

Figure 7.12   An analysis of the application of Freirean principles to primary healthcare (PHC) using Frankena's model

However, in accordance with the ever-present threat of false consciousness, a greater challenge to Freirean ideology and practice is the suggestion that Freire's ideas have been co-opted and thus emasculated (Kidd and Kumar, 1981; Zacharakis-Jutz, 1988). Kidd and Kumar refer to the co-option threat in terms of the emergence of a 'pseudo-Freirean' perspective that appears, superficially, to have radical credentials but, in fact, does not significantly challenge the status quo and its power structure. Referring to adult education (in all its many aspects), Kidd and Kumar (1981: 28) identify the following features of pseudoradical education:

- naming the central problem as 'poverty' rather than as 'oppression' (that is, ignoring the primacy of power)
- identifying the cause of poverty as the self-inflicted deficiency of the poor rather than oppression (that is, the problems of the poor are acknowledged but considered to be due to a 'culture of poverty' created by the shortcomings of the poor themselves)

- proposing, as treatment, to change the behaviour of the poor by means of a transmission of information and skills
- converting Freire's method into a 'neutral', apolitical classroom technique (for example, the use of group discussion – any kind of group discussion – rather than true dialogue leading to praxis, and the conversion of 'problem posing' into 'discovery learning' where the learner is helped to 'discover' the correct, predetermined answer to the problem)
- defining 'action' as coping activity (that is, the acquisition of personal competences other than those associated with political challenges to authority).

Freirean practice – difficult and dangerous

It should be stated that the emancipatory practices associated with critical consciousness-raising and praxis are difficult to achieve and there is clearly a temptation to follow 'pseudo-practices'. In certain circumstances (as Freire himself acknowledged), the pedagogy of the oppressed can be physically dangerous to both educator and learner. We are reminded of a cartoon embodying advice to would-be radical educators that showed an ostrich with its head in the sand. The novice educators are counselled not to ignore reality in that way, but an accompanying picture showing the ostrich on the receiving end of a fusillade of rifle fire also advises them not to stick their heads above the parapet!

The effectiveness of the approach may be increased and the risks reduced if the oppressed and powerless could enlist the support of an alliance of those who possess both goodwill and power – see the empowerment model in Chapter 1. Moreover, the process of praxis may be facilitated and, again, the element of risk reduced if consciousness can be supplemented by the acquisition of key 'protective' skills and those that facilitate the attainment of power. We will now, therefore, examine this latter suggestion and consider the role of life skills and action competences as part of critical health education.

Life skills, action competences and health

Life skills teaching enjoyed a good deal of popularity in the UK, originally for personal and social education in schools and, subsequently, for health education generally (see Hopson and Scally, 1980–2, 1981). At this point, we will concern ourselves with the application of life skills teaching and action competences to critical education – inside or outside the school sector. We will further consider the relevance of life skills and action competences to the health-promoting school in Chapter 10.

Hopson and Scally (1981) summarized the key elements of life skills teaching in terms of providing a 'survival and growth kit for an age of future shock':

> a school should provide a basic survival kit for young people … they need to be taught skills like values clarification, decision making, how to cope with crises, intellectual and emotional problem solving, helping, assertiveness, relationship building, how to find appropriate information and use personal and physical resources which are available in the community. They need to be made aware of themselves, others and the world around them, in order to become more self-empowered people.

The reference to *self*-empowerment is perhaps revealing. Critics of a radical persuasion saw the reference to self as evidence that the life skills approach was effectively blind to socioeconomic circumstances. While it is true that many life skills do indeed refer to individual empowerment and sometimes to an acceptance of the social status quo (for example, skills such as how to present yourself at interview in order to get a job), the following points should be noted:

- Many skills are indeed concerned with individual growth and development and include, for example, preventive health skills, such as stress management.
- The armamentarium of life skills includes large numbers of transferable skills that may be applied to a wide variety of situations – both conformist and revolutionary! Indeed, we noted earlier that lack of literacy skills is essentially de-powering and intimately associated with Freire's adult education approaches. Again, skills involved in working with groups could be used in taking action to achieve changes in health policy.
- A number of what might be called 'skills for radicals' are incorporated in Hopson and Scally's life skills menu.

Hopson and Scally identified the skills needed in different contexts, as shown in Figure 7.13.

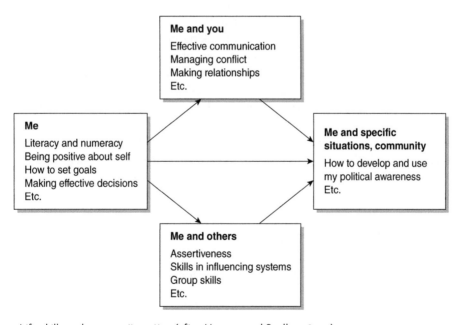

Figure 7.13   Life skills and community action (after Hopson and Scally, 1980-2)

There is a good deal of overlap and congruence of purpose between life skills and action competences. Although Hopson and Scally's work is firmly committed to Freirean principles, the action competence approach is, on the face of it, somewhat more radical. This is doubtless due to its overt commitment to critical theory and, thus, critical education. The work on action competences is very much associated with the Danish School of Education (see, for example, Jensen, 1991, 2000) and its emphasis on education for democracy in school and community. Jensen and Schnack (1997) also argue that it is central to environmental education. They see environmental problems as having their origin in society and ways of living, and that the solution requires developing the capacity to envisage alternatives and to act at a societal as well as an individual level. Fien refers to the notion of political literacy that has parallels with Freire's formulation of critical thinking and praxis, as can be seen in the following definition:

> The ultimate test of political literacy lies in creating a proclivity to action, not in achieving more theoretical analysis. The politically literate person would be capable of active participation (or positive refusal to participate) … The highly politically literate person should be able to do more than merely imagine alternatives … The politically literate person must be able to devise strategies for influence and for achieving change. (Crick and Lister's, 1978: 41, use of the term, as cited by Fien, 1994: 43)

Wals and Jickling (2000) also support this view in their comprehensive discussion of the role of environmental education, which they consider should be essentially emancipatory with reference to social, political and economic matters and concerned with 'recognizing, evaluating and potentially transcending social norms' (see also Fien and Trainer, 1993).

Mogensen (1997) describes praxis and critical thinking in environmental education as a holistic combination of feeling and reason – a dialectical process of examining situations from multiple perspectives and 'constantly challenging, querying, criticizing, breaking down parts of existing practice with the aim of reconstructing a new and alternative practice'.

According to Schnack (2000), critical thinking and praxis are essential in the context of what he calls 'the dissolution of tradition'. He also makes the point that action competence for health and environmental education should include the traits associated with C. Wright Mills's (1959) concept of 'sociological imagination' – that is, 'the capability of shifting perspective backwards and forwards between the individual, personal level, which is often seen as the purely private sphere, and the social, structural level'.

THE PRIMACY OF EDUCATION

In this chapter, we have reiterated and emphasized the point that, following the 'formula':

> health promotion = healthy public policy × health education

education is a *sine qua non* for contemporary health promotion. Indeed, it is challenging to find a situation in which education cannot be identified as being a major component in health promotion.

The importance of education for achieving sustainable development is recognized in the following quotation:

> Ethical values are the principal factor in social cohesion and, at the same time, the most effective agent of change and transformation. Achieving sustainability … will need to be motivated by a shift

in values. Without change of this kind, even the most enlightened legislation, the cleanest technology, the most sophisticated research will not succeed in steering society towards the long-term goal of sustainability. *Education in the broadest sense will by necessity play a pivotal role in bringing about the deep change required in both tangible and non-tangible ways.* (UNESCO-EPD report, 1997: 32, cited in Fien, 2000: 47)

This is equally applicable to the contribution of health education to health promotion and public health, not only in relation to their need to engage with environmental concerns, but also in relation to achieving other health goals – notably empowerment.

KEY POINTS

- Effective communication is central to health education and requires consideration of source, message and audience factors.
- The development of health education interventions requires clear specification of intended learning outcomes – cognitive, affective, conative and skills.
- The selection of methods also requires consideration of the characteristics of the teacher and learner.
- The use of participatory methods is consistent with the principles of empowerment. It is also more effective and less likely to induce reactance among learners.
- Methods such as creative arts, which have a multidimensional impact, can achieve confluence between different learning dimensions.
- The use of targeting and tailoring can increase the effectiveness of large-scale programmes by making messages more relevant to individuals.
- A power imbalance between teacher and learner can be a barrier to learning. Peer education can enhance learning by capitalizing on the shared characteristics of teacher and learner.
- Factors to consider in the design of messages to influence attitudes include sidedness, implicit versus explicit conclusions, inoculation and refutational pre-emption, and the use of affect – either positive or negative.
- The use of fear appeal is controversial from an ethical standpoint and can backfire. However, fear can be a useful motivator provided individuals both believe that they can and are able to do something to protect themselves.
- Health education can raise awareness of the factors influencing health and can empower individuals and groups to take action to tackle these factors.
- Within the critical theory tradition and in line with Freirean approaches, health education can be involved with critical consciousness-raising in relation to oppressive social structures and enabling learners to seek solutions.

CHAPTER 7: INTERNATIONAL CASE STUDIES

The following case studies on the online resources website are relevant to the content of this chapter: 1, 5, 8 and 9.

CRITICAL REFLECTION AND APPLICATION TO PRACTICE

This chapter has considered a range of factors in education for health and the contribution of education to health promotion. Which of these factors have more relevance to the work that you do? What aspects of the communication are most pertinent and why? Why is learning so central to health education and health promotion? What type of learning is most important in the context in which you work? What factors influence the learning climate? In your experience, what are some of the challenges of methods that persuade, coerce or induce fear? How might issues of equity and social justice be addressed through education in the context within which you work?

ONLINE RESOURCES

Please visit https://study.sagepub.com/greentones5e for all the online resources for the book, including recommended further reading on each chapter subject, useful weblinks (both introduced by the authors), as well as the abovementioned case study material.

8 MASS COMMUNICATION

Nothing is easier than leading the people on a leash. I just hold up a dazzling campaign poster and they jump through it.

Joseph Goebbels, cited in Rhodes (1976)

OVERVIEW

This chapter focuses on the use of mass media in health promotion. It will:

- consider the potential and limitations of mass media interventions for health promotion
- note the incidental effects of mass media as part of the wider environmental influences on health
- identify pathways through which mass media exert an effect on the individual
- consider theoretical and technical issues involved in planning mass media interventions
- identify the key elements of social marketing
- explore the use of media for advocacy purposes
- explore the use of social media within health promotion.

INTRODUCTION

This chapter begins by considering the more conventional role of mass media in persuading individuals to adopt healthy behaviours. Despite their potential to reach large numbers of people, mass media are not without their limitations in achieving behaviour change. Social marketing attempts to address these by applying marketing principles to the design of programmes and we will examine its contribution to health promotion. We will also turn our attention to a less widely acknowledged role of mass media, but one which is central to our view of health promotion – that is, its contribution to the development of healthy public policy. Finally, the role of social media in promoting health is discussed.

MASS COMMUNICATION AND HEALTH PROMOTION

The term 'mass communication' is often used interchangeably with 'mass media'. In the interest of clarity, it is worth giving brief consideration to the use of the terms 'communication' and 'media'.

Applying our earlier definition of 'communication' as the business of transmitting messages from a source to a receiver would limit the scope of 'mass communication' in a way that is certainly not intended by those who use it. The intended meaning is more in line with 'education' – as we have used it in Chapter 7, but with an emphasis on its persuasive dimension. The educational messages are, however, mediated by the use of a range of electronic, print and social media that have the advantage of being able to contact very large numbers of people at any one time. Their limitations derive from the fact that, as the messages are mediated, interpersonal contact is not possible. It is, therefore, very difficult precisely to tailor communications to the audience and impossible to react immediately to people's reactions to the mediated messages.

What exactly is a mass audience? It is meaningless to refer to precise numbers as it is not so much the actual numbers that are important but the one-way, top-down nature of communication. For instance, a typical 'block' lecture to the public or a student group has more in common with mass media than with interpersonal education, despite relatively small numbers.

Schramm and Roberts (1972: 392, cited in Reardon, 1981: 195) refer to the 'latitude of interpretation and response' that characterizes mass media:

> Characteristics of the mass communication situation, such as the receiver's freedom from many of the social constraints which operate in interpersonal communication, greatly attenuated feedback, and lack of opportunity to tailor messages for specific people allow any individual receiver a good deal more latitude of interpretation and response than he [*sic*] has when speaking face-to-face with friend, colleague or acquaintance.

Issues for health promotion

There are four main areas of interest and debate for health promotion in respect of mass media:

- the unhealthy influence of mass media generally, for example, encouraging health-damaging behaviours such as excessive alcohol consumption, or copycat violence, or even reducing the stock of social capital – see Putnam's (1995) suggestion that the decline in social capital is substantially due to the increase in television viewing
- the specific marketing of unhealthy products using mass media
- the acceptability of using mass media to achieve health promotion goals and associated debate about the relative effectiveness of mass media compared with alternative interpersonal approaches
- debate about the use of persuasive messages and/or coercive means to 'sell health' rather than empower choice.

Mass media

The variety of available media is substantial, including television and radio; print media such as newspapers, magazines, billboards and mass mailshots; and the plethora of communication channels opened up by modern information and communication technology such as social media. However, despite the shared characteristics mentioned above, it is unwise to treat mass media as completely homogeneous. It is obvious that there are differences between, for example, advertisements that deliver a health promotion message, coverage of health issues in documentary and news programmes, and the inclusion of health issues in drama or soap operas – so-called 'edutainment'. Equally, paying for media time (or space) for advertising one's message is different from using public service announcements (PSAs) that are delivered by mass media channels without charging.

It is also important to make a clear distinction between mass media and superficially similar devices, such as videos that are used to trigger discussion and involve interpersonal interaction with a teacher. A video endlessly repeated in a shopping mall is an example of mass media; the same video used as an aid to discussion and learning is a 'learning resource' or visual aid.

We should also be aware of rapidly evolving possibilities offered by interactive digital media, including websites, chat rooms, email lists, newsgroups, mobile phones, CD-ROMs and a variety of social media (Facebook, Twitter, TikTok, Instagram and so on) that continues to expand. While some usage may exhibit the characteristics of mass communication, these media also have the potential to tailor messages to suit the user's needs and include opportunities for feedback (Bernhard, 2001). In addition, as Vassallo et al. (2022) point out, these types of media are hugely popular and can be used to engage directly with specific target groups moving well beyond the possibilities of more traditional mass media channels.

The advantages and disadvantages of various channels are summarized from a practical perspective by the National Cancer Institute (undated) (see Table 8.1).

MASS MEDIA – CAPABILITIES AND FUNCTIONS

What, then, can we expect from mass media? Implicit in such a question is frequently an expectation of mass behaviour change – especially when posed by politicians and practitioners. However, such expectations – either in pursuit of profit or social welfare and health goals – will typically fail to materialize. Mass media are not a 'magic bullet' that will generate dramatic and widespread success, despite the hopeful expectations of some decision-makers. These unrealistic expectations reflect a model of mass media that is now rather disparagingly referred to as the 'direct effects' model or 'hypodermic model'. It derives from the assumptions that:

- mass media have a direct effect on the audience
- mass media act like a hypodermic syringe – advertisers fill it with a powerful message and inject it into the population at large
- if it does not achieve the desired result, a bigger syringe is needed (more intensive media blitz) with a more powerful content (new, more persuasive message)!

Mendelsohn (1968) challenged the direct effects model, preferring to use the metaphor of an aerosol spray, arguing that, as the mass media message was sprayed on to the target population, most of it

Table 8.1 Advantages and disadvantages of selected media channels

Mass media channels	Activities	Pros	Cons
Newspaper	Ads Inserted sections on a health topic (paid) News Feature stories Letters to the editor Op-ed pieces	Can reach broad intended audiences rapidly Can convey health news/breakthroughs more thoroughly than TV or radio and faster than magazines Intended audience has chance to clip, reread, contemplate and pass along material Small circulation papers may take PSAs	Can be costly, time-consuming to establish May not provide personalized attention Organizational constraints may require message approval May lose control of message if adapted to fit organizational needs
Radio	Ads (paid or public service placement) News Public affairs/talk shows Dramatic programming (entertainment education)	Range of formats available to intended audiences with known listening preferences Opportunity for direct intended audience involvement (through call-in shows) Can distribute ad scripts (termed 'live-copy ads'), which are flexible and inexpensive Paid ads or specific programming can reach intended audience when they are most receptive Paid ads can be relatively inexpensive Ad production costs are low relative to TV Ads allow message and its execution to be controlled	Reaches smaller intended audiences than TV Public service ads run infrequently and at low listening times Many stations have limited formats that may not be conducive to health messages Difficult for intended audiences to retain or pass on material

Mass media channels	Activities	Pros	Cons
Television	Ads (paid or public service placement) News Public affairs/talk shows Dramatic programming (entertainment education)	Reaches potentially the largest and widest range of intended audiences Visual combined with audio good for emotional appeals and demonstrating behaviours Can reach low-income intended audiences Paid ads or specific programming can reach intended audience when most receptive Ads allow message and its execution to be controlled Opportunity for direct intended audience involvement (through call-in shows)	Ads are expensive to produce Paid advertising is expensive PSAs run infrequently and at low viewing times Message may be obscured by commercial clutter Some stations reach very small intended audiences Promotion can result in huge demand Can be difficult for intended audiences to retain or pass on material
Internet	Websites Email mailing lists Chat rooms Newsgroups Ads (paid or public service placement)	Can reach large numbers of people rapidly Can instantaneously update and disseminate information Can control information provided Can tailor information specifically for intended audiences Can be interactive Can provide health information in a graphically appealing way Can combine the audio/visual benefits of TV or radio with the self-paced benefits of print media Can use banner ads to direct intended audience to your programme's website	Can be expensive Many intended audiences do not have access to Internet Intended audience must be proactive – must search or sign up for information Newsgroups and chat rooms may require monitoring Can require maintenance over time

Source: National Cancer Institute (undated)

'drifted away', only a small amount actually hit the target and only a very small proportion 'penetrated'. Klapper (1960, cited in Wallack, 1980: 15) made a similar point in relation to its effect:

> Within a given audience exposed to particular communications, reinforcement, or at least constancy of opinion, is typically found to be the dominant effect, minor change as in intensity of opinion is found to be the next most common, and conversion is typically found to be the most rare.

Nonetheless, mass media can have dramatic repercussions, sometimes unintended! The global COVID-19 pandemic provided several good examples of this and has been called the 'first social media *infodemic*' (Ahmad and Murad, 2020). During the first stages of the pandemic huge amounts of (often contradictory) information were shared via various channels including mass media and social media, resulting in the spread of panic and fear among different populations. Evidence from different countries shows that this was not peculiar to specific contexts but was the case in many places including, for example Iraqi Kurdistan, where social media use and the spread of panic about coronavirus were significantly correlated (Ahmad and Murad, 2020). The lockdowns that took place in many countries contributed to the spread of (mis)information via different media. Another study in Egypt had similar findings, also concluding that social media played a significant role in the spread of panic and anxiety during the pandemic; although the authors acknowledge that this varied according to gender, level of education and occupation (Shehata and Abdeldaim, 2022). Without mass media and social media and these widespread means of communication, anxiety and fear would not have spread so quickly through different populations during the pandemic.

There is some evidence that mass communication can be effective in increasing awareness of health risk although it is acknowledged that mass media *alone* are not necessarily the most effective approach to health communication; rather, as Deane (2018) argues, it more is likely have impact when combined with other types of intervention. However, the WHO (2002a: 42) notes that:

> Although newspapers, magazines, radio and television are often criticized for inaccurate and biased reporting, in industrialized countries they remain the most influential sources for everyday information on risks to health. The rapid spread of these media in developing countries, together with improvements in literacy, mean that this is increasingly true in low and middle income countries.

Several systematic reviews have examined the effects of mass media campaigns on different health-risk issues such as driving under the influence of alcohol (Yadav and Kobayashi, 2015), reducing illicit drug use (Allara et al., 2015) and alcohol consumption and harm (Young et al., 2018). A considerable challenge is the heterogeneity of the studies that are examined and inconsistency of findings, which can lead to a lack of firm conclusions. In addition, people often remember details about mass media campaigns but there is little impact on how they behave as a result of them. Young et al.'s (2018: 302) systematic review on mass media and alcohol consumption concluded that 'mass media campaigns about alcohol are often recalled by individuals, have achieved changes in knowledge, attitudes and beliefs about alcohol but there [was] little evidence of reductions in alcohol consumption'. However, Wakefield et al. (2010: 1261) systematically examined the results of several mass media campaigns designed to address a range of health-risk behaviours and concluded that 'mass media can produce positive changes or prevent negative changes'. More recently, Stead et al. (2019) carried out a systematic review on the use of mass media across six health topic areas and concluded that there was mixed evidence of effectiveness – please see Abstract 8.1 for more details.

ABSTRACT 8.1

Mass media to communicate public health messages in six health topic areas: a systematic review and other reviews of the evidence. Stead, M., Angus, K., Langley, T., Katikireddi, S.V., Hinds, K., Hilton, S. et al. (2019)

Background: Mass media campaigns can be used to communicate public health messages at the population level. Although previous research has shown that they can influence health behaviours in some contexts, there have been few attempts to synthesize evidence across multiple health behaviours.

Objectives: To (1) review evidence on the effective use of mass media in six health topic areas (alcohol, diet, illicit drugs, physical activity, sexual and reproductive health and tobacco), (2) examine whether or not effectiveness varies with different target populations, (3) identify characteristic of mass media campaigns associated with effectiveness and (4) identify key research gaps.

Design: The study comprised (1) a systematic review of reviews, (2) a review of primary studies examining alcohol mass media campaigns, (3) a review of cost-effectiveness evidence and (4) a review of recent primary studies of mass media campaigns conducted in the UK. A logic model was developed to inform the reviews. Public engagement activities were conducted with policy, practitioner and academic stakeholders and with young people.

Results: The amount and strength of evidence varies across the six topics, and there was little evidence regarding diet campaigns. There was moderate evidence that mass media campaigns can reduce sedentary behaviour and influence sexual health-related behaviours and treatment-seeking behaviours (e.g. use of smoking quitlines and sexual health services). The impact on tobacco use and physical activity was mixed, there was limited evidence of impact on alcohol use and there was no impact on illicit drug behaviours. Mass media campaigns were found to increase knowledge and awareness across several topics, and to influence intentions regarding physical activity and smoking. Tobacco and illicit drug campaigns appeared to be more effective for young people and children but there was no or inconsistent evidence regarding effectiveness by sex, ethnicity or socioeconomic status. There was moderate evidence that tobacco mass media campaigns are cost-effective, but there was weak or limited evidence in other topic areas. Although there was limited evidence on characteristics associated with effectiveness, longer or greater intensity campaigns were found to be more effective, and messages were important, with positive and negative messages and social norms messages affecting smoking behaviour. The evidence suggested that targeting messages to target audiences can be effective. There was little evidence regarding the role that theory or media channels may play in campaign effectiveness, and also limited evidence on new media.

Conclusions: Overall, the evidence is mixed but suggests that (1) campaigns can reduce sedentary behaviour, improve sexual health and contribute to smoking cessation, (2) tobacco control campaigns can be cost-effective, (3) longer and more intensive campaigns are likely to be more effective and (4) message design and targeting campaigns to particular population groups can be effective.

Dale and Hanbury's (2010) work on using mass media health campaigns to promote healthy eating emphasizes the importance of role models and vicarious learning in promoting behaviour change, an approach that is supported by Bandura's social cognitive theory (Bandura, 1986). However, their intervention also used techniques such as goal setting. Notwithstanding the view that mass media are more effective when combined with other methods than when used alone as stated earlier, Wakefield et al. (2010: 1261) make the point that, although mass media are frequently used to expose populations to messages about health, this exposure is 'generally passive'. Yanovitzky and Stryker (2001) suggest that the direct model fails to account for alternative pathways of influence that might lead to behaviour change. They argue that paying ever more attention to improving the persuasive appeal of messages ignores the well-recognized knowledge–behaviour gap – that is to say the fact that knowledge alone is rarely sufficient to motivate behaviour change. Drawing on an analysis of media coverage of youth binge drinking, they propose two additional pathways of influence:

1. the influence of mass media on social norms and the acceptability (or otherwise) of behaviours mediated through social influence
2. the effect of policy changes in response to the issue.

Wellings and Macdowall (2000: 23) distinguish these approaches as the 'risk factor model', which is concerned with changing individual behaviour; and the 'social diffusion model', which sees mass media as activating the forces for social change.

Furthermore, Katz and Lazarsfeld (1955) described the influence of mass communications on the audience as a two-step process. Communications instigated by national leaders and transmitted via mass media (in those days, chiefly radio and the press) were 'intercepted' by opinion leaders (see the diffusion of innovations theory, Chapter 3). Opinion leaders were, almost by definition, more open to, and receptive of, mass media information. They also tended to be sought out for advice by what Katz and Lazarsfeld rather archaically called the 'rank and file'.

It is interesting to note that, nearly 60 years ago, Lazarsfeld and Merton (1955), in challenging simplistic views of mass communication effects, identified three conditions for mass media effectiveness:

1. **Monopolization** – the success of any given influence attempt was most likely where there was no opposition or counter-messages (and, arguably, where there was a limited overall volume of media activity).
2. **Canalization** – success was most likely to occur where persuasive messages were consistent with the audience's existing motivation and could be 'plugged in' to these existing prejudices, desires and wishes.
3. **Supplementation** – mass communication would be more likely to succeed when this supplemented, and was supported by, interpersonal influences.

The potential for health communication, as identified by the US National Cancer Institute, is shown in Box 8.1 and could equally apply to mass media communication.

BOX 8.1   THE ROLE OF HEALTH COMMUNICATION

Communication alone can:

- Increase the intended audience's knowledge and awareness of a health issue, problem, or solution
- Influence perceptions, beliefs and attitudes that may change social norms
- Prompt action
- Demonstrate or illustrate healthy skills
- Reinforce knowledge, attitudes or behaviour
- Show the benefit of behaviour change
- Advocate a position on a health issue or policy
- Increase demand or support for health services
- Refute myths and misconceptions
- Strengthen organizational relationships.

Source: National Cancer Institute (undated: 3)

The strengths of mass media lie in their ability to reach large audiences and groups who would be difficult to reach through more interpersonal methods. They have limited capacity to develop skills and achieve sustained attitude and behaviour change unless they form part of a more comprehensive programme. However, well-planned and executed mass media interventions of sufficient intensity can raise awareness of health issues and risks and lend credibility to local programmes. Furthermore, mass media can raise the profile of health issues on the public agenda and take on an advocacy function in relation to social and political change – as we discuss in more detail later in this chapter. Over and above more 'traditional' usage, mass media can, therefore, contribute to empowerment and social change and the model of critical health education set out in the previous chapter. Overall, the health promotion role of the media can be summarized as:

- general information dissemination
- specific focused campaigns, either through direct influence on individuals or indirectly through influencing social and cultural norms
- countering the advertising and marketing of 'unhealthy' products
- advocating for policy change.

The National Social Marketing Centre (2006: 99) identifies 10 situations when mass media use is most appropriate:

1. When wide exposure is desired.
2. When the time frame is urgent.

3. When public discussion is likely to facilitate the educational process.
4. When awareness is a main goal.
5. When media authorities are 'on-side'. Where journalists, editors and programmers are 'on-side' with a particular health issue, this often guarantees greater support in terms of space and editorial content.
6. When accompanying on-the-ground back-up can be provided.
7. When long-term follow-up is possible.
8. When a generous budget exists.
9. When the behavioural goal is simple.
10. When the agenda includes public relations.

Theoretical considerations

Murphy and Bennett (2004) noted that many mass media campaigns have been criticized for being atheoretical or relying on inappropriate theories and models. The Communication Evaluation Expert Panel (2007: 233) endorsed:

> the use of explicit program logic models that incorporate theoretical constructs into descriptions of the causal pathways through which program effects are expected to come about. They found that theory-based logic models help to keep message strategies linked to psychosocial predictors and performance measures on mark.

However, Stead et al.'s (2019) more recent systematic review (see Abstract 8.1) found little evidence of the role that theory plays in public health mass media campaigns. Klapper (1995) emphasizes that in order to understand and use media effectively, it is important to view mass communication in the context of broader theories of the individual and society. The problem, then, becomes, not a shortage of theory, but rather which theories to select from the plethora of theories available.

Clearly, no single model or theory will suffice. The design of mass media interventions should conform with the principles of health promotion planning and include:

- definition of goals and specific objectives for the mass media programme
- specification of the audience and identification of audience characteristics including any subgroups
- development of the message and pre-testing with the target group
- selection of channels that will maximize reach
- selection of a 'source' to maximize appeal and credibility with the target audience
- implementation
- evaluation – both formative and summative.

The development of mass media campaigns will also need to consider theory at a number of different levels. By way of example, these might include the following.

At the individual level:

- behavioural theories such as health action model, health belief model, theory of reasoned action, protection motivation theory
- communication theory
- theories concerning persuasion and attitude change (including the use of fear appeal)
- stage models of change.

At the interpersonal level:

- social cognitive theory.

At the organizational/community/societal level:

- organizational change theory
- diffusion of innovations theory.

These various theories have been discussed at some length earlier in this text and, notwithstanding their undoubted relevance to the development of mass media campaigns, we do not propose to reiterate them here. We will, however, consider at this point some additional theoretical insights.

Berger (1991) identifies four separate analyses that can be applied to mass communication:

- a Marxist analysis
- a semiological analysis
- psychoanalytic criticism
- sociological analysis.

A Marxist perspective

Marxist media theory demonstrates the ways in which capitalism exercises control over the proletariat by, among other means, the use of mass media. Many of the key concepts of Marxism can be applied to the analysis of mass media. McQuail (2010) highlights the following:

- Mass media are owned by a ruling class.
- Media are operated in the interest of a class.
- Media promote working-class false consciousness reproducing exploitation.
- Media access is denied to political opposition; media are unbalanced.

The notion of 'hegemony' is one of several key Marxist notions that Berger thought relevant to the role of mass media in society. This position is also adopted by critics such as Dutta (2020), who argues that hegemony is central to the control exercised by those in power. Berger (1991: 49) defines hegemony as:

a complicated intermeshing of forces of a political, social, and cultural nature [that] transcends but also includes two other concepts – culture, which is how we shape our lives, and ideology, which, from a Marxist perspective, expresses and is a projection of specific class interest … Ideology may be masked and camouflaged in films and television programmes and other works carried by mass media but the discerning Marxist can elicit these ideologies and point them out.

Unsurprisingly, mass media would provide an invaluable tool for creating false consciousness and reducing potential threats to the status quo. Similarly, and in relation to the key notion of alienation, Berger (1991: 43–4) argued that:

the media play a crucial role. They provide momentary gratifications for the alienated spirit, they distract the alienated individual from his or her misery (and from consciousness of the objective facts of his or her situation) and, with the institution of advertising, they stimulate desire, leading people to work harder and harder. (Advertising has replaced the Puritan ethic in America as the chief means of motivating people to work hard.)

And, in respect of the consumer society:

people must be driven to consume, must be made crazy to consume, for it is consumption that maintains the economic system. Thus the alienation generated by a capitalist system is functional, for the anxieties and miseries generated by this system tend to be assuaged by impulsive consumption … Advertising generates anxieties, creates dissatisfactions, and, in general, feeds on the alienation present in capitalist societies to maintain the consumer culture. There is nothing that advertising will not do, use, or co-opt in trying to achieve its goals, and if it has to debase sexuality, co-opt the women's rights movement, merchandise cancer (via cigarettes), seduce children, or terrorize the masses, all of these tactics and anything else will be attempted. One thing that advertising does is divert people's attention from social and political concerns into narcissistic and private concerns. Individual self-gratification becomes an obsession and, with this, alienation is strengthened and the sense of community weakened.

Bearing in mind our early comments on policy and the WHO's imperative to deal with inequity in particular and social issues in general, the implication of the above analysis for fostering healthy public policy needs no further comment!

Insights from semiology

'Semiology' is the science of signs (from the Greek *semeion*, which means 'sign') and derives originally from linguistics. Its founding father was de Saussure (1915). Semiology is used virtually interchangeably with 'semiotics' – a term devised by the American Charles Sanders Peirce (1839–1914). Although language was the original sign system subjected to semiotic scrutiny and 'discourse analysis', the methods of study were increasingly applied to signs of all kinds.

One especially relevant application of discourse analysis to mass media is embodied in the concept of 'myth'. Despite the sense in which it is used in everyday parlance, 'myth' does not necessarily mean false beliefs. Chapman and Egger (1983: 167) define it as:

any real or fictional story, recurring theme or character type that appeals to the consciousness of a group by embodying its cultural ideals or by giving expression to deep, commonly felt emotions.

They provide a revealing demonstration of the ways in which myth frequently figured in cigarette advertising in its embodiment of major interests and concerns in a given society. An example of an Australian advertisement for Winfield cigarettes is provided in Case study 8.1.

CASE STUDY 8.1 CREATING THE MYTH OF THE WINFIELD SMOKER

Some key features of the advertising campaign:

- It used Paul Hogan – a comedian who later enjoyed international fame for his movie portrayal of *Crocodile Dundee*. Hogan was originally a painter on the Sydney Harbour Bridge and was discovered in a talent show prior to becoming 'Winfield Man'. He personified the anti-hero 'rags-to-riches' myth of the working-class male who had made it to the top from humble beginnings without losing the common touch – and thus appealed to the market segment targeted by this particular brand of cigarettes.
- The word 'anyhow' was used in all Winfield advertising – 'Anyhow, Have a Winfield!' This word is allegedly associated in Australian minds with another expression, 'she'll be right', which connotes a fatalistic outlook on life (and death), but with a touch of optimism in the face of adversity. As Chapman and Egger indicate, 'the word "anyhow" is probably intended to act as a pat on the back to people on low incomes, with high mortgages, with bad marriages, with bleak prospects, etc. It is saying "yes, we know your life is dull/bleak/wearying/unrewarding, but … anyhow …"'

Source: Chapman and Egger (1983)

Mass media, in all their forms, may also perpetuate other types of myths and can (unwittingly perhaps) promote negative and damaging stereotypes even when used in the name of health promotion. For example, O'Hara et al. (2015) undertook a critical discourse analysis of multimedia used in the 'war on obesity' in Australia. They examined the content with respect to the ethics of health promotion and concluded that the methods and language used comprised labelling, coercive and paternalistic approaches to notions of choice, which were not aligned to the ethical values and principles of health promotion.

Sociological and psychoanalytic insights

We have already noted that social and cultural factors will influence the acceptability of messages, their wider dissemination through social channels and the extent to which they might ultimately influence behaviour.

At a practical level, it is possible to 'prescribe' key elements of effective, persuasive messages. Nicholson (2007) summarizes these as including grabbing attention, being easy to understand, personally relevant, provoking the audience to think about or discuss the message/campaign and ultimately motivating action. However, she goes on to raise the question of what actually contributes to the appeal of campaigns such as the highly successful 'truth' anti-smoking campaign. Notwithstanding criticism and legal action, the 'truth' campaign (see Case study 8.2) has produced a substantial decline in youth smoking (Farrelly et al., 2005). In contrast, exposure to the Philip Morris 'Think. Don't Smoke' campaign, aired around the same time, was not only ineffective in reducing youth smoking, but was associated with more positive beliefs and attitudes about the tobacco industry (Farrelly et al., 2008). She quotes Salovey's comments:

> If the principles of psychology were a series of main effects – meaning that x works better than y – rather than more qualified statements that reflect interactions between variables, then we wouldn't need a science of human behavior to deduce them. They'd be obvious.

She speculates that the unprecedented success of the 'truth' adverts was because they 'simply tapped into what motivates teenagers'. In particular, their 'anarchistic vibe', taking on big corporations and fast-paced 'gritty' style, was thought to appeal to free-spirited rebellious teens. In contrast, the Philip Morris advert spoke down to teenagers, telling them what to do. Over and above message factors, it should also be evident that there are differences in source factors, too. Notably, the 'truth' campaign capitalized on peer influence, homophily and source credibility:

> We're a dependable source of real facts and information. The minute we lose that quality and start bending and manipulating facts to our gain, then we're no better than the tobacco industry. (Truth, undated)

CASE STUDY 8.2 THE TRUTH CAMPAIGN

The truth campaign started in 2000 and was run by the American Legacy Foundation, funded under the terms of the 1998 Tobacco Master Settlement Agreement against the four largest US tobacco companies.

'Truth' is a hard-hitting media campaign that uses edgy television, radio and print ads featuring youth-led activism against tobacco companies and exposing the industry's deceptive marketing techniques. Some examples of the campaign's advertisements include a commercial that features 'a youth piling body bags outside a tobacco company's headquarters and another that exposes how the industry purposefully markets towards young people' (Krisberg, 2005).

The emphasis is NOT on telling young people what to do but on 'exposing how the tobacco industry has been manipulating our generation and others before it' (see www.thetruth.com/aboutUs.cfm).

The latest campaign, 'The Sunny Side of Truth', uses heavy irony to present positive messages about tobacco:

Sure, truth has been tough on Big Tobacco. And for good reason: they make a product that kills over 1200 people a day, so someone has to say something. But after all these years, we thought we'd give Big T a break and look at the sunnier side for once. Like if every 1 of every 3 youths who smoke will eventually die from it, that means 2 live! See how easy that is. (See www.thetruth.com)

The website also provides access to popular elements of contemporary youth culture – blogs, videos, games and free music remixes.

Uses and gratification theory

Uses and gratification theory provides some insight into the appeal of messages and also into the limitations of the 'hypodermic model' of media operation and the reason why so little of the contents of the 'aerosol' manage to penetrate. Rather than seeing the audience as homogeneous passive recipients, uses and gratification theory asserts that individuals interact selectively with messages according to different needs such as 'information, relaxation, companionship, diversion or escape' (McQuail, 2010: 423).

Those watching a television programme may or may not focus on the message. Even if they do concentrate, there is absolutely no guarantee that they will interpret the message in the ways intended by the programme's producers, indeed quite the opposite may occur in practice. Moreover, they will not only actively select what they watch, but they will also interpret it in accordance with the principles of wish fulfilment.

According to uses and gratification theory, people *use* the media to *gratify* their desires and satisfy their prejudices. Berger (1991) provides a comprehensive list of a wide range of typical gratifications offered by the media that clearly illustrates this particular theory of mass media use – see Box 8.2.

BOX 8.2 TYPICAL GRATIFICATIONS

- To be amused
- To see authority figures exalted or deflated
- To experience the beautiful
- To have shared experiences with others/sense of community
- To satisfy curiosity and be informed
- To identify with the deity and the divine plan
- To find distractions and diversion
- To experience empathy

(Continued)

- To experience, in a guilt-free and controlled situation, extreme emotions, such as love and hate, the horrible and the terrible, and similar phenomena
- To find models to imitate
- To gain an identity
- To gain information about the world
- To reinforce our belief in justice
- To believe in romantic love
- To believe in magic, the marvellous and the miraculous
- To see others make mistakes
- To see order imposed on the world
- To participate in history (vicariously)
- To be purged of unpleasant emotions
- To obtain outlets for our sexual drives in a guilt-free context
- To explore taboo subjects with impunity
- To experience the ugly
- To affirm moral, spiritual and cultural values
- To see villains in action.

Source: Berger (1991: 86–91)

More recently, there has been a burgeoning of research exploring uses and gratification theory as applied specifically to social media. For example, in exploring why adolescents use Facebook Tanta et al. (2014) found that they used it to socialize, to communicate with their friends, to make social arrangements and find out what was happening among their friends. The authors argued that Facebook 'primarily gratifie[d] adolescents' need for integration, social interaction, information and understanding of their social environment' (Tanta et al., 2014: 86). Similarly, in a Nigerian study exploring students' use of social media Musa et al. (2015) found that almost all the students in the study used social media for 'communication, collaboration, sharing news and research, expressing their opinions, maintaining contact with others, and making friends with people from other countries' (p. 83). The authors concluded that, whilst uses and gratification theory might seem like a rather dated concept, social media were breathing 'new life' into it.

Elaboration likelihood model

The elaboration likelihood model (Petty and Cacioppo, 1986) considers the extent to which a person is likely to think about (or 'elaborate' on) a message (McQuail, 2010). The model suggests that there are two routes through which messages might change attitudes – the central route and the peripheral route. The central route involves messages being subjected to considerable thought and scrutiny, that is to say high levels of elaboration. The peripheral route does not involve the same level of critical thinking and relies more on the general appeal of the message and the way in which it is conveyed, including the credibility and attractiveness of the source. A large proportion of the research that has been carried out using the ELM has been in advertising and consumer behaviour (Li, 2012). The way in which campaigns are branded would also exert an influence.

The route taken is influenced by both motivational and ability factors. The former include the relevance of the message and compatibility with previously held beliefs and attitudes. The latter include the ability to process information logically and having time to do so. While both routes can influence attitudes and, indeed, behaviour, the high elaboration central route is more likely to achieve enduring attitude change. There is some empirical support for the ELM with adult populations; however, research using the ELM to establish how messages are received by adolescents is less conclusive, particularly for those who are less academically able (Flynn et al., 2011). Notably, research carried out in Israel on young people aged 4–15 years concluded that young people do not use either route for changing attitudes (Te'eni-Harari et al., 2007). Given the changes that have taken place in communication since the ELM was first introduced, Kitchen et al. (2014) revisited the model and suggested that the validity and relevance of it should be reconsidered, particularly in the light of the increasing use of the online environment. They concluded that 'researchers should consider further elaboration of the ELM' (2014: 2045).

Prospect theory – framing the message

Prospect theory (Kahneman and Tversky, 1979) indicates that the choices that people make are influenced by whether messages are conveyed in terms of benefits (gain framed) or negative consequences (loss framed) and the level of uncertainty about each. People appear to be less likely to accept risks and uncertainty when choosing between options when they have something to gain and more likely when they have something to lose. Rothman and Salovey (1997) have applied this thinking to health education. They propose that preventive messages should be framed positively to focus on gains. In contrast, where there is a high level of uncertainty associated with going for a screening procedure, such as a mammogram, messages that focus on potential losses appear to be more effective (Toll et al., 2008). Despite some mixed findings in the literature, research on framing messages to promote physical activity appears to support these theoretical assumptions. In a study carried out in the USA by Latimer et al. (2008), gain-framed messages resulted in higher rates of participation in physical activity than loss-framed messages. Other factors in relation to the message may also be important. For example, further research by Chien (2011) on the willingness of young Taiwanese to be vaccinated against HNV1 found that, alongside the framing of the message, the colours used (background and text) were also significant. However, a systematic review carried out by Penţa and Băban (2018) on message framing and vaccine communication introduces a note of caution, concluding that 'it should not be assumed that a generic emphasis on gains or losses will, by itself, have a major impact on outcomes and will solve the challenge of vaccine communication' (p. 312).

Mass media and supportive environments for health

As we observed above, in addition to the specific use of mass media to influence individual attitudes and health behaviour, they can also have more general health-enhancing or damaging effects. The mass media, therefore, are part of the wider environmental influences on health. From a health promotion perspective, the action implication is to control and minimize harmful effects and to maximize any beneficial effects.

The general health-damaging consequences of mass media have been well documented and range from Putnam's view that they undermine 'social capital' (as noted above) to specific effects, such as glorifying the use of firearms. However, there is considerable debate about the alleged *direct* effects of, say, the portrayal of violence on film or television and, for example, copycat killings. Indeed, uses and gratification theory would suggest that negative inclinations are already present, that mass media events are merely used as an adjunct to trigger negative behaviour and perhaps shape the form it takes. Nonetheless, mass media clearly exert a 'normative effect', as we noted in Chapter 3. Even if they do not exactly exert pressure on individuals to adopt behaviour that they would not otherwise have adopted, they often signal that such behaviour is normal and acceptable. Before commenting further, it is important to note that at this point we are not discussing deliberate persuasive advertising. Rather, we are concerned here with 'incidental' effects exerted via a variety of media. For example, the portrayal of harmful health behaviours in movies such as smoking and drinking alcohol has been shown to have a negative effect on adolescent behaviour (Hanewinkel et al., 2012). Indeed, researchers and those working in health promotion and public health have typically recommended that television companies should adopt a healthier and more responsible approach to alcohol use, specifically, and health issues, more generally. Callister et al. (2012) argue a similar point with regard to the portrayal of sexual content in novels written for the adolescent market. While this is a relatively neglected area in the research on mass communication, the authors note that such content 'rarely dealt with issues of abstinence, safe sex practices, and the health risks associated with sex' (p. 477). Rannamets (2015: 127) notes that, in relation to dietary behaviour, unhealthy lifestyles are 'portrayed on screens through extensive consumption of food items especially high in sugars' and this influences people's behaviour; movies and television programmes typically have high incidences of branded unhealthy food product placements (driven by commercial interests) which, in turn, increases the likelihood that the people watching them will 'develop the same kind of view of the world that is depicted on the screens'.

As we have noted, over and above deliberate attempts to use the media to convey health messages or advertise products that can affect health, the media have more subtle effects. Not only do they exert an influence through the foreground narrative or theme, the background content is also important. Furthermore, in addition to such incidental coverage, some companies have deliberately attempted to exploit the potential of these background influences through product placement, as discussed by Rannamets (2015) in relation to the product placement of high sugar, high fat foods.

What can be done to minimize this negative influence? On the one hand, the capacity of the public to engage with the media more critically can be developed by improving *media literacy*. Media literacy includes the skills needed to deconstruct media messages and, where relevant, 'identify the sponsor's motives' (National Cancer Institute, undated: 248). Such awareness, it might be assumed, would offer some protection against clandestine attempts to persuade.

On the other hand, these media influences are pervasive and it would be unrealistic to expect people constantly to engage in critically appraising them – notwithstanding the peripheral effects that bypass critical scrutiny (see the elaboration likelihood model) and indirect effects through influences on social norms. In the interests of developing supportive environments for health, it is important that the media's potentially negative influence on health is recognized and steps taken to ameliorate it.

In an attempt to explore and conceptualize the ways in which Canadian (and other) adolescents interact and critically engage with health messages in different types of media, Wharf-Higgins and Begoray (2012) have arrived at the term 'critical media health literacy'. This, they argue, draws (although not exclusively) on understandings and definitions of other terms such as 'health literacy', 'critical health literacy', 'media literacy', 'critical media literacy', 'media activism' and 'critical viewing'. They provide the following working definition:

> Critical media health literacy is a right of citizenship and empowers individuals and groups, in a risky consumer society, to critically interpret and use media as a means to engage in decision-making processes and dialogues; exert control over their health and everyday events; and make healthy changes for themselves and their communities. (Wharf-Higgins and Begoray, 2012: 142)

The parallels with this and the WHO definition of health promotion (WHO, 1986) are, we trust, self-evident.

Despite the implied responsibility on the individual's behalf to be 'literate' rather than on the media to take ownership, there is some reluctance to take action to control the media – often linked to support for the freedom of the press. Defoe and Breed (1989) have argued for a compromise approach involving 'collaborative consultation', in which health promoters work with media and persuade them to adopt a responsible approach to their programming:

> [The] massive growth of health information on the Internet; the global nature of the Internet; the seismic shift taking place in the relationship of various actors in this arena, the absence of real protection from harm for citizens who use the Internet for health purposes are seen to be real problems. (Risk and Dzenowagis, 2001: e28)

In recognition of this, many organizations have established codes of conduct in an attempt to address the quality of health information. Such issues are important in light of increasing use of the Internet and other new media for promoting health (Atkinson et al., 2011).

A number of codes of practice have been developed, for example in relation to junk food and alcohol. However, they tend to focus on explicit advertising rather than on more incidental coverage. Nevertheless, the Television Advertising Standards Code, developed by the British Broadcast Committee of Advertising Practice (2011), specifically refers to food and soft drink advertising and children. The first requirement relates to diet and lifestyle with a single statement that: 'Advertisements must avoid anything likely to encourage poor nutritional habits of an unhealthy lifestyle in children.' Subsequent sections set out requirements in relation to 'pressure to purchase' and 'promotional offers'. There are also further requirements for specific advertisements about alcohol, especially in relation to limiting their appeal to young people. In relation to the promotion of soft drinks, the GULP campaign (Give Up Loving Pop) likens the tactics of energy drink companies to that of big tobacco (using celebrities to endorse products and creating addiction – to caffeine) (see www.giveuplovingpop.org.uk) and calls for tighter regulation and greater responsibility.

Soap operas and edutainment

There is considerable evidence for the impact of soap operas. They illustrate, par excellence, the uses and gratification theory in practice. Viewers identify with the characters, the characters reappear in other media, such as popular magazines, and so fiction and reality appear to blend seamlessly. Clearly, soap operas are not real – indeed, analysis demonstrates that they caricature reality (for example, in the amount of alcohol apparently consumed and the high incidence of unnatural deaths and criminality!). They do, however, mirror viewers' constructions of reality and focus on common concerns, interests and prejudices. The portrayal of alcohol and alcohol consumption by the media has been subjected to substantial research. For example, Barker et al. (2021: 595) analysed tobacco and alcohol content in UK soap operas and they found that 'whilst tobacco content was rare, alcohol content was common'. They point out that this is a potential driver of alcohol consumption in viewers, particularly among young people.

Soap operas can also be used more directly to convey health messages. The use of entertainment media for educational purposes has become referred to as 'edutainment' – defined in the *American Heritage Dictionary of the English Language* (2000) as 'The act of learning through a medium, particularly media-based, that both educates and entertains' (see also Zeedyk and Wallace, 2003).

An example of a highly successful edutainment initiative is provided by Soul City (Soul City Institute, 2008), which is a multimedia project in South Africa that tackles a range of health and development issues. Many other examples exist, such as East Los High – see Case study 8.3.

CASE STUDY 8.3   EAST LOS HIGH

East Los High is a culturally sensitive transmedia edutainment project aimed at Latina/o Americans in the United States at high risk for sexually transmitted infections.

It includes an online drama series and several narrative extensions (such as extended sequences, a website and vlogs) across multi-platforms targeted at young Latina/o Americans. It aims to tackle sexual and reproductive health issues such as sexually transmitted infection, pregnancy and rape through the narratives of a number of different Latina/o characters.

Since 2013 East Los High has been rated as a top show on Hulu attracting 1 million visitors per month to the Hulu Latino homepage.

East Los High has resulted from an extensive network of collaborative partnerships including media-based companies and non-governmental organizations. An evaluation of the first season of East Los High concluded that 'pioneering transmedia edutainment interventions such as East Los High are tremendously promising for health promoters and educators' (Wang and Singhal, 2016: 1009).

Advertising and counter-advertising

Freudenberg (2005) identifies advertising as one of the corporate behaviours that promote disease if the product is harmful in itself or can be used in ways that damage health. Advertising, therefore, makes up part of the wider environmental influences on health. Controls on advertising and voluntary agreements have been used to limit the effects – for example, banning tobacco advertising in many countries. However, there are concerns about the effectiveness of voluntary agreements (see, for example, Munro, 2006).

Efforts to counter the negative influence of advertising include using the media to deliver alternative messages. These frequently rely on humour to undermine the original message or the use of shock tactics to expose the reality of negative health consequences of products being marketed. They also adopt similar styles to the original advertisements – indeed, campaigns such as the BUGA UP campaign, which we will discuss in more detail later, use graffiti to modify billboard advertising and change tobacco marketing messages into anti-tobacco messages.

Warning labels on products have also been used. These have generally taken the form of written warnings about the health hazards associated with using the product. Canada was one of the first countries to introduce picture warnings. In the UK, from 1 August 2008, tobacco manufacturers were required to include picture warnings covering 40% of the back of packs of cigarettes or tobacco products as well as having an approved written warning on the front. These warnings are selected in rotation from a set of 14. A study by Hammond et al. (2007) found that the effectiveness of warnings on cigarette packs was influenced by the design and 'freshness' of the warning. Prominent warnings were more likely to be effective and this was further enhanced by the inclusion of pictorial images.

MASS MEDIA IN PRACTICE

The two case studies that follow illustrate how mass media campaigns have been used with some degree of success to influence attitudes and behaviour with regard to weight-loss lifestyle change and HIV/AIDS.

CASE STUDY 8.4   THE 'LIVELIGHTER' HEALTHY WEIGHT AND LIFESTYLE MEDIA CAMPAIGN

Location: Western Australia.

Target audience: Adults aged between 25 and 64 years.

Aim: To increase weight reduction in overweight adults through motivation to lifestyle change.

Campaign: The LiveLighter campaign is a mass media campaign that uses 'graphic anatomical images of visceral fat to illustrate negative health effects of overweight alongside recommending alternatives to obesogenic behaviours' (Morley et al., 2016: 121). The campaign had two 'waves' and used multiple methods including paid television advertising, a campaign website and paid cinema, radio, print media and online advertising. The advertising was part of a broader strategy

(Continued)

involving stakeholder engagement and media advocacy aimed to generate supportive policy and environmental changes through community, media and political support. The campaign had two key messages 1. Why change? – using images of visceral or 'toxic' fat around an overweight person's internal organs 2. How to change – showing how small changes in lifestyle, such as increasing activity levels and changing diet, can make a difference.

Effect: After the first wave of advertising, 54% of the population surveyed were aware of the LiveLighter campaign. Adults who were overweight were more likely to recall the campaign and perceive it as personally relevant. There were also some population-level improvements in proximal and intermediate markers of campaign impact such as change in attitude, increases in self-efficacy and reported changes in behavioural intentions.

Conclusions: The authors concluded that the LighterLife campaign achieved strong penetration and 'cut-through' amidst a substantial amount of mass media messages about obesity.

Source: See Morley et al. (2016)

CASE STUDY 8.5 MASS MEDIA COMMUNICATION AND HIV TESTING

Location: South Africa.

Target audience: Young people aged 16–24 years.

Aim: To increase uptake of HIV testing in young people.

Background: Young people are amongst the most vulnerable to HIV infection worldwide and less likely to be tested than adults. HIV infection continues to be a significant public health challenge in the South African context. In 2010 the South African government started a huge campaign aimed at reducing HIV infection which emphasized HIV testing.

Campaign: HIV-related mass media communication programmes on HIV testing, which included the use of different types of media such as the radio, magazines, newspapers, the Internet, and advertisements and television programmes aired on the three main South African television channels.

Effect: There was evidence of an indirect effect of exposure to HIV-related mass communication on being tested for HIV through its influence on encouraging young people to talk about HIV testing with their sexual partners and friends (Do et al., 2016). Being exposed to mass media communications increased the likelihood that a young person would engage in discussion about HIV testing which, in turn, increased the likelihood that they would be tested; however, there was no significant direct effect of mass media communication on HIV testing.

Conclusions: The authors concluded that the 'findings suggest that continued investment in communication programs [was] likely to have a long-term effect on positive structural factors that are conducive for behavior change' (p. 2042).

Source: Do et al. (2016)

The case studies in context

The two examples share common features, including having clear objectives, a straightforward aim, adaptation of the message to suit the audience and the intensity of the campaign involving several channels.

It is interesting to note commonalities with the principles set out by Aldoory and Bonzo (2005) for the development of injury prevention campaigns. These were identified following a review of the research literature and theoretical perspectives. In their view, campaigns should:

- be multi-component multichannel – incorporating interpersonal, mass media and printed sources
- use a mix of voices to spread campaign messages – both authority figures and peers
- focus on simple steps to injury prevention – i.e. on changes that are easy to make
- encourage the confidence to change
- emphasize benefits over risks
- address and reduce constraints/barriers to action – perceived and real
- work with opinion leaders
- consider mediating factors in message design such as age, sex, ethnicity, level of education.

In addition:

- the success of fear appeals depends on the amount of efficacy information.

Overall, it appears that what you get out depends on what you put in, in terms of planning, understanding the audience, involving the audience and having adequate resources to implement a campaign of sufficient intensity. Even so, the achievements are relatively modest. Probably the most systematic and comprehensive approach to achieving behaviour change has been provided by 'social marketing'.

Evaluation is discussed in greater depth in Chapter 11; however, it is worth noting that there are some key challenges associated with mass media approaches to promoting health. As Wakefield et al. (2010) point out, it is of course inherently difficult to isolate the direct effects of mass media interventions to promote health given that a plethora of other influential factors come into play. Wellings and Macdowall (2000) advocate for a systematic approach to evaluating mass media techniques, arguing that it is difficult to determine the cost-effectiveness of such approaches. They assert that formative, process and outcome evaluation is required as well as a combination of non-experimental and experimental approaches. Getachew-Smith et al. (2022) more recently emphasized the importance of process evaluation in health communication media campaigns as a result of their systematic review, concluding that 'process evaluation provides insights about mechanisms and intervening variables that could meaningfully impact interpretations of outcome evaluations' (p. 367). These various aspects of evaluation are explored in more detail in Chapter 11, as previously mentioned.

ABSTRACT 8.2

A social marketing perspective of young adults' concepts of eating for health: is it a question of morality? Brennan, L., Klassen, K., Weng, E., Chin, S., Molenaar, A., Reid, M., Truby, H. and McCaffrey, T.A. (2020)

Background: Poor dietary choices are a risk factor for non-communicable diseases. Young adults have low levels of engagement towards their health and may not see the importance in the adoption of healthy eating behaviours at this stage in their lives. In this study the authors utilize social marketing principles, digital ethnography and online conversations to gain insights into young adults' attitudes and sentiments towards healthy eating.

Methods: Young Australian adults who use social media at least twice a day were recruited by a commercial field house. Using a mixture of methods, combining online polls, forums and conversations, participants (*n* = 195, 18–24 years old) engaged in facilitated discussions over an extended four-week period about health and eating-related topics. Data were analysed using a thematic analysis constant comparison approach. A post-hoc conceptual framework related to religion was theorized and used as a metaphor to describe the results.

Results: Findings demonstrate that different segments of young adults with varying attitudes and interest towards healthy eating exist. The authors developed a conceptual framework based on consumer segmentation which adopted religious metaphors as a typology of 'consumers'. Some young adults practise and believe in the message of healthy eating (*saints*), whilst some oppose these messages and are not motivated to make and change (*sinners*), another segment are both aware of and interested in the issues but do not put healthy eating behaviour as a current priority (*person in the pew*).

Conclusions: Consumer segmentation and social marketing techniques assist health professionals to understand their target audience and tailor specific messages to different segments. The typology presented may be a useful tool for health professionals and social marketers to design strategies to engage young adults in healthy eating, particularly those *in the pew* who are contemplating a change but lacking the motivation. The utilization of marketing segmentation in health promotion has the potential to enhance health messaging by tailoring messages to specific segments based on their needs, beliefs and intentions and therefore drive the efficient use of resources towards those most likely to change.

SOCIAL MARKETING AND HEALTH PROMOTION

A cursory glance at the wider literature reveals an increasing use of social marketing to promote health. By way of some global examples social marketing has been used to address mental illness stigma in the USA and also in the UK (Collins et al., 2019; González-Sanguino et al., 2019); to promote smoking cessation in France (Djian et al., 2019); to address co-morbid physical and mental health in rural populations in Australia using digital and social media (Mehmet et al., 2020); to explore determinants of workplace health promotion in Iran (Kaveh et al., 2021); to promote family planning in Pakistan (Agha et al., 2019) and Nigeria (Liu et al., 2018); and for sanitation and hygiene in Malawi (Cole et al., 2015).

According to Solomon (1989), 'The field of social marketing was probably born in 1952, when Wiebe (1952) raised the question, "Why can't you sell brotherhood like you sell soap?"' He reviewed four examples of what would now be called health promotion campaigns and concluded that their effectiveness was proportional to the extent that they were similar to commercial product marketing. Kotler et al. (2002) identified further seminal events and landmarks in the rise of social marketing. These included an article by himself and Zaltman (1971) and the formation of the Social Marketing Institute in 1999.

Kotler et al. (2002: 19–20) define social marketing as follows:

> Social marketing is the use of marketing principles and techniques to influence a target audience to voluntarily accept, reject, modify, or abandon a behaviour for the benefit of individuals, groups, or society as a whole … [it] is largely a mix of economic, communication, and educational strategies … As a last resort, the social marketer may turn to the law or courts to require a certain behaviour.

Rather more succinctly, Brocklehurst et al. (2012: 81) state that social marketing:

> uses the principles of [commercial] marketing to understand health-related behaviour and tailor appropriate and effective interventions to population subgroups … [relying] on stimulating behavioural change for future health gain.

While it would be generally accepted that mass media campaigns utilize communication and educational strategies, reference to economics and legal measures moves beyond the preserve of traditional mass communications. Social marketing, therefore, is more than mass communication and can also involve interpersonal and policy development. Katz and Lazarsfeld's principle of 'supplementation' mentioned earlier is relevant here. Mass media are more effective when supplemented by additional interpersonal strategies.

Much of the early development of social marketing was in the USA. In England, social marketing began to receive more attention following the publication of the *Choosing Health* White Paper (Department of Health, 2004) and is now a key part of UK government strategy aimed at improving health and tacking inequalities (Crawshaw and Newlove, 2011).

Kotler et al. (2002: 20) identify several differences between commercial and social marketing:

> Social marketers focus on selling behaviours, whereas commercial marketers position their products against those of other companies, the social marketer competes with the audience's current behaviour and associated benefits. The primary benefit of a 'sale' in social marketing is the welfare of an individual, a group, or society, whereas in commercial marketing the primary benefit is shareholder wealth.

Drawing on work by Solomon (1989) and Webster (1975), Windahl et al. (2009: 123–4) also highlight a number of differences, as follows:

- there is less competition
- clients do not always have to pay in money for products and services
- powerful interest groups are often challenged
- the product or behaviour being advanced is often not desired by the receiver (e.g. adhering to a low-fat diet)
- increased demand may be dysfunctional due to a lack of resources.

Kotler et al. (2002: 21–2) also:

> resent the notion that social marketing has the same motivations and therefore the same processes as those found in organizations for profit. Commercial ventures are 'in it' for the shareholders. We're in it for the public good. We don't like the association.

The National Social Marketing Centre (2005) makes the point that social marketing does not merely 'import' commercial marketing techniques, but also draws on non-governmental and community sector expertise. In its broadest sense social marketing for health is about applying the principles of marketing to health using techniques proven to promote commercial products (Evans and McCormack, 2008), such that a healthy lifestyle has now become a 'desirable and marketable commodity' (Scally, 2017: 285).

Key features of social marketing

Lefebvre and Flora (1988: 301) identify eight essential characteristics of social marketing:

1. A consumer orientation
2. An emphasis on voluntary exchanges of goods and services between providers and consumers
3. Research in audience analysis and segmentation strategies
4. The use of formative research in product or message design and the pre-testing of these materials
5. An analysis of distribution (or communication) channels
6. Use of the marketing mix
7. A process tracking system with both integrative and control functions
8. A management process that involves problem analysis, planning, implementation and feedback functions.

There are clearly commonalities with Solomon's 10 key concepts (see Box 8.3) and the model developed by the National Social Marketing Centre (see Figure 8.1, which shows the element of social marketing clearly placing the consumer at the middle of the triangle and indicating the relationship between 'behaviour and behavioural goals', 'audience segmentation' and 'intervention and marketing mix'). We will briefly consider the most significant elements.

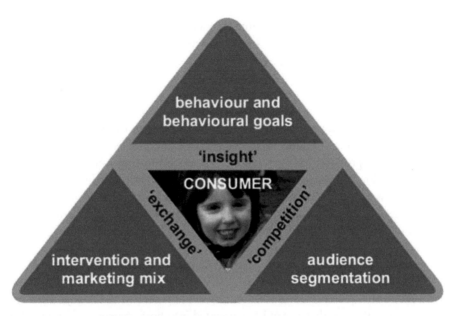

Figure 8.1 Elements of social marketing (French and Blair-Stevens, 2007: 35)

'Customer triangle' adapted from the National Consumer Council © 2006

BOX 8.3   TEN KEY CONCEPTS OF SOCIAL MARKETING

- Marketing philosophy
- The marketing mix
- A hierarchy of communication effects
- Audience segmentation
- Understanding relevant markets
- Information and rapid feedback systems
- Interpersonal and mass media interactions
- Utilization of commercial resources
- Understanding the competition
- Expectations of success.

Source: Solomon (1989)

Consumer orientation

The core feature and underlying philosophy of social marketing is its consumer or customer orientation. Figure 8.1 graphically places the consumer at the heart of the enterprise. The consumer can be the public, professionals or policy-makers. The key issue is understanding them within their social context – what is important to them, what motivates them and what factors influence their behaviour (National Social Marketing Centre, 2007). Grier and Bryant (2005) emphasize that social marketing should identify and address clients' needs and interests.

Exchange

The 'primary operational mechanism is based on exchange theory' (Lefebvre and Flora, 1988: 302). This involves an exchange of something valued by two or more parties. In commercial marketing, it is typically a consumable product that is exchanged for money. In social marketing, it more typically involves ideas or behaviour. Similarly, costs can include time and effort rather than money. Lefebvre and Flora (1988) stress that the approach should encourage voluntary exchange and reject the use of high-pressure persuasion. While the notion of profit tends to be alien to social programmes, the concept can equally embrace social benefits such as health and well-being.

Audience segmentation

Meeting the needs of the 'audience' in relation to the development of either a product or a message will clearly be enhanced if the audience can be segmented into homogeneous subgroups that share key characteristics. Segmentation can be based on a range of variables, including traditional geographical and demographic factors. However, greater precision can be introduced by considering so-called psychographic factors such as lifestyle, personality, stage of readiness for change, and perceptions of costs and benefits. Although not strictly the intended audience, the views of any gatekeepers may also be important.

Channel analysis

This involves identifying which channels or combination of channels will be most effective in conveying the message to the target audience. Consideration will need to be given to the reach and credibility or persuasive appeal of different channels. These would include opinion leaders as well as mass media and the identification of what Lefebvre and Flora (1988) refer to as 'life path points' such as grocers, restaurants, bus stops, hairdressers. Maximizing interaction between media and interpersonal interventions is likely to increase effectiveness in line with Lazarsfeld and Merton's key principle of 'supplementation' (Lazarsfeld and Merton, 1955).

Financial constraints may encourage social marketers to use commercial resources by working with commercial agencies. For instance, Solomon (1989) suggests that advertising agents might be persuaded to lend their support to enhance their own agency's brand image of social responsibility. Such tactics should be approached with caution as association with certain commercial ventures might well undermine the integrity and credibility of health promotion. For instance, to accept support from manufacturers of powdered baby milk for antenatal education would be unwise.

The marketing mix

The so-called 'marketing mix' refers to the classic four 'Ps' – Product, Price, Place, Promotion – that have obvious roots in commercial marketing (Upton and Thirlaway, 2014).

The main principle for marketing health is that health *products* should be tangible, attractive and accessible. Certainly, a major problem with many health promotion 'products' is that they can be intangible and their accessibility is limited – for instance, a lack of exercise facilities or, more importantly, access to a decent job, money and respect. As for attractiveness, several traditional health promotion goals may look distinctly unappealing to the potential customer! As Windahl et al. (2009: 124) point out, 'a product may be a thing, an idea, a practice, or a service'. Kotler et al. (2002) describe three levels of product. These are core products (benefits), actual products (behaviour) and augmented products (tangible objects or services).

Price is clearly important for all marketing. This may involve actual financial expense but, typically, includes social, psychological and environmental 'costs'. Reference to the health belief model indicates that preventive behaviour will only occur if the perceived benefits outweigh the costs. The implication for social marketing is, in Kotler et al.'s words, 'managing the costs of behaviour change'. Kotler et al. provide examples of the costs of tangible objects (bike helmets, condoms, sunscreen, earthquake preparedness kits) and services (swimming classes and family planning services). Non-monetary costs include time, effort and energy – for instance, parking one's car before using a mobile phone or using public transport. A third category of non-monetary cost is labelled 'psychological risks and losses', such as embarrassment or fear of rejection. Kotler et al. specifically refer to:

- finding out whether or not a lump is cancerous
- saying 'no' to a second glass of wine
- having a cup of morning tea without a cigarette
- using sunscreen and returning from Hawaii looking pale.

The cost associated with physical discomfort includes activities such as having a mammogram, suffering nicotine withdrawal or taking exercise. Windahl et al. (2009) also refer to what might be referred to as 'social' cost – such as that which might be attached to attending sexual health screening in a small community.

Hastings (2007) draws on Rangun et al. (1996) to propose systematically assessing the level of cost in relation to the production of tangible or intangible benefits (see Table 8.2). He suggests that change is relatively easy for low cost/tangible benefits and communication would be the key element of a social marketing strategy. In contrast, the high cost/intangible benefits quadrant is the most difficult and may need to rely on moral persuasion and social influence rather than marketing. When both

Table 8.2 Cost-benefit assessment

	Tangible personal benefits	Intangible societal benefits
Low cost	Using the stairs rather than lifts to increase personal fitness	Separating household rubbish for separate collection and recycling
High cost	Giving up smoking	Stopping taking holidays which involve air flights to reduce carbon emissions

the cost is high and benefits are tangible and personal, 'push marketing' approaches may be needed providing support and augmented products to reduce the cost to the individual. For the remaining quadrant, low cost/intangible benefits, convenience should be emphasized along with the benefits to the individual and society.

Place in commercial marketing would generally refer to distribution channels for goods: for example, retail outlets. In social marketing, place refers to where tangible products or services are provided or where the behaviour occurs. However, it also includes where people might receive information.

Promotion is rather wide-ranging. It includes campaign publicity and, more importantly, the complexities of message design and dissemination, together with monitoring and modification. It also refers to the methods or activities that might be used to create awareness of a particular 'product' (Windahl et al., 2009: 243). As Solomon (1989: 94) notes:

> Promotion is far more than simply and superficially placing advertisements. It is actively reaching out to the right people with the right message at the right time in order to obtain the right effects. And this is not easy to achieve, especially with the large number of competing messages and media.

Clearly, it depends on detailed understanding of other elements of the marketing mix, the audience and communication channels.

Positioning is sometimes added as a fifth 'P'. It is substantially concerned with the psychological location of products or 'how a receiver perceives a product relative to other products' (Windahl et al., 2009: 256). It involves framing products or social issues so that target groups will perceive certain characteristics, and believe and remember them rather than alternative, less desirable frames.

While the marketing mix provides a useful starting point, the National Social Marketing Centre (2007) contends that it may not be sufficient to fully address complex behaviours.

Understanding the competition

Anti-health competition is not difficult to find – as the running battle between public health and the tobacco industry over many years has demonstrated. As well as direct anti-health messages, there may be other 'competing offers' – either external such as competition for time and attention, or internal such as addiction, habit or pleasure (National Social Marketing Centre, 2007: 36).

Planning and implementation

One of the undoubted strengths of marketing in general and social marketing in particular is its commitment to systematic planning. There is no fundamental difference between the approach to health promotion planning set out in this book and the various planning strategies that appear in social marketing practice – see, for instance, the Montana Model of Systematic Coordination (Linkenbach and D'Atri, 1998) or the Total Process Planning Model (National Social Marketing Centre, 2006).

The initial stage involves a thorough assessment of needs. The National Social Marketing Centre (2007) refers to this as scoping. It involves behavioural analysis, developing insight into the customer's perspective and audience segmentation as well as bringing together stakeholders and developing partnerships. It culminates in agreeing which ideas to take forward for further development. Although scoping is critical to success, the National Social Marketing Centre notes that in practice there has been a tendency to sidestep efforts to fully understand what would 'move and motivate' the audience (2007: 129).

Programme development should be based on *formative research* that involves the 'consumer'. Formative research allows ideas to be pre-tested prior to implementation and enables consumers' views to be incorporated into the development of products and services and the design of messages.

Grier and Bryant (2005) argue that continuous monitoring and revision is paramount and should begin at the start of the planning process. Such monitoring systems allow checks to be made on programme delivery and the progress of campaigns. They provide important evaluation data and also the opportunity to adjust the programme. In our later discussions of evaluation (see Chapter 11), we use the more conventional terms of 'process' and 'formative evaluation'.

Clearly, evaluation is an integral part of the planning process – including summative as well as formative and process elements. The key question is: what level of success can be expected? The emphasis in social marketing is on achieving behavioural goals including preventing the emergence of problem behaviours, sustaining existing desired behaviours, and changing existing problem behaviours (National Social Marketing Centre, 2005). However, the hierarchy of communication effects would indicate several intermediate outcomes beginning with awareness of the programme through to the final stage of the hierarchy, which would be adoption of the behaviour. Perhaps one of the most useful lessons to be learned from commercial marketing is its recognition that behavioural goals are difficult to achieve, even with the expenditure of large sums of money. Expectations must be realistic if they are to be achievable. Realistic expectations derive from research, previous experience and a sound theoretical understanding of what is involved in achieving results of a particular kind with the specified target group.

The relationship between health promotion and social marketing

Notwithstanding their separate origins, there are clear commonalities between social marketing and health promotion. Nonetheless, there are technical lessons to be learned from social marketing's close adherence to systematic planning, especially detailed analysis of the determinants of the behaviour in question, understanding the audience and its motivations, developing messages that tap into these motivations and pre-testing all materials.

The early development of social marketing for health focused on achieving specific behavioural goals. The emphasis on individual behaviour made it vulnerable to criticisms of victim-blaming in the same way as the preventive model of health promotion. Social marketing has responded by acknowledging the importance of considering and addressing the social determinants of health behaviour. It attempts to understand individuals within their wider social context and gain insight into the reality of people's lives (see National Social Marketing Centre, 2007). This strand has become more evident as social marketing has developed over time, along with its contribution to tackling inequality. Further, its role in policy development has been recognized. For example, the National Social Marketing Centre distinguishes between *operational social marketing* that 'is applied as a process and worked through systematically to achieve specific behavioural goals' and *strategic social marketing*, where the approach is used 'to inform and enhance strategic discussions, and guide policy development and intervention option identification' (2006: 24).

This clearly echoes health promotion's concern to address the wider determinants of health. The territory of social marketing appears to be expanding and becoming remarkably similar to health promotion itself. Moreover, the promise that it offers for achieving designated behavioural outcomes is attractive to public health managers and those responsible for achieving defined health targets (see, for example, Department of Health, 2008). This raises several key questions. Is social marketing an alternative to health promotion? What, if any, are the differences?

While there are undoubted similarities, there are also distinct differences in emphases and values. The primary focus for social marketing is on achieving behavioural goals, whereas for health promotion – and certainly the model espoused by this book – it is on empowering individuals and communities to achieve control over their health. Health promotion would, therefore, have a wider remit in working towards individual and community empowerment, in seeking to create supportive environments for health and tackling power imbalances. For some critics, this has been at the expense of supporting individual behaviour change. However, comprehensive health promotion should include enabling individual behaviour change – not as an end in itself, but as instrumental to achieving the wider goal of empowerment.

Notwithstanding social marketing's claims to be consumer-led, there appears to be an element of top-down paternalism both in defining the agenda and in addressing all the requisite variables to achieve desired behavioural outcomes. Health promotion, in contrast, is more concerned with facilitating choice rather than securing adherence to prescribed behaviours. This is reflected in ways of working that include engaging individuals and communities, participation, building individual and community capacity and addressing the structural determinants of health and health-related behaviour.

Social marketing recognizes the importance of tackling structural factors and advocacy is included within its repertoire of activity. However, advocacy in this context tends to be undertaken on behalf of client groups rather than involving individuals and communities and enabling them to take action, which would be more typical of an empowerment approach.

The development of social marketing has confounded early concerns that marketing approaches are inappropriate for health and inconsistent with health promotion. Social marketing methods can clearly be successful in achieving designated behavioural outcomes. The wisdom of extending its remit beyond this is debatable. We contend that it is not an alternative to health promotion. However, to see health promotion and social marketing as competitors is unhelpful. Social marketing methods can have an important place within health promotion, provided, of course, that they facilitate voluntary adoption of behaviours. Equally, locating social marketing within health promotion capitalizes on the synergy between the two, enhancing the capacity to achieve both behavioural and empowerment goals. In an analysis of the relationship between health promotion and social marketing, Griffiths et al. (2008: 3) concluded that:

> By coming together, specialised health promotion and social marketing for health can ensure that health improvement strategies and practice are as effective as they possibly can be.

Social marketing is used a lot to promote health, as a cursory glance at the wider literature shows. The approach has been used to address many types of public health issues such as, for example, alcohol use and smoking; however, there is a notable 'western' bias within the so-called American-centric nature of social marketing that is reflected in the research and literature (Lindridge et al., 2013). Despite this social marketing is also used in low- and middle-income countries (LMIC). For example, Varquez and Pastrana (2022) point out how social marketing has been used for the past four decades in Latin America and argue that it still has huge potential as an approach to social and behaviour change. A review of social marketing interventions in LMIC found that they are effective in addressing many issues related to the Sustainable Development Goals, all of which link back to health in some way (Schmidtke et al., 2021).

The importance of 'upstream' social marketing has been emphasized, distinguished as follows by Gordon (2013: 1525) – 'downstream social marketing focuses on behavior change at the individual level while upstream social marketing focuses on behavior change at policy-maker level'. That is, upstream social marketing focuses on influencing structural and environmental factors that shape the way that an individual behaves (Cross et al., 2017b). Clearly the more upstream efforts are, the more closely they will be aligned with the intentions of health promotion which seeks to move attention from the individual level to the wider determinants of health.

ADVOCACY FOR HEALTHY PUBLIC POLICY – THE ROLE OF MASS MEDIA

Traditionally, mass media have been associated with attempts to inform, influence and persuade. One of the more vitriolic condemnations of the persuasive use of mass communication has been provided by Rakow (1989: 169–70) in her discussion of critical theory and information campaigns. She reiterates a point that we made earlier in our discussions of ideology when she comments that:

> Bureaucratic organizations are … selective about the information they provide, which exposes the myth that simply providing information is a commendable activity. Organizations control which information will be made available to whom because their goal is not really to inform but rather to control … That one can presume to have even the *right* to persuade someone else, let alone the *responsibility* to do so is never questioned … [this] cultural preoccupation with persuasion reflects a conquest mentality that justifies the 'violence' [invasiveness] of strategies to change others, reflecting a larger cultural – masculine – propensity to dominate and conquer.

Rakow (1989: 169–70) also forcefully challenges the downstream tendency to utilize media in the service of individual behaviour change, rather than addressing the root causes and determinants of unhealthy outcomes:

> What information is a potential client of a social service agency going to be given? How to beat the system that put her in the situation in the first place? Why are behaviours such as drug use or teenage pregnancy portrayed as the country's most important problems and not militarism, violence against women, or homelessness? Why is the medical profession targeting individuals with health messages such as restriction of cholesterol intake rather than targeting government and industry who are responsible for the actions and policies that put carcinogens in our food, pollute our planet, determine whose health problems get research attention, and the like?

The alternative strategies advocated by Rakow involve community development and participation. Wallack et al. (1993) concur but also consider that mass media may make a substantial contribution, in tandem with community work, in advocating for healthy public policy. However, before examining this role more closely, we will consider how mass media might address the fundamental health issue of inequalities.

The health divide – contributions of mass media

In 1997, a working group was established by the English Health Education Authority to consider the most efficient use of mass media for tackling inequality in health (Hastings et al., 1998). Two conflicting approaches to addressing this fundamental issue for health promotion were identified.

The first of these centres on the use of audience segmentation and careful targeting of health messages to reach disadvantaged groups. The techniques involved are exemplified by the tobacco industry's practice of directly marketing brands to specific target groups on the basis of characteristics such as their socioeconomic status and personal traits, particularly by direct mail. Strategies used include 'relationship marketing' – that is, the attempt to build a relationship with customers. As Hastings et al. (1998: 49) explain:

> Loyal customers … buy more … products, are easier to satisfy, are less price-sensitive and make positive recommendations to their friends and family … acquiring new customers through research, promotion and other marketing is up to five or six times more expensive than retaining existing ones. Similarly, research indicates that the average company loses 10 per cent of its customers each year … by contrast unhappy customers are a considerable liability – they stop buying the company's products – usually without warning – often support the competition and complain to their friends and family.

'Emotional branding' is also considered to play a major part in selling commercial or social products. As Hastings et al. (1998) note, 'customers buy products to satisfy not only objective, functional needs, but also symbolic needs'.

Social marketers should, therefore, ensure that product 'tonality' matches the needs of their target audience and particularly lower socioeconomic status and disadvantaged groups (Hastings et al., 1998: 52):

> There is also evidence that branding may be a particularly effective way to reach people in deprived communities. Research into how working-class populations use cultural symbols in advertising found that these groups are often poorly informed about the objective merits of different products and therefore tend to rely more heavily than other groups on 'implicit meanings' – context, price, image – to judge products (Durgee, 1986) … de Chernatony (1993) and Cacioppo and Petty (1989) found that people in deprived communities are less likely to evaluate products on a rational objective basis, but look for clues as to the product's value in terms of its price or its image. They argued that the symbolic appeal of brands is particularly effective in targeting those individuals who do not have the time, skills or motivation to evaluate the objective attributes and benefits of a particular campaign.

The alternative strategy to address the 'health divide' is to use media advocacy to challenge the social and political system that results in the disadvantage in the first place!

Defining media advocacy – social justice and market justice

The Health Communication Unit (2000: 1) defines media advocacy as:

> the strategic use of media (usually the news media) to shape public opinion, mobilize community activists, and influence decision makers to create a change in policy.

Freudenberg (2005) also refers to its role in changing corporate practices that impact negatively on health.

Wallack et al. (1993), in their classic text, challenge individualistic, victim-blaming approaches and assert that advocacy:

> is necessary to steer public attention away from disease as a personal problem to health as a social issue … [It] is a strategy for blending science and politics with a social justice value orientation to make the system work better, particularly for those with the least resources.

Wallack et al. (1993: 7) make a succinct and coherent distinction between market justice and social justice in a number of observations that chime with our discussion of voluntarism in Chapter 1:

> Market justice suggests that benefits such as healthcare, adequate housing, nutrition, and sustainable employment are rewards for individual effort (on a level playing field), rather than goods and services that society has an obligation to provide. Market justice depends on enlightened self-interest as a guarantor of the distribution of necessary goods and services to those in need.

Wallack illustrates this philosophy, which is so deeply embedded in the USA (and, indeed, many European societies), by citing Galbraith's (1973: 5–6) classic and maverick approach to economics and his critique of large American corporations:

> The corporate economic is not responsible – or is only minimally responsible – for what it does … If the goods that it produces or the services it renders are frivolous or lethal or do damage to air, water, landscape or the tranquility of life, the firm is not to blame. This reflects public choice. If people are abused, it is because they choose self-abuse.

Social justice, on the other hand, 'is concerned with whether conditions in society are fair and whether resources are distributed equitably. Too often they are not' (Galbraith, 1973).

A healthy society is a democratic society founded on social justice (Krieger, 1990: 414, cited in Wallack et al., 1993: 15):

> Democracy is about having a stake because you are a real participant. It is about knowing whom to hold accountable, and it is about having the power to hold them accountable. Democracy is not

about letting priorities be set by a bureaucratic or technocratic élite, or by the 'blind forces' of the market (which always turn a blind eye toward human suffering); it is about constructing a social agenda, based on human need, through informed and active popular participation at every level.

Subscribing to the 'religious mystique' of individualism and market forces is uncontroversial, so social marketing is entirely acceptable within the dominant ideology. The use of media advocacy is not!

BOX 8.4 ADVOCACY - THE STRUGGLE

If there is no struggle, there is no progress. Those who profess to favour freedom, and yet deprecate agitation, are men who want crops without ploughing up the ground. They want rain without thunder and lightning. They want the ocean without the awful roar of its many waters. This struggle may be a moral one; or it may be a physical one; or it may be both moral and physical; but it must be a struggle. Power concedes nothing without a demand.

Source: Frederick Douglass (1857), cited in Wallack et al. (1993: 39)

DISTINCTIONS BETWEEN TRADITIONAL MEDIA USE AND MEDIA FOR ADVOCACY

Media advocacy shifts the focus from individual responsibility to social responsibility and the goal away from individual behaviour to social and environmental change (Health Communication Unit, 2000). The main differences between traditional media practices in health promotion and the practice of media advocacy are summarized as follows (which draws on Wallack et al., 1993: 60–75).

Traditional mass media direct messages from a central source to a mass audience. They involve one-way communication and, typically, limit audience involvement to pre-testing and segmentation. Media advocacy, on the other hand, has close links with communities and 'seeks to provide community groups with skills to communicate their own story in their own words'. Accordingly, media advocacy has been considered to involve 'narrow-casting' rather than broadcasting and is targeted at relatively small audiences and individual decision-makers. Community members are viewed as potential advocates and change agents. The focus of traditional mass communication is on *individual* attitude and behaviour change, whereas media advocacy seeks to develop 'healthy public policy'. Its role can therefore include, in ascending order of radicalism:

- gaining unpaid advertising by providing newsworthy information
- agenda setting about health issues as a precursor to later action
- consciousness-raising to stimulate actions having a focus on disease and inequalities in health
- critical consciousness-raising about social, economic and environmental issues which influence health and equity.

Although advocacy addresses short-term, pressing issues, the goal is to set this within the broader context of general policy change designed to address social and environmental determinants of health. A particular feature of media advocacy is its concern with agenda setting and critical consciousness-raising. Media advocates are health activists who confront social rather than individual 'pathogens'. They, therefore, seek to make full use of news channels by reacting to news and creating it. They present themselves as 'partners in the news-making and gathering processes'. The use of news may be supplemented by appropriate use of paid media placements. However, public service announcements (PSAs) are viewed with suspicion as they rarely have access to prime-time programming and controversial issues are likely to be censored. In short, media advocacy aims to fill the 'power gap' rather than the 'information gap'.

Agenda setting

Our earlier comments about the 'aerosol model' and mass media strengths and limitations have received support over the years from many distinguished theoreticians and practitioners. Cohen (1963: 13), for example, commented on the power of the press as follows:

> [the press] may not be successful much of the time in telling people what to think, but it is stunningly successful much of the time in telling people what to think *about*. [An observation also attributed to Ed Murrow, the distinguished American journalist and radio reporter.]

Cohen continues with an apt observation that both supports the uses and gratification theory and indicates the role of media producers in shaping opinion:

> the world looks different to different people, depending not only on their personal interests but also on the map that is drawn for them by the writers, editors, and publishers of the papers they read.

A major function of media advocates is thus to 'draw particular maps' that highlight key social issues following the now well-recognized strategy of 'agenda setting'. In this sense, media advocacy may be also be concerned with seeking policy solutions to tackle specific health issues (Dorfman and Krasnow, 2014) and is about promoting system change (Cross et al., 2017a). Wallack et al. (1993: 61) offer a nice image (from Lippmann, 1965) of the process of agenda setting as 'directing the searchlight':

> Mass media are like the beam of a searchlight that moves restlessly about, bringing one episode and then another out of darkness into vision.

The short-term goals are, therefore, to generate increased media coverage of the issues and to 'frame the coverage in ways that support policy solutions' (Niederdeppe et al., 2007: 47).

The empowerment model of health promotion, discussed in Chapter 1, emphasized the importance of agenda setting. It placed particular emphasis on the process of 'critical consciousness-raising' (CCR) as a more potent device than simple agenda setting – one that often seeks to bring about quite radical political change. CCR will be revisited in our discussion of community development in Chapter 9. As Cross et al. (2017a) argue, mass media can promote the development of healthy public policy through public debate.

Narrow-casting

Reference was made above to media advocacy's 'narrow-casting' approach (providing specific messages for specific target audiences; see Atkin and Rice, 2013). This is an important characteristic of advocacy's employment of media. It asserts that, although the general population is the ultimate beneficiary, the primary goal will typically be decision-makers, legislators, community leaders and community groups. As Wallack et al. (1993: 78) observe:

> Media advocacy isn't about a mass audience. It's not about reaching everybody. It's about targeting the two or three per hundred who'll get involved and make a difference. It's about starting a chain reaction.

They also illustrate the narrow-casting function of media advocacy in relation to attempts to challenge the impact of the giant McDonald's chain on the nation's diet. They describe a radio spot produced by Schwartz that:

> addressed the CEO of McDonald's by name and told him he could be a hero to children all over the world if he just changed the way his company fried its food … when people hear their names or the names of their organizations mentioned in a spot, they not only pay attention but imagine everyone else hearing the spot is paying attention as well. Schwartz wanted to change the behaviour of only one man; his radio message had an intended audience of one. (Wallack et al., 1993: 118–19)

Media advocacy and civil disobedience – the case of BUGA UP

BUGA UP was an Australian movement that followed a particularly vigorous and radical pathway, adopting tactics that were, on occasions, of dubious legality and included civil disobedience.

The acronym stands for Billboard Utilizing Graffitists Against Unhealthy Promotions and activists set out to alter advertising messages on billboards and other displays with spray cans to replace them with more appropriate healthy messages. Examples of the finished products included changing the messages on a very large billboard located on top of a building at one of Sydney's crossroads. The original was an advertisement for Marlborough cigarettes. After the 'spray can surgery', it read 'It's a Bore'. A rather more risqué facelift was given to a poster advertising Winfield cigarettes, which incorporated the emblematic term 'Anyhow' (see Case study 8.1). After the improvements, it read, 'anyhow … have a Wank IT'S HEALTHIER'.

The activists were accused of defacing private property. They claimed that they were 're-facing' it. Chesterfield-Evans and O'Connor (1986: 241) indicate the effects of this 'civil disobedience':

> The group has attracted hundreds of people of all ages. Among about fifty arrests there have been five doctors and a university professor. The charges have generally been along the lines of 'malicious damage'. But the definition of 'malicious' involves 'indifference to human life and suffering' and this has been used by the graffitists to deny malicious intent and maintain that the advertisement was malicious prior to its message being altered. Hence the graffiti 'improved' the ad.

The quotation from Chesterfield-Evans and O'Connor indicates two of the main strengths of BUGA UP's approach. The activists were eminently respectable people and their facing up to the giant tobacco corporations was readily 'framed' in terms of the myth of David and Goliath. Chapman's description of the origins of BUGA UP (Chapman, 1994) reveals that the reasons for its members' dissatisfaction was that existing health education approaches to smoking were having little effect and they felt that they should 'refocus upstream'.

It is important to note at this point that media advocacy is one particular strategy within the general armamentarium of public health advocacy (see Chapter 6). However, as with all effective mass media use, it is important to supplement media with interpersonal methods. Chapman and Lupton (1994), in their 'A–Z of public health advocacy', describe a full range of detailed tactics that can be employed (see Box 8.5).

BOX 8.5 TEN TACTICS FROM AN A–Z OF PUBLIC HEALTH ADVOCACY

- Be there! The first rule of advocacy
- Crank letters (or how to put your opposition's worst foot forward)
- Demonstrations
- Gatecrashing
- Jargon and ghetto language
- Media cannibalism (how media feed off themselves)
- Networks and coalitions
- 'Piggybacking'
- Shareholders
- Talkback (access) radio.

Source: Chapman and Lupton (1994)

Chapman and Wakefield (2001) summarize some of the techniques used by the Australian anti-tobacco movement to attract media attention. These include:

- test cases involving ordinary individuals suing employers, airlines and nightclubs for not providing smoke-free areas
- making passive smoking an occupational health issue by equating it to asbestos exposure
- publication of expert reports and the views of international experts
- use of sound bites such as 'a non-smoking section in a restaurant is about as much use as a non-urinating section in a swimming pool'

- commissioning of opinion polls
- challenging misleading press statements on environmental tobacco smoke made by the tobacco industry and reports produced by their scientists that downplayed the risk.

Some of the 'highlights' of the advocacy campaign against tobacco advertising included:

- the six-year civil disobedience billboard graffiti campaign
- finding and supporting sports and cultural celebrities to speak out against the use of their sport for tobacco sponsorship
- picketing the tobacco-sponsored Australian Open Tennis Championship
- levying of a 5% state tobacco tax used to replace sponsorship with public health messages.

Maintaining media interest over a sustained period is undoubtedly challenging. Reflecting on 30 years' experience of tobacco control advocacy in Australia, Chapman and Wakefield (2001: 276) conclude that 'properly conducted advocacy rests on analytic precision drawn from both theoretical perspectives and empirical trial-and-error experience'. Further, effective public health advocates have the capacity to frame issues in ways that attract public and political support. They note, for example, tapping into myths such as David and Goliath – the small person taking on the might of the tobacco industry; and the Pied Piper – the tobacco industry leading children to take up a dangerous habit.

The use of social media for health promotion

Social media have burgeoned since the first edition of this book was published in 2004. The potential for the use of social media in promoting health is huge. Social media offer 'exciting ways' to improve people's health, 'new ways of reaching people' as well as increased access to information and support (Abroms et al., 2019: 9S). Even in the poorest countries, high numbers of people use social media and engage in social networking (Novillo-Ortiz and Hernández-Pérez, 2017). The global COVID-19 pandemic saw social media being used very widely for health-related purposes in all corners of the globe (Chen and Wang, 2021). As Ratzan (2011: 803) argues, 'there is a great potential to leverage new communication technologies and tools in this era of convergence with social media'. In short, Ratzan's point is that new methods of communication open up huge opportunities in health promotion. Uses range from 'tweeting' up-to-date, 'hot-off-the-press' health-related research findings to using text messaging to improve attendance at outpatient clinic appointments. A study carried out in Kenya found that the use of an SMS (short message service or text message) intervention with HIV-infected adults increased adherence to anti-retroviral treatment (Lester et al., 2010). This type of finding has huge implications for promoting health in relatively resource-poor settings – a point that is picked up by Kubheka et al. (2020), who argue that social media present significant opportunities for health promotion in South Africa. More broadly however, they caution that 'there is a need to take into account country specific socio-economic issues, which may perpetuate unintended consequences related to the digital divide, data costs and varying levels of health literacy' (p. 2071). In a different context, the Los Angeles County Department 'Sugar Pack' health marketing campaign (Barragan et al., 2014) included messaging via social media (Twitter, Facebook, YouTube and e-cards) in order to increase awareness and motivation among the general public so as to reduce excess calorie consumption from sugar-sweetened beverages.

Social networking sites may provide a form of social support and reduce feelings of social isolation that are long since known to impact negatively on individual health experience (Cattan and Tilford, 2006). The Anderson Cancer Center in Houston, Texas, uses various types of social media for educational purposes, hosting user-generated images and video, for example. Visitors to the host website can also download podcasts and information content to pursue later in their own time (Shea, 2009).

Using the same format as the table containing information about the advantages and disadvantages of selected mass media channels (from the National Cancer Institute – see Table 8.1), we can consider the pros and cons of social media as shown in Table 8.3.

Table 8.3 Advantages and disadvantages of social media

Mass media channel	Activities	Pros	Cons
Social media (including social networking sites, Twitter, YouTube, blogging, vlogging, etc.)	Ads inserted into Facebook pages; newsfeeds and alerts; virtual social support (online groups, etc.)	Has broad reach to potentially very large audiences Can convey up-to-the-minute information with immediate effect Audiences can re-circulate or pass on information very quickly Use of a range of audio and visual techniques, including feedback mechanisms Relatively cheap and accessible to many Potential for interactivity	Sometimes difficult to target a specific 'audience', depending on the type of social media Potential for 'information overload' or 'message clutter' Requires a degree of information/media literacy

BOX 8.6 QUESTIONS FOR HEALTH PROMOTION

- How do we conduct health promotion in the context of social media?
- How do we structure social media sites so that they are more health promoting?
- What are the tangible opportunities for collaboration across the public and private sectors in applications of digital technology to improve public health?
- What kinds of oversight and regulatory actions are needed, especially around public health topics like suicide and the spread of health-related misinformation that lead, for example, to vaccine hesitancy?

Source: Abroms et al. (2019)

Health promotion has little choice but to engage with social media. Norman (2012) acknowledges the opportunities and challenges that this brings. Likewise, Abroms et al. (2019) suggest that we are faced with many questions about how to utilize social media for better health (see Box 8.6). Social media provide an opportunity to review 'traditional' practices within health education and to adapt to new approaches to health communication. However, the use of social media also raises questions about the quality of health information that is available which, in practice, varies hugely (Afful-Dadzie et al., 2023) and Schillinger et al. (2020) argue that public health and health communication practitioners have 'lagged' behind in terms of making sense of the many ways that social media can be used to influence people's health. They advocate for a coherent framework 'for integrating core elements from communication and public health sciences' that can be used to guide practice (p. 1396). A study in the USA by Hanson et al. (2011) concluded that many health educators are already using a variety of social media in their day-to-day work – most commonly, social networking sites (34.8%), podcasts (23.5%) and media sharing sites (18.5%). However, there were also some 'laggards' and people who were willing but whose efforts were curtailed by those in management. The authors concluded that 'social media use holds promise as a supporting methodology to enhance health education practice' (Hanson et al., 2011: 197). Nevertheless, Condran et al. (2017) argue that, in relation to promoting sexual health, health promotion has not fully realized the potential of social media. Indeed, 'figuring out how to make our digital technologies health promoting is', Abroms et al. (2019: 9S) argue, 'one of the key public health challenges of the 21st century'. It is worth noting that successful engagement with social media in health promotion will ultimately depend on the application of theoretical principles and lessons learned from using other mass media channels. Similarly, the use of social media to promote health would need to conform with the ethical principles of health promotion as explored within this book.

MASS MEDIA AND HEALTH PROMOTION

The mass media are still frequently seen as a panacea and can give the illusion that action is being taken – even if it may not always be effective action! However, properly planned mass media interventions can have a place in health promotion, ideally as part of comprehensive programmes that also include interpersonal influences.

The use of mass media for advocacy is entirely consistent with an empowerment model of health promotion. In addition to achieving the primary goal of social and policy change, media advocacy can also help to mobilize communities and contribute to community development – an issue that will be discussed in the next chapter. In conclusion, it is useful to turn to a set of policy recommendations made by Wakefield et al. (2010: 1268):

- Mass media campaigns should be included as key components of comprehensive approaches to improving population health behaviours.
- Sufficient funding must be secured to enable frequent and widespread exposure to campaign messages continuously over time, especially for ongoing behaviours.
- Adequate access to promoted services and product must be ensured.
- Changes in health behaviour might be maximized by complementary policy decisions that support opportunities for change, provide disincentives for not changing, and challenge or restrict competing marketing.

- Campaign message should be based on sound research of the target group and should be tested during campaign development.
- Outcomes should undergo rigorous independent assessment and peer-reviewed publication should be sought.

KEY POINTS

- Mass media can successfully raise awareness, transmit relatively simple information and influence attitudes. However, they are less successful in developing complicated understandings, teaching the skills needed to support health-related behaviour, or promoting the adoption of beliefs and attitudes that are inconsistent with existing value systems and motivations.
- Mass media are more effective when combined with methods that use personal interaction and as part of comprehensive, community-wide programmes.
- In addition to being a channel for specific campaigns, the media offer other (no-cost) opportunities for health promotion such as inclusion of health issues in entertainment programmes like soap operas or in news coverage.
- Over and above the deliberate use of mass media to persuade, the media also have a considerable background influence on social norms.
- Drawing on the principles of social marketing, mass media work should follow tried and tested marketing principles, in particular:

  o systematic planning
  o understanding the target group and its needs, motivations and priorities
  o analysing the cost–benefit implications for the individual as a basis for constructing messages and putting strategies in place to deal with barriers
  o audience segmentation
  o designing and pre-testing messages which appeal to the audience and are simple, clear and appropriately branded
  o using an appropriate source who is credible and attractive
  o ensuring that the programme is delivered through appropriate channels and is of sufficient intensity in relation to number of individuals reached, number of times individuals are exposed to the message, and duration of the programme
  o using multiple media is more likely to be effective. Repetition is useful – provided it does not become boring!

- Media advocacy can shape public opinion and bring about policy change through its direct influence on decision-makers and/or by creating a groundswell of public opinion.
- Health promotion needs to recognize the potential of social media and to engage with modern communication technologies in line with appropriate theoretical underpinnings and ethical principles.

CHAPTER 8: INTERNATIONAL CASE STUDIES

The following case studies on the online resources website are relevant to the content of this chapter: 5, 8 and 9.

CRITICAL REFLECTION AND APPLICATION TO PRACTICE

This chapter has focused on the use of conventional, and more contemporary, mass media in health promotion. Why are mass media so central to promoting public health? How do the contents of this chapter apply to the work that you are involved in? What aspects of mass media are most relevant, and why? Reflect on your use of mass media including social marketing approaches and different types of social media – what has worked well? Or not so well? Why is this? What could be improved? How might social media be utilized for advocacy purposes in the context in which you work?

ONLINE RESOURCES

Please visit https://study.sagepub.com/greentones5e for all the online resources for the book, including recommended further reading on each chapter subject, useful weblinks (both introduced by the authors), as well as the abovementioned case study material.

9 WORKING WITH COMMUNITIES

Go to the people

Live with them

Learn from them

Love them

Start with what they know

Build with what they have

But with the best leaders

When the work is done

The task accomplished

The people will say

'We have done this ourselves'

Lao-Tzu, 604–531 BC

OVERVIEW

This chapter considers ways of working with communities. It will:

- consider the meaning of community
- identify different types of community health work
- focus particularly on community development and empowerment as approaches consistent with the values of health promotion
- discuss aspects of good practice in working with communities
- consider some of the challenges in aligning the rhetoric of community development and empowerment with practice.

INTRODUCTION

Throughout this text, we have emphasized the centrality of community participation to health promotion and have referred to the WHO's repeated endorsement of the primacy of equity and the importance of active participating communities. We have also argued in favour of an empowerment model of health promotion. This chapter focuses on ways of working with communities and developing their capacity to participate, and particularly on community development as a means of achieving community empowerment.

WORKING WITH COMMUNITIES: DEFINITIONS AND CONCEPTS

The concept of community

Involving communities is regarded as being a central pillar within health promotion and continues to be recommended in international declarations (WHO, 2012). However, 'community' is a contested and 'fuzzy' concept that has long been debated (Warwick-Booth and Foster, 2021).

While understandings of community as linked to place are common in both popular conceptions and in policy initiatives (for example in the UK Government's 'Levelling Up' agenda; HM Government, 2022), it can be misleading to conflate 'community' simply with 'neighbourhood', 'pride of place' or a geographical boundary. In the early days of community development, understanding of community tended to be associated with 'communities of place' (South et al., 2013: 11) and traditionally much community development work operated within relatively small and self-contained geographical locations of similar size to a neighbourhood.

Boutilier et al. (2000) and more recently Warwick-Booth and Foster (2021) note the absence of clear definitions of community in both health promotion policy initiatives and in more general bureaucratic usage, together with the tendency to infer the existence of community in the occupation of a geographic space, rather than other aspects such as collective identity, sense of belonging, shared values and network membership. The term itself is often tagged on as a descriptor (for example, 'community health initiatives') or vague references are made to the 'community' as a solution; for example, in such phrases as 'we just need to work more with the community' (Boutilier et al., 2000: 252). Such imprecise and abstract notions of community can give them an idealized quality that fails to address the 'realities of citizen participation' (Boutilier et al., 2000: 252). The assumption is that communities are homogeneous and inclusive, whereas in fact there may be disparate groups, vested interests and conflict, and some groups will be more able to participate than others.

Commentators have long suggested that community is not exclusively related to place, but rather the interconnections and communication arrangements between individuals (de Leeuw, 2000). From this perspective, the term 'community' relates to a web of social connections, both formal and informal (Fairbrother et al., 2013). Broader conceptualizations of 'community' have been put forward that suggest that the term is a shorthand for the relationships, bonds, identities and interests that join people together or give them a shared stake in a place, service, culture or activity (Public Health England, 2015).

New types of interaction are emerging to challenge traditional ideas of community. The development of modern communication technology has in many ways removed the geographical constraints that formerly limited communication and opened up a range of 'virtual communities'. For example, virtual communities are constantly forming on social media sites (Woodall and Cross, 2021). De Leeuw (2000) is critical of any distinction made between real and virtual communities, contending that virtual communities are real to those who feel that they belong.

Over and above issues of location and communication, social bonds and a sense of connectedness are central to the concept of community. Recent evidence has demonstrated the power of community during periods of crisis – such as the COVID-19 pandemic – showing how strong community connections can increase well-being and reduce depression and anxiety (Bowe et al., 2022). A community is characterized by the existence of a network of vertical and horizontal relationships and a shared sense of identity, predicament and, in some instances, purpose. Adopting this outlook, Brint (2001: 8) defines community as:

> aggregates of people who share common activities and/or beliefs and who are bound together principally by relations of affect, loyalty, common values, and/or personal concern.

Community health work

The initial challenge in discussing ways of working with communities is terminology, a point recently made by South et al. (2019). There is considerable semantic confusion stemming from the variety of different terms (see Box 9.1), subtle differences, the absence of universal definitions, the tendency to use terms interchangeably, differences in terminology in different parts of the world and changes in terminology over time. The review by the National Institute for Health and Care Excellence (NICE) (2008: 12) noted that 'no two definitions of the same approach are the same' and that different terms have been used to describe very similar approaches.

BOX 9.1 COMMUNITY WORK AND HEALTH: TERMS IN COMMON USE

- Citizenship
- Community action
- Community activity
- Community capacity-building
- Community development
- Community empowerment
- Community engagement
- Community involvement
- Community mobilization
- Community organization
- Community participation
- Social action.

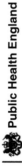 **Public Health England**

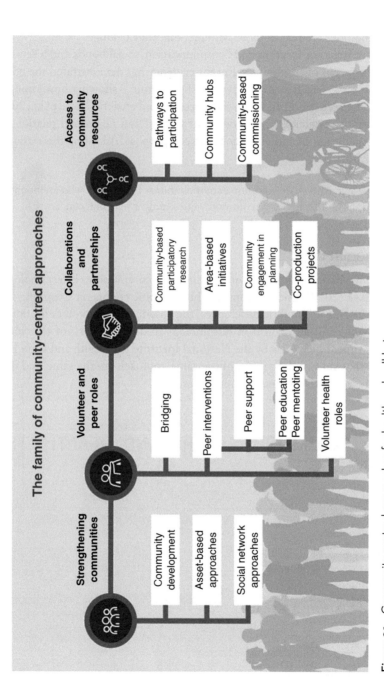

The family of community-centred approaches

Strengthening communities
- Community development
- Asset-based approaches
- Social network approaches

Volunteer and peer roles
- Bridging
- Peer interventions
- Peer support
- Peer education
- Peer mentoting
- Volunteer health roles

Collaborations and partnerships
- Community-based participatory research
- Area-based initiatives
- Community engagement in planning
- Co-production projects

Access to community resources
- Pathways to participation
- Community hubs
- Community-based commissioning

Figure 9.1 Community-centred approaches for health and well-being

Reproduced with permission under the terms of the Open Government Licence.

In the UK, South et al. (2019) offered a framework for mapping and understanding the myriad of strategies purporting to take a community-centred approach to health. Their conceptual map, described as a 'family' of approaches, categorized community-centred approaches under four areas: (1) strengthening communities; (2) volunteer and peer roles; (3) collaborations and partnerships; and (4) access to community resources. This is depicted in Figure 9.1.

The family of community-centred approaches for health and well-being

It is clear, therefore, that community-level health promotion interventions are of many and various types – although some have suggested some common factors linking the interventions together. This includes: community-based interventions not depending on the professional healthcare system; those interventions being able to potentially reach a wide range of individuals; and community-level interventions focusing on tackling environmental factors that shape lifestyle (Nickel and von dem Knesebeck, 2020). A major point of distinction is between *working in communities* and *working with communities*. The former refers to a location or target for health promotion activity to address an externally defined agenda – and frequently behavioural targets. It is, therefore, often referred to as 'community-based' and associated with 'top-down' interventions. In contrast, the latter signals a commitment to involving communities in developing their own agenda and working collectively to improve the health of the community.

An example that shows processes of working both 'in' and 'with' communities is shown in Case study 9.1.

CASE STUDY 9.1 'COMMUNITY HEALTH CHAMPIONS'

The term 'community health champion' is a relatively new addition to the already burgeoning array of terminology related to community work and health. However, the concept has distinct similarities to other types of community and volunteer health roles. NICE (2008: 40) defined health champions as:

> individuals who possess the experience, enthusiasm and skills to encourage and support other individuals and communities to engage in health promotion activities. They also ensure that the health issues facing communities remain high on the agenda of organisations that can effect change. Health champions offer local authorities and community partnerships short-term support as consultants, encourage them to share good practice and help them develop activities to improve the health of local people.

Community health champions are individuals who are engaged, trained and supported to volunteer and use their life experience, understanding and position of influence to help their friends, families and work colleagues lead healthier lives. Community health champions may also be involved in advocacy work or lobbying to change local services and organizations. Engaging community members in promoting health within their own communities is backed up by a solid

(Continued)

body of evidence that this work is effective. For example, there is very good evidence on the effectiveness of lay health workers or volunteers in:

- increasing knowledge and awareness of health issues in communities
- helping people access health services, including increasing uptake of preventive measures such as immunization
- supporting positive behaviour changes, particularly when working with disadvantaged, low-income or minority ethnic communities
- physical activity and nutrition, where reported outcomes include increased physical activity, increased consumption of fruit and vegetables, lower intake of dietary fat, and better food safety knowledge and skills
- improving health status, including better mental health and improved disease management where programmes are focused on helping people with long-term conditions
- supporting appropriate use of healthcare services, including reducing barriers to access and decreasing hospital admissions.

Source: South et al. (2010)

Evaluation of programmes show that the community health champion role can be a catalyst for change for both individuals and communities. Indeed, community health champions have the potential to be instrumental in creating a cultural shift in communities towards healthier and more integrated living (Woodall et al., 2012b).

In a general sense, this type of approach has been referred to as 'community development'. The term 'community organization' is also common in the health promotion discourse, particularly in the North American context, and was defined in the Younghusband Report (1959) as:

> primarily aimed at helping people within a local community to identify social needs, to consider the most effective ways of meeting these and to set about doing so, in so far as their available resources permit. (Cited in Smith, 2016)

Community organization is a planned process to activate a community to use its own social structures and any available resources to accomplish community goals that are decided on primarily by community representatives and that are generally consistent with local values. Purposive social change interventions are organized primarily by individuals, groups or organizations from within the community in order to attain and sustain community improvements and/or new opportunities.

The focus on the collective rather than the individual is emphasized in the Global Consortium on Community Health Promotion's view that community health promotion refers to 'health promotion action initiated with community members by community members and for community members' (Ritchie, 2007: 96). Further, a core principle is that:

> Community participation is essential and must drive every stage of health promotion actions – setting priorities, making decisions, planning strategies and conducting evaluation. (Nishtar et al., 2006: 7)

Some time ago, Rothman (1979) developed a typology of different types of community intervention that provides a useful framework. The types of intervention are:

- **locality development** – self-help, community capacity and integration (process goals)
- **social planning** – problem-solving with regard to community problems (task goals)
- **social action** – shifting of power relationships, achievement of social change (task/process goals)
- community development – proper
- **political action** – similar to Alinsky's social action approach
- **social planning** – collaboration between voluntary bodies and the state to change and improve services.

Social planning, on the one hand, is generally led by organizations external to the community and involves the community, to a greater or lesser extent, primarily in order to increase effectiveness in solving the community's problems and improving service provision. Social action, on the other hand, attempts to shift the distribution of power and resources and influence policy and practice in the public or private sector. It is a movement embodying protest and often associated with the work of Alinsky (1969, 1972). Kirklin and Franzen (1974: 5) offer a succinct description:

> Large numbers of people are organized to bring into being a new power aggregate (or community organization) to force the existing political/economic power structure to change public and private policies. The battle is classically seen to be between the 'power haves' and the 'power have nots'.

Laverack (2013) lists the various forms of protest and demonstration used in community activism. Some of these include: protest marches; demonstrations and rallies; picketing; street protesting; 'bulldozer-diving', involving individuals using their bodies to stop machinery; and sit-ins. Other approaches have also been recently highlighted: a study by Freeman (2019) outlined how Indigenous young people used 'culture-based activism' to call for change regarding the sociopolitical and environmental issues that impact on Indigenous communities.

The terms 'locality development', 'community development' and 'community organization' have, in the past, been used to describe ways of working that are concerned with developing the capacity of the community to identify its own priorities and work towards them. These approaches tend to be based on collaboration with statutory organizations and authorities.

However, for some, community development is more political in intent and has a more overarching meaning encompassing developing the capacity – and, indeed, the motivation – to take social action. Some have suggested that more radical forms of community development encompass social change that move beyond local or shared areas of concern to challenging broader power and political structures in society (Ledwith, 2020).

The extent to which individuals participate and are involved in community-based efforts to improve health will, of course, vary. These levels can vary from minimal engagement where individuals have limited commitment or participation, to more substantive levels with higher control.

Laverack (2007) identifies three roles for practitioners that reflect these different levels: directive, telling communities what to do; facilitative, supporting communities to identify and achieve their own goals; working with communities, to achieve social and political change. Some of these issues are reflected in Table 9.1.

Table 9.1   Key differences between community-based and community development approaches

Issue	Community-based	Community development
Community organizing model	Social planning	Locality development; social action
Root metaphor	Individual responsibility	Empowerment
Approach/orientation	Weakness/deficit	Strength/competence
	Solve problem	Capacity-building
Definition of problem	By agencies, government or outside organization	By target community
Primary vehicles for health promotion and change	Education, improved services, lifestyle change, food availability, media	Building community and control, increasing community resources and capacity, economic and political change
Role of professionals	Key, central to decision-making	Resource
Role of participation by target community members and institutions	Providing better services, increasing consumption and support	To increase target community control and ownership, improve social structure
Role of human service agencies and formal helpers	Central mechanism for service delivery	One of many systems to respond to needs of a community's members
Primary decision-makers	Agency representatives, business leaders, governmental representatives, 'appointed' community leaders	Indigenous elected leaders
View of community	Broad site of the problem, technically and externally defined, consumers	Specific, targeted source of solution, internally defined, subjective, a place to live
Target community control of resource	Low	High
Community member ownership	Low	High

Source: Boutilier et al. (2000), based on Felix et al. (1989)

In practice, 'pure' forms of the various approaches referred to rarely exist. Regardless of the label used to describe different ways of working, a number of key conceptual strands emerge. These are the extent to which approaches:

- are controlled by external agencies or from within the community
- meet community or externally defined goals
- enable communities to participate
- build capacity and empower communities
- challenge power relationships
- seek social and political change.

Figure 9.2 provides an overview of different types of community health work.

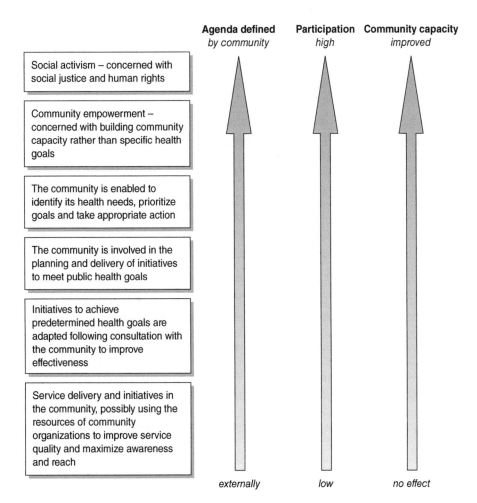

Figure 9.2 Typology of community health work

Contemporary definitions

Latterly, the terms 'community participation' and 'community engagement' have come into more frequent use and have some commonalities with 'community development'.

Community participation, although a term where standard definitions have become elusive and contentious (Haldane et al., 2019) it is referred to as:

> a process by which people are enabled to become actively and genuinely involved in defining the issues of concern to them, in making decisions about factors that affect their lives, in formulating and implementing policies, in planning, developing and delivering services and in taking action to achieve change. (WHO, 2002b: 10)

Community engagement has been similarly defined as:

> the process of getting communities involved in decisions that affect them. This includes the planning, development and management of services, as well as activities which aim to improve health or reduce health inequalities. (Popay, 2006, cited in NICE, 2008: 5)

Community development as a term predates the use of community participation and community engagement. It was defined by the Calouste Gulbenkian Foundation (1984) as:

> a strategy for the attainment of social policy goals. It is concerned with the worth and dignity of people and the promotion of equal opportunity … [it] is most needed in communities where social skills and resources are at their weakest. [It] involves working with those most affected by poverty, unemployment, disability, inadequate housing and education, and with those who for reasons of class, income, race or sex are less likely than others to be, or to feel, involved and significant in local community life.

This definition draws attention to the focus on disadvantaged and excluded communities and the need to increase their capacity to participate. Over and above developing skills and motivation among the community, tackling power imbalances is clearly a key issue, as emphasized in the following definition.

> Community development is about building active and sustainable communities based on social justice and mutual respect. It is about changing power structures to remove the barriers that prevent people from participating in the issues that affect their lives. (Standing Conference for Community Development, 2001: 5)

Community development is accordingly based on a number of core values and commitments (see Box 9.2).

BOX 9.2 COMMUNITY DEVELOPMENT – VALUES AND COMMITMENTS

Values

- Social justice
- Participation
- Equality
- Learning
- Cooperation.

Commitments

- Challenging discrimination and oppressive practices within organizations, institutions and communities

- Developing practice and policy that protects the environment
- Encouraging networking and connections between communities and organizations
- Ensuring access and choice for all groups and individuals within society
- Influencing policy and programmes from the perspective of communities
- Prioritizing the issues of concern to people experiencing poverty and social exclusion
- Promoting social change that is long term and sustainable
- Reversing inequality and the imbalance of power relationships in society
- Supporting community-led collective action.

Source: Standing Conference for Community Development (2001: 5)

The role of community development in enabling community action is recognized in Henderson et al.'s (2004: 6) definition:

Community development: the process of change in neighbourhoods and communities. It aims to increase the extent and effectiveness of community action, community activity and agencies' relationships with communities.

Asset-based approaches

Key principles in community development see a shift from the deficits in communities (such as unemployment, high crime rates, etc.) towards a focus on people and their capabilities, skills and strengths to participate in things that affect their lives (Warwick-Booth et al., 2013a). This resonates with assets-based approaches to working in communities that have attracted a great deal of interest, even a level of evangelism (Friedli, 2013), in the UK and USA. Asset-based approaches are a popular intervention strategy in health promotion and seen as a legitimate way to addressing health inequalities by empowering people in more disadvantaged communities to use local resources and increase control over health and its determinants (Cassetti et al., 2020).

The evidence base for asset-based approaches is in its infancy, with few empirical studies existing that demonstrate the effectiveness of the approach (Cassetti et al., 2020). Moreover, the outcomes and benefits of such strategies are not always explicit (Rippon and South, 2017), although the approach is frequently underpinned by the idea of salutogenesis with a reorientation towards positive health outcomes and factors that promote resilience (South et al., 2013).

The popularity of asset-based approaches in health promotion is perhaps characterized by the numbers of community projects that adapt the core principles and philosophy. One variation is 'positive deviance' (PD), a form of asset-based community development that aims to build on strengths using the existing skills of the community. PD has a small, but emerging evidence base with effect results shown in countries worldwide (Marsh et al., 2004) and has been shown to build confidence and self-esteem on issues as diverse as female genital mutilation, reintegrating child soldiers back into communities and overcoming under-nutrition in Vietnamese children. It is based on the recognition that in every community there are certain individuals or groups whose uncommon behaviours and strategies enable them to find better solutions to problems than their peers, while having access to the same resources and facing similar challenges (Marsh et al., 2004). The approach is based on the PD four-step process (Bradley et al., 2009):

1. Define the problem.
2. Determine common practices (what people generally do about the problem).
3. Discover individuals or communities who have found successful ways of dealing with the problem.
4. Design a means of sharing these successful ways.

A recent application of PD was applied to fathers in a deprived community in England to enhance family well-being (Robertson et al., 2016). From this research it was apparent that when positive, salutogenic approaches are taken that value views of communities (in this case men), solutions to entrenched health and social issues can be discovered. By identifying positive deviants, or assets, in communities it was clear that fathers were better able to cope and address health and social factors in their lives.

An asset-based philosophy is certainly in vogue, but it is not new and can be traced back to the values enshrined in the Ottawa Charter (Brooks and Kendall, 2013; Cassetti et al., 2020). Strengthening community action is one of the five action areas identified by the Ottawa Charter (see Box 9.3), which also identifies community development as the means of increasing the capacity to take action. Community action is interpreted here as the range of actions needed to achieve change that will improve the health of the community. This contrasts with the narrower interpretation as political activism, aligned with the notion of social activism mentioned above.

BOX 9.3   OTTAWA CHARTER: STRENGTHEN COMMUNITY ACTIONS

Health promotion works through concrete and effective community action in setting priorities, making decisions, planning strategies and implementing them to achieve better health. At the heart of this process is the empowerment of communities – their ownership and control of their own endeavours and destinies. Community development draws on existing human and material resources in the community to enhance self-help and social support, and to develop flexible systems for strengthening public participation in and direction of health matters. This requires full and continuous access to information, learning opportunities for health, as well as funding support.

Source: WHO (1986)

Community development is not new (for a review of its history, see Ledwith, 2020). Bivins (1979) described it as an old and reliable grassroots approach to health education and gave examples of its use in the 1940s, although its principles and applications were in use at a much earlier date. For instance, Hilton (1988: 3–4), using the synonym 'community organization', sees its origins in the Antigonish movement of the 1920s. The movement's principles, set out below, are entirely consistent with community development and the emphasis on the importance of adult education is of particular interest:

- Each person is endowed by God with intellectual, volitional (act of will) and physical faculties that must be developed to obtain full and abundant life for all.
- Major social institutions of society must be transformed to guarantee equal opportunity and full development of all people.
- Adult education and group action are the most effective means whereby the common people themselves will be able to transform social institutions and this will be done by defining and controlling the nature and direction for social change.
- The process begins when common people use adult education and group action to solve their immediate social and economic problems.

Community organization first appeared in US social work textbooks in the 1920s and 1930s; however, not until the War on Poverty in the sixties did the concept and its application receive much attention. [Its] purpose is to enable communities to improve and change their socio-economic milieu and/or their position in that milieu. [It] developed largely as a response to the conditions of poor people in Western urban settings, but is now practised in a variety of forms in urban and rural locales, in Third World as well as technologically advanced contexts. (Kindervatter, 1979: 71)

In many countries, governments support the rhetoric of community engagement (Brunton et al., 2017; HM Government, 2022) but this has often been undermined by broader policy matters. Indeed, community development has had an indifferent history across the world, with practice often falling out of favour with funders and those in power, when people become empowered and question the status quo (Warwick-Booth and Foster, 2021). The philosophy of community development also sits awkwardly besides the current focus in many countries on achieving narrow targets around disease reduction and behaviour change set by managers and politicians, not communities (Warwick-Booth et al., 2013a).

Conceptualizations of community development generally encompass the notion of empowerment. Indeed, the participation of communities forms 'the backbone of empowering strategies' (Wallerstein, 2006: 9). The premise, as articulated by Tengland (2016), is that the more empowered individuals and communities are the more healthy they become. Even when empowerment strategies are not focused on health *per se* health outcomes often derive as people feel a greater sense of control and security over their life and situation.

Ideology

There are clear similarities between community development and an empowerment model of health promotion. For many, the empowering potential of community development makes it the strategy of choice for health promotion. The very existence of a genuine community is frequently seen as a desirable goal in its own right – that is, a social system where there is a shared sense of purpose, a coherent network of social relationships and the capacity to work together to achieve collective goals. Where a community possesses an additional fund of competences such that it can offer social support to its members, it can also be said to be healthy. The currently popular description of this 'fund of competences' is, of course, social capital.

As we observed in Chapter 2, there is considerable evidence that social support contributes not only to health and well-being, but also to disease prevention. It could reasonably be argued, therefore, that the mere fact of creating or building communities having social capital where none existed before is quintessentially health promoting. However, the ultimate ideological goal of health promotion and community development is the achievement of equity and the reduction of inequalities in health. Particular attention, therefore, needs to be paid to ensuring that marginalized and disadvantaged groups are able to participate and that their needs are met. Furthermore, commitment to empowerment demands that individuals and communities are able to establish control over factors which influence their health. This idea is exemplified by Rappaport (1987), who defined empowerment as a process whereby individuals and communities gain 'mastery' over their affairs.

Braunack-Mayer and Louise (2008) contend that community empowerment is aligned with bottom-up approaches and favoured as an alternative to top-down paternalistic approaches whether or not they are coercive. Community empowerment has similarities with, but is still different from, other terms like community capacity and social capital. Community empowerment, however, concerns power relations and intervention strategies that ultimately focus on challenging social injustice through political and social processes (Wallerstein, 2006). The overall aim is to allow people to take control of the decisions that influence their lives and health (Woodall et al., 2010). Community empowerment has been described as both a process and an outcome; it is, however, most consistently seen as a process in the form of a continuum (Laverack and Wallerstein, 2001). As a process, community empowerment can be regarded as a series of actions that progressively contribute to more organized community and social action (Laverack, 2004). Starting with an individual's concerns about a given issue, the process of community empowerment begins with the development of small mutual groups, then community organizations, partnerships and ultimately to groups of people taking political and social action to create social change through the redistribution of resources and power (Laverack, 2006; Wallerstein, 2002). Each point along the continuum represents a progression towards the goal of community empowerment (see as an example the paper by Sardu et al. [2012] that reports the development of community empowerment in a Sardinian village, Ulassai). However, marginalized and disadvantaged communities may lack the power to exercise autonomous choice or, indeed, influence policy. Braunack-Mayer and Louise (2008: 6) argue that this may 'create a licence for paternalistic intervention' or for an alternative form of paternalism that is concerned with developing community capacity. That said, some evidence suggests that empowerment processes can be fostered in marginalized populations who face some of the most coercive situations. People residing in maximum-security prisons, despite legitimate coercive and disempowering processes, can still be enabled to take control over their situation through engagement in democratic processes and by enabling skill-development to tackle the social determinants influencing their health (Woodall, 2020b). There is, obviously, a stark tension between security and 'top-down' processes and attempts to support 'bottom-up' community organization. Laverack and Labonte have made this point previously (2000) and have argued for the inclusion of community empowerment as a parallel track in all health promotion programme planning, even top-down behaviourally orientated programmes (see Figure 4.6).

Despite the endorsement of empowerment approaches in health promotion by the authors of this text, there are several very legitimate critiques of empowerment strategies. Tengland's (2016) critique, for example, highlights how empowerment can sometimes lead to 'power-over' certain groups or communities, which may be counterproductive. Others have been more critical and have argued that the radical discourse of empowerment, whereby communities work together to increase the control that they have over events that influence their lives and health, has been lost within health promotion practice. The political and radical overtones of community empowerment have to some extent been diluted by a neoliberal ideology underpinning contemporary health promotion (Woodall et al., 2012a).

Ends and means

There may be a variety of different motivations underpinning the use of community- based strategies to improve health. At one extreme, it may involve little more than cosmetically concealed top-down, authoritarian attempts at persuasion to achieve externally defined goals. It may also serve to shift responsibility from the state to the community. For example, the community can become the scapegoat for problems that are the product of wider social, economic and environmental factors – victim-blaming at the collective level! Alternatively, the community can be seen as a resource to respond to inadequacies in state provision. Boutilier et al. (2000) comment critically on the use of community rhetoric as a response to fiscal crises in the North American context and a means of legitimizing the transfer of responsibility to the community.

Clearly, such cynical misappropriation is entirely inconsistent with the definition of community development set out above and its attendant values. Other, more consistent goals, range in intent from the conservative to the more radical, for example:

- improving service delivery to meet the community's needs
- developing self-reliance and the capacity for self-help in the community
- enabling people to achieve their personal health goals
- activism to tackle the structural determinants of health and create healthier environments
- activism to defend the rights of disadvantaged groups and challenge oppression and oppressive practices.

Gilchrist (2000: 2) notes the inherent tension in community development 'between the goals of the state and the aspirations of the "target" community, with no guarantee that they would necessarily be aligned'. Even at the community level, there may be tensions between achieving the collective goals of the community as opposed to meeting the needs of specific groups or vocal individuals.

CASE STUDY 9.2 COMMUNITY DEVELOPMENT PROJECTS (CDPS) 1969–77

The Community Development Project (CDP) was set up as a Home Office initiative in 1969 to identify ways of meeting the needs of local people in areas of high social need.

Many, although not all, CDPs developed radical critiques of the economic and political policies underlying poverty and deprivation. Some came into conflict with the local authorities because of their involvement in tenants' and other local community groups that opposed council policies on housing and other issues. There was also conflict with the Home Office, who closed down the central unit in 1976 and became increasingly concerned at what was going on. Some projects closed early after government and local authority pressure. There were also internal conflicts within some CDP teams.

Source: Working Class Movement Library (undated); see also Smith (2016)

Elements of tokenism in regard to engaging the community is counterproductive. Indeed, commentators have suggested that, to date, the potential of community-led health promotion has not been fully realized – this is for a range of reasons, including the poor methodological rigour in evaluating such strategies (Nickel and von dem Knesebeck, 2020). It is clear though, that approaches in which communities are partners, or have delegated or total control, result in more positive effects on health and other aspects of people's lives, such as sense of community and social capital, along with empowerment and enhanced well-being.

Claims about the contribution of community participation to health promotion include:

- increasing democracy
- combating exclusion
- empowering people
- mobilizing resources and energy
- developing holistic and integrated approaches
- achieving better decisions and more effective services
- ensuring the ownership and sustainability of programmes. (WHO, 2002b: 12)

The outbreak of the Ebola virus in West Africa, particularly in Guinea, Liberia and Sierra Leone, between 2014 and 2016, demonstrated the value of community engagement and participation in efforts to control the virus transmission. Observers commented that community engagement offered an added value through the self-management of quarantines, control of cross-border movement, safe and dignified burials, and the siting of Community Care Centres. Nonetheless, there was a view that during the crises there was a tendency to adopt 'pre-packaged and top-down approaches' which may have potentially worsened the effects (Laverack and Manoncourt, 2016).

There are often complex and reciprocal relationships between participation and its anticipated effects. Figure 9.3 shows that the process of participation can be empowering, but equally empowerment can enhance participation.

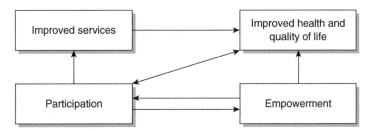

Figure 9.3   Pathways to community empowerment

From a pragmatic perspective, those involved in planning health promotion interventions should be explicit about what their ultimate goal is and the change pathway leading towards it – that is to say, what the intended outcome is and what the strategy for achieving it is. Is developing active participating communities a goal in its own right or a strategy for increasing the likelihood of adopting healthy behaviours? Is participation a way of improving service provision or a means of empowering individuals and communities?

Moreover, it is important to be clear about the approach being used and its underpinning values (Woodall and Cross, 2021). Commitment to the principles of community development requires critical attention to process as well as outcomes to ensure that it is empowering. The Global Consortium on Community Health Promotion states that:

> it is the participatory, empowering and equity focused *process* that forms the fundamental bedrock of community health promotion. (Nishtar et al., 2006: 7)

Furthermore, processes should ensure that members of the community are able to participate on an equal footing with professionals.

There are obvious differences between consultation that seeks the opinion of local people, participation that involves mobilizing people to become involved, and empowerment that strengthens individuals and communities – this creates a whole spectrum of ways in which participation of communities can occur (Woodall and Cross, 2021). Communities may become involved in a number of different ways that will vary in relation to the amount of power and control that they have. These various levels of participation are usually depicted as ladders, ascending from being told nothing, up to being informed, consulted, advising, planning jointly, having some delegated responsibility and, finally, the highest stage of having control (for example, Arnstein, 1969; Brager and Specht, 1973; see also Figures 5.6 and 5.7, respectively).

We noted in Chapter 1 that greater levels of participation are linked to higher levels of empowerment (see Figure 1.6). These levels are also incorporated into the framework in Figure 9.4 showing the pathways from participation to empowerment and health.

The use of ladders as a form of representation implies a hierarchy and the superiority of higher levels over lower. While this may be the case in relation to their empowering potential, there may equally be situations when it is appropriate to use information-giving approaches (NICE, 2008).

There is some debate about whether empowerment is an end in itself or the means to improving other health outcomes. Braunack-Mayer and Louise (2008) challenge the view of 'empowerment

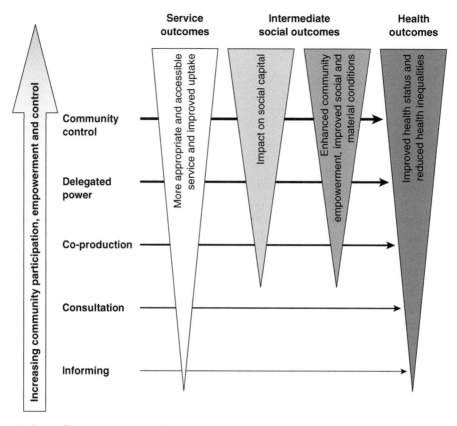

Figure 9.4 Pathways from community participation, empowerment and control to health improvement (NICE, 2008: 8, based on Popay, 2006)

as an end' on two grounds. First, improved health outcomes are often invoked as justification for empowerment approaches. Second, health promotion's concern to address 'social, political and economic powerlessness' (2008: 7) stems from the fact that they have a bearing on health.

We have argued in Chapters 1 and 3 that empowerment is central to definitions of health and is a primary goal of health promotion. We do not see any contradiction with the fact that having power and control can at the same time be a means of enabling individuals or communities to achieve other health outcomes.

GOOD PRACTICE IN COMMUNITY HEALTH PROMOTION

While communities may come together spontaneously to tackle a health issue (see, for example, the Entabeni project in Case study 9.4), it is more common for an external agent to be involved in initiating community involvement and activity. Efforts to involve communities in health promotion may fail for a number of different reasons – not least poor past experience of involvement. It is important that those involved in community health promotion are aware of standards of good practice (see Table 9.2)

Table 9.2 Good practice for community development and health work

	Good practice requires
Clear and realistic role and remit	• Projects to work within a wide definition of health and to establish health as an important community issue • Clarity and consensus about participatory principles and values and their implications • Community participation at all stages of a project • Changes in the culture and ways of working with the statutory sector • A realistic remit for community projects and initiatives based on the time and resources available and the needs and history of the community/users • Respect for minority and different needs and the need for mainstream as well as specific project work
Adequate and appropriate resources to meet the project remit	• Secure, adequate and long-term funding • Accessible and appropriate premises • Experienced, long-term staff with community development skills • Reliable, committed and properly supported volunteers and activists
Adequate and appropriate management and evaluation to support the project	• Effective and supportive project management (through a management committee or line management model) by people with appropriate time, skills and experience • Clearly defined structural arrangements between projects and key agencies to avoid relying too heavily on individuals and to feed in community needs and concerns • Community involvement in project management and decision-making • Appropriate monitoring and evaluation to inform project planning and development
Recognition of the importance of the wider environment within which projects operate	• Building on the past history and experience of communities and local agencies and developing new projects within that context • Harnessing the support of local politicians and linking projects to new national policies that endorse community participation • Effective inter-agency and sector links and partnership at local and district or city-wide levels
Building in long-term sustainability	• Linking community health projects into agendas for change that are emerging in the health and social policy fields • Projects achieving real change and gains, and promoting these to communities, funders and agencies • Building community capacity in terms of skills, information access points, networks and groups • Making sure that local agencies and professionals have the skills, knowledge and commitment to support local community participation work, to build community needs and views into their planning, policy and prioritizing and to respond appropriately to community identified needs for change • Seeing sustainability as an integral part of project work, not a final stage.

Source: Henderson et al. (2004)

and incorporate these into their initial planning and as a frame of reference for ongoing reflection and evaluation of the process. Not only is this a fundamental ethical requirement, it is also likely to lead to more successful practice.

National standards for community engagement to ensure quality and improve the experience of all involved have also been developed in a number of countries (Communities Scotland, 2005), with some based on the following principles:

- Fairness, equality and inclusion must underpin all aspects of community engagement, and should be reflected in both community engagement policies and the way that everyone involved participates.
- Community engagement should have clear and agreed purposes, and methods that achieve these purposes.
- Improving the quality of community engagement requires commitment to learning from experience.
- Skill must be exercised in order to build communities, to ensure practice of equalities principles, to share ownership of the agenda and to enable all viewpoints to be reflected.
- As all parties to community engagement possess knowledge based on study, experience, observation and reflection, effective engagement processes will share and use that knowledge.
- All participants should be given the opportunity to build on their knowledge and skills.
- Accurate, timely information is crucial for effective engagement. (Communities Scotland, 2005)

More recently, it has been proposed that community engagement comprises of a cycle of 'initial actions, further actions, then evaluation, reflection and further actions' (Hubley et al., 2021: 211). First, however, the importance of the entry stage involves finding out about the community so that you can plan appropriate activities. This can comprise a whole myriad of activities, such as: being knowledgeable about the community in terms of its economic conditions, political structures, informal (or formal) leadership structure, norms and values, demographic trends, history and experience with engagement efforts. The initial action stage is also important: the overarching goal is to encourage actions on issues that most people agree are problems, are held widely as felt needs, and can unite people in a common purpose. 'Further actions', as suggested by Hubley et al. (2021), are where momentum and self-confidence may be built in communities and where individuals from the community may emerge as leaders and take on more extended roles in community activities. In parallel, this stage often involves mobilizing local resources and communities (discussed below). Finally, within community engagement processes the concept of evaluation as an ongoing 'iterative' process of determining impact, learning lessons and using insights gained to redefine activities is absolutely critical (Hubley et al., 2021).

Mobilizing communities

One of the major challenges in community health promotion is mobilizing the community and ensuring that all groups are represented; yet there is evidence that public health interventions using community engagement strategies for disadvantaged groups are effective in terms of changes to health behaviours, health consequences, health behaviour self-efficacy and perceived social support (O'Mara-Eves et al., 2015).

ABSTRACT 9.1

The effectiveness of community engagement in public health interventions for disadvantaged groups: a meta-analysis. O'Mara-Eves et al. (2015)

Background: Inequalities in health are acknowledged in many developed countries, whereby disadvantaged groups systematically suffer from worse health outcomes such as lower life expectancy than non-disadvantaged groups. Engaging members of disadvantaged communities in public health initiatives has been suggested as a way to reduce health inequities. This systematic review was conducted to evaluate the effectiveness of public health interventions that engage the community on a range of health outcomes across diverse health issues.

Methods: The authors searched the following sources for systematic reviews of public health interventions: Cochrane CDSR and CENTRAL, Campbell Library, DARE, NIHR HTA programme website, HTA database and DoPHER. Through the identified reviews, they collated a database of primary studies that appeared to be relevant, and screened the full-text documents of those primary studies against the inclusion criteria. In parallel, the authors searched the NHS EED and TRoPHI databases for additional primary studies. For the purposes of these analyses, study design was limited to randomized and non-randomized controlled trials. Only interventions conducted in OECD countries and published since 1990 were included. The authors conducted a random effects meta-analysis of health behaviour, health consequences, self-efficacy and social support outcomes, and a narrative summary of community outcomes. They tested a range of moderator variables, with a particular emphasis on the model of community engagement used as a potential moderator of intervention effectiveness.

Results: Of the 9467 primary studies scanned, 131 were identified for inclusion in the meta-analysis. The overall effect size for health behaviour outcomes is $d =.33$ (95% CI.26,.40). The interventions were also effective in increasing health consequences ($d =.16$, 95% CI.06,.27); health behaviour self-efficacy ($d =.41$, 95% CI.16,.65) and perceived social support ($d =.41$, 95% CI.23,.65). Although the type of community engagement was not a significant moderator of effect, the analysis identified some trends across studies.

Conclusions: There is solid evidence that community engagement interventions have a positive impact on a range of health outcomes across various conditions. There is insufficient evidence to determine whether one particular model of community engagement is more effective than any other.

However, community engagement policies often do not take sufficient account of the diversity of communities. Groups least likely to have their views heard are often ethnic minority groups, carers, the LGBTQ + community, people with mental or physical disabilities, refugees and asylum seekers, people experiencing homelessness and young people (Blake et al., 2008; Harrison et al., 2022). The literature suggests a number of barriers to 'getting heard':

- practical barriers such as lack of information and understanding of relevant decision-making processes, lack of transport to meetings and lack of childcare
- personal barriers such as lack of confidence and/or feelings of discomfort in formal meetings and/or difficulties in the use of English

- socioeconomic barriers including the lack of rights for asylum seekers and the reality of refugees needing to have several jobs to try to support themselves and families back home
- motivational barriers such as scepticism as to whether involvement is likely to make any difference, cynicism as a result of previous negative experiences, or simply doubts as to whether the desired outcomes could be achieved via local structures of governance at all rather than via some other route (such as through the local MP)
- barriers relating to legitimacy, recognition and acceptance – recognition that is sometimes gained from established organizations or council officers and in other instances by the fact of moving from informal organization towards formal constitution. (Blake et al., 2008; Harrison et al., 2022)

Burton et al. (2004) noted that the types of people involved in area-based initiatives vary according to the nature of the initiative. Strategic level involvement tends to place greater reliance on 'proxy representatives' (2004: 32), such as community leaders or community development workers. In contrast, grassroots initiatives involve local residents to a greater extent. Burton et al.'s review of area-based initiatives found that involvement could be better planned in relation to approach, structures, roles, processes, methods and resources. In particular, the role of the community needs to be 'clearly articulated at the outset' (2004: 30) and the diversity of the community recognized. Flexibility is also needed to allow 'strategic goals to be changed in the light of community involvement' (2004: 30). Too strong a central commitment to particular policies could lead to alternative community suggestions being dismissed as intransigent.

Some of the barriers to community involvement included structures such as partnership boards run along formal lines characterized by formal agendas, limited opportunity for discussion, rapid decision-making and the use of jargon. Clearly, attention needs to be given to ensuring that processes, rather than being intimidating, encourage involvement (see Case study 9.3). Lack of commitment to community involvement among some public sector partners was also an issue and the importance of respecting the 'different but equally valuable contributions of different partners' (Burton et al., 2004: 31) was emphasized. The review noted that effective involvement requires capacity-building among all members – not just parts of the community.

CASE STUDY 9.3   ENABLING COMMUNITIES TO PARTICIPATE

A structured literature review was undertaken to assess the challenges and barriers to community-driven decision-making in urban development and moreover to identify the potential solutions to overcome them. The study found 48 barriers and challenges – the most salient challenges were an absence of meaningful community engagement, and poorly-defined aims and purpose of community engagement activities. The review concluded with several practical solutions to improve the communities' involvement in inclusive decision-making processes. These included:

- scheduling community engagement events at convenient times and places
- offering childcare and other facilities such as wheelchair access and transport

- bringing community engagement *to* the community to avoid any financial costs and constraints
- using venues which are familiar to the community and creating an informal atmosphere to make communities feel at ease
- using plain language and avoiding jargon
- being clear on the purpose of the community's participation, what form of participation is appropriate, and when to involve participants.

Source: Geekiyanage et al. (2020)

Coalitions, community partnerships and community collaboratives are increasingly being seen as a viable vehicle to create population-wide, macro-level changes (Woodall and Cross, 2021). However, involving communities in coalitions and partnerships with statutory agencies is generally premised on the view that problems in relation to involvement are likely to be due to reluctance on the part of the community. Nair and Campbell (2008), importantly, remind us that the converse can be the case. The Entabeni project (see Case study 9.4), for example, experienced difficulty in mobilizing external partners and found that:

> Most often it is the external partners – particularly those in the public and private sectors – that lack the capacity or skills or organisational systems that would enable them to support the community responses. Our experience is directly in contrast to that presented in the general literature about community development, which often depicts willing and able partners battling to mobilise reluctant communities. (Nair and Campbell, 2008: 51)

CASE STUDY 9.4 THE ENTABENI PROJECT

The Entabeni project was conceived by local people in a remote rural community in South Africa. Local health volunteers provided assistance to the large numbers of people with AIDS in this deprived community. A three-year project was set up with an NGO to strengthen the community's response.

It aimed:

to empower local volunteers to lead HIV-prevention and AIDS-care,

and

to make public services more responsive to local needs. (Nair and Campbell, 2008: 45)

The role of the external change agent was to 'facilitate grassroots community responses to AIDS' (2008: 50). They also provided bridging social capital.

The project was successful in providing training for health volunteers in home-based care, peer education, project management and procedures for obtaining grants and services.

One year into the project, attempts to mobilize public and private organizations as partners was proving to be more challenging.

Source: See Nair and Campbell (2008) for more details

Progress was assessed using Campbell's (2003) criteria for effective partners:

- commitment to HIV/AIDS management and partnership
- conceptualization of HIV/AIDS as a social/developmental issue
- mechanisms for partner accountability to target communities
- incentives to be involved in partnership
- agency capacity.

Particular difficulties included the absence of formal systems to ensure accountability to service users, along with limited capacity due to shortages of funding and trained personnel. Over and above addressing these issues, Nair and Campbell identify the need for positive morale and confidence among prospective partners and the institutionalization of partner roles.

COMMUNITY HEALTH PROJECTS: EXAMPLES

There are clearly numerous different types of community projects. By way of example, we will briefly consider two drawn from opposite ends of the spectrum of participation.

Community-wide health worker interventions

One of the main resources in community health projects are the community members themselves. Community projects aim to involve local people and tap their interest, expertise and enthusiasm. This involvement could emerge spontaneously, or it can come about through a deliberate programme of recruitment of volunteers (Hubley et al., 2021). There is increasing interest within health promotion in community-based health worker (CHW) programmes (Scott et al., 2018). While these types of interventions have always been a mainstay of health promotion activity, there is increasing recognition of the importance of such approaches to tackle health inequalities (Woodall and Cross, 2021).

A systematic review (Scott et al., 2018) assessed the evidence and impact of CHW programmes looking at evidence spanning a 12-year period in low-, middle- and high-income countries. Most of the literature identified was focused on LMICs and a range of primary healthcare, child health, and maternal and child health interventions. The evidence within high-income countries focused on non-communicable diseases and reaching specific underserved groups. Interventions tended to be categorized into six modes of delivery:

1. Deliver diagnostic, treatment, and other clinical services.
2. Assist with appropriate utilization of health services.
3. Provide health education and behaviour change motivation to community members.
4. Collect and record data.
5. Improve relationships between health services and communities.
6. Provide psychosocial support.

Supervision and training were consistently recognized as key mechanisms for the success of CHW programmes, but the evidence did not always report specific or sufficient examples of how either of these activities were undertaken. A further aspect which increased the likelihood of success of the programmes was the 'embeddedness' of CHWs and their abilities to build rapport and connect within the community. CHWs who were trusted and respected as well as identifying from the same community as the recipients of the intervention were particularly powerful.

The review concluded that CHW programmes in high-, middle- and low-income countries contribute to improving a range of health outcomes for individuals and community groups. That said, the outcomes were not always clear and robust (Scott et al., 2018). It may not be unreasonable to speculate that the limited success of some of these well-designed interventions has something to do with failure to address fundamental structural issues and the root social and political determinants of the problem.

Social action and health activism

At the other end of the spectrum are social action and health activism projects, which were touched upon earlier in the chapter. Health activism encompasses community development models of community participation, but is also an example of a social movement and, in some instances, an attempt to build a new social order (Warwick-Booth and Foster, 2021). Health social movements (HSMs) vary considerably in their focus and form. In health promotion, there has been interest in constituency-based HSMs such as the women's health movement, or grassroots-based organizations and community development projects addressing local health problems (Warwick-Booth and Foster, 2021). There are several examples of health activism and community mobilization to effect social and political change. Analysis undertaken by Ribero-Almandoz and Clua-Losada (2021) focused on Marea Blanca (White Tide) in Madrid and Keep Our NHS Public in Greater Manchester – two activism initiatives aimed to foster community mobilization and to prevent healthcare privatization. The research showed how these movements focused on local contexts and individual healthcare sites, bringing their campaign closer to local communities. This created a tangible recognition of the potential impact of privatization in local areas and was effective in garnering more support and more mobilization of individuals. Keep Our NHS Public launched Health Campaigns Together (HCT), which was an alliance of over 100 local campaign groups, trade union branches and political parties opposed to NHS privatizations, budget cuts and closures. The alliance established solidarity and heightened awareness about the impact on public health and social care services due to underfunding and privatization processes. The authors concluded that both campaigns:

> developed localised and territorially rooted forms of mobilisation, which have been useful means for the construction and strengthening of community relations by connecting workers, activists and neighbours through their everyday needs and demands, and have allowed for the experimentation with forms of grassroots organisation, collective deliberation, and horizontal decision making. (Ribero-Almandoz and Clua-Losada, 2021: 190)

Catalani et al. (2012) describe a project implemented in New Orleans after Hurricane Katrina had left much of the region in a state of disarray. The New Orleans Videovoice project was a community-based participatory research (CBPR) project and documentary film response to growing demands from communities for voice, leadership and action based on their needs while reflecting their assets. Using a videovoice method, a community–academic–filmmaker partnership engaged members of the community, who took part in an 18-week training and community assessment. The partnership produced a 22-minute film that was premiered before more than 200 city leaders and residents and reached more than 4000 YouTube viewers during its first two months online. Viewing the film further helped mobilize the community for action on three priority issues: affordable housing, education and economic development.

CHALLENGES AND DILEMMAS

We have argued that health initiatives that actively engage communities in partnership are consistent with the principles of health promotion and particularly the empowerment model that we have advocated. However, in practice, a number of challenges arise.

A key issue is the role of community health workers. The rhetoric of community development would support the use of non-directive approaches whenever possible. Yet there are situations when more directive approaches may be called for, either to meet the needs of the target group, to suit the stage of the project, or to achieve externally or professionally defined outcomes. For example, the most marginalized and powerless groups may not have their voice heard unless health workers adopt an advocacy or activist role or focus on capacity-building. The important issue is that directive approaches should not further disempower these groups by creating dependency, but rather that they should actively contribute to empowering them.

Boutilier et al. (2000) point out that community development workers may initially occupy a position of power vis-à-vis those with whom they are working by virtue of greater income, professional status and their ability to influence political agendas. However, exercising this power becomes 'transformative' if the process enables community members to acquire power as a consequence. As the authors note, this transfer of power classically results in community workers working themselves out of a job. Their role will change through the course of an initiative from being directive at the outset to becoming progressively non-directive as the community assumes control. Indeed, a review of empowerment and its impact on health and well-being suggests that practitioners can help to create situations where empowerment is likely through helping people build confidence or by facilitating groups and that efforts need to be made to promote equal relationships between professionals and communities (Woodall et al., 2010).

Clearly, it is incumbent on community health workers to ensure that all members of the community and diverse interest groups are represented. Their ability to do so will depend on their understanding of the community and insight into the factors that would encourage the participation of different groups – issues that should inform initial planning. Some groups will be more able to participate than others. Ongoing critical reflection to assess the extent to which initiatives are successful in engaging different groups is essential and strategies should be put in place to reach out to under-represented groups. Nonetheless, the views of more powerful groups may come to dominate. NICE (2008: 23) notes the need to:

> Recognise that some groups and individuals (from the public, community and voluntary sectors) may have their own agendas and could monopolise groups (so inhibiting community engagement).

Situations may also arise when the priorities and needs expressed by the community may differ from those of professionals. Bolam (2005: 447) notes that while lay people have a complex understanding of health, there is a tendency, especially in lower social groups, to focus on 'agency and strength of character' rather than structurally orientated explanations of health inequalities. Furthermore, there is concern among these groups about the 'potential stigma associated with being seen as a victim'. Clearly, then, there may be a conflict of interest between professionals seeking to engage in social action to tackle the upstream structural determinants and some community groups that may prefer more downstream solutions. Commitment to evidence-based practice may also prove to be problematic if the evidence conflicts with the community's views.

There is no easy answer to resolving these issues. Bolam suggests that media advocacy may be needed at the outset to raise awareness of the social determinants of health among such community groups. Yet again, this implies the need for initial paternalistic interventions and assumes that professionals have greater overall strategic insight. We will consider the issue of professionals attempting to subtly influence the agenda to conform with their own views – so-called facipulation – in the following subsection. Commitment to the principles of community development would demand that all positions are respected, fully discussed, additional information sought and a collective decision reached by democratic processes.

There is a view that collective decisions and action can militate against individual freedom of choice and action. We argued in Chapter 1 that an unbridled free-for-all is inconsistent with the values of health promotion. While individuals have the right to self-fulfilment, this should not be at the expense of the rights of others and the well-being of the community more generally. The overarching principle is that fundamental human rights must be respected, whether or not they are recognized by specific groups. Clearly, prejudice and discriminatory practice in all its forms should be challenged.

Gilding the ghetto? Some limitations of community development

Although criticisms have been directed at community-based health work that operates in a top-down fashion with predetermined agendas, it cannot be assumed that community development is a panacea for addressing social-structural health problems. Indeed, although an advocate of community development, Constantino-David (1982) provides a very thoughtful critique, listing the following limitations and potential threats:

- Community members are at risk of becoming dependent on the community workers and when the workers withdraw and/or funding is withdrawn, the project collapses.
- A new elite might be created from indigenous workers/opinion leaders recruited by change agents.
- Community workers may face a dilemma: the community's felt needs may be relatively insignificant in the long term and more fundamental goals, such as empowerment or political change, may be deferred or ignored.
- Following on from this last point, community workers must be on their guard to avoid imposing their own political agenda on the community. They therefore face a 'facilitation vs manipulation' dilemma. Their role is to facilitate community decision-making in the interest of empowerment. They may, however, yield to the temptation to manipulate or subtly steer the community in the direction of their own choosing. Constantino-David refers to this process as 'facipulation'.

A more important question mark hanging over community development is whether or not it can really have any significant influence on major structural problems such as inequality. The activities of communities and their successes have been described by such metaphors as 'rearranging the deck-chairs on the *Titanic*'. Loney (1981), for example, makes this point when referring to the report of the Community Development Project (1977) (referred to in Case study 9.2), which was aptly titled 'Gilding the Ghetto'.

Rahman (1995: 32) discusses the problems associated with the failure of successive approaches to Third World development initiatives and comments specifically on what he describes as a 'new worldwide culture of development action termed "popular participation in development" or simply "participatory development"'. He has strong reservations about small-scale participatory efforts that 'seem to be serving the purpose mainly of providing a "safety net" and do not promise fundamental movement toward people's liberation' and do not reflect 'the values of social activism, building towards a more genuinely participatory approach to transformation'.

Serrano-Garcia (1984) discusses the effect of a community development programme in Esfuerzo, a poor rural community in Puerto Rico, and asks the questions, 'Did our intervention facilitate the empowerment of the residents of Esfuerzo? What are the limits of empowerment efforts within our colonial context?' Serrano-Garcia (1984: 197) concludes that:

> the community members had gained new skills, feelings of competency, and insights that should enable them to achieve greater control over some aspects of their community life. [They would probably have] … a different, more affirmative, perspective on their role in their community.

Her writing, however, reflects concern that they might have 'fostered the illusion' that their society enables empowerment. She then questions the possibility of creating real social change using community development techniques. Her (1984: 197–8) review of the nature of the society, its power structure and barriers to change is illuminating and iterates the recurring observations we have made throughout this book:

> I am convinced that our society does not allow [empowerment]. Ours is a society which, along with the economic and political facts previously presented, is characterized by an ideology of conservatism and pro-American values. These emphasize (a) an electoral definition of democracy, (b) the prevalence of a conservative vision of law and order, (c) uncritical acceptance of United States dominance over Puerto Rico, (d) rigid value stances that acknowledge only clear-cut definitions of right and wrong, (e) individualism, (f) veneration of the right to private property, (g) the belief in the governmental duty to protect this right, (h) protection of the free market, and (i) intolerance toward dissidence … demonstrated through the constant and active persecution of pro-independence group members.

In higher-income countries, considerable support has been expressed for the potential contribution of participation to tackling inequality in health. The particular relevance of participation of communities to tackling health inequalities includes:

1. Developing an understanding of priorities for health and well-being.
2. Enabling people to take greater control of their health, both individually and collectively.

3. Taking part in decision-making can help the most excluded groups feel that they have more con-
    trol, decrease their sense of loneliness and isolation and enhance self-esteem.
4. Policy-makers can draw on local expertise to achieve better decisions and make genuine and
    meaningful relationships with local people.
5. Using the expertise of community and voluntary groups to deliver some public services can be
    more successful in reaching vulnerable and excluded groups. (Hill-Dixon, 2019; Smith, 2007)

Bentley (2008) includes in the 10 major lessons learned to date about tackling health inequalities the
need to 'capitalise on community engagement' and specifically to:

> Support local authority partners in the development of neighbourhood and community infrastruc-
> tures to engage residents, particularly those 'seldom seen, seldom heard' in services. Use [community
> engagement] to ensure that services are responsive to needs, but also to help motivate and support
> appropriate health-seeking behaviour. Establish effective links with frontline services, utilising the
> potential of VCF [voluntary, community and faith] sector agencies as valuable catalysts for dialogue,
> mutual understanding and empowerment. (2008: 5)

While in no way undermining the undoubted value of participation and engagement, the general
tenor of all of these documents is located within the mainstream and lacks the radical edge required
to address the primary determinants of health inequalities. Ledwith (2020) argues that those involved
in community development are allowing themselves to be redefined as a tool of government policy
at the expense of their transformative purpose. As Dixon (1989: 84) observed some time ago, unless
it can be redefined to become more politically aware and radical, community development is unlikely
to bring about necessary fundamental change in society to address 'class, race or gender struggles to
transform the existing economic and power structures' – such sentiments might equally be applied to
health promotion more generally (Woodall et al., 2012a). Bridgen (2007: 257) notes that any attempt
to genuinely empower communities, as opposed to capacity-building or developing social capital,
must involve 'some attempt to increase the influence of the community over the external policy developments that affect it'. Attention must, therefore, be paid to '(i) the relationship between community
empowerment programmes and their external political environment, and (ii) the types of processes
that would be required if the former was significantly to alter the latter' (2007: 263).

It is our intention below to consider how community health programmes can contribute to wider
development and social action goals.

DEVISING COMMUNITY PROGRAMMES FOR DEVELOPMENT AND SOCIAL ACTION

We noted above the importance of shared awareness of health issues for mobilizing communities and,
indeed, potential partners. Bracht et al. (1999: 85) describe stimulation or activation as the process by
which a community:

- becomes aware of a condition or problem that exists within a community
- identifies that condition as a priority of community action

- institutes steps to change the condition
- establishes structures to implement and maintain programme solutions.

A Freirean perspective

As we noted in our general discussion of critical education in Chapter 7, Freirean approaches provide quite detailed suggestions for practice and these are consistent with community development principles.

Kindervatter (1979) asks if it is really possible to empower, 'in political settings not committed or even antagonistic to a more equitable sharing of power and resources?' She also raises the important question of the 'balance of power between conflicting parties' and the need for confrontation by less powerful parties. She (1979: 240) makes an important cultural point, too – namely, that cultural norms in the two projects that she studied were inimical to confrontation:

> Confrontation has been employed by some groups in Asian contexts, such as squatters in the Philippines, but only in reaction to grossly oppressive conditions. In most cases, people would probably seek other means to solve a problem, and if that failed, possibly leave the problem unsolved.

She observes that although some gains were achieved in the Thai and Indonesian projects, 'these gains were not those which significantly altered existing power structures or relationships'. In those countries:

> people know that posing real challenges to the political or economic system can have serious consequences [and] people themselves must balance the possible risks and sacrifices with achieving a particular gain, and decide what course of action to follow.

An expanded model of community development is needed to take account of these several difficulties. It also needs to emphasize the importance of identifying ways to actively support community members' commitment to action. Figure 9.5 seeks to identify key elements of this expanded model.

In short, community workers act as catalysts and occupy a kind of combined counselling and catalyst role. They employ such typical counselling skills as active listening and providing reflective feedback and act in accordance with the 'holy trinity' of counselling – demonstrating respect, empathy and genuineness. Their credibility and perceived status is clearly important. As we noted in our earlier discussion of communication of innovations theory, the quality of homophily is important in establishing a trusting relationship.

The major feature of this expanded model of community development centres on the kinds of support provided to the dialogic process of consciousness-raising and praxis. Before the action plans resulting from praxis can be translated into successful actions, community members will need a range of appropriate life skills and action competences if they are to work effectively in groups, act as lobbyists and deploy a range of other confrontational techniques.

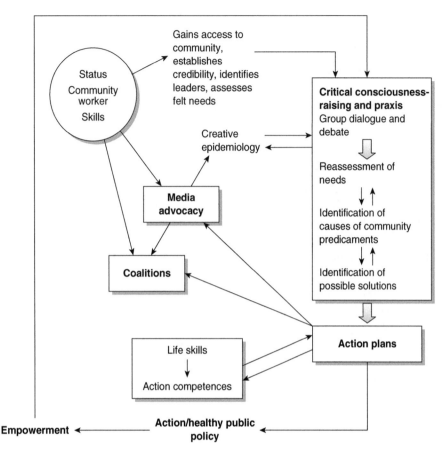

Figure 9.5 An expanded model of community development to include advocacy, praxis and healthy public policy

Media advocacy – following the precepts described in Chapter 8 and associated with Wallack's (1980) formulation – enables community activists to raise consciousness in the community as a whole. They might, for instance, use media messages based on creative epidemiology or, as described by Wang and Burris (1994), create their own images of community life and predicaments using photography. As Wallack and others have demonstrated, media advocacy is typically associated with the development of coalitions of like-minded people, both within and outside the community. Although the main focus of action might be on a relatively small scale, such as the development of food cooperatives or credit unions, by collaborating with broader-based coalitions, local communities may contribute to a more substantial movement for addressing issues such as health inequalities. As Taylor (1995: 109–10) remarks:

> it is likely that in a more fragmented 'postmodern' environment, networks and alliances will be the foundation on which empowerment is built. Community work needs to develop a practice which can work with allies across the institutional map to find the possibilities for change in an increasingly turbulent environment.

BOX 9.4   THE EXPERT'S TASK

Experts should be on tap not on top!

Source: Kindervatter (1979)

The educational dimension

One of the main themes of this book is our assertion that education (broadly defined) is at the epicentre of health promotion. Its contribution to community development and its variants are probably self-evident. However, Kindervatter's philosophy and practice is of particular interest as she more or less equates community development/organization with what she calls 'non-formal education'. She (1979: 87–8) defines community development as:

- attempting to build local capability by nurturing grassroots organizations and creating coalitions of organizations
- utilizing natural groups or structures
- starting from people's interests and moving at their pace
- emphasizing the identification and development of 'native' leaders – that is, opinion leaders
- promoting peer support and mutual help
- having an open-ended agenda and aiming to activate people to work together
- building cooperative community problem-solving capacity and a power base from which existing power relationships can be confronted
- emphasizing discussion methods, democratic procedures and action
- having an organizer who serves as a 'process guide' and resource person
- enabling the transfer of initiative and responsibility from community worker to the people to achieve local autonomy.

The *raison d'être* of non-formal education (NFE) is identical to the WHO's definition of empowerment as people gaining control over their lives (and their health) or, in Kindervatter's words, gaining 'understanding of and control over social, economic, and/or political forces'. Its methodology includes small group 'teaching' with a community worker as a facilitator rather than instructor, the transfer of responsibility from teacher to participants and an emphasis on participant leadership, as well as the integration of reflection and action (praxis).

We have already discussed the radical philosophy of Freire's empowering educational approach and its imperative for sociopolitical change in pursuit of equity. Kindervatter (1979: 149) incorporates Freire's principles and practice, together with those of Charnofsky (1971), Curle (1972) and Wren (1977), and summarizes them under the rubric 'education for justice' (see Box 9.5):

- development of critical consciousness
- small group discussion (culture circles)

- utilization of a problem stimulus for circle members to decode
- utilization of tools, such as games, to help people reflect on their realities
- a focus on 'system blame' rather than 'person blame' as a cause of problems
- the aim to achieve conflict resolution with a win–win outcome
- emphasis on non-hierarchical methods and relationships, dialogue and shared leadership
- utilization of facilitators who are committed to liberation, have faith in people, are humble and who act primarily as problem and question posers.

BOX 9.5 EDUCATION FOR JUSTICE

Justice calls for the establishment of a society on both a global and national scale where each person has an equal right to the most extensive basic liberties compatible with a like liberty for all, where social and economic inequalities are so arranged that they are to the greatest benefit of the least advantaged, and where they are linked with position and appointments which are open to all through fair equality of opportunity.

Source: Wren (1977: 55)

Ledwith (2007) emphasizes the need for community development to be both critical and vigilant to retain its radical edge and concern for social justice rather than 'slipping into some feel-good, ameliorative, sticking plaster on the wounds of injustice'. She argues that:

> the full collective potential of community development is threatened by a resistance to praxis, a theory–practice divide which results in 'actionless thought' on one hand, and 'thoughtless action' on the other (Johnston, cited in Shaw, 2004: 26). If we fail to generate theory in action, and move towards a unity of praxis where theory and practice are synthesised, we give way to anti- intellectual times which emphasize 'doing' at the expense of 'thinking'; we react to the symptoms rather than root causes of injustice – and leave the structures of discrimination intact – dividing people through poverty, creating massively different life chances by blaming the victims of an unjust system.

KEY POINTS

- Understanding the nature of community and the characteristics of specific communities is fundamental to community health work.
- Community health work can be broadly divided into working in communities to achieve externally defined targets or working with communities to enable them to identify their own targets and the best means of achieving them.
- Notwithstanding problems with terminology, we have identified a number of features that characterize community health work. Key among these is the extent to which communities actively participate in decision-making and whether the focus is on achieving social action to address the structural determinants of health.

- Efforts to engage communities should pay particular attention to ensuring that disadvantaged and socially excluded groups are able to participate and have their voices heard.
- Initiatives that involve communities can serve a range of purposes, from improving service provision and achieving behaviour change through to tackling the structural determinants of health and radical social change.
- Practitioners working with communities should have a clear view of their goals and should reflect critically on the process, particularly in respect to power relationships.
- Education has a central role in community development/empowerment that includes increasing the capacity to participate and consciousness-raising leading to praxis.
- Community development is an important means of achieving empowerment, equity and tackling social injustice. It requires a critical approach, rooted in the core values of mutual respect and cooperation.

CHAPTER 9: INTERNATIONAL CASE STUDIES

The following case studies on the online resources website are relevant to the content of this chapter: 1, 2, 4, 8 and 9.

CRITICAL REFLECTION AND APPLICATION TO PRACTICE

This chapter has emphasized the importance of working with communities as an essential strategy for health promotion practice. The notion of 'community' is continually evolving – evident none more so than through virtual environments. To what extent does or has your practice evolved to capture less traditional (geographic) ideas of community? How could current health promotion practice shift to encompass this? One of the salient threads through the chapter has been the idea of empowerment as a cornerstone of working with communities. In what ways have the radical roots of empowerment been diluted and is this problematic? In what ways have empowerment approaches been superseded in practice by behavioural or lifestyle approaches?

ONLINE RESOURCES

Please visit https://study.sagepub.com/greentones5e for all the online resources for the book, including recommended further reading on each chapter subject, useful weblinks (both introduced by the authors), as well as the abovementioned case study material.

10 SETTINGS FOR HEALTH

Change is not made without inconvenience, even from worse to better.

Samuel Johnson (1780–4)

OVERVIEW

This chapter focuses on the settings approach. It will:

- identify key elements of the settings approach, drawing on examples from a range of different settings
- consider factors supportive of the successful implementation of the settings approach
- focus on the health-promoting prison to exemplify the settings approach in more depth
- make further observations about different settings for health.

INTRODUCTION

We have already considered macro-level strategies for influencing health, notably policy and mass media. At the meso level, we have also considered community-based approaches. While the community might well be regarded as a setting for health, in Chapter 9, we focused on issues relating to community development and empowerment. We now turn our attention to the settings approach itself.

The emergence of the 'settings approach' has generally been attributed to the Ottawa Charter's (WHO, 1986) assertion that: 'health is created and lived by people within the settings of their everyday life; where they learn, work, play and love' (redefined as: 'created in the settings of everyday life – in the neighbourhoods and communities where people live, love, work, shop and play' [WHO, 2016a]). The approach has been purported to be one of the most successful strategies to emerge from the Ottawa Charter (Torp et al., 2014) and one of the 'fundamental international foundations of health promotion' (Kokko et al., 2014: 495). It has most recently also been argued to be a viable vehicle to addressing the challenges and recovery from COVID-19 (Woodall, 2020a). The settings approach involves a shift from individual behavioural approaches towards considering the contribution of major settings to health. Not only do settings impact directly on health and well-being, but individual choices about health and health behaviour are taken in the settings encountered in day-to-day life – the home, community, workplace and school (WHO, 1999). As Kickbusch (1996: 5) notes, the settings approach shifts 'the focus from the deficit model of disease to the health potentials inherent in the social and institutional settings of everyday life', reiterating the fact that health is produced outside of illness (health) services and that effective health improvements require investment in social systems (Dooris, 2004).

Commitment to the settings approach has been both explicitly and implicitly evident in several WHO conferences on health promotion. For example, it was strongly endorsed by the Jakarta Declaration (WHO, 1997), in the Nairobi Call to Action (WHO, 2009) and the global health promotion conference in Shanghai (WHO, 2016a) where there was a reaffirmation that health was created in everyday settings.

THE SETTINGS FOR HEALTH APPROACH

It is self-evident that access to individuals or groups is a fundamental requirement for health education. The opportunity afforded by different settings for gaining entry has, therefore, been of considerable interest. The vast majority of settings do not have 'health' as their main mission or *raison d'être* – indeed we have observed this in the COVID-19 pandemic where settings were having to trade off between their primary goal (perhaps economic growth) and health (Dooris and Baybutt, 2021). It is therefore pertinent to think carefully about access to the setting prior to any engagement. Key questions for assessing a setting are provided in Box 10.1.

BOX 10.1   KEY QUESTIONS FOR WORKING IN SETTINGS

Regarding access

- What kind of target group is accessible via this setting?
- How many people will be reached?
- How easy will it be to reach them?

Regarding the philosophy and purpose

- Has the institution with which the strategy is associated a particular philosophy or goal?

Regarding commitment

- How committed are the institution and its members to the preventive philosophy underpinning the aims (of health education)?

Regarding credibility

- How credible are the institution and the people in it who will act as health educators? How will the public respond to them?

Regarding competence

- Irrespective of commitment, do the potential health educators have the necessary knowledge and communication/education/training skills to promote efficient learning?

Source: After Whitehead and Tones (1990: 19–20)

However, there is an important distinction to be made between seeing a setting merely as a location that offers opportunities for delivering health education – that is, 'health education in a setting' – and the 'settings for health approach', which involves a more comprehensive and coordinated response. A key feature of the settings approach is that it involves ensuring that the ethos of the setting and all the activities are mutually supportive and combine synergistically to improve the health and well-being of those who live, or work, or receive care there. It involves adopting an ecological approach in which the whole environment and culture are committed to promoting health in a coherent and integrated manner (Tones, 2001).

To illustrate the difference, Table 10.1 provides a comparison of health education provided in a school and the health-promoting school.

Table 10.1 Moving from traditional school health education to the health-promoting school

Traditional health education	The health-promoting school
Considers health education only in limited classroom terms	Takes a wider view, including all aspects of the life of the school and its relationship with the community - for example, developing the school as a caring community
Emphasizes personal hygiene and physical health to the exclusion of the wider aspects of health	Based on a model of health that includes the interaction of physical, mental, social and environmental aspects
Concentrates on health instruction and acquisition of facts	Focuses on active pupil participation with a wide range of methods, developing pupils' skills

(Continued)

Table 10.1   (Continued)

Traditional health education	The health-promoting school
Lacks a coherent, coordinated approach that takes account of other influences on pupils	Recognizes the wide range of influences on pupils' health and attempts to take account of pupils' pre-existing values, beliefs and attitudes
Tends to respond to a series of perceived problems or crises on a one-off basis	Recognizes that many underlying skills and processes are common to all health issues and that these should be pre-planned as part of the curriculum
Takes limited account of psychosocial factors in relation to health behaviour	Views the development of positive self-image and individuals taking increasing control of their lives as central to the promotion of good health
Recognizes the importance of the school and its environment only to a limited extent	Recognizes the importance of the physical environment of the school in terms of aesthetics and also direct physiological effects on pupils and staff
Does not consider actively the health and well-being of staff in the school	Views health promotion in the school as relevant to staff well-being and recognizes the exemplar role of staff
Does not involve parents actively in the development of a health education programme	Considers parental support and cooperation as central to the health-promoting school
Views the role of school health services purely in terms of health screening and disease prevention	Takes a wider view of the school health services, which includes screening and disease prevention, but also attempts actively to integrate services within the health education curriculum and helps pupils to become more aware as consumers of health services

Source: Young and Williams (1989: 32)

Extending and moving the arguments forward in health promotion efforts in schools, Ewert (2017) has compared the health-promoting school principle with recent efforts to use 'nudge tactics' (see Chapter 3) in school to influence the health and behavioural choices (see Table 10.2). Ewert (2017) notes the shortcomings in 'nudging' and concludes that more holistic, participatory and inclusive approaches to address health in schools – characterized by settings-based health promotion – are better suited.

Creating health-promoting settings remains a crucial strategy for achieving the United Nations Development Agenda 2030 and its Sustainable Development Goals (WHO, 2016a). Cities were particularly cited as one of the key settings for achieving population health and well-being. The healthy cities movement is perhaps the longest-standing and most researched of all the settings. The idea emerged almost simultaneously with the establishment of the Ottawa Charter in the mid-1980s, with cities regarded as one of the key ways in which the pillars of the Ottawa Charter could be operationalized (Woodall and Cross, 2021). In short, the rationale for establishing healthy cities is that 'people's physical, mental and social wellbeing is the core business of cities' (International Institute for Global Health, 2018: 150). There are Healthy Cities Networks in all six WHO regions – in the European region, for example, there are now over 1400 healthy cities and towns as members and in Asia, the

Alliance for Healthy Cities (AFHC) coordinates information exchange and good practice in this region (Hu and Kuo, 2016). The principles of the approach have been applied to other settings – some of them linked internationally via WHO networks (see Box 10.2).

Table 10.2 Comparison of the settings approach versus nudge in health promotion (adapted from Ewert, 2017)

	The health-promoting school	Nudge tactics in school
Definition of health	Open - up to collective deliberation; depending on the particularities of the respective setting	Predefined by policy-makers and largely in line with biomedical concepts
Scope of health issues to be addressed	Holistic (including political, administrative, economical, sociocultural and spatial layers of health)	Selective (addressing single behavioural health issues)
Strategy of health promotion	Applying behavioural and structural change through collective action within (a) predefined setting(s)	Changing individual behaviour by modifying environment-bound health choices
Conception of subjects	Reasonable citizens able to learn, reflect and deliberate collectively	Duped consumers prone to erroneous decisions and non-reflective behaviour
Role of policy-makers	Facilitators and mediators, creating new spaces for multi-stakeholder and citizen participation	Experts and choice architects, exercising 'governance by stealth'

BOX 10.2 EXAMPLES OF SETTINGS FOR HEALTH

- Healthy cities
- Healthy villages
- Healthy islands
- Health-promoting hospitals
- Health-promoting schools
- Health-promoting prisons
- Healthy marketplaces
- Workplace health promotion
- Virtual settings.

Dooris (2006) notes that settings occupy different levels that may be nested within each other or have cross-links with other settings. A setting is not a discrete entity, but exists as part of a wider interconnected system (Corcoran and Bone, 2007; Naidoo and Wills, 2000) as demonstrated within the ecological theory of development proposed by Bronfenbrenner (1977). For example, health-promoting schools may exist within healthy cities and be linked to healthy communities, operating somewhat like 'Russian dolls' (Dooris, 2006: 3). Broadly speaking, there are two categories of settings: 'contextual settings' – cities, communities, families – those seen as being difficult to define with fluid boundaries and undefined structures; and 'elemental settings' – marketplaces, schools, workplaces, hospitals, prisons, universities, nightclubs, sports clubs, airports – which often have more easily defined physical boundaries, rules and structures (Woodall and Cross, 2021).

A range of terms have been used to identify settings-based health promotion with much of the semantic differences being unintentional, and with terms often used interchangeably (Woodall and Cross, 2021). The terms used for health promotion in higher education has differed internationally, for example. Europe and Latin America use the phrase 'health-promoting universities', in the UK 'healthy universities' and in the USA a mixture of 'healthy campus' or 'healthy campus community' is used (Sarmiento, 2017). While the semantic differences may seem trivial, commentators have argued for greater clarity on the etymology (Barić, 1998; Dooris, 2006; Kokko et al., 2013). Kokko et al. (2014: 499), for example, argue for an examination of the differences between a 'healthy setting' and 'health-promoting setting'. The former term, they suggest, gives the indication of a static or ideal setting; however, in their view, no such setting can be continuously healthful. In contrast, the term 'health-promoting setting' invokes 'the dynamic and conditional nature of health promotion activities and conditions and the process of making them healthful' – it does not assume a permanent healthy state but, rather, considers the actions necessary continuously to adapt the setting to changing circumstances.

A key consideration is who is left out of a settings approach and recent concerns have again been raised in relation to the potential for settings approaches to increase inequities (Newman et al., 2015). Clearly, settings have limited potential for reaching the unemployed, those who do not or cannot attend school (and, even within schools, those who feel alienated are less likely to be influenced) and the homeless – that is, the most disadvantaged groups in society and those who have the greatest health needs. Green et al. (2000: 25) contend that:

> health promotion has chosen to privilege some settings (e.g. workplaces, schools, communities) as being more 'legitimate' sites of practice than others (e.g. bingo halls, nightclubs, street corners, public washrooms and other 'sites of resistance').

If the settings approach is to avoid the risk of increasing the health gap in society, it will need to address the needs of marginalized groups and include unconventional and challenging settings. This would potentially offer those once marginalized by a settings approach to have an opportunity to address key determinants of their health. The exponential growth of the Internet, and social media particularly, has created opportunities for health promotion to locate in 'virtual' settings (Cross et al., 2017a). Technological enhancements and online communication have revolutionized the way many of us live our lives. Work, education, leisure and social interaction have increasingly moved away from geographically bounded locations to the virtual world. Indeed, research shows that people spend more time interacting each day virtually than in person (Verduyn et al., 2017). Many people now work from home, enrol on distance learning courses, or spend leisure time in online communities (Loss et al., 2014). The reality is that we now live in a fast-paced, 24-hour world, where people demand instantaneous information via their smartphones, tablets, laptops and computers. Given this context, it is clear that health promoters must embrace this and consider the virtual space as a legitimate setting for health. Social media may also have the advantage of reaching those who may not easily access 'traditional' health information in crisis situations. Research is showing, for example, the advantage of social media for disease surveillance and control – particular examples include the use of social media to communicate information regarding Ebola, natural disasters, Avian Bird Flu and influenza. This approach provides real-time information and support that can easily be followed using the newsfeed on social media sites (Woodall and Cross, 2021).

A setting has been defined as:

> where people actively use and shape the environment and thus create, or solve problems relating to, health. Settings can normally be identified as having physical boundaries, a range of people with defined roles, and an organizational structure. (Nutbeam, 1998a: 362)

Green et al. (2000: 23) draw on critical theory to provide a broader conceptualization. They caution against taking a simple, instrumental view of settings as neutral, self-contained environments that have 'target audiences' and argue that settings are more than 'physically bounded space–times in which people come together to perform specific tasks (usually oriented to goals other than health)'. A good example is the increased use of online settings for health and social connection as discussed earlier (Newman et al., 2015). Dooris (2013), through his research with an elite sample of interviewees pivotal to the evolution of the settings approach, has perhaps further extended the concept of a setting. His research suggests that settings must connect 'outwards', 'upwards' and 'beyond' health if the approach is to be successful. Connecting 'outwards' relates to settings working in joined-up ways in order to appreciate the interconnectedness between the places where individuals live their lives and to embrace the complexity of health issues that do not respect physical boundaries. To date, work between settings has not been successful and this is perhaps best exemplified in the criminal justice system, where research suggests that the transition that individuals make from the prison setting to the community can be potentially complex and often detrimental to health (Woodall et al., 2013a). Connecting 'upwards' is ensuring that broader political, economic and social factors are being addressed through settings programmes effectively developing advocacy and lobbying roles (Dooris, 2013). St Leger (1997: 101), for example, argues that when adopting a settings framework, there is a requirement always to stay with 'the big picture' and indeed health-promoting schools have been involved in local planning and national decision-making on issues related to health. Finally, connecting 'beyond health' concerns settings making connections with parallel agendas to maximize their contribution to health and well-being; for example, a greater understanding of the way in which settings can link to sustainable development agendas and the interconnections between settings and the health of the planet (Poland and Dooris, 2010):

> Global issues are fundamental for settings-based health promotion as well; climate change, peak oil and environmental degradation are concerns of everyone. (Kokko et al., 2014: 502)

The variability of activity under the rubric of health-promoting settings poses the question: 'What then is enough for a setting to be called health promoting?' (Kokko et al., 2014: 500). Barić (1993) suggests that, in order to achieve the status of a health-promoting setting, the following conditions should be met:

- the creation of a healthy working and living environment
- the integration of health promotion into the daily activities of the setting
- the creation of conditions for reaching out into the community.

The settings literature does not suggest one underpinning theory informing the approach (Dooris, 2013), but it is clear that settings-based health promotion is consistent with an ecological view of health. Bronfenbrenner (1977) proposed an ecological theory of development that has been relevant to the design of ecological models applied in health promotion. In this framework, behaviour is viewed as being affected by, and affecting, multiple levels of influence (McLeroy et al., 1988). Bronfenbrenner describes these multiple levels as the micro-, meso-, exo- and macrosystem levels. The microsystem refers to face-to-face influences in specific settings, for example, the home, school or workplace. The mesosystem is the system of microsystems and pertains to the interrelations among the various settings in which the individual is involved (McLeroy et al., 1988). The exosystem refers to forces within the larger social system in which the individual is embedded. Finally, the macrosystem refers to the overarching institutional patterns of the culture or subculture that influence both the microsystem and the mesosystem (Bronfenbrenner, 1977). Green et al. (2000: 16) contend that the settings approach sees health as dependent on the interaction between 'individuals and subsystems of the ecosystem'. The settings approach, therefore, offers the potential for shaping these elements to maximize health gain. It shifts the goals away from specific behaviour change towards creating the conditions that are supportive of health and well-being more generally, with a corresponding shift in focus of activity from risk factors and population groups towards organizational change. In this respect, the settings philosophy challenges a neoliberal, individualistic view of health promotion and, when executed in a way that is consistent with the original theoretical roots, is 'explicitly determinants focused' (Dooris, 2013: 46).

Denman et al. (2002) locate the settings approach within Beattie's (1991) model (referred to in Chapter 5) by characterizing it as having a collective focus and negotiated style of working. Similarly, drawing on Caplan and Holland (1990), they see it as concerned with radical change rather than social regulation and based on the view that knowledge is subjective rather than objective – that is, it is consistent with a radical humanist position.

Shareck et al. (2013: 46), drawing on Poland and Dooris (2010), identify six guiding principles of the approach. They are:

- adopting an ecological and whole system perspective
- starting where people are and respecting people's lived experiences
- rooting practice in the social context of settings
- deepening the sociopolitical analysis in order to locate action in the broader context of power relations
- building on assets and successes already prevailing in settings
- building resilience and capabilities for sustained change.

Consideration of the respective contributions of behaviour and environment to health – or alternatively agency and structure – has been a major concern of health promotion, as we have noted on a number of occasions. Green et al. (2000) draw attention to the reciprocal determinism between environment and behaviour that is integral to ecological perspectives of health promotion and the settings approach. In short, behaviour is influenced by environment and the behaviour of individuals and groups shapes the environment. The settings approach does not, therefore, subscribe to a simple input–output view of intervention and effect, but, rather, presupposes a complex web of interaction between multiple layers of inputs. Poland et al. (2000: 346) identify the key characteristics of settings for health projects as 'integrated, comprehensive, multifaceted, participatory, empowering, partnership, responsive, and tailored'. Whitelaw et al. (2001: 341) suggest that activity in the settings approach is concerned with:

- development of personal competences
- policies
- reshaping environments
- building partnerships
- bringing about sustainable change by means of participation
- developing empowerment
- ownership of change throughout the setting.

There have been consistent critics of the settings approach in health promotion. Wenzel (1997) contends that, despite the rhetoric, the settings approach has amounted to little more than a rebadging of traditional health education and that settings are simply a vehicle for individualistic health promotion. Schools, for example, frequently purport to be embracing holistic 'whole-systems' approaches to tackling the health of children; however, in reality, 'topic-based' interventions are often implemented which focus heavily on the individual at the expense of broader social or environmental efforts (Thomas and Aggleton, 2016). Dooris (2006: 2) also notes that despite a high level of support, the settings approach has 'not gained as much influence as it might have – in terms of either guiding wider international policy or driving national-level public health strategy'. Others have similar concerns, especially in relation to the current lack of commitment of global organizations, like WHO, in regard to settings-based health promotion (Woodall, 2016) and the general lack of momentum and drive that has led to a stalled start for settings-based health promotion (Woodall and Freeman, 2020).

Green et al. (2000) suggest that any failure to achieve full health-promoting setting 'status' may derive not so much from the inherent sophistication of the concept and the lack of comprehension on the part of practitioners, but from practical limitations within the setting. These include the 'competing interests, agendas and interpretations of key "gatekeepers"' (2000: 24). Whitelaw et al. (2001) attribute the relatively modest achievements to health promotion being only one element within the context of wider organizational development and identify a number of practical difficulties:

- competing forces
- translating the philosophy of the approach into practical activity within the setting
- the credibility and status of health promoters as agents of change
- lack of sufficient support.

Kokko et al. (2014) note how history is also a determinant of a setting's openness to health promotion. As an example, schools have long been seen as viable settings for reaching children and influencing their health choices (Hubley et al., 2021), but in contrast it is only very recently, because of political and ideological tensions, that prisons have been open to health promotion approaches (Woodall, 2016).

Whitelaw et al. (2001) note the variation in what is being attempted under the settings banner and the difficulty faced by practitioners in moving beyond a focus on projects and towards achieving broader change across the setting and sustaining activity over a significant period. Johnson and Baum (2001: 286), for example, demonstrated a variety of practice under the health-promoting hospital banner. They suggest that:

> Some hospitals do little more than move beyond providing health information and education to patients, while other initiatives achieve a significant re-orientation of their activities and institute significant organizational reform supported by strong policy and leadership.

Whitelaw et al. (2001) raise the issue of whether or not there should be a consensus on what constitutes a settings approach – a one size fits all – given the differences in:

- the scale of what is attempted
- the nature of the setting – from nation-states to prisons
- the range of outcomes and emphases.

While a consensus contributes to achieving a common vision, Whitelaw et al. (2001: 341) note that allowance should be made for practical reality failing to live up to the theoretical ideal. Poland et al. (2000: 346) also suggest that 'a one size fits all approach (the use of identical protocols in similar settings)' may be inappropriate and that local autonomy may be required in relation to adaptation to suit specific needs and circumstances.

Whitelaw et al. (2001: 342–4) identify five broad types of settings activity by considering the ways in which problems are framed and solutions identified – in particular, the respective weight attached to the contributions of agency and structure:

- **The passive model**: the problem and solution are dependent on the behaviour and actions of individuals. Traditional health education activity takes place within the setting – the setting itself merely has a subservient role.
- **The active model**: the primary problem and part of the solution lie with the behaviour of individuals and part of the solution with the setting. The contribution of the setting is therefore needed to facilitate change in behaviour and the achievement of goals.
- **The vehicle model**: the problem lies with the setting and the solution with learning from individually based projects. The primary goal shifts from the individual to changing features of the setting. Working on specific topic- focused projects is the 'vehicle' for achieving this – for example, beginning with an issue such as sun protection as a basis for considering the wider health-promoting potential of the organization.
- **The organic model**: the problem is seen to lie with the system and the solution with the processes and practices that make up the whole. It focuses on the development of individuals and groups

throughout the organization, premised on the assumption that overarching systems are the product of individual actions. The overall aim is to improve the ethos or culture of the setting and strengthen collective participation.

- **The comprehensive model**: this aims to change the structure and culture of the setting with the assumption that individuals are relatively powerless to do anything about it. It takes more of a deterministic view that systems change is dependent on 'powerful levers', so the emphasis is on policies and strategies for achieving change.

The last two are clearly more consistent with the 'ideal' interpretation of the settings approach. However, Whitelaw et al. (2001) suggest that the distinctions between these five types of activity should be viewed loosely and that they may overlap in a complementary way or operate sequentially to facilitate progression within an organization.

Variations in practice may, therefore, arise from the extent to which organizations aspire, and are able, to achieve the 'ideal'. The particular characteristics of organizations will also undoubtedly influence the way in which the settings approach is operationalized. Denman et al. (2002) observe that differences in the size and complexity of settings will influence the mode of operation of the settings approach. For example, they refer to healthy cities as macro settings that rely heavily on intersectoral collaboration to achieve their goals. Schools, in contrast, are held to be more self-contained and self-sufficient. While collaboration has undoubted benefits (and is a core principle of the approach), schools will be less dependent on this aspect.

Variation also occurs within settings. There is a broad division into types of schemes – prescriptive and needs-led. The former involve working towards predefined criteria, whereas needs-led approaches are more flexible and responsive to local priorities. The WHO position has been to acknowledge – indeed welcome – diversity in implementation of the settings approach, both between and within settings, provided it is consistent with core principles. In line with notions of subsidiarity, this affords considerable local autonomy and the opportunity to respond to local needs while maintaining the integrity of the approach and commitment to its underpinning values.

Carrots and sticks

A range of factors will impinge on an organization's decision to become a health-promoting setting – at the most basic level, these could be the latitude for making change and the resources available. A critical issue is the momentum created by external pressure (or incentives!) and internal motivation. In some instances, formally structured international or national programmes or networks may be in place that may help to create that momentum.

International networks can fulfil an important advocacy role. The Health in Prisons Project (HiPP), for example, coordinated by the WHO, encourages cooperation and establishes integrated work between public health systems, international non-governmental organizations and prison health systems to promote public health and reduce health inequalities. Prior to the establishment of the HiPP, prison health services throughout Europe were of limited interest to prison management and national health services (Gatherer and Møller, 2009).

The concept of the health-promoting school (HPS) was largely developed by the European HPS Network in the 1990s. It has been highly successful and has since been replicated throughout the world. In the USA and Canada, this has resulted in the Comprehensive School Health Program (Gugglberger, 2021).

Barnekow Rasmussen (2005) notes that the European Network of Health Promoting Schools (ENHPS) launched in 1991 enlarged from an initial small group of seven countries to include 43 countries a decade later. It encouraged commitment from and cooperation between relevant government departments – in this instance, education and health. Such high-level support and cooperation are key factors in developing national initiatives. International networks can also establish core principles and quality standards and be a means of encouraging innovation and disseminating good practice.

Drawing on the experience of involving countries in the ENHPS, Barnekow Rasmussen identifies a number of stages between initial pilot and ultimate incorporation into mainstream policy, which could equally apply to other settings. These are:

- positive identification by decision-makers
- disseminating information
- building credibility
- demonstrating relevance
- demonstrating feasibility
- incorporation into government policy. (Barnekow Rasmussen, 2005: 171)

The development of 'healthy' settings in the private sector is, perhaps, less amenable to regulation and national or local control than it is in the public sector and, therefore, tends to rely on convincing organizations about the potential benefits. For example, with regard to workplace health promotion, it is possible to regulate health and safety issues. However, the move towards consideration of positive health and addressing the factors that would improve health demanded by the settings for health approach relies more on gaining the commitment of individual employers.

The origins of workplace health promotion lie in the reorientation of traditional occupational health and safety legislation and practice supported by the European Framework Directive on safety and health (Council Directive 89/391/EC), together with recognition of the workplace as an important setting for health (European Network of Workplace Health Promotion [ENWHP], 2007). The Luxembourg Declaration 1997 provided the first definition of workplace health promotion:

> the combined efforts of employers, employees and society to improve the health and well-being of people at work. This can be achieved by a combination of improving the work organisation and the working environment, promoting active participation and by encouraging personal development.

In the early 1980s workplace health promotion programmes were criticized as being overly focused on individual issues and risk factors, neglecting broader structural determinants. Since the 1990s, a more sophisticated and interdisciplinary approach has been widely adopted as a result of the myriad of factors impacting on employee health – in short, interventions have become more holistic and based not only on individual risk-factors but on broader issues like culture and policy design and implementation. A healthy workplace has been described as:

one in which workers and managers collaborate to use a continual improvement process to protect and promote the health, safety and well-being of all workers and the sustainability of the workplace by considering the following, based on identified needs:

- health and safety concerns in the physical work environment
- health, safety and well-being concerns in the psychosocial work environment, including organization of work and workplace culture
- personal health resources in the workplace; and
- ways of participating in the community to improve the health of workers, their families and other members of the community. (WHO, 2010: 6)

Clearly, different settings will vary both in their commitment and capacity to prioritize health goals. Again, this might be expected to be a more realistic proposition within the public than the private sector, notwithstanding Kickbusch's (1998: 2) assertion that 'almost all organizations have not only a vested interest, but also a social responsibility, in maintaining and improving their members' health'. This was indeed highlighted recently during the COVID-19 pandemic where many workplaces acted swiftly and decisively to protect their employees and wider community.

The literature suggests a myriad of positive effects as a result of workplace health promotion, including improvements in the status of employees' health; increased health consciousness; changes in health behaviour; better working atmosphere; better communication and cooperation among employees; and reduction of risk factors that affect health (Bandenburg, 2012). Notwithstanding these effects, there are many barriers to health promotion in the workplace. Some of these have been identified by Rojatz et al. (2016) in their qualitative systematic review, including:

- external conditions (e.g. global economic downturns) hindering the likelihood of workplaces engaging in workplace health interventions
- limited managerial support and an unfavourable health-promoting 'organizational culture/ climate'
- lack of 'resources' to implement interventions (time, money, staff and infrastructure)
- the incompatibility of the intervention with staff working hours/processes
- the workplaces' lack of 'experience with health promotion'
- poor staff participation rates, especially when interventions are scheduled during holiday periods.

Beyond health and safety requirements, workplace health promotion is unlikely to be a priority for most employers and managers. However, commentators have discussed whether workplaces should adopt a more salutogenic approach, focusing more on issues such as: joy, growth, self-actualization and flourishing (Bauer, 2022). Convincing arguments will, therefore, be needed to justify investing resources of both time and money in developing the health-promoting potential of organizations. Such arguments are frequently couched in economic terms emphasizing the monetary return on investment (see Box 10.3). While purists might be critical of the narrow focus on servicing the needs of productivity, from the perspective of persuasive communication, framing the argument in this way means that it is likely to appeal to the primary motivation of those working in industry and the private sector.

BOX 10.3 THE ECONOMIC BENEFITS OF WORKPLACE HEALTH PROMOTION

- Research suggests that it is possible to influence work-related outcomes, especially absenteeism, positively through health promotion efforts (Grimani et al., 2019).
- While estimates on savings as a result of implementing workplace health promotion vary, WHO (2016b) estimates that every US$1 of investment results in a return of $4-6.
- Research has shown a link between high-performing, well-managed companies and the amount of investment in workforce health and well-being (Grossmeier et al., 2016). This suggests that health, productivity and performance are interlinked.
- Recent systematic review evidence in Europe suggests that the methodological quality of studies restricts the conclusions that can be made on the economic value of workplace health promotion. To this extent, the economic value of health-promoting workplaces remains uncertain (Lutz et al., 2019).

An alternative conceptualization of benefits might include improved working relationships, the opportunity to improve the health and well-being of the workforce and enhance the corporate image – echoing the tradition of nineteenth-century British industrial philanthropists such as Salt, Cadbury and Rowntree! The report by de Greef and Van den Broek (2004) for the ENWHP emphasizes the need for business to combine 'technical and economic innovation with social innovation' and outlines a broader set of arguments to support workplace health promotion that it is claimed:

- leads to an improved working situation
- improves health-related outcomes
- generates an enhanced image
- improves human resources management
- boosts productivity
- increases health awareness and motivation
- leads to healthy workers
- generates more job satisfaction. (2004: 54)

The report identifies the following main drivers for the business case for workplace health promotion:

- corporate values that recognize the social and economic relevance of a participatory workplace culture
- social and demographic trends with significant impacts on the labour market as external drivers
- the impacts of workplace health investments along the employee–customer–profit chain also highlighting the role of workplace health investments for improved business processes. (2004: 55)

De Greef and Van den Broek argue that the case for workplace health promotion needs to be aligned with companies' goals and strategies. This is equally true for settings more generally. Within the educational context, there is clear recognition of the reciprocal relationship between health and education. Children who are healthy are more able to take advantage of education and education contributes to health.

For most settings, health and health promotion do not form part of their core business. It might be anticipated that an organization's motivation to become a health-promoting setting would be influenced by the level of compatibility with:

- its primary goals
- its core values
- its modus operandi.

Hospitals, for example, might appear to be obvious contenders in that the core business of hospitals could loosely be defined as being concerned with health. However, the move to becoming a health-promoting hospital (see Box 10.4) would require traditional organizations to undergo a major reorientation – from curing disease to promoting health, from patient compliance to empowerment, from a narrow concern with patients to including relatives, staff and the wider community, and from being inward-looking to being outward-looking. Such developments have again been supported by international networks – initially European, but a global network has more recently been established. The definition of a health-promoting hospital used in the WHO glossary emphasizes the need to include health promotion in the corporate identity:

A health promoting hospital does not only provide high quality comprehensive medical and nursing services, but also develops a corporate identity that embraces the aims of health promotion, develops a health promoting organizational structure and culture, including active, participatory roles for patients and all members of staff, develops itself into a health promoting physical environment and actively cooperates with its community. (Nutbeam, 1998a: 11)

BOX 10.4   HEALTH-PROMOTING HOSPITALS (HPHS)

Fundamental principles: the Vienna Recommendations

Within the framework of the Health for All strategy, the Ottawa Charter for Health Promotion, the Ljubljana Charter for Reforming Health Care and the Budapest Declaration on Health Promoting Hospitals, a health-promoting hospital should:

1. Promote human dignity, equity and solidarity, and professional ethics, acknowledging differences in the needs, values and cultures of different population groups
2. Be orientated towards quality improvement, the well-being of patients, relatives and staff, protection of the environment and a realization of the potential to become learning organizations
3. Focus on health with a holistic approach and not only on curative services

(Continued)

4. Be centred on people providing health services in the best way possible to patients and their relatives, to facilitate the healing process and contribute to the empowerment of patients

5. Use resources efficiently and cost-effectively, and allocate resources on the basis of contribution to health improvement

6. Form as close links as possible with other levels of the healthcare system and the community.

Standards for health promotion

- Management policy
- Patient assessment
- Patient information and intervention
- Promoting a healthy workplace
- Continuity and cooperation.

Source: Groene (2006)

In contrast, while at first sight schools are primarily concerned with educational rather than health goals, commitment to education as a means of developing the whole person has much in common with a positive, holistic view of health. Furthermore, the emergence of the 'whole school approach' to education in the 1980s was entirely consistent with the settings approach and prepared the ground for the emergence of the health-promoting school concept. The 'whole school approach' recognized that a child's learning at school is the product not just of what is taught through the planned formal curriculum, but also their total experience at school, which would include the environment, relationships and practices in the school (the hidden curriculum), the activities organized by the school (the informal curriculum) and contact with the school health service (the parallel curriculum).

We have made some general observations about the key features of the settings approach. We will now consider the health-promoting prison in more detail as an example. Although there are substantial contextual differences between settings, as we have noted, there are still some parallels to be drawn. We will then conclude by making some brief points of comparison with other settings.

THE HEALTH-PROMOTING PRISON

Previous editions of this book have provided a detailed critique of the health-promoting school and a great deal continues to be written about this setting from various international perspectives (Chen and Lee, 2016; Wang et al., 2015). Settings have progressed at varying rates with some working at a global level (for example, cities), others at continent level (for example, prisons) and some at a national level (for example, sports club) (Kokko et al., 2014). Some settings-based initiatives have had over three decades of activity while others are still in their embryonic stage. This section looks briefly at one of those settings in their infancy, the health-promoting prison.

As noted earlier, the WHO, through various international declarations, has been largely responsible for the historical development and leadership of a settings approach within health promotion, although this has been far more apparent in Europe than in other parts of the world such as the USA (Woodall, 2016).

Prisons have been regarded as the most 'unpopular' of the settings-based environments as prisons generally work within hierarchical, disempowering and penalizing structures that are fundamentally antithetical to the core values of health promotion (Smith, 2000; Whitehead, 2006; Woodall, 2010). While the discourse and ideology of health promotion is incongruous in a setting that curtails individual freedom and choice, there are clear opportunities for health promotion work, even in the most restrictive security contexts (Woodall, 2020b).

ABSTRACT 10.1

Health promotion co-existing in a high-security prison context: a documentary analysis. Woodall, J. (2020b)

Purpose: There is interest in promoting health in prison from governmental levels, but, to date, understanding how best to do this is unclear. This paper argues that nuanced understanding of context is required in order to understand health promotion in prison and examines the potential for empowerment, a cornerstone of health promotion practice, in high-security prison establishments.

Design/methodology/approach: Independent prison inspections, conducted by Her Majesty's Inspectorate of Prisons for England and Wales (HMIP), form a critical element in how prisons are assessed. Documentary analysis was undertaken on all eight high-security prison reports using framework analysis.

Findings: Analysis revealed elements of prison life which were disempowering and antithetical to health promotion. While security imperatives were paramount, there were examples where this was disproportionate and disempowered individuals. The data show examples where, even in these high-security contexts, empowerment can be fostered. These were exemplified in relation to peer approaches designed to improve health and where prisoners felt part of democratic processes where they could influence change.

Practical implications: Both in the UK and internationally, there is a growing rhetoric for delivering effective health promotion interventions in prison, but limited understanding about how to operationalize this. This paper gives insight into how this could be done in a high-security prison environment.

Originality/value: This is the first paper which looks at the potential for health promotion to be embedded in high-security prisons. It demonstrates features of prison life which act to disempower and also support individuals to take greater control over their health.

Indeed, there are some compelling arguments for promoting health in prison. First, prisoners' health tends to be poor and it is now widely acknowledged that the prevalence of ill health in the prison population is higher than that reported in the wider community (Baybutt et al., 2019). Mental health problems (WHO, 2008b), long-standing physical disorders (Plugge et al., 2006; Stewart, 2008) and drug and alcohol issues (Centre for Social Justice, 2009; Social Exclusion Unit, 2002; Woodall, 2012b) are commonplace. Second, there is a humanitarian argument that people in prison are 'citizens' who have rights to health. Third, there is a growing evidence base that demonstrates how well-coordinated health-promoting interventions have the potential to reduce health inequalities and address the health needs of those who are the most marginalized in society (Baybutt et al., 2010; Woodall and South, 2012). Fourth, there is a public health imperative, an argument originally made by penal reformer John Howard in the eighteenth century (Ross, 2013), as those in prison often serve multiple and relatively short-term sentences, meaning that prisoners' health and the public's health are strongly interconnected. Fifth, the health-promoting prison concept does not only concern prisoners who '(temporarily) live' there, but can also be used as an opportunity to address staff health (Woodall, 2013). It is axiomatic that for prisoners to be rehabilitated and released into the community as law-abiding, healthy citizens, prison staff need to feel valued and in good physical, mental and psychosocial health (Bögemann, 2007).

The concept of a health-promoting prison is guided by several key principles. Prisoners' rights are at the core of the health-promoting prison – in 1966, the United Nations in its International Covenant on Economic, Social and Cultural Rights (UN, 1966) stated that every citizen has the right to the highest attainable standard of physical and mental health and, in 1990, they declared that prisoners should have access to health services available in the country without discrimination based on their legal status (UN, 1990). Linked to prisoners' rights is the principle of healthcare equivalence. The premise is that individuals detained in prison must have the benefit of care equivalent to that available to the general public (Niveau, 2007).

ABSTRACT 10.2

Health-promoting prisons: theory to practice. Baybutt, M. and Chemlal, K. (2016)

As a setting, prisons offer a unique opportunity to invest in the health of disadvantaged and marginalized populations and address health inequalities and social exclusion – thereby achieving sustainable improvements in well-being for offenders and their families and in turn, helping to reduce rates of re-offending. This article draws on English and French experiences and doctoral research to advocate a shift from a pathogenic model towards a salutogenic model of health as a helpful way to address inequalities and thus, by promoting joined-up working across justice and wider systems, impact positively beyond 'health' for the effective resettlement of prisoners. The paper utilizes examples from horticulture to further argue the powerful role of nature in the prison setting in mediating aspects of culture particularly relating to processes of socialization. Critical success lies in bridging across systems and a commitment to joined-up working at all levels across and beyond prison.

While the health-promoting prison is a relatively new concept, a definition has been proposed that reflects the rights and equivalence agenda. It states that the health-promoting prison is:

a place of compulsory detention in which the risks to health are reduced to a minimum; where essential prison duties such as the maintenance of security are undertaken in a caring atmosphere that recognizes the inherent dignity of all prisoners and their human rights; where health services are provided to the level and in a professional manner equivalent to what is provided in the country as a whole; and where a whole-prison approach to promoting health and welfare is the norm. (Gatherer et al., 2009: 89)

The health-promoting prison should include all facets of prison life, from addressing individual health need through to organizational factors and the physical environment (see, for example, Baybutt and Chemlal's [2016] work on access to green space and horticulture and its effect on prisoner health and well-being).

The Ottawa Charter (WHO, 1986) is a useful framework to envisage these facets of prison life (see Figure 10.1) and has been used by others to map settings-based work in prisons (Ramaswamy and Freudenberg, 2007; Woodall and South, 2012; Woodall et al., 2014).

Conceptual challenges

Critics of the health-promoting prison have described it as a 'contradiction in terms' (Smith, 2000), 'an oxymoron' (de Viggiani, 2006a), 'simply incompatible' (Greenwood et al., 1999) and, according to de Viggiani (2006b), at best a vision and at worst, a dream. Authors have argued that there are several fundamental challenges that have inhibited the development of the health-promoting prison. The first challenge concerns the concept of 'prison health' that has, in the main, been clearly aligned to a biomedical perspective (Sim, 1990). Morris and Morris (1963: 193), in their study of Pentonville Prison, encapsulated the predominant discourse that surrounded prison health:

For the prison, health is essentially a negative concept; if men are not ill, de facto they are healthy. While most modern thinking in the field of social medicine has attempted to go further than this, for the prison medical staff it is not an unreasonable operational definition.

In the American correctional system, the concept of health had been underpinned in a similar way. When the Medical Center for Federal Prisoners in Springfield was opened in 1933, it was 'dedicated solely' to caring for the diseased and the 'broken bodies and minds of offenders' (Bosworth, 2002: 79). Through this lens, health is conceptualized in a reductionist, rather than holistic, way and viewed in terms of pathology, disease, diagnosis and treatment (Warwick-Booth et al., 2013a). This has notable implications, as health is defined by its absence of disease and not the attainment of positive health and well-being. Moreover, the medical model of health tends to focus on physical dimensions of health (such as physical fitness and functionality) rather than on mental (such as having a sense of purpose and meaning) and social dimensions of health (such as feeling connected to the community).

The second challenge is that health promotion interventions within prison settings have been consistently criticized because they frequently focus on the symptoms of the problem rather than tackling the root causes of poor health, such as the social determinants of health (Woodall et al., 2021).

Finally, whether values central to the health promotion discourse – namely empowerment – can be applied to the context of imprisonment is debatable (Woodall, 2020b). Empowering prisoners has never been an accepted pursuit in prison systems, even regarded as 'morally questionable and politically dangerous' (Aldridge Foundation and Johnson, 2008: 2). However, if a settings approach

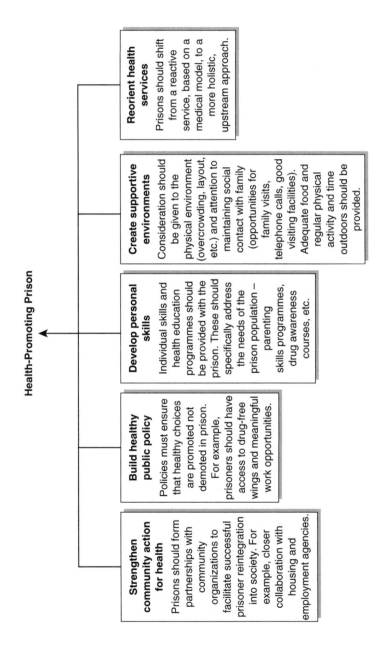

Health-Promoting Prison

Strengthen community action for health

Prisons should form partnerships with community organizations to facilitate successful prisoner reintegration into society. For example, closer collaboration with housing and employment agencies.

Build healthy public policy

Policies must ensure that healthy choices are promoted not demoted in prison. For example, prisoners should have access to drug-free wings and meaningful work opportunities.

Develop personal skills

Individual skills and health education programmes should be provided with the prison. These should specifically address the needs of the prison population – parenting skills programmes, drug awareness courses, etc.

Create supportive environments

Consideration should be given to the physical environment (overcrowding, layout, etc.) and attention to maintaining social contact with family (opportunities for family visits, telephone calls, good visiting facilities). Adequate food and regular physical activity and time outdoors should be provided.

Reorient health services

Prisons should shift from a reactive service, based on a medical model, to a more holistic, upstream approach.

Figure 10.1 The Ottawa Charter as a framework for action within the health-promoting prison

in prison is truly to move forward, both conceptually and practically, then health promoters should seek ways to embed the key values of health promotion within the prison setting. Practically, this could include considering architecture, policies, structures, prisoner–staff relationships and how these impact on the health of individuals. For example, ensuring that sufficient occupational activities are provided in prison; regular contact is maintained with families; and opportunities for accessing fresh air, exercise facilities and nutritious food are available.

In summary, developing the health-promoting prison is not easy and those who are currently working to deliver successful interventions in this setting are doing so within an environment of paradoxical values and philosophies. Approaches to health, particularly health promotion, have developed considerably within prisons but there is still a way to go.

OTHER SETTINGS FOR HEALTH

Within this section we do not propose to consider the full range of settings in detail, but rather to draw some brief points of comparison. Some of the key features of different settings are provided in Table 10.3.

Table 10.3   Settings – points of comparison

	Examples	
	High	**Low**
Scale	Healthy cities Healthy islands	Healthy prisons
Supportive national/international networks	Healthy cities Health-promoting schools	Beauty salons
Opportunity for regulation	Health-promoting schools	Healthy stadia
Alignment with core purpose	Health-promoting hospitals	Manufacturing industry
Reach	Health-promoting schools	Beauty salons
Access to disadvantaged groups	Health-promoting prisons	Health-promoting universities
Funding	Variable, but generally not generous	

Three short examples will be presented to show how it remains possible to apply the principles of the settings approach across different settings. This adaptability is perhaps testament to the value of the approach.

Health-promoting sports clubs are becoming more globally prominent with examples of good practice reported across many parts of the world (Johnson et al., 2020; Kokko et al., 2016). The theory of a health-promoting sports club is that it embraces the macro, meso and micro influences on individuals' health – drawing on socioecological principles of health promotion (Kokko et al., 2016). Given the centrality of many sports clubs within the community, they are considered a prime site for addressing health inequalities and may be particularly effective at addressing the issues facing young people (Lane et al., 2017). Moreover, there have been recent drives with professional sports clubs, particularly football clubs, to embrace healthy settings ideals and this has been effective in reaching sub-sections of the community where engagement with health promotion has traditionally failed (Pringle et al., 2013).

ABSTRACT 10.3

Health promotion orientation of GAA sports clubs in Ireland. Lane, A., Murphy, N., Donohoe, A. and Regan, C. (2017)

In Ireland, a Gaelic Athletic Association (GAA) sports club exists in almost every community. The purpose of this analysis is to present the health promotion orientation of clubs who have been recruited to a project run in partnership with the GAA and the Irish Department of Health. Clubs completed a questionnaire and took part in a focus group to explore why they were willing to take part in this initiative. Clubs viewed health promotion as a natural progression of their existing work. They scored low in relation to policy and coaching activities specific to health promotion, and higher for their ideology and environmental considerations. GAA sports clubs are already engaging in some health-related activities and are eager to engage further. Clubs require support to ensure health promotion is embedded into their core business.

Interest in healthy food markets has also been considerable in the past decade. Healthy food markets have been implemented in all WHO regions, although were launched and remain concentrated in the WHO Western Pacific Region (WHO, 2019). The WHO (2019) suggest that a healthy food market is one that seeks to protect health by eliminating disease and other hazards at all places along the farm-to-consumption continuum. The food market also serves as the centre of community life and people use markets with the expectation that the food they buy is safe and nutritious. Nevertheless, in some instances, markets have also become associated with the spread of a number of emerging diseases. One example of the development of a healthy food market is Buguruni Market in Dar es Salaam, Tanzania. Prior to work to develop the healthy market, Buguruni Market had a single pit latrine and one water standpipe. The market lacked central administration and maintenance, there was no pest control programme and moreover food inspections were infrequent. Vendors from the market, alongside governmental and non-governmental organizations, established the Buguruni Healthy Marketplaces Task Force. As a consequence of the task force there have been significant developments, including:

- improvement in road access
- construction of a solid waste storage bay
- construction of toilet and handwashing facilities
- development of a system for the collection and sorting of solid waste for subsequent disposal.

The success of the Buguruni Market has been seen in the development of the healthy market concept being introduced into several other markets in Dar es Salaam and other cities in Tanzania (WHO, 2006b).

Finally, although under-theorized and under-researched in relation to other settings, there is capacity for the family setting to be harnessed to support the development of healthy children, families and societies (Panter-Brick et al., 2014; Soubhi and Potvin, 2000). Traditional family structures are now being accompanied by structures that are more diverse and heterogeneous. Children may be raised by married parents, cohabiting parents, single parents, step-parents or same-sex parents (Golombok, 2015) and many children move in and out of these varied forms during their childhood years. Despite these changes, recent research has shown how the focus of the family can be a practical and effective setting for health promotion (Robertson et al., 2016). Novilla et al. (2006: 29) suggest that the 'ecological perspective serves as the unifying framework for defining family health' and McLeroy et al.'s (1988) ecological model of health promotion, drawing prominently on the work of Bronfenbrenner (1977), acknowledges that tackling health and health inequalities is relatively futile without acknowledging micro, meso and macro processes that impact on family dynamics and well-being. While structural determinants of health are crucial factors in tackling health inequalities, the contributory role that family relationships and systems play in supporting health within this multilevel context is critical. However, it is arguable if health promotion practice or policy has fully utilized or embraced families as a viable setting for health promotion interventions (Novilla et al., 2006).

THE SETTINGS APPROACH – FUTURE POTENTIAL

Organizations and social systems have an enormous impact on health. The settings approach aims to harness that potential to promote health and well-being. The advantages offered by the settings approach are that it:

- offers opportunities for working at least some way upstream to develop conditions supportive of health
- embeds consideration for health within organizational structures
- has a holistic orientation rather than a focus on problems, risks or specific groups.

However, there are also numerous challenges:

- Less obvious settings should be considered as well as large-scale mainstream ones to avoid further marginalization of some disadvantaged groups.
- The settings approach demands organizational change and commitment – it is not merely a vehicle for more traditional approaches.
- It requires a delicate balance between top-down managerial support and the creation of an overall sense of direction on the one hand and, on the other, participation and a sense of ownership at grassroots level.
- It demands new ways of working.

The shift in emphasis from behaviour or policy change to organizational change will necessarily draw on a different combination of professional skills and insights (see Box 10.5).

BOX 10.5 REQUIREMENTS FOR ACHIEVING ORGANIZATIONAL CHANGE

- Understanding the influence of organizations on the health and illness of their clients and members
- Understanding the special logic and dynamics of organizations in different sectors
- Skills in analysing social structures and processes in organizations
- Ability to shape their own role within the organizations
- Social skills for teamwork and team leadership
- Skills for intervening in organizations.

Source: After Scala (1996)

Poland et al. (2000: 347) provide a useful summary of key factors contributing to the success of the settings approach that depend on a 'reflexive reading of the particular setting and one's role in it'. These include:

- the institutional organizational culture
- the expectations, attitudes and beliefs of key players – workers, management, patients and physicians, students and teachers, parents and children, community groups and state officials
- the nature of the practice environment – such as incentives and disincentives for undertaking health promotion, such as reward structures, pace of work, competing demands, scepticism, regarding the value or relevance or effectiveness of health promotion, training of key staff
- historical developments in the setting – trends in the organization of work, composition of the family or organization of healthcare
- internal politics, leadership (formal and informal), past successes and failures
- who controls access to the setting, who has influence within the setting
- broader social, economic and political context – non-setting factors.

Dooris (2006) identifies the main challenges in taking the settings approach forward and seeking to increase its influence: first, clarifying the theoretical base of the settings approach and, second, developing the evidence base. On this latter point, commentators almost 10 years on argue that the evidence base for settings remains weak and requires further funded research (Newman et al., 2015). Dooris also points out the need to keep an eye on the bigger picture, that is to say the social, economic and environmental influences on health.

The emergence of the settings approach acknowledged the interplay of factors that influence health. It moved forward from seeing settings merely as a means to providing access to a target population towards harnessing the potential offered at all levels within a setting – policy, environment (in its widest sense, including social relationships and interaction), along with opportunities for education. Furthermore, the settings approach sees the boundaries of settings as permeable, with opportunities to interact in a mutually beneficial way with the wider community and other settings.

The ultimate indicator of the success of the settings approach will be when giving consideration to health is so firmly embedded into the structure and ways of working of organizations, that the qualifying term 'healthy' is no longer needed.

KEY POINTS

- The settings approach shifts the focus of interventions from the individual to creating the conditions supportive of health and health behaviour.
- The settings approach involves considering how all aspects of the setting influence the health of all those who come into contact with it.
- It is important to identify which population groups are reached by specific settings and which are not.
- Innovative approaches may be needed to ensure that disadvantaged and excluded groups are reached so that the settings approach can contribute to a reduction in health inequalities.
- The implementation of the settings approach is enhanced by the existence of local, national and international networks.
- Internal motivation is a key factor in implementing settings for health approaches.
- Compatibility with the core purpose of the setting, or appreciation of the potential advantages to the setting, increases motivation and favours the development of healthy settings.
- The settings approach involves organizational change and requires new ways of working and associated professional competences.
- Changing organizational culture and ways of working takes time.
- Recognition and celebration of early successes can help to generate and sustain motivation.
- As with all health promotion initiatives, the settings approach should be based on clear, realistic objectives and sufficient resources, including staffing, should be allocated to achieving them.
- The evidence base for the settings approach needs to be improved by generating evidence relating to the totality of the setting. It therefore requires attention to process as well as outcomes.

CHAPTER 10: INTERNATIONAL CASE STUDIES

The following case studies on the online resources website are relevant to the content of this chapter: 2, 3, 8 and 9.

CRITICAL REFLECTION AND APPLICATION TO PRACTICE

This chapter has discussed the settings approach, a critical strategy in tackling health issues and addressing inequalities. What advantages do settings-based approaches present and is it an appropriate strategy for health promoters in all cases? Which setting(s) relate best to your professional practice? What other settings could be identified to improve the reach of your role? In what ways can settings-based approaches be evaluated effectively? What do you see as the future of settings-based health promotion? Which 'new' settings do you envisage being prominent in your practice?

ONLINE RESOURCES

Please visit https://study.sagepub.com/greentones5e for all the online resources for the book, including recommended further reading on each chapter subject, useful weblinks (both introduced by the authors), as well as the abovementioned case study material.

11 EVALUATION

When God made Heaven and God made Earth

He [*sic*] formed the seas and gave them birth;

His heart was full of jubilation;

But he made one error – no EVALUATION!

'Oh!' He said, 'That's good!' and He meant it too,

But now we know that that won't do.

Even something that we know is best,

We've got to PROVE by a PRE-POST test.

Apocryphal wisdom from a NASA newsletter

Evaluation is a vast, lumbering, overgrown adolescent. It has the typical problems associated with this age group too. It does not know quite where it is going and it is prone to bouts of despair. But it is the future after all ...

Pawson and Tilley (1997: 1)

OVERVIEW

This chapter addresses evaluation for health promotion and the importance of understanding the effectiveness of interventions in order to develop evidence- informed policy and practice. It will:

- consider the influence of values on evaluation
- discuss the implications of different research paradigms for health promotion evaluation and the limitations of the randomized controlled trial (RCT)
- emphasize the need to look at process and context as well as outcomes
- consider the various types of indicator required
- propose the judicial principle as a means of establishing validity.

INTRODUCTION

Fundamental to all evaluation research is the question of validity – the need to 'prove' that any claims made about the effectiveness and efficiency of interventions are robust and justifiable. It is essential, therefore, to identify appropriate methodology for evaluating health promotion interventions. Traditionally, the randomized controlled trial (RCT) has been viewed as the 'gold standard' for assessing effectiveness. However, there has been considerable debate about its relevance for health promotion. This debate has been characterized by an intense clash of ideologies – earning the description of 'paradigm wars'. In this chapter, we are critical of the use of RCTs for health promotion evaluation and propose a new gold standard based on the 'judicial principle'. We also consider the type of information needed to build an evidence base that can inform future practice and policy.

WHY EVALUATE?

At its simplest, the purpose of evaluation is to assess the extent to which interventions have achieved their goals and potentially the extent to which interventions can be transferred or generalized elsewhere (Fleming and Baldwin, 2020). In a climate where there is increasing pressure to ensure that public funds are being used to good effect, evaluation is frequently a means of demonstrating accountability and value for money (Woodall and Cross, 2021). However, it can have a much broader role. Lewis (2001) recognizes the current emphasis on evaluation for accountability and calls for a 'campaign for more evaluation for learning – of both process and impact' (2001: 392).

As we have argued earlier, evaluation is a key element of good health promotion practice and an essential component of the health promotion planning cycle. It allows those implementing interventions to keep a check on progress and introduce any necessary modifications. Importantly, given health promotion's commitment to equity, it can assess whether the benefits reach the most disadvantaged and contribute to a reduction in health inequalities.

Clearly, the development of evaluation evidence is essential for building the evidence base for health promotion and improving practice (Fleming and Baldwin, 2020). Over and above establishing what works, it is important that such evidence provides insight into how interventions work and under what conditions and in what contexts they succeed or fail.

From an ethical standpoint, evaluation can help to ensure that interventions do no harm either directly, or, in the case of ineffective interventions, indirectly 'by squandering limited resources' or alienating community groups and making them 'more resistant to other attempts to bring about change' (Green and South, 2006: 5).

The purposes of evaluation can, therefore, be summarized as:

- evaluation for accountability
- evaluation for programme management and development
- evaluation for learning
- evaluation as an ethical obligation. (Green and South, 2006: 5)

VALUES AND EVALUATION

Evaluation is by no means a neutral, technical activity – it is saturated with values, ideological debate and, sometimes, vitriolic argument concerning what should be regarded as evidence of success and the means of assessing it.

The WHO (1995) noted that health promotion is an investment and evaluation is concerned to address the costs and benefits of this investment. More specifically, evaluators might measure programme outcomes and processes in order to assess one or more of the following results of this investment:

- contribution to knowledge base/theory of health promotion
- insights that will result in more effective health promotion practice
- relative costs and benefits in financial terms
- levels of stakeholder satisfaction
- evidence to influence policy-makers in respect of:

  o development of health policy
  o continued employment of researchers and health promotion departments

- impact on individual and public health.

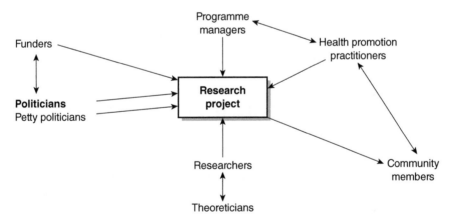

Figure 11.1   The stakeholder community

However, different stakeholders may well differ in their aspirations for health promotion programmes. There is often substantial variation in the views of stakeholders about what would constitute success and, indeed, about the purpose of the evaluation enterprise itself. Figure 11.1 provides an overview of the dynamics of the stakeholder community.

In theory at least, the various stakeholders may all influence evaluation, although the amount of influence different groups bring to bear will vary. Funders are clearly key stakeholders. As the adage reminds us, 'he who pays the piper calls the tune'. Funder power can operate at both ends of the evaluation enterprise, sometimes explicitly but often in implicit ways. Allocation of funding can be used to control the evaluation research agenda. Funders can also act as gatekeepers in relation to the dissemination of research findings – to the extent of withholding unpalatable findings. Some of the less reputable approaches to evaluation are summarized in Box 11.1.

BOX 11.1   PSEUDO-EVALUATIONS

- **Eyewash** – focus on surface appearances
- **Whitewash** – covering up programme failure
- **Submarine** – political use of evaluation to undermine a programme
- **Posture** – ritual use of evaluation without any intention to use the findings, for example where evaluation is necessary to secure funding
- **Postponement** – as a means of avoiding or at least postponing action.

Source: Newburn (2001: 9), drawing on Suchman (1967), cited in Robson (1993)

It is, perhaps, not unreasonable that funders should wish to exercise some degree of control. Pawson and Tilley (1997) quote a Department of Health Code of Practice (see Box 11.2) to illustrate this phenomenon.

BOX 11.2   IS THE CUSTOMER ALWAYS RIGHT? THE ROTHSCHILD PRINCIPLE

The main principle governing any Government funding of R&D is the Rothschild principle, laid down in Cmd 4814 and reiterated in the White Paper 'Realising Our Potential: A Strategy for Science, Engineering and Technology': ' … the customer says what he [*sic*] wants, the contractor does it, if he can, and the customer pays'.

Source: Code of Practice, Department of Health (1993), cited in Pawson and Tilley (1997: 14)

The authors also refer to Stufflebeam's concern about the 'standards' produced by the US Joint Committee on Standards for Educational Evaluation:

[these have] four features … utility, feasibility, propriety and accuracy [in that order] … and evaluation should not be done at all if there is no prospect for its being useful to some audience. Second, it should not be done if it is not feasible to conduct it in political terms, or practicality terms, or cost-effectiveness terms. Third, they do not think it should be done if we cannot demonstrate that it will be conducted fairly and ethically. [If it has utility, feasibility and propriety] … they said we could turn to the difficult matters of the technical accuracy of the evaluation. (Stufflebeam, 1980: 90, cited in Pawson and Tilley, 1997: 13)

The authors object to this kowtowing to customer demands, which, in their view, is characteristic of what they call 'pragmatic evaluation'. This mode of evaluation is criticized as 'methodologically rootless'. Epistemologically speaking, knowledge is considered to be valid only to the extent that it is pragmatically acceptable, so, ontologically, the social world centres on 'power play'. Political astuteness and technical proficiency rule (Pawson and Tilley, 1997: 14).

The political dimension

The question of power is central to the dynamics of the stakeholder community. Evaluation is inherently political – it is rooted in some stakeholders' concerns to achieve change (and, of course, to justify preferred policies and actions!). In many instances, the political agenda is writ large. For example, a critical theory stance in health promotion is manifestly concerned to bring about social change involving, ultimately, a challenge to many aspects of capitalist economies. However, most programmes – even those having a radical agenda – tend to operate within systems rather than directly challenge them. For instance, community development might typically concentrate on creating food cooperatives rather than developing a popular movement designed to confront the power of the web of agencies and government departments involved in food production or, indeed, the retail profit motive. Pawson and Tilley (1997) have coined the term 'petty political' to refer to the operations involved in the former, limited pressure for change. We have retained the term in Figure 11.1 and expanded its meaning somewhat to refer to the various minor processes and all actors involved in jostling for power at different levels of influence.

Health promotion values – the seal of approval

While there may be conflicting values, both explicit and implicit, in the stakeholder community, it is worth emphasizing the research-related values that must be upheld if an evaluation is to follow ideological commitments to an empowerment model of health promotion. For example, research carried out on rather than with individuals and the community would be antithetical to the participation imperative inherent in empowerment. Woodall et al. (2018) reiterate the importance of health promotion values in research-related activities, suggesting the importance of upholding key issues – participation, empowerment, as illustrative examples – in research and evaluation practice.

ABSTRACT 11.1

What makes health promotion research distinct? Woodall, J., Warwick-Booth, L., South, J. and Cross, R. (2018)

(Continued)

There have been concerns about the decline of health promotion as a practice and discipline and alongside this, calls for a clearer articulation of health promotion research and what, if anything, makes it distinct. This discussion paper, based on a review of the literature, the authors' own experiences in the field, and a workshop delivered by two of the authors at the 8th Nordic Health Promotion Conference, seeks to state the reasons why health promotion research is distinctive. While by no means exhaustive, the paper suggests four distinctive features. The paper hopes to be a catalyst to enable health promotion researchers to be explicit in their practice and to begin the process of developing an agreed set of research principles.

Further to this, Green and South (2006) set out 10 key principles for evaluating public health interventions (see Box 11.3).

EVALUATION AND PROGRAMME DESIGN

Evaluation is often overlooked in programme design and this can be for a myriad of reasons according to Fleming and Baldwin (2020), including:

- limited time, expertise or resource in the programme team
- a belief that the programme is successful and an evaluation is unnecessary
- fear that an evaluation would highlight adverse outcomes
- the costs of external evaluation.

However, as a key element of systematic programme planning, evaluation should be considered from the outset and integrated at all stages. The model adopted here centres on the key elements described in Figure 11.2.

BOX 11.3 KEY PRINCIPLES FOR EVALUATING PUBLIC HEALTH INTERVENTIONS

1. Purpose: evaluation should have a clear purpose.
2. Practicality: evaluation should have practical relevance.
3. Process: evaluation should include attention to process as well as outcomes.
4. Peripheral (contextual) factors: evaluation should consider the effect of contextual factors.
5. Probing: evaluation should go further than attempting to offer simple input–output explanations to provide more complex understanding and contribute to the development of theory.
6 Plural: evaluation should use multiple methods to collect information.
7. Participation: evaluation should involve all stakeholders

8. Plausibility: findings should reflect the experience of stakeholder groups, i.e. they should make sense.
9. Power: evaluation should recognize the power structures within which it operates, but not be restricted by them. It should include the lay perspective and contribute to empowerment
10. Politics: evaluation is essentially political, informing decisions at different levels – project, organization, local policy, national policy.

Source: Green and South (2006: 33)

Three varieties of evaluation are included in Figure 11.2 – summative, formative and process. 'Summative' refers to an assessment of the extent to which the programme has achieved its purpose. It is primarily concerned with the achievement of outcomes. The term 'impact' is generally used to refer to immediate changes that lead to longer-term 'outcomes'. However, there is inconsistency in the literature with some authors referring to outcomes leading to impacts. For simplicity, our preference is to use the single term 'outcome' and, if necessary, distinguish short-, medium- and long-term outcomes.

'Process' evaluation consists of recording information collected throughout the programme and will be used for 'illumination'. 'Formative' evaluation also involves using information acquired throughout the programme. However, this information is used during the programme to make changes designed to maximize outcomes.

The construction of objectives formulates specific goals based on intended outcomes and information about the 'client group' or community. The actual selection of research methodology and methods

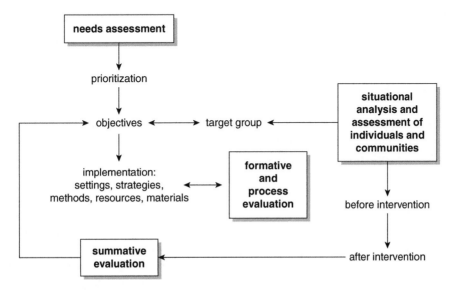

Figure 11.2 Programme planning – the place of research

will depend on the nature of the evaluation task and, of course, the ethical/ideological appropriateness of that methodology. At this juncture, we will consider the ideological issues associated with the choice of research methodology. In essence, this will involve discussing approaches that have competing value positions and which have been the subject of considerable debate.

BOX 11.4 PARADIGM – A DEFINITION

Paradigms are preferred ways of understanding reality, building knowledge and gathering information about the world.

Source: Tracy (2013)

PARADIGM WARS – POSITIVISM AND ITS ALTERNATIVES

Conflicts between different paradigms (see Box 11.4 for definition) not only apply to the nature and philosophy of health promotion, but are reflected in the stance taken about what should or should not constitute appropriate and ethical evaluation. The major debate centres on the battle between positivism and a collection of approaches associated with qualitative methodology.

'Epistemology' is at the very centre of disagreements about which research approach and its concomitant methods are acceptable. Epistemology is concerned with beliefs about knowledge and what constitutes evidence. It is associated with the concept of 'ontology'. Denzin (1994: 99) succinctly describes the relationship between paradigms and the abovementioned concepts, along with their specific application in methodologies:

> A paradigm encompasses three elements: epistemology, ontology and methodology. Epistemology asks, how do we know the world? What is the relationship between the enquirer and the known? Ontology raises basic questions about the nature of reality. Methodology focuses on how we gain knowledge about the world.

Accordingly, some approaches to evaluation would be considered inherently flawed and incapable of revealing the 'truth'. Furthermore, advocates of some approaches might argue that there are different forms of truth, while others might deny that truth exists.

The positivist paradigm

By way of simplifying a complex field of philosophical analysis and criticism related to conceptualizations of research and practice, three different paradigms will be discussed briefly below. These are positivism, interpretivism and a 'third way' that espouses critical realism and a utilization-focused perspective. The major debate has been between advocates of interpretivism and what has been until recently the dominant paradigm of positivism – notwithstanding the fact that interpretivism itself embraces a number of research traditions. The 'third way' might be subject to challenge, largely because of its alleged compromise position. For health promotion, however, the positivism vs interpretivism debate is of special importance as a positivist approach has characterized the medical model and underwritten the alleged 'gold standard' for evaluating programmes – the randomized controlled trial (RCT).

Positivism defined

The positivist paradigm is often espoused as the 'scientific' approach to research (Hennink et al., 2011). Positivist philosophy can be traced to Auguste Comte (1798–1857), who compared and contrasted three constructions of reality – theological, metaphysical and positive. Positivism was equated with science, which was seen as the sole way forward to gaining a true understanding of the world. Comte's ideas were adopted by the logical positivists, whose philosophy rested on the assumption that we could gain an accurate representation of the world through our senses (and various devices that would increase the power of our senses); this 'scientific knowledge' would form the basis for progressive and cumulative advances in knowledge that would be free from partial interpretations and superstitious interpretations of reality.

Positivist science was viewed as having a value-free, 'neutral' status. It was objective rather than subjective. Moreover, the positivist approach was more than mere empiricism – a procedure, 'involving the production of accurate data – meticulous, precise, generalisable – in which the data themselves constitute the end for the research. It is summed up by the catchphrase "the facts speak for themselves"' (Bulmer, 1982). While accurate data collection and generalizability are also characteristic of positivist research, unlike empiricism, it is theory driven. The ultimate goal is the construction of general laws.

Experiment is central to positivist methodology, although Popper has challenged its capacity to achieve verification. His centrally important concept of falsifiability is now inevitably considered to be at the heart of 'scientific method'. In other words, a theory holds until disproved, so the logical method of science is falsification and continual checking of claims to knowledge. In short, the key features of Popper's perspective are as follows:

- it is critical of 'induction'
- it is impossible to verify a universal theory with any degree of certainty, but it is possible to disprove a theory and therefore only one convincing 'disproof' will result in the rejection of theory regardless of how much supporting evidence already exists
- therefore, theory (a set of hypotheses) only survives until disproved
- accordingly, the method employed by 'science' must be falsification
- therefore, the 'gold standard' results of a properly constructed randomized controlled trial would also only hold until disproved.

Knowledge is, therefore, always provisional. As the procedure involves deduction rather than induction and is based on the confirmation or falsification of hypotheses, the scientific model adopted has been described as 'hypothetico-deductive' (Popper, 1945, 1959).

Perhaps unsurprisingly, social and behavioural scientists seeking an objective truth looked to the natural sciences and positivism as the way forward. As we have noted, such an approach is central to the medical model. However, its relevance for health promotion has been subject to intense criticism associated with the mounting challenge to medical hegemony.

Interpretivism – an alternative to positivism

While positivism is relatively easy to define, it is much more difficult to pick one's way through the plethora of methodologies and methods that constitute the opposition! Perhaps the most frequently used overarching terms are 'interpretivism' and 'constructivism'.

'Interpretivism' – a concept virtually identical to 'constructivism' (Guba and Lincoln, 1989) – centres on people's ways of interpreting/making sense of reality. It is essentially inductive – theory tends to be generated from data rather than data being used to test theory.

As Hennink et al. (2011: 14) note, interpretivism:

> means that the approach seeks to understand people's lived experience from the perspective of people themselves, which is often referred to as the emic perspective or the inside perspective.

One of the main traditions within the interpretivist approach has been termed 'hermeneutics' (from the Greek god Hermes, the messenger, who interpreted messages from Zeus to human beings). Holloway (1997: 87) notes that:

> Researchers … gather data from language, texts and actions. They have to return to the data frequently, and ask the participants what the data mean to them.

Guba and Lincoln (1989) emphasize the importance of a 'dialectic' approach that involves questioning assumptions. As Schwandt (1994: 128) explains:

> They believe that the best means of achieving researcher and client constructions of reality is the 'hermeneutic-dialectic' process, so called because it is interpretive and fosters comparing and contrasting divergent constructions in an effort to achieve a synthesis of same. They strongly emphasize that the goal of constructivist enquiry is to achieve a consensus (or, failing that, an agenda for negotiation) on issues and concerns that define the nature of the enquiry.

Apart from the constructions of the research reality embodied in this latter constructivist approach, it will be apparent that 'subjects' of the research are not 'objects' but, rather, participants. This commitment is also apparent in what Guba and Lincoln (1989) called 'fourth generation evaluation', which entails stakeholder involvement, exploration of different perspectives and issues, negotiation to achieve consensus, development of reports communicating the nature of consensus and proposed actions to participants, and an iterative process of reviewing and revisiting the evaluation to address perceptions, concerns and issues that have not been resolved.

This emphasis on the experience and perspectives of individuals is central to phenomenological enquiry – another major strand within the interpretivist tradition associated with the work of Husserl and later Heidegger. It draws on Hegel's philosophy and particularly the centrality of conscious experience. A key feature of phenomenological research is that it attempts to be free from assumptions, preconceptions and preformed hypotheses.

By way of a résumé of the key features of the paradigms opposed to positivism, we might usefully summarize the 'manifesto' of new paradigm research, according to Reason and Rowan (1981) as shown in Box 11.5.

BOX 11.5   A MANIFESTO OF NEW PARADIGM RESEARCH

- Research is never neutral – either it accepts or rejects the status quo.
- Research may be beneficial, but it may also be harmful.
- A close relationship between researcher and researched is essential. Both are equal in the research process. They are partners in defining the scope and nature of the research.
- Researcher and researched should have equal ownership of the products of the research.
- Research should be particularly concerned with knowledge having a practical, action-orientated outcome.
- Research should encourage people to take action – new paradigm research supports the politics of self-determination.
- New paradigm research rejects a traditional 'objective' approach and associated quantitative methods. It seeks a new kind of synthesis of subjectivity and objectivity.
- New paradigm researchers are committed to a holistic view of people and the environments and contexts in which they live their lives.

Source: After Reason and Rowan (1981)

Pawson and Tilley (1997: 19) provide a useful graphic summary of constructivist research and its rationale (see Figure 11.3).

Participatory research

As we noted earlier, the participative convictions of interpretivism chime with health promotion's ideological commitment to involving client and community. Participatory approaches fit well with health promotion's core values, which privilege the idea of individuals and communities taking greater control of their situation (Hubley et al., 2021). Participatory approaches are an important cornerstone of health promotion research and are a useful way of understanding issues faced by communities and militate against any perceived power imbalances between evaluators and communities. A closer recognition of power in the research endeavour is perhaps in sharper focus in health promotion research and evaluation, given the broader goals to reduce health inequalities and frequently because health promotion research engages with marginalized groups in society (Woodall et al., 2018). Eakin et al. (1996), for example, outline how power is a salient issue for health promotion research, with the inclusivity and participation of individuals and the community in health promotion research processes as important. Participatory evaluation approaches are therefore often favoured in health promotion as

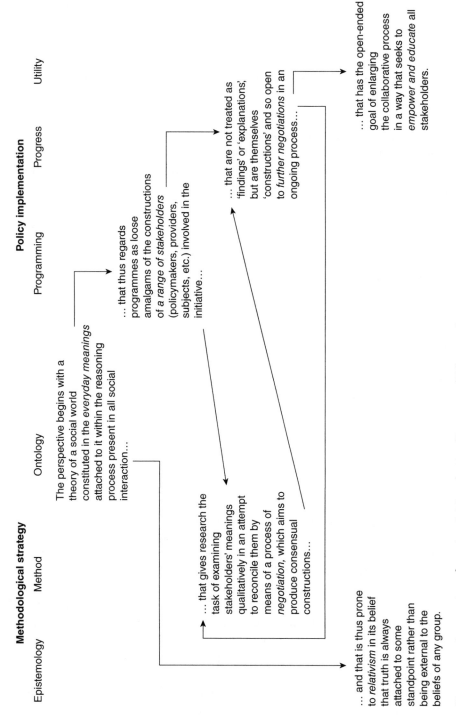

Figure 11.3 An overview of constructivist evaluation (Pawson and Tilley, 1997)

they can potentially offer greater illumination of issues with findings more likely to be considered and implemented (Woodall and Cross, 2021).

While the meaning of participatory research varies, as noted by Mantoura and Potvin (2013), it is most often defined in relational terms describing the interaction between those conducting research and those whose lives are the focus of the research (Wright et al., 2010). Whyte (1997) provides an interesting historical slant on the development of 'participatory research' and 'action research'. He notes the possible confusion between the terms 'action research', 'participatory research' and 'participatory action research' and proceeds to remind us that it is possible to have action research without participation and participatory research without action. Moreover, participation and action can 'emerge' from social research and Whyte recalls how, in his classic research on Street Corner Society (Whyte, 1943), two participants, Doc and Sam Franco, 'became in a very real sense participant observers'. Moreover:

> We all hoped that publication of the book would eventually be helpful to the district and to others like it … (although there were no specific action or policy recommendations). Certain individuals begin as informants, then become key informants and ended up as co-participant observers, helping the professional field worker to interpret what they are learning from interviewing and observation.

Whyte (1991: 20) defined 'participatory action research' (PAR) as follows:

> In participatory action research (PAR), some of the people in the organization or community under study participate actively with the professional researcher throughout the research process from the initial design to the final presentation of results and discussion of action implications.

He subsequently felt that it was necessary to expand this definition to take account of emancipatory values (which he considered had always been implicit in the first definition). The addendum (Whyte, 1997: 111–12) states:

> The social purpose underlying PAR is to empower low-status people in the organization or community to make decisions and take actions which were previously foreclosed to them.

Realistic vs utilization-focused evaluation

Pawson and Tilley (1997) have launched a vigorous, and influential, challenge to both traditional, positivist research paradigms and, at the same time, to the constructivists' equally constraining insistence that, in the words of Guba and Lincoln (1989: 17), 'no accommodation is possible between positivist and constructivist belief systems as they are now formulated'. To do this, they felt, was to throw out the evaluation baby with the positivist bathwater! However, they questioned what they describe as a purely 'pragmatic approach', which they felt was exemplified in Patton's (1982: 49) alleged lack of interest in the epistemological basis of research and his overemphasis on an all-purpose methodological 'toolbox'. They disapprovingly cite the following statement:

> If a funding mandate calls for a summative outcomes evaluation, then the evaluator had better be prepared to produce such an animal, complete with a final report that includes that terminology right there on the front page, in big letters in the title.

This is perhaps rather unfair. Patton (1997), in a text on 'utilization-focused evaluation', acknowledges the value of both positivist and interpretivist paradigms. He considers that discussions about paradigm wars 'are now primarily about philosophy rather than methods'. He (1997: 296) adds:

> I disagree, then, that philosophical assumptions necessarily require allegiance by evaluators to one paradigm or the other. Pragmatism can overcome seemingly logical contradictions … the flexible and open evaluator can view the same data from the perspective of each paradigm and can help adherents of either paradigm interpret data in more than one way.

From our particular perspective on the inherently political nature of health promotion, we should note Patton's belief that evaluation is not value-free and 'politics is omnipresent in evaluation' (see Box 11.6).

Patton also adds that, as utilization-focused evaluation is pragmatic (and 'useful'), it can be applied to a variety of situations having different ideological commitments. Accordingly, he (1997: 103) states that: 'Using evaluation to mobilize for social action, empower participants, and support social justice are options on the menu of evaluation process uses.'

An interesting indicator of Patton's 'pragmatic paradigm' is provided by his apparent affection for Rudyard Kipling's (*Just So Stories*, 1902) well-known aphorism:

> I keep six honest serving men, (They taught me all I knew);
>
> Their names are What and Why and When and How and Where and Who.

He translates this as:

- Who is the evaluation for?
- What do we need to find out?
- Why do we want to find that out?
- When will the findings be needed?
- Where should we gather information?
- How will the results be used?

Further consideration of the philosophy and ideology of pragmatism requires much more space than is at our disposal here and, we have, no doubt, not seen the end of the debate!

BOX 11.6 WHEN IS EVALUATION NOT POLITICAL?

Evaluation is not political under the following conditions:

- no one cares about the programme
- no one knows about the programme

- no money is at stake
- no power or authority is at stake
- and no one in the programme, making decisions about the programme, or otherwise involved in, knowledgeable about, or attached to the programme, is sexually active.

Source: Patton (1997: 352)

Realistic evaluation

Pawson and Tilley's approach to 'realistic evaluation' has been particularly influential in evaluating 'social programmes' and, thus, is especially relevant to the complex interventions and collaborations characteristic of health promotion. The approach can be termed 'post-positive' and recognizes the existence of realities that can be investigated in robust fashion and used to implement social policy. At the same time, the narrow positivist approach epitomized by RCTs is determinedly discarded. The authors approvingly quote Guba and Lincoln's observation that true experimental design 'effectively strips away the context and yields results that are valid only in other contextless situations' (1989: 60, cited in Pawson and Tilley, 1997: 22). Realistic evaluation rejects this 'successionist' logic and argues for a 'generative logic'. The essence of realistic evaluation is to be found in a simple formula:

Outcome = mechanisms + context

Part of the rationale for Pawson and Tilley's rejection of the simplistic causal underpinning of the RCT is based on the recognition of a 'stratified reality' and inherently complex 'mechanisms'. Observations of 'regularities' in both physical and social science can be understood and influenced only by understanding these mechanisms. We will later, in discussing health promotion programmes, make reference to the 'black box' that must be illuminated if understanding is to be gained and efficient programmes achieved. Moreover, the individual choices resulting from the interplay of 'mechanisms' take place within 'contexts' – in other words, within various settings and their associated sets of norms and social rules. Accordingly:

Evaluators need to acknowledge that programmes are implemented in a changing and permeable social world, and that programme effectiveness may thus be subverted or enhanced through the unanticipated intrusion of new contexts and new causal powers. Evaluators (also) need to focus on how the causal mechanisms which generate social and behavioural problems are removed or countered through the alternative causal mechanisms introduced in a social programme … (Pawson and Tilley, 1997: 216–18)

Before leaving our brief description of realistic evaluation, it is worth noting that qualitative/interpretivist methodology is central to its philosophy and practice. One particularly interesting aspect is the authors' argument that a central part of the collaboration of researcher and participants involves a 'teaching-learning' process: stakeholders are 'taught' by the researchers so that they gain understandings of programmes and their attributes in order to participate fully in (empowered) decision-making. Also, of course, the researchers need to be taught by the stakeholders to gain maximum insight into the social and psychological realities and constructions of reality.

Before proceeding to consider the factors associated with selecting indicators of programme success, we should perhaps end this section on paradigm wars by asking where we stand. Which paradigms and ideologies and methodologies would seem to be most appropriate to health promotion? Should the emphasis be on agency or structure? Should we aim to seek an objective truth or recognize that there are different interpretations of reality?

Springett draws on the work of Habermas and Heidegger to identify important considerations for health promotion:

> the relationship between organism and the environment, on context, on the whole being greater than the sum of the parts; on connexions and synergy; on emergent systems, complexity and non-linear causality. (2001: 142)

The 'realist' perspective recognizes the existence of structures and institutional factors which are 'independent of the individual's reasoning and desires' (Pawson and Tilley, 1997: 23). At the same time, it acknowledges the importance of including a constructivist or interpretivist perspective in relation to exploring individual experience. Similarly, interpretive approaches are central to critical theory, but they also accept the existence of structures and processes that shape individual experience (Connelly, 2001) and that could be explored by other forms of enquiry.

We would wish to avoid postmodern pessimism and consider that it is, in fact, possible to develop general understandings of the world. However, we recognize that multiple interpretations occur as a result of psychological and social constructions of reality. Our stance is thus consistent with the realist and critical theory positions. Life and health are complex and we must gain in-depth understandings drawing on multiple methodologies if we are to exert influence over the development of health promotion – indeed, the expansive methodological toolkit that health promotion researchers have at their disposal can and should be drawn upon in their practice (Woodall et al., 2018). We are firmly committed to participative, emancipatory research designed to empower and address social injustice and health inequalities. Health promotion is inherently interdisciplinary and not dogmatically tied to a fixed research paradigm, view or perspective. Health promotion research and evaluation should be flexible and diverse to address the issue being explored or investigated and it is our view that such a position is upheld, especially given the range and types of work carried out under the health promotion banner.

EFFECTIVENESS, EFFICIENCY AND EFFICACY

In the last analysis, evaluation is concerned with whether or not an intervention has been successful notwithstanding alternative conceptualizations and debate about what constitutes success. Two standards are typically used in assessing the extent of success – or failure. These are 'effectiveness' and 'efficiency'. The former term simply refers to the extent to which a programme has achieved its goals, while 'efficiency' is a measure of relative effectiveness – that is, how successful a programme has been in comparison to competing strategies or methods. For instance, if a course of drugs could lower population cholesterol levels more quickly, completely and safely than dietary change, then it would be more efficient (although possibly less cost-effective) to prescribe that drug.

The efficacy paradox

The concept of efficacy has also been used, albeit less commonly, as a measure of effectiveness. It describes effectiveness and efficiency when interventions operate under ideal conditions: 'Effectiveness has all the attributes of efficacy except one: it reflects performance under ordinary conditions' (Brook and Lohr, 1985: 711).

The concept of efficacy relates to the notion of programme fidelity, which means the extent to which an intervention is delivered in accordance with recommended best practice. It has particular significance for evaluating health promotion programmes in relation to what we describe here as the 'efficacy paradox'. For instance, if an intervention has been shown to be effective when it has been constructed according to an ideal specification and implemented with complete fidelity, the chances are that ordinary practitioners working under average conditions will not be able to achieve the same degree of success. Indeed, the programme might fail. Conversely, when such a programme has not met its objectives and, consequently, has been considered ineffective, that evaluation judgement is flawed as the programme was doomed to fail due to inadequate implementation. We will consider the implications of such flawed judgement when discussing the question of validity later in the chapter. For now, we should merely note that programme design must clearly identify what might be achieved within existing limitations and set the objectives accordingly. If these limited results are judged to be not worthwhile, the proposed programme should be scrapped. In the last analysis, the decision is grounded in health economics – do the programme gains justify the expenses incurred?

On cost-effectiveness

One of the most important criteria for appraising the efficiency of health promotion programmes involves calculating the relative financial costs of competing interventions. That said, there are a plethora of methodological problems relating to economic evaluations of health promotion interventions and how economic analysis captures benefits for the individual and broader effects on the family, community or society as a whole (Huter et al., 2018). There are several types of analyses relating to intervention costs and the choice is broadly down to whether one or more interventions are under consideration and whether costs or costs and effects are being included (Issel, 2009). Godfrey (2001) notes the tendency for using 'partial' economic assessments – for example, merely describing the cost of an intervention. Clearly, this situation would be seen as far from satisfactory by health economists and Godfrey lists four different types of 'full' economic evaluation:

- Cost-minimization – the costs of two or more interventions assumed to achieve identical outcomes are calculated. The intervention that minimizes costs is judged to be the intervention of choice.

- Cost-effectiveness analysis – in addition to measuring the cost of programmes, benefits are assessed in quantifiable terms, such as the numbers of individuals exercising regularly or uptake of immunization against childhood diseases. It would, of course, be meaningless to make judgements about relative value for money unless indicators of health common to all programmes are employed (for instance, life years gained).
- Cost-utility analysis – this mode of analysis seeks to measure the utility or values attached to particular health gains. Quality adjusted life years (QALYs) are typically used to assess utility.
- Cost–benefit analysis (CBA) – this not only states the costs in monetary terms, but also seeks to place a price tag on the benefits accruing from the programme. A calculation of the cost per given benefit is then possible, typically expressed as a cost–benefit ratio.

Following these observations, it is both clear and logical – and indeed ethical – that if two or more programmes prove to be equally effective and acceptable, then the intervention that costs least should be selected. This is in line with Godfrey's (2001) view that the primary purpose of economic evaluation is to maximize what can be achieved by a given budget. Box 11.7 provides examples of the calculated benefits against costs of selected health promotion measures.

Although at first sight this type of analysis may be very seductive for those keen to demonstrate effectiveness and cost-effectiveness, there are both technical and ideological concerns. While costing 'input' is relatively unproblematic, the appropriateness of costing 'output' – that is, assessing and assigning a value to life and quality of life – poses major ethical problems, as discussed in Chapter 2. Indeed, the relevance of cost–benefit analysis to more holistic interpretations of health and interventions operating at interpersonal, community, social and environmental levels that are more typical of health promotion, is very challenging to cost with accuracy and precision (Huter et al., 2018). Moreover, Green and South (2006) argue that if cost-effectiveness is the sole criterion, then interventions targeted at easy-to-change groups would be favoured over those that focused on groups more resistant to change or coping with adverse social circumstances. This would ultimately result in widening health inequalities. Attention, therefore, needs to be given to 'goals such as equity, regeneration, social inclusion and social justice' (2006: 41).

Furthermore, costing studies are highly technical activities and there may be clear difficulties in translating findings for a variety of audiences (see the last section of Chapter 12 on 'Evidence into practice'). Issel (2009: 519), therefore, urges practitioners to become 'savvy consumers of economic evaluations', and while we would partially agree, we would also suggest an imperative for the research community to disseminate findings in appropriate ways.

BOX 11.7 HEALTH PROMOTION – INSTANCES OF ECONOMIC EFFECTIVENESS

- Compañeros en Salud Programa de Enfermedades Crónicas (CESPEC) – a novel community-based model of diabetes care in rural Mexico is a comprehensive model that integrates community health workers, provider education, supply chain management and active case finding.

A study sought to compare the cost-effectiveness of CESPEC with usual care. The economic cost of the CESPEC diabetes model was US$144 per patient per year, compared with US$125 for usual care. That said, CESPEC was associated with 0.13 additional years of health-adjusted life expectancy compared with usual care and 0.02 additional years in the first five years of treatment (Duan et al., 2021).

- The Community-based Hypertension Improvement Project (ComHIP) in Ghana is an intervention with multiple components, including: community-based education on cardiovascular disease (CVD) risk factors and healthy lifestyles; community-based screening and monitoring of blood pressure. ComHIP was compared against standard hypertension care in Ghana. The research concluded that ComHIP failed to develop a model of delivery that achieved sufficient levels of retention and outcomes were not impactful enough to achieve cost-effective implementation (Pozo-Martin et al., 2021).

- Smoke-free prison policies – that prevent smoking in any part of the prison setting – were found to be cost-effective because of health benefits after reductions in smoking and exposure to second-hand smoke (Hunt et al., 2022).

- A Danish smoking-cessation telephone service 'quitline' that offers counselling on smoking cessation, showed a total of 511 ex-smokers gaining 2172 life years based on continued abstinence over 12 months. The costs per life years saved were estimated at €213 for ex-smokers using the service (Rasmussen, 2013).

DISENTANGLING COMPLEXITY – SELECTING INDICATORS OF SUCCESS

The purpose of indicators is 'to capture key aspects of a programme and its effects' (Green and South, 2006: 45). They provide insight into whether programme objectives have been achieved or whether progress is being made towards them. However, the selection of indicators is essentially political and influenced by values and ideologies. Hubley et al. (2021) suggest that indicators will reflect the extent to which programmes focus on the use of medical and social models and individualistic and structuralistic approaches.

We noted in Chapter 4 the centrality of objectives to programme planning. The identification of appropriate indicators will be more straightforward if programme objectives are well defined and comprehensive. Rigorously formulated objectives provide a secure basis for identifying indicators of success – particularly if they set out standards and conditions. SMART objectives should lead to SMART indicators (specific, measurable, appropriate, relevant and time related). The acronym SPICED has also been used and incorporates some of the key principles referred to above:

Subjective

Participatory

Interpretable

Cross-checked

Empowering

Disaggregated.

Figure 11.4 provides an overview of a hypothetical, large-scale health promotion programme.

First, it is assumed that the programme has been designed according to the principles of systematic planning discussed earlier in this book. It is launched at a particular time (T1) and will achieve its final goals (if ever) at another point in time (T4). Temporal progress is indicated by a proximal–distal spectrum – that is, activities occurring at T1 are proximal to the start of the programme, whereas final outcomes at T4 and all other events in between will be more or less distal.

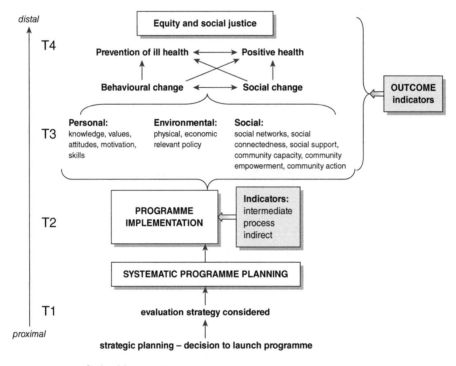

Figure 11.4   An overview of a health promotion programme

Two kinds of final outcomes are shown in Figure 11.4. They include, on the one hand, the traditional goals of a preventive model – namely, primary, secondary and tertiary prevention – and, on the other, the outcomes of a strategy seeking to address 'positive health'. The emphasis on the former in many evaluations reflects their respective ease of measurement. However, from a health promotion perspective, it is important to address the challenge and include the positive dimension. The label 'positive health' is used to refer to any outcomes related to 'quality of life' or, even more broadly, 'the good life'. These are not, of course, completely discrete as the quality of life is typically damaged by disease and enhanced by its prevention. Moreover, as has also been clearly demonstrated, the achievement of well-being, and, more demonstrably, the reduction of inequalities, may have a major impact on preventive outcomes.

There is frequently a substantial time gap between particular health promotion inputs and what might be seen to be final outcomes. For example, it may take many years for the benefits of a school-based healthy eating and exercise programme to become apparent in reduced mortality from coronary heart disease – the gap between T1 and T4 in such a case could well be 30 or 40 years. The use of morbidity and mortality data as indicators to assess the effectiveness of the teaching programme would thus be entirely unrealistic! The goal of the health promotion programme would be to alter the known risk factors.

A further objection is based on the fact that many successful health education/promotion interventions may be necessary, but not sufficient to influence final outcomes. Typically, a complicated web of inputs over time would be needed. For instance, effective life skills training, together with an efficient sex education programme in schools, might only have an impact on sexual risk-taking if policy measures have been implemented to ensure ready access to condoms and, say, a user-friendly drop-in centre for young people.

Intermediate, indirect and process indicators

The myriad of activities and interventions under the rubric of health promotion, and the multiple levels of operation, create challenges for its evaluation and measurement (Thorogood and Coombes, 2010). As an example, Cross et al. (2017b) in their commentary paper discuss the challenges in 'measuring' empowerment, arguing that the lack of clear guidance is problematic given that it is a fundamental value of the discipline.

ABSTRACT 11.2

Empowerment: challenges in measurement. Cross, R., Woodall, J. and Warwick-Booth, L. (2017b)

Empowerment is core to health promotion; however, there is a lack of consensus in the wider literature as to how to define it and at what level it may occur. Definitional inconsistency inevitably leads to challenges in measuring empowerment; yet if it is as important as is claimed, this must be addressed. This paper discusses the complexities of measuring empowerment and puts forward a number of recommendations for researchers and policy-makers as to how this can be achieved, noting some of the tensions that may arise between theoretical considerations, research and practice. The authors argue that empowerment is a culturally and socially defined construct and that this should be taken into account in attempts to measure it. Finally they conclude that, in order to build up the evidence base for empowerment, there is a need for research clearly defining what it is and how it is being measured.

Green and South (2006) emphasize that it is important to have realistic aspirations for what might reasonably be achieved within the time frame of a programme when defining outcome indicators. For example, these might include a change in health-related behaviour, or the introduction of a workplace health policy to achieve environmental change, or development of social capital within a community. To reiterate our earlier point: if strong evidence already exists about the link between such factors and disease reduction or positive health goals, there is no need to revisit this. If there is no such robust relationship with mortality and morbidity – or positive health – then there is no ethical justification for the introduction of the programme in the first place!

Intermediate indicators identify antecedents of the outcomes. They relate to the various stages in the causal pathway between the intervention and the outcomes. Intermediate indicators contribute, in various degrees, to the outcome. Hubley et al. (2021) point out that the classification of indicators as intermediate or outcome is to some extent a matter of definition. Furthermore, this could well vary from programme to programme. For example, self-empowerment and social capital may be deemed to be outcomes worth pursuing in their own right, so evidence of achievement in this regard, provided by measures of confidence and control, could rightly be called outcome indicators. However, it seems increasingly clear that empowerment is a major determinant of adopting behaviour consistent with preventive outcomes. In this latter case, evidence of empowerment would provide intermediate indicators of success.

Process indicators would be used to record the fidelity and quality of the programme and identify any need for improvement and refinement. Understanding which elements of the process contributed to success – or equally to failure – is also important in relation to the wider dissemination and uptake of programmes.

Implementing a programme may involve a number of subsidiary activities such as the development of leaflets or the training of staff. Indicators relating to these are referred to as indirect indicators – for example, pre-testing leaflets to assess their suitability or assessing the capacity of teachers to provide drug education following training. Although necessary to the success of the intervention, these indirect indicators do not form part of the direct causal pathway linking intervention and outcome. Again, the distinction can be blurred. Barnes et al. (2004) recognize the difficulty of separating process, outcomes and systems indicators. For example, the development of good partnerships may be an essential element of the process and also a positive outcome.

Opening the black box

One of health promotion's major requirements is illumination. In other words, we need to know not just whether or not a programme has been effective, but to identify key elements of the process and how these link to outcomes. In line with realist evaluation, we need to understand how an intervention works and why it works, or fails to work, within a particular context. The more complicated the programme, the greater the need for illuminative insights.

Again, the significance of illumination in evaluation is not a discovery of health promotion. Workers in the field of educational research who questioned the value of experimental design also argued the case for gaining insights through illumination. Parlett and Hamilton (1972), for example, proposed an 'illuminative, social-anthropological paradigm' that took account of the wider contexts in which educational programmes function. They used an analogy with the theatre to point out that, without such insights, evaluators risk being 'rather like a critic who reviews a production on the basis of the script and applause-meter readings, having missed the performance'!

Figure 11.5 illustrates what might be called the 'black box problem'. It simulates an experimental evaluation of a school-based programme designed to reduce the incidence of unwanted pregnancies by comparing its long-term results with one of a number of control schools lacking such an intervention. An evaluator would need detailed information about the intervention and its dynamics. Figure 11.6 shows the kinds of complexity that might be revealed if the black box were opened.

In short, we would expect to observe a complex web of synergistic elements. It also demonstrates that a number of additional, cumulative inputs would be needed over quite a lengthy period of time if success were to be achieved. Moreover, as a school setting might be only one component of a comprehensive community-wide programme, Figure 11.6, in fact, substantially underestimates the level of complexity that there could actually be.

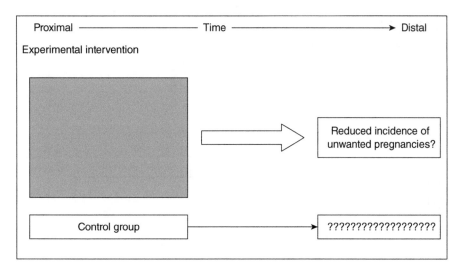

Figure 11.5   The black box problem

Theory of Change and the selection of indicators

Reference to relevant theory and models that shed light on the anticipated change process will help with the identification of appropriate indicators. For example, the use of the health action model (HAM) will shed light on the various factors that inform behavioural intention and those that will affect whether that intention is put into action.

As we have noted above, indirect, intermediate and outcome indicators should be selected to provide evidence at various stages along the complex and often convoluted pathway leading from proximal interventions to ultimate outcomes. Yet, in many instances, the assumptive logic linking an intervention with anticipated effects is either missing or poorly articulated, leading to problems with

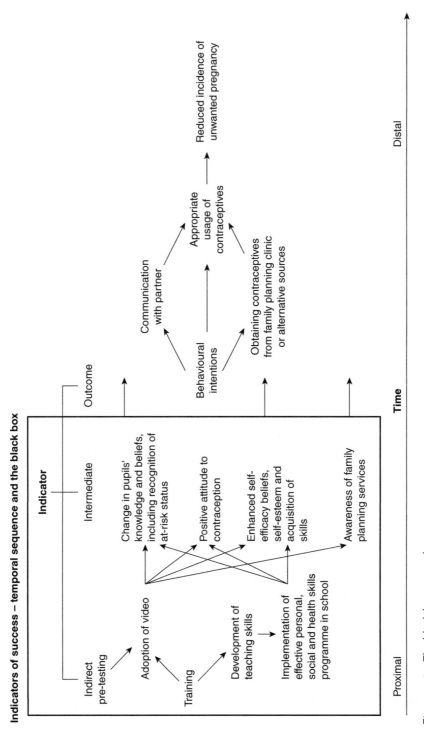

Figure 11.6 The black box opened

evaluation as well as compromising the success of an intervention. This is particularly so in the case of complex community initiatives.

> A key reason complex programs are so difficult to evaluate is that the assumptions that inspire them are poorly articulated ... stakeholders of complex community initiatives typically are unclear about how the change process will unfold and therefore place little attention to the early and mid-term changes that need to happen in order for a longer term goal to be reached. The lack of clarity about the 'mini-steps' that must be taken to reach a long term outcome not only makes the task of evaluating a complex initiative challenging, but reduces the likelihood that all of the important factors related to the long-term goal will be addressed. (ActKnowledge, undated a)

The Theory of Change Approach was developed by the Aspen Institute Roundtable on Community Change to respond to the challenge of evaluating comprehensive community initiatives (CCIs), also referred to as complex community initiatives (see Connell et al., 1995; Fulbright-Anderson et al., 1998). These involve interventions with multiple components leading to multilevel outcomes. The Theory of Change Approach provides a means of unpicking the steps along the pathways of change – or indeed the complex networks. It involves 'surfacing' the latent theory that outlines stakeholders' expectations about the various steps along the pathway linking activities to the achievement of goals. This is done through a guided process that draws on existing knowledge and theory and also the insight of practitioners and other stakeholders. Evaluators and stakeholders work together to 'co-construct' the Theory of Change for an initiative. The stages are summarized in Box 11.8. They start with the identification of long-term goals as, in practice, it has proved easier to reach agreement about these and then work back to intermediate outcomes and activities. The development of indicators for each stage makes the theory testable.

BOX 11.8 STAGES IN THE THEORY OF CHANGE

1. Identification of long-term goals and the assumptions behind them
2. Backwards mapping to connect to the preconditions or requirements needed to achieve the goal
3. Identification of the actions undertaken to achieve the desired change
4. Developing indicators to measure outcomes to assess the performance of the initiative
5. Writing a narrative explaining the logic of the initiative.

Source: ActKnowledge (undated b)

The characteristics of a good theory are held to be that it is:

* plausible
* doable
* testable. (Connell and Kubisch, 1998)

The use of logical frameworks for programme planning is consistent with the Theory of Change. As we noted in Chapter 4, logical frameworks help to ensure that all necessary elements of a programme are in place and also make explicit the assumptions about the way programmes will work. As with the Theory of Change, they help to ensure that programmes are successful as well as identifying key indicators to assess progress. An example of a Theory of Change linking the rationale for the activity (in this case, participatory action research) with anticipated short-, medium- and longer-term outcomes that provide the basis for the development of indicators comes from the Children's Fund evaluation (see Figure 11.7).

Theory of Change has been a popular approach for evaluating complex social policy programmes. This includes a whole range of programmes and initiatives, such as: anti-poverty tourism (Phi et al., 2018); web-based counselling and support for children and young people (Hanley et al., 2021); dementia care, treatment and support in middle-income countries (Breuer et al., 2022); and Figure 11.7 demonstrates how it was applied by the Children's Fund in their work with traveller children (see Barnes et al., 2004).

Mason and Barnes (2007) distinguish between those programmes that have involved evaluators from the initial stages of programme planning, more typical of the USA where the approach was developed, and those that have not involved evaluators until programmes are under way, more typical of the UK experience. In the latter situation, it is not uncommon for the theory to be constructed retrospectively and, indeed, to be influenced by the need to justify actions.

RELIABILITY, VALIDITY AND THE RCT

Having considered the various types of indicator to include in evaluation, it is important to ensure that resulting evidence is valid. In other words, if the combined results of the indirect, intermediate and outcome indicators demonstrate a certain level of effectiveness, we must be satisfied that the evidence is robust and any claims of success can be justified.

The two standard criteria for assessing the quality of research measures are reliability and validity. Reliability is concerned with consistency and replicability – that is, the extent to which research techniques will produce consistent results, regardless of how, when and where the research is carried out. For example, a completely reliable questionnaire should yield identical scores, whoever administers the questionnaire. Moreover, if individuals are retested, they should provide the same response (provided, of course, that they have not actually changed during the time that elapses between test and retest). Similarly, if individuals or groups are interviewed or observed, then different interviewers or observers should draw the same conclusions.

Validity is, quite simply, the extent to which investigators and their instruments actually measure what they intend to measure – and nothing else. It describes the truth and authenticity of research findings. An unreliable evaluation cannot be valid. Equally, an evaluation might demonstrate highly reliable results, but lack validity – it might merely have measured the wrong things, but done so very consistently.

In the context of evaluation of research, two varieties of validity are distinguished – internal and external. 'Internal validity' refers to the degree of certainty that the results of an evaluation are due to the intervention under investigation and not to other factors.

Problem/context	Activity	Rationale	Outcomes		
			short term	medium term	long term
Poor educational performances. Poorly integrated into schools and local communities. Poorer than average health. Lack of understanding of travellers in statutory agencies. Absence of culturally appropriate services and resources.	Participatory action research involving traveller and non-traveller children, their parents and front line workers from different agencies.	The 'problem' is one of relationships – collective activity is a good means of breaking down barriers. Limited evidence of interventions specific to traveller children, but positive experiences of the impact of PAR on participants. Involving ranges of service providers who will increase their skills and maximize sustainability. Learning from the research can inform service and policy developments.	Police, health service and education staff working together. Traveller and non-traveller children working together. Parents of traveller and non-traveller children involved. Different statutory agencies contributing resources to work with traveller children.	Increased skills and understanding amongst front line staff. Enhanced self-esteem amongst traveller children. Less bullying of traveller children. Development of more culturally appropriate services. Fewer complaints from non-traveller parents.	Better educational outcomes. Improved health. Less conflict within schools and in the local community.

Figure 11.7 A Theory of Change for work with traveller children (derived from Barnes et al., 2004)

'External validity' describes the generalizability of the results – that is, the extent to which a given intervention can be expected to produce similar results in other populations and, therefore, be of use to other practitioners and planners. A health promotion intervention might have been successful in one context, but the same success might not be achieved in another, where the local community may have a different cultural background or there are other differences in levels of community identity or active local organizations and faith-based groups, for example (Hubley et al., 2021). A recent review of RCTs examining mindfulness-based programmes for mental health promotion in adults in non-clinical settings concluded that while this intervention can promote mental health in the 'average nonclinical setting' it cannot be expected to work in every setting (Galante et al., 2021). It is clear how such a conclusion can leave health promotion practitioners with serious consideration as to whether such an approach should be implemented or not!

As we will see, on the one hand, the classic RCT is strong on internal validity, but weak on external validity. On the other hand, interpretivist approaches are, perhaps arguably, more likely to generate results that can be used by other practitioners. However, special efforts must be made to ensure rigour.

The RCT – strengths and limitations

The RCT conforms to the principles of true experimental design. The RCT is considered methodologically strong to assess cause and effect relationships and evidence of the effectiveness of interventions because of several features embedded in its design (Woodall and Rowlands, 2021). Within the domain of medicine, the popularity of the RCT – and the current movement for evidence-based medicine – have been ascribed to the influential work of Cochrane (1972, cited in McPherson, 1994: 6), who argued that evaluation of effectiveness should be the first priority of the NHS in the UK and decided 'to concentrate on one simple idea – the value of randomized controlled trials in improving the NHS – and to keep the book short and simple'.

Cochrane's rationale was certainly convincing, as was his demonstration that many routinely performed medical interventions were not based on evidence of effectiveness. The argument for evidence-based practice – and the use of experimental method – was by no means confined to medicine. Indeed, as Shacklock Evans (1962) points out, the use of experimental designs of the kind Cochrane espoused can be attributed primarily to Fisher (1949) and the field of agricultural biology and later applied to education by Lindquist (1940). The emphasis of the experimental approach on avoiding threats to internal validity can be seen in Fisher's (1949: 19) observation:

> Whatever degree of care and experimental skill is expended in equalizing the conditions, other than the one under test, which are liable to affect the result, this equalization must always be to a greater or less extent incomplete and in many important practical cases will be grossly defective.

Let us begin by noting some of the obvious limitations of claims that programmes have been effective where the validity of the results can be severely challenged!

Inadequacies in judging programme effectiveness

Situation 1 in Figure 11.8 is so limited in its utility that it cannot really be called a research design, as there is no indication of the status of the group before the intervention (X). The result of the assessment (observation 'O') might therefore be due to a positive effect of the intervention. Alternatively, the intervention might have had no effect at all. Indeed, it might have made things worse!

Situation 2 – a simple pre–post test design – provides more information. However, although it would be possible to record any changes occurring between the pre-test and post-test, it would not be possible to demonstrate with any degree of certainty that the changes were due to the intervention.

Situation 3 uses a control group that does not receive the intervention and, so, assuming that there is a statistically significant difference between pre- and post-test and no such difference in the control group, it is reasonable to conclude that the intervention did have an impact. Unfortunately, there can be no certainty that the experimental and control groups were identical in all key respects before the intervention. Accordingly, the apparently superior performance of the experimental group might, by chance, have been due to differences between the groups rather than the effectiveness of the intervention.

Situation 4, however, is a TRUE experimental design. This is symbolized here by the use of the traditional 'OXO' terminology initiated and elaborated by Campbell and Stanley (1963) and Cook and Campbell (1979). The essential difference is that 'subjects' are randomly assigned to experimental and control situations, thus partialling out differences of any kind. Randomization is the key to the superior status of the RCT and the justification for its gold standard accolade.

Furthermore, the rigour of RCT versions of true experimental design have been enhanced by the use of additional measures, such as the 'double blind trial', in which neither researchers nor subjects know who is receiving the active, experimental ingredient. This helps to minimize researcher bias and avoid placebo effects.

Type 1 and 2 errors and true experimental design

The major strength of true experimental designs is their capacity to avoid 'Type 1 error'. In other words, to avoid claiming that a given intervention has been effective when apparent differences between experimental and control groups might have resulted from extraneous factors. The success of the research design lies in its capacity to eliminate alternative causes so that the effects attributable to the intervention can be identified.

This particular virtue may be achieved at the expense of incurring a 'Type 2 error' – that is, drawing an erroneous conclusion that an intervention was ineffective when it may, in fact, actually have had an effect. For instance, a programme may actually have had an impact on the target group, but the instruments might have been insufficiently sensitive to discriminate between the effect on experimental and

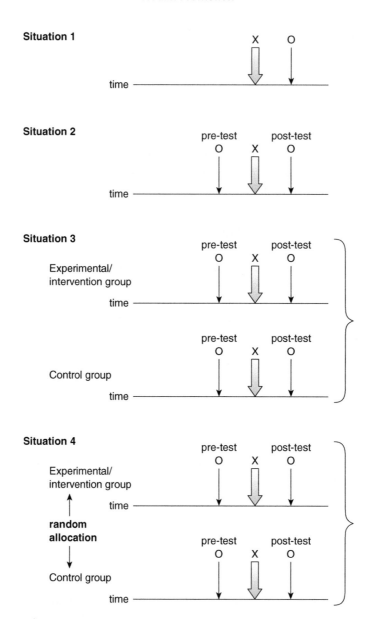

Figure 11.8   Evaluation designs

control groups. Similarly, failure to detect change may also occur when there are mixed populations and the positive effect of an intervention in one section of the population is diluted by a zero effect in the rest of the population or even a negative 'reactance' effect. An overview of different types of error is provided in Box 11.9.

BOX 11.9 FIVE TYPES OF ERROR

Type 1 error

An erroneous conclusion that an intervention has achieved significant change when, in fact, it has failed to do so.

Type 2 error

An erroneous conclusion that an intervention has failed to have a significant impact when, in fact, it has actually done so.

Type 3 error

Asserting that an intervention has failed to achieve successful results when it was so poorly designed that it could not possibly have had a desired effect.

Type 4 error

Conducting an evaluation of a programme that no one cares about and is irrelevant to decision-makers. Evaluation for the sake of evaluation is central to this error.

Type 5 error

An intervention is shown to produce a genuine statistically significant effect, but the change is so slight as to have no practical significance.

Source: After Basch and Gold (1986: 300–1)

Green and Lewis (1986: 264–7), while cautioning evaluators against the 'fallacy of assuming inexorable forward movement', list the following situations that may also distort understanding of the effectiveness of interventions and contribute to Type 1 and 2 errors.

- Delay of impact (or sleeper effect) – an intervention actually has an impact, but this does not emerge until later – perhaps quite a long time after the evaluation when circumstances are favourable.
- Decay of impact (or backsliding effect) – the intervention produces an effect, but this decays more or less rapidly. Without continuing measurement, the programme might have been judged a success when it had, for all practical purposes, been a failure.
- Borrowing from the future – the intervention triggers changes in behaviour that would have happened anyway, the programme merely hastening the inevitable.

- Secular trends – a positive secular trend may result in overestimating programme effects, while a negative secular trend may result in discounting an influence that had delayed the decline.
- Contrast effects – premature termination of a programme may create a backlash resulting in a slowing or reversal of behavioural outcomes that would have occurred had the programme continued.

Although accepted as standard practice for testing drugs, the limitations of the RCT have been recognized even within a biomedical context. Charlton (1991: 355) argued that the RCT was:

> vital but of restricted applicability to medicine … it should only be employed in conditions of clinical unpredictability. When an obviously effective treatment emerges there is no need for a controlled trial to establish its usefulness.

However, he noted that:

> Gain in objectivity is achieved by simplification and at the cost of completeness … the patient is depersonalized, the doctor is deskilled. (1991: 356)

Are RCTs ever relevant for evaluating health promotion?

Rigorous evaluation of studies is, of course, vitally important but this does not mean that the RCT is the best approach in all circumstances (Britton, 2010). In fact, our response to the question posed 'Are RCTs ever relevant for evaluating health promotion?' would be 'Well, not never, but hardly ever!' More particularly, we might say that the RCT or, more properly, the true experimental design, is only likely to be useful to the extent that the health promotion intervention approximates to the clinical trial. In other words, that, first, the intervention is simple and, second, we do not know the answer already nor have better ways of finding it. This is rare within the overall complexity of the health promotion enterprise. Furthermore, following our earlier discussion of realistic and utilization-focused evaluation, if the trial strips away consideration of contextual factors, the findings will have little relevance to other situations. Our views seem to resonate with others:

> RCTs are not a tool suitable for determining effectiveness of health promotion programs because their restrictive nature does not capture the complexity, community responsiveness, and wide scope present in many health promotion programs. (Groot, 2011: 510)

We have considered above some of the epistemological concerns about the use of RCTs for health promotion evaluation. There are also technical and practical issues.

Establishing an adequate control group presents a number of difficulties. Interventions are generally complex, frequently multisectoral and usually targeted at groups of various size rather than individuals. The allocation of individuals to intervention and control groups, as required by true experimental designs, is therefore simply not practicable. Random assignment of whole groups such as communities or schools is more feasible (see, for example, the effectiveness of a health-promoting schools approach using a cluster-randomization of Australian schools [Waters et al., 2017]). However, inherent differences between groups may compromise their use as controls. Such studies are generally held to have a 'comparison group' or 'reference group' rather than a proper control. Studies in which random allocation to control and intervention group is not possible are usually referred to as quasi-experimental; because of this they are often, but not always, regarded as being less reliable than RCTs (see Britton, 2010, and the hierarchy of experimental research evidence). Some of the large-scale community intervention trials such as the Community Intervention Trial for Smoking Cessation (COMMIT) matched communities with regard to key characteristics before randomly allocating them to intervention and comparison groups (COMMIT Research Group, 1991) in order to minimize this problem.

Furthermore, when the impetus for an intervention comes from the community itself, it is virtually impossible to provide an adequate control (Mackenbach, 1997). Similarly, McPherson (1994: 12) notes that the pursuit of objectivity fails to acknowledge the potential influence of volition and decision-making. He concludes that 'choice itself can dramatically affect important measures of outcome'. Choice and control are both recognized as central to the health promotion endeavour. Removing these elements by random allocation would, therefore, systematically introduce bias by reducing effectiveness.

Contamination of the reference or control group can also be a problem and difficult to avoid (Britton, 2010), especially in large-scale interventions. For example, Nutbeam et al. (1993) reported that reference areas used by the 'Heartbeat Wales' heart disease prevention programme rapidly became independently involved in establishing their own heart health initiatives, thus compromising their value as controls. Moreover, an RCT investigating the effectiveness of a mobile phone text message intervention to promote safer sex and sun safety for young people conceded that text messages may have been inadvertently sent to those in the control group (Gold et al., 2011).

Although not unique to RCTs, the emphasis in evaluation design is on assessing outcomes rather than the quality of the intervention itself. A 'Type 3 error' occurs when an intervention could not possibly succeed because of its inherent inadequacy. The Type 3 error relates to the concept of efficacy that was defined earlier in this chapter. Key considerations in relation to the quality of the programme include:

- it has been systematically planned
- it addresses all key determinants derived from theoretical analysis and research into the needs of the target group
- fidelity of implementation
- adequate resources – financial and staffing
- sufficient intensity
- sufficient reach
- supportive materials have been pre-tested with the target group
- staff are properly trained and have the competences needed to implement the programme.

The 'Type 5 error' is a well-known phenomenon, but not normally labelled in this way. It is not unknown for research to yield very respectable p-values by simply using very large numbers of subjects! Practical significance is undoubtedly of more relevance to those working in the field than such artificially constructed statistical significance.

Furthermore, we should emphasize that health promotion does not conform with a simple input–output model. There may be a range of outcomes – anticipated and unanticipated – that are the product of complex pathways of change. The capacity of RCTs to unpick that complexity is open to question – however sophisticated the design and statistical tests. Lang's acerbic comment about using 'statistics as a drunken man uses lampposts – for support rather than illumination' (cited in Cohen and Cohen, 1960) encapsulates over-reliance on statistics. Equally, the complex social interventions needed to tackle contemporary public health problems are not amenable to RCT design. Green and South (2006) conclude that experimental and quasi-experimental methods have limited utility for informing public health policy and practice.

Our concerns about the relevance of the RCT for health promotion evaluation are summarized in Box 11.10 and we concur with the conclusions of the WHO European Working Group on Health Promotion Evaluation (WHO, 1998a: 3):

> Conclusion 4: The use of randomized control [*sic*] trials to evaluate health promotion initiatives is, in most cases, inappropriate, misleading and unnecessarily expensive.

For a better understanding of the impact of health promotion initiatives, evaluators need to use a wide range of qualitative and quantitative methods that extend beyond the narrow parameters of randomized controlled trials.

BOX 11.10 LIMITATIONS OF RCTS FOR HEALTH PROMOTION EVALUATION

- Inability to cope with the complexity of health promotion programmes
- Do not pay sufficient attention to process and the quality of interventions
- Practical difficulties in relation to randomization
- Contamination of control or reference groups
- Statistical significance may be achieved at the expense of practical significance
- Do not provide illumination of the pathways linking intervention and outcomes and the ways in which these are influenced by the various components of complex interventions
- Do not include formative evaluation, which is essential to improving the success of programmes
- Are ideologically incompatible with health promotion in relation to:

  o   commitment to 'active' individual and community participation in the research process
  o   contributing to its empowering and 'emancipatory' role
  o   the use of research as a tool for achieving political and social change.

A NEW GOLD STANDARD – THE JUDICIAL PRINCIPLE

We have asserted the need for adopting a particular kind of post-positivist paradigm for health promotion research. The rejection of a positivist approach, together with its gold standard RCT design, does not mean that we should abandon the pursuit of reliability and validity. Quite the reverse. A critical realist model, as we have seen, has no difficulty in addressing Type 2 and 3 errors, but it is imperative that it replaces the techniques intrinsic to true experimental design with robust alternatives that will maximize internal validity – that is, provide strong evidence that will substantiate claims that programmes or parts of programmes have produced change.

Reliability, replicability, dependability and validity

As qualitative methodology is central to the interpretivist aspects of critical, realistic evaluation, it makes sense to give some thought to the methods recommended by qualitative researchers to achieve reliability and validity.

Reliability and validity are often assessed simultaneously and qualitative researchers tend to use such terms as 'replicability', 'dependability', 'confirmability', 'trustworthiness', 'transferability' and 'authenticity' to assess the consistency of interventions and the extent to which their results actually measure the constructs that they are claiming to measure.

According to Denzin (1994: 508):

> The foundation for interpretation rests on triangulated empirical materials that are trustworthy. Trustworthiness consists of four components: credibility, transferability, dependability, and confirmability (these are the constructionist equivalents of internal and external validity, reliability and objectivity).

Various specific techniques have also been devised to provide a basis for demonstrating credibility and providing transparent results that allow judgements to be made about reliability and validity. Some examples will be discussed below.

Member checks

Member checking is frequently used in qualitative research as a means to maintain the overall trustworthiness of a study. In general, the rationale for this technique is testing results of research against the perceptions of audience members. 'Member checks' tends to be the preferred term used for this process in the USA; elsewhere, particularly within the UK, 'respondent validation' is often the term deployed in the literature (Torrance, 2012). Member checking is a way for the researcher to ensure the accuracy of participant voices by allowing participants the opportunity to confirm or deny the interpretations of data – this could be after a single interview with a participant or after analysing several interviews with participants (Candela, 2019; Rolfe et al., 2018).

Thick description

Denzin (1994: 505) compares 'thin description' to 'thick description'. The former:

> simply reports facts, independent of intentions or circumstances. A thick description, in contrast, gives the context of an experience, states the intentions and meanings that organized the experience, and reveals the experiences as a process. Out of this process arise ... claims for truth, [and its] verisimilitude.

In short, thick, rich detail makes it possible to gain illuminative insights and allow others to check a researcher's claims. Thick description, as an example, often provides details of the social, demographic and health profile of participants (e.g. gender, education, health conditions), as well as the setting and context of their experiences (i.e. where they live, what access to healthcare they have). In this way, thick description can aid research transferability to other contexts and settings (Rolfe et al., 2018).

Audit trails

This interpretivist research technique is designed to provide a detailed account of how researchers/ evaluators have reached their decisions about the categories that they have constructed from raw data and the conclusions they have reached and, perhaps, about the theories they have derived from these. In short, an audit trail is a record of how a study was carried out and how conclusions were arrived at by researcher. Undertaking such processes ensures the rigour and transparency of research processes (Carcary, 2020).

Transferability

This is the alternative version of external validity. Again, thick descriptions can provide sufficiently detailed information for people to make judgements about the relevance of findings to different but related situations and to know how to proceed.

'Purposive/purposeful sampling' is considered to yield the most useful data. Situations and/or individuals are deliberately selected in the expectation that they will prove to be a rich source of relevant data. Deliberate selection implies choosing from alternatives. Choices should be made on the basis of both previous research and, of course, sound theoretical understandings.

Authenticity

Lincoln and Guba (1985) offer authenticity as an alternative concept to validity. Research is not only authentic when the strategies it uses will ensure true reporting of participants' feelings and ideas, it should also demonstrate that it is consistent with these ethical and ideological principles. The components of authenticity would typically include:

- notions such as fairness and equity
- ontological authenticity – that is, participants gain some insight into their human condition
- understandings that help with insight and relating to other people
- catalytic authenticity/validity – the research method itself should achieve its substantive ideological goals so that, for example, in participative health promotion research, it should contribute to empowerment.

The judicial principle – assessing the validity of evidence

The business of evaluating health promotion, with all its complexities, requires a new approach – a new gold standard. Decisions must, of course, still be made on the basis of evidence, but the criteria for making the vigilant decisions that would be used by real people in real life when addressing problems and making policy must be reassessed.

Accordingly, we propose here the use of a 'judicial principle'. As the words suggest, we draw a parallel with the judicial system and argue that decisions should be made on the basis of a potpourri of evidence derived from different sources. Two degrees of judicial certainty should be employed. Where the level of certainty for action must be of a higher order, the criterion used in criminal law should be used – that is, it must be beyond reasonable doubt. Where the consequences of decision-making are less serious and the demand for evidence is, therefore, less stringent, the criterion employed in civil law might be used – that is, take into account the balance of probabilities.

These two levels of probability could loosely be compared with their quantitative equivalents – p-values of $p < 0.01$ (or less if the evidence is especially compelling) and $p < 0.05$ for balance of probability estimates.

Evidence and causality

Although Pawson and Tilley (1997) questioned the utility of assumptions based on a successionist logic – that is, the notion that whatever follows an event is presumed to have been caused by it – cause and effect evidence is important in applying the judicial principle. As we noted in Chapter 2, several criteria are generally accepted as providing evidence of causality in the medical arena. In addition to identifying strong, specific, consistent associations that are temporally correct, health promotion research would, ideally, seek evidence that better results were achieved when interventions were relevant, comprehensive and of sufficient intensity – and theoretically plausible.

The question of triangulation

In the last analysis, the question of causality and internal validity rests on the nature and quality of the evidence that has been assembled by the evaluation research. It is our view that the judicial principle should make substantial use of triangulation of evidence to maximize researchers' and decision-makers' conviction that cause has been demonstrated to at least the level of a balance of probabilities.

Triangulation is of central significance for qualitative research methodology. Essentially, triangulation is a technique derived from surveying or navigation. It involves two or more sightings of a particular target to then accurately establish its geographical position. In the same way, using different 'research sightings' should contribute to valid interpretations of reality or realities. The idea is both attractive and has the virtue of common sense – two or more 'research sightings' are better than one and potentially provide a fuller picture of what is going on (Torrance, 2012). However, some researchers have struck a cautionary note based on pragmatic, epistemological and ontological arguments (Noble and Heale, 2019).

To provide an extreme illustration, consider a situation in which one group of researchers believes that it is not possible to know the world, but only a variety of different interpretations of it, whereas another group believes that the world is real and knowable. If these contradictory beliefs are well founded, then it has to be admitted that using evidence based on one perspective could not be used to support evidence based on the other! However, as Blaikie (1991) suggests, researchers adopting a post-positive realist position can legitimately accumulate evidence from many different sources and, in principle, these sources of data can all offer valid insights into whatever issue or problem is under investigation. As is hopefully clear by now, we concur with the realist position. Accordingly, we believe that a considered use of triangulation is justified. A number of varieties have traditionally been identified (Denzin, 1970):

- data triangulation
- investigator triangulation
- theory triangulation
- methodological triangulation.

In short, our confidence in the validity of observations and findings is proportional to the extent that information from different sources is congruent and compatible. For instance, from: different data sources (such as GP records of drug use over a period of time; interview data from patients and data from observations of patients in social settings); reports of different investigators (such as interview reports from other investigators); consistency between analyses of findings derived from different (and appropriately selected) theories (such as consistency between communication of innovations theory and the health belief model); and achieving similar results from different methods (such as questionnaire data, semi-structured interviews and sources of 'unobtrusive measures').

Producing conclusive evidence about what works in relation to tackling complex and enduring social problems such as health inequality is undoubtedly challenging. Judge and Bauld (2006) argue that there are often unrealistic expectations about evaluation and the speed with which findings can be generated. This is particularly so when initiatives are driven by political agendas rather than the need to plan interventions rigorously with sufficient attention to evaluation from the outset to be able to generate robust evidence. The emphasis on outcomes and the pressure to know rapidly whether complex initiatives work can also obscure important learning. As Judge and Bauld (2006: 343) comment:

> The challenge when evaluation opportunities arise in this way is to negotiate the best possible research approach that acknowledges inter alia that incontrovertible measures of impact are not the only useful products that can be generated. The value of throwing light on complex processes in reflective and scholarly ways should not be underestimated even if it falls short of what is ideally required.

KEY POINTS

- Evaluation is an essential component of the health promotion planning cycle – evaluation and dissemination should, therefore, be considered from the very first stages of planning.
- Health promotion evaluation should conform with the key principles, values and ideology of health promotion – notably participation and empowerment
- RCTs are rarely, if ever, applicable to health promotion evaluation.
- The judicial principle, based on the notion of triangulation, has been proposed as a means of assessing evidence that can cope with the complexity of health promotion and public health interventions.
- Evaluation should address process as well as outcomes.

- The selection of appropriate evaluation indicators is easier if programme objectives are well defined and the anticipated pathway between intervention and the achievement of outcomes is explicitly stated – the so-called Theory of Change.
- Evaluation should not only demonstrate whether an intervention has been successful, but should also identify how the various intervention components lead to outcomes and how contextual factors influence programme delivery and its success – or failure.

CHAPTER 11: INTERNATIONAL CASE STUDIES

The following case study on the online resources website is relevant to the content of this chapter: 11.

CRITICAL REFLECTION AND APPLICATION TO PRACTICE

Evaluation is a key competency for health promoters, but there remain challenges in developing a strong evidence base. To what extent should evaluation in health promotion adhere to key values, such as participation and empowerment, and to what extent should they be abandoned to conform to traditional evidence hierarchies? How can evaluation skills and competencies be embedded more effectively in the training and support of the health promotion workforce? How can the dissemination of evaluation evidence be encouraged? To what extent should dissemination modes such as blogs, tweets and online communication be supported alongside traditional academic publishing approaches?

ONLINE RESOURCES

Please visit https://study.sagepub.com/greentones5e for all the online resources for the book, including recommended further reading on each chapter subject, useful weblinks (both introduced by the authors), as well as the abovementioned case study material.

12 EVIDENCE-BASED HEALTH PROMOTION

The plural of anecdote is not data.

Raymond Wolfinger

OVERVIEW

This chapter addresses the development of an evidence base for health promotion. It also looks at the translation of evidence into practice. It will:

- identify the types of evidence relevant to evidence-based practice
- consider the contribution of systematic reviews to the evidence base
- consider how evidence informs practice.

INTRODUCTION

A credible discipline requires an evidence base on which practitioners and decision-makers can base their practices (Deehan and Wylie, 2010). This then relies on two key components – good quality research and evidence being produced *and* this research and evidence being understood and applied in appropriate contexts (Homer et al., 2022). Health promotion has strived to legitimize itself against more medical approaches to prevention through gathering evidence of what works. Given the diversity of health promotion activity, such evidence has come in a variety of forms – some of which is perceived in some professional domains as being more legitimate than others. Despite many contemporary health challenges which could be addressed using health promotion approaches, the evidence base to deploy effective health promotion strategies is limited (Schwarzman, 2019). For some time, there have been discussions about how health promotion strategies and approaches can best show their 'worth' and 'value' to funders and service commissioners, but consistently health promotion has faced numerous challenges in establishing a firm and credible evidence base (Cross et al., 2017b). Some have even suggested 'hostility' towards health promotion interventions by medical professions through the discipline not having a robust evidence base (South and Tilford, 2000). Such a portrayal of health promotion can be problematic for its 'image':

the image and lack of an evidence base for health promotion are fundamentally interrelated as they tend to feed off each other: the lack of an evidence base leads to a poor image; a poor image means the spotlight is on demonstrating effectiveness. (Nettleton and Burrows, 1997: 41)

The movement towards evidence-based practice in health promotion has been heavily influenced by evidence-based medicine, the origins of which Sackett et al. (1996) trace back to mid-nineteenth-century Paris. Its basic tenets are summarized in Box 12.1.

BOX 12.1   THE BASIC TENETS OF EVIDENCE-BASED MEDICINE

- Clinical decisions should be based on the best available scientific evidence.
- The clinical problem determines the evidence to be sought.
- Identifying the best evidence involves epidemiological and biostatistical ways of thinking.
- Conclusions based on the available evidence are useful only if put into action for individual patients or for population healthcare decisions.
- Performance should be constantly evaluated.

Source: Davidoff et al. (1995), in Jacobson et al. (1997: 449)

As we noted in Chapter 5, there is increasing recognition of the importance of evidence-based practice within the wider public health arena and considerable current interest in evidence-based health promotion. Nutbeam (1999) points to the significant inclusion of the words 'evidence-based' in the call for member states to 'adopt an evidence-based approach to health promotion policy and practice' in the Resolution on Health Promotion passed at the 51st World Health Assembly (WHO, 1998a). He takes this to imply the need to justify health promotion activity with greater reference to research evidence on effectiveness in achieving 'predetermined outcomes'. Moreover, Groot (2011) notes the consistency with which 'evidence' is mentioned in WHO declarations on health promotion – the exception being the Ottawa Charter – with this becoming more apparent in later conferences. She continues, however, to note the absence within the WHO declarations about how evidence should be produced or what should be considered as 'evidence'. The Nairobi Call to Action, for example, states to use:

> the existing evidence to prove to policy-makers that health promotion is fundamental to managing national and global challenges such as population ageing, climate change, global pandemic threats, maternal mortality, migration, conflict, and economic crises. (WHO, 2009)

Although some have persuasively argued that the notion of evidence is a redundant idea in health promotion given that it is a values-based activity (Seedhouse, 1997), the increasing emphasis on evidence-based practice derives, in part, from 'economic rationalism' and the need to justify expenditure and ensure that funds are deployed to maximum effect (Li et al., 2015; Raphael, 2000). In recent times, governments in high-income countries and low- and middle-income countries as well as donor agencies have had fewer resources in recent times and, therefore, budgetary allocations for public health and health promotion interventions need to be based on solid evidence (Owusu-Addo et al., 2017; Smith et al., 2016).

ABSTRACT 12.1

Evidence-based practice in local public health service in Ghana. Owusu-Addo, E., Cross, R. and Sarfo-Mensah, P. (2017)

While the role of evidence-based public health in improving health outcomes is frequently touted, there remains a dearth of research examining the use of evidence in public health service particularly in low- and middle-income countries. Therefore, the aim of this research was to examine the use of evidence in local public health service in Ghana, a lower middle-income country. Semi-structured in-depth interviews were conducted with local health managers from 11 District Directorates of Health in Ashanti Region. Three organizing themes emerged from the interview transcripts: understanding of evidence-based public health; the process of using evidence; and the value of evidence in public health practice. The study suggests that though evidence-based practice was not new to the local health managers, its application was very low. The process of using evidence commenced with making a decision about the direction of a programme which had been already prioritized and planned by other high-level actors and then various sources of information, including available research evidence, were used to justify the decision. The study has revealed that there is an urgent need for pre-service and in-service training programmes that build and maintain common skill sets and language among local public health practitioners in Ghana to accomplish evidence-based public health goals. Similarly, giving local health managers flexibility to prioritize and make decisions would result in increased uptake of evidence in local public health service.

There is also a strong ethical imperative to adopt the principles of evidence-based practice to ensure that health promotion does no harm – either directly or indirectly by wasting limited funds on ineffective or inappropriate interventions or by raising unrealistic expectations about what might be achieved. Health promotion practitioners, in a study by Li et al. (2015: 196), stressed the value of evidence for this reason – one participant noted: 'I do firmly believe that we need some evidence before we launch into things. I think the prospect of doing harm is too great to not have some inkling of where it is going to go.' Incorporating evidence into decisions about practice is a key aspect of 'reflective practice' and fundamental to the provision of quality health promotion. Indeed, if practitioners are to successfully implement change then they must draw on the evidence base to aid logical decision-making (Dixey et al., 2013). The basic premise of this is that the systematic planning of health promotion requires a series of decisions to be made at each stage and that these should be informed by a thorough appraisal of available evidence. However, recent evidence from the UK (Homer et al., 2022) suggested significant challenges for public health and health promotion practitioners working in local government to apply evidence to their practice as this could be influenced and shaped by political factors. Indeed, evidence that the political and policy environment directly affects evaluation approaches and funding in health promotion has been established (Schwarzman, 2019). Furthermore, increasing demands and limited capacity and resources impact on even the most research-engaged practitioners' ability to do and apply research in their practice (Homer et al., 2022). These findings are not unique and apply beyond the UK (Schwarzman, 2019).

Reiterating this, Perkins et al. (1999: 4) noted that, 'like motherhood and apple pie', evidence-based health promotion has come to be seen as a good thing. However, they identify a number of tensions in implementing it. The first of these is the tension between reflection and action and the issue of how much evidence is required before action can be taken and what level of uncertainty can be tolerated.

Second is the tension between evidence and practice and the theory–practice gap that arises from failure to translate research findings into practice. This, they suggest, can have a number of origins, which include shortcomings on the part of practitioners in accessing, interpreting and acting on relevant evidence or on the part of researchers in addressing relevant issues and disseminating their findings in ways that meet practitioners' needs. On the former point, it has been suggested that training for practitioners in interpreting research evidence is a necessary competency to aid professional judgements (Owusu-Addo et al., 2017). Latterly, both Li et al. (2015) and Owusu-Addo et al. (2017) have demonstrated that practitioners in health promotion value evidence from researchers that is context-bound and relates directly to their own practice, rather than evidence which is more abstract or out-of-context.

Third, there is the tension between different types of knowledge – not only between different research paradigms, which we have discussed above, but also between empirical evidence and professional judgement.

Fourth, there is the tension between values and evidence and the complex interplay between the two, particularly in relation to the selection and interpretation of evidence. Commentators such as Seedhouse (1997) have explored this issue is great detail.

Finally, Perkins et al. note the tension between inspiration and evidence and the relative emphasis on tried and tested methods in contrast to innovative and creative solutions to problems.

A particular area of contention concerns attempts to apply the principles of evidence-based medicine to health promotion. This derives from a conceptualization of evidence-based medicine as being associated with the use of the RCT as the gold standard of evaluation and taking a narrow biomedical view of outcomes – an interpretation that has been challenged even by the proponents of evidence-based medicine. The key issues that we will consider at this point are what evidence of effectiveness is relevant to health promotion practice and how that evidence can be accessed – in particular via systematic reviews.

WHAT IS EVIDENCE?

This section broadly concerns what evidence means in a health promotion context – currently a 'hotly contested' issue as noted elsewhere (Woodall and Rowlands, 2021). The relationship of health promotion with 'evidence' has been an uncomfortable one because of the constant comparison with the principles of evidence-based medicine (Van den Broucke, 2012). Some have even suggested that the inability to have a coherent understanding of what evidence is and means for health promotion has been a significant barrier for practitioners in undertaking evaluation of their practice (Fleming and Baldwin, 2020). Despite this, evidence-based health promotion has been defined (Wiggers and Sanson-Fisher, 1998: 141) as: 'the systematic integration of research evidence into the planning and implementation of health promotion activities'.

Thorogood and Coombes (2010) argue that there has been a tradition in health promotion to emphasize outcomes in evaluation, often at the expense of paying sufficient attention to process and context in the construction of the health promotion evidence base. McQueen (2007) suggests that this may have been influenced by the prominence of 'medical public health' that, like evidence-based medicine, relies on experimental designs as a fundamental principle when determining effectiveness. We have questioned the utility of experimental methods for assessing the effectiveness of health promotion and many others have largely shared our position (for example, Kelly et al., 2010). MacIntyre and Pettigrew (2000) suggest that resistance to applying the principles of evidence-based medicine – and by this they are essentially referring to systematic reviews and experimental designs – to social or public health settings derives from a number of misconceptions:

- Systematic reviews and experimental designs have a biomedical provenance.
- The real world is too complex for evidence-based medicine principles.
- Social and public health interventions do not have the capacity to do harm.
- It is sufficient to know that an intervention does good in a general sense without the necessity of analysing how much, for which subgroups and at what cost.
- Plausibility is an adequate basis for policy-making.
- Experimental methods define outcomes narrowly and use too short a time frame.

A particular concern is the capacity to do harm. The authors cite a study by Carlin and Nolan (1998) that demonstrated that a bicycle safety education programme doubled the risk of injury in boys. Furthermore, they note that plausibility is not necessarily sufficient justification. For example, putting babies to sleep in the prone position would seem to make sense in that it resembles the recovery position, but it has been shown to be associated with increased risk of sudden infant death syndrome. They argue that systematic evaluation offers the opportunity to identify the wider effects of interventions, both positive and negative. While agreeing with these concerns and upholding the need for rigour in evaluation research, our contention is that this is best achieved by means of triangulation and the judicial principle. Furthermore, evaluation needs to remain open to unanticipated outcomes.

There is a growing consensus that the best evidence in relation to health promotion interventions includes both quantitative and qualitative research and addresses process and context as well as outcomes – such a position is now very well established in health promotion circles (Woodall and Rowland, 2021). The answer to the simple question 'Does it work?' is not enough and evidence is needed in relation to process as well as outcomes. Interestingly, however, a study that interviewed a purposive sample of 39 members of three NICE advisory groups found that participants' views on the nature and definition of evidence in a public health context were not consistent. For some, evidence was still defined in 'scientific' terms, underpinned by evidence-based medicine, but for others a broader recognition of the value of professional and lay experience and drawing on a wider range of sources were noted (Atkins et al., 2013). Using a range of evidence within health promotion decision-making is now broadly accepted and this recognition has meant an abandonment of hierarchies of evidence towards typologies of evidence (Dixey et al., 2013) or evidence that is fit for purpose. Wharf-Higgins et al. (2011: 291) note that:

> Evidence comes in many types of formats, including academic research, informal or formal evaluations of community-based programs and policies, stories and experiences of public health staff and community leaders. Diverse types of evidence are used by staff to shape programs and make policy decisions, and all should be considered valid.

Indeed, a whole series of supplementary questions require answers that often cannot be achieved simply by experimental designs. For example:

- How does it work?
- Were there any unanticipated outcomes?
- What components are essential for success?
- What components are redundant?
- Why does it work in this context (or, equally importantly, not work)?
- Can it be replicated?
- Is this an appropriate and acceptable way of tackling the problem?

Liamputtong (2016) suggests the value of qualitative evidence for public health and health promotion, outlining the value of such approaches in exploring, understanding and disentangling complexity and identifying unanticipated effects of interventions or programmes. There is a plethora of other 'non-traditional' forms of evidence that may also be drawn on in health promotion decision-making processes as part of a judicial review process. Contemporary research with children has used methods as diverse as 'photo-elicitation' and 'draw and write' to gather the views of children to develop the evidence base in certain areas (Carter and Ford, 2013). These methods resonate less with positivist traditions and more with participatory modes of gathering evidence of 'what works'. For example, 'draw and write' has been used effectively in understanding children's views on road safety (Green et al., 2007) and toothbrushing in the home (Woodall et al., 2013c).

Raphael (2000) suggests that even when there is a strong accumulated evidence base, decision-making should still draw on local evidence. On the one hand – and particularly at the needs assessment stage – this helps to secure local ownership. On the other hand, it ensures and checks out local relevance. This was exemplified in a study by Jack et al. (2010: 662), whereby traditional knowledge from Canadian Aboriginal communities was regarded as being critical in 'providing interpretations of scientific data that make sense to the local community'.

Wiggers and Sanson-Fisher's (1998) definition referred to previously presupposes that evidence derives from research. However, Sackett et al.'s (1996: 71) discussion of evidence-based medicine, while calling for the 'conscientious, explicit and judicious use of current best evidence in making decisions about the care of individual patients', also recognizes the importance of integrating evidence with clinical expertise (1996: 72):

> Without clinical expertise, practice risks becoming tyrannized by evidence for even excellent external evidence may be inapplicable or inappropriate for an individual patient. Without current best evidence, practice risks becoming rapidly out of date to the detriment of patients.

They see the application of professional expertise as a means of avoiding evidence-based medicine becoming merely 'cookbook' medicine. Equally, professional judgement that incorporates familiarity with the context and constraints is important in relation to assessing what health promotion interventions are likely to be successful in particular situations and with specific groups. Indeed, it is recognized that expert knowledge – defined as 'substantive information on a particular topic that is not widely known by others' (Martin et al., 2012: 30) – can offer valuable information in terms of understanding the process and mechanisms of implementing an intervention (Petticrew and Roberts, 2003). It is particularly useful when accessing more 'traditional' types of empirical data may be insufficient or too challenging (Caley et al., 2014). For example, expert opinion was used to understand the process and delivery of peer interventions in prison settings to improve health (Woodall et al., 2015); while gathering expert evidence complemented a systematic review also being conducted on the subject, the authors were confident that expert views offered a unique insight into peer interventions that would not have been gathered through systematic literature searching (South et al., 2012). Indeed, Wharf-Higgins et al. (2011) also highlighted how public health practitioners' tacit knowledge was often effectively combined with academic evidence when making decisions. Nonetheless, the use of expert evidence to understand practice is controversial and there are concerns about relying solely on this form of evidence for decision-making (Martin et al., 2012). Part of the concern is not only based on what experts say, which may potentially be biased or self-serving, but also on the methodology used to gather these perspectives which are still in their relative infancy (Woodall et al., 2015).

Finally, in this section, it is important to highlight the value of lay perspectives in evidence generation, as this is increasingly being extolled as an essential component of developing a broader conceptualization of evidence in health promotion (South et al., 2013). Lay understandings of health are often complex and multifaceted, often extending beyond the views of medical or professional 'experts'. Moreover, lay evidence allows a greater understanding of the 'real' issues that people face and provides a more nuanced understanding of the factors contributing to health-damaging and health-enhancing behaviours (Henderson, 2010; Springett et al., 2007). While we agree wholeheartedly with the incorporation of lay evidence, there is little doubt that a default position of many decision-makers continues to be an under-appreciation of this form of evidence, largely because of the extent to which this knowledge can be generalized beyond the experiences of a given individual (Henderson, 2010; Rychetnik et al., 2004). We would echo Springett et al.'s (2007) view that different types of evidence, including lay perspectives, need to be viewed in a more equal way than at present.

EVIDENCE THEORY AND VALUES

Green (2000: 125) has argued that empirical evidence alone is 'insufficient to direct practice and that recourse to the explanatory and predictive capability of theory is essential to the design of both programmes and evaluations'. When there is no empirical evidence available, then recourse to theory will be the only option. However, even when there is ample empirical evidence, the application of theoretical principles remains important for a number of reasons. Identification of appropriate indicators of outcome and process is reliant on theory. Reference to theory, as we have noted, can also ensure that all the necessary elements of a programme are in place and, therefore, reduce the risk of intervention failure and Type 3 errors in evaluation. Consideration of the extent to which they are based on theory therefore becomes an essential criterion in assessing the quality of interventions and evaluation designs. Not only should evaluation be informed by theory, but the findings of evaluations should contribute to the further development and refinement of theory in a constantly evolving cycle.

Without the extraction of general theoretical principles, empirical evidence of effectiveness risks offering little more than a menu of, often context-specific, proven interventions. General principles will be of more relevance to practitioners in that they allow adaptation to suit specific situations. Yet, too often, theory is disregarded as either being too abstract or removed from practice, with some arguing that health promotion research is largely a-theoretical in nature (Van den Broucke, 2012). Breton and de Leeuw's (2011) study may in fact confirm this assertion, as they examined the application of policy theory in policy research in health promotion. Their findings were that from the 119 articles reviewed, only 39 applied a theoretical framework and only 21 referred to a theory from the political sciences. The authors' conclusions were clear:

> the field [health promotion] has yet to acknowledge critical concepts that would help to shed light on the policy process, and that validated rigorous theoretical frameworks to inform research and practice are hardly applied. (Breton and de Leeuw, 2011: 82)

Clearly, the interpretation of evidence may be value-laden – note, for example, the different interpretations of ways to achieving better health in Box 12.2. Raphael (2000: 355) argues that, given the commitment of health promotion to enabling and empowerment, evidence relevant to health promotion should encompass consideration of whether or not these goals have been achieved, contending that 'ethical health promotion practice requires explicit recognition of the interactions among ideologies, values, principles and rules of evidence'.

BOX 12.2 ALTERNATIVE INTERPRETATIONS OF THE ROUTE TO BETTER HEALTH

Ten tips for better health (Donaldson, 1999)

1. Don't smoke. If you can, stop. If you can't, cut down.
2. Follow a balanced diet with plenty of fruit and vegetables.
3. Keep physically active.
4. Manage stress by, for example, talking things through and making time to relax.
5. If you drink alcohol, do so in moderation.
6. Cover up in the sun and protect children from sunburn.
7. Practise safer sex.

(Continued)

8. Take up cancer-screening opportunities.
9. Be safe on the roads: follow the Highway Code.
10. Learn the First Aid ABC – airways, breathing, circulation.

An alternative 10 tips for better health (Gordon, 1999)

1. Don't be poor. If you can, stop. If you can't, try not to be poor for long.
2. Don't have poor parents.
3. Own a car.
4. Don't work in a stressful, low-paid, manual job.
5. Don't live in damp, low-quality housing.
6. Be able to afford to go on a foreign holiday and sunbathe.
7. Practise not losing your job and don't become unemployed.
8. Take up all the benefits that you are entitled to, if you are unemployed, retired or sick or disabled.
9. Don't live next to a busy major road or near a polluting factory.
10. Learn how to fill in the complicated housing benefit/asylum application forms before you become homeless and destitute.

Source: Raphael (2000: 362)

It is interesting to note the Cochrane Collaboration's (2002) disclaimer about Cochrane Reviews that acknowledges interpretations of the evidence may vary:

> The results of a Cochrane Review can be interpreted differently, depending on people's perspectives and circumstances. Please consider the conclusions presented carefully. They are the opinions of review authors, and are not necessarily shared by the Cochrane Collaboration.

Nutbeam (2000b) and more recently Homer et al. (2022) notes that different stakeholders have different perspectives on what constitutes success and may have different views about the evidence needed:

- Policy-makers and budget managers may be concerned about the likely short-term achievement of returns on the level of investment in relation to health gain.
- Health promotion practitioners need to assess the feasibility of achieving defined objectives within particular contexts.
- The population that is to benefit from health promotion intervention may be concerned about whether or not the programmes address recognized priorities and felt needs and are participatory.
- Academic researchers may be concerned with epistemological considerations and methodological rigour in making judgements about success.

EVIDENCE OF EFFECTIVENESS

A key requirement for getting evidence into practice involves access to evidence. It is worth noting at this point that there may be a mismatch between the needs and interests of those generating research evidence and the end-users of that evidence. Furthermore, comparatively little attention has been given to the dissemination of research findings.

It is widely acknowledged that searching for literature is now easier than ever as a result of the Internet and electronic databases; for example, the Internet revolution has meant that hand searching for literature has become almost a thing of the past (Aveyard and Sharp, 2012):

> digital content delivery has, within a relatively short time-span, shifted the landscape of scientific publishing considerably and opened up the market for alternative ways of distributing scientific literature. At the same time the process of finding, acquiring, and consuming scholarly content has been revolutionized by technology. (Laakso et al., 2011: 1)

Recent bibliometric research has highlighted the numerous journals that publish papers on relevant issues and the variety of different databases that cover health promotion literature (Merigó and Núñez, 2016). The disparate nature of research in health promotion can cause challenges and while there are many useful guides for literature searching (see Aoki et al., 2013, for a brief overview), locating all published papers on a particular health promotion topic can be problematic and indeed research shows that health promotion practitioners cannot always access what they require (Homer et al., 2022).

Analysis by Merigó and Núñez (2016) identified the most 'influential journals' within health promotion and health behaviour based on the number of papers published in the journal, total citations, journal impact factor and other measures; their research worryingly demonstrated the dominance of medical and preventive medicine journals. Such findings may potentially preclude individuals from searching within social science fields, for example, where there is also a plethora of high-quality health promotion research studies.

Clearly, journal editors and peer reviewers of articles occupy key gatekeeper positions. Not only do they control quality standards for published material and establish what would be regarded as minimal reporting criteria, but they also arbitrate on matters of current interest.

Even presupposing that information is readily available, coping with the amount of published material can be problematic for practitioners – this often results in health promotion practitioners engaging with literature in more *ad hoc* than systematic ways (South and Tilford, 2000). Research from Ghana, for example, suggested that those working in health promotion and public health roles only used published research when they were writing project proposals to seek funding from external organizations, rather than it being seen as part of informing commissioning decisions or programme delivery (Owusu-Addo et al., 2017).

It is not surprising that increasing emphasis is being placed on reviews of evidence that attempt to synthesize the literature – given the barriers that health promotion practitioners face to accessing high-quality material (Homer et al., 2022), being able to locate a synthesis of the evidence base is potentially time consuming and resource intensive. Tones and Tilford (2001) distinguish between commentary reviews and systematic reviews. The former bring together the findings of available studies and, hence, are subject to the vagaries of access to and selection of information and, in some instances, interpretation. There is clearly a risk that, consciously or unconsciously, such commentaries will be based on studies selected to suit a particular agenda or argument – the politics of research and evaluation can therefore come into play and must be an important part of assessing the quality of the work (Fleming and Baldwin, 2020). Clearly, objectivity would demand that an attempt is made to seek out and, if appropriate, discount contradictory findings. Over-reliance by commentators on a few key studies can inflate their importance in influencing decisions about practice.

Cummins and MacIntyre (2002) use the term 'factoids' to refer to assumptions or speculations that are reported and repeated until they are considered to be true. This can be seen in policy circles, where small pockets of evidence can be taken out of context or amplified in order to make a political point – this can cause tensions between academic rigour and the political need to get things done (Homer et al., 2022). Some of these tensions were seen at various points in decisions concerning public health in relation to the COVID-19 pandemic where evidence could be distorted or magnified to make policy decisions. Cummins and MacIntyre (2002: 438) conclude that:

> The over interpretation of a few small-scale studies undertaken up to ten years ago could end up being used to make policy decisions supported by major central government groups and agencies, because the findings are understood to fit in with the current way of thinking …

Their paper illustrates how factoids can easily and uncritically become part of the apparatus of government health policy when they fit in with broader policy objectives. The key problem is that the burden of proof, or demand for evidence, may vary according to a policy's perceived fit with the prevailing collective worldview about issues of popular topical interest. One of the main messages of the evidence-based movement needs to be emphasized: when making any health policy (or other) decisions, we need to move away from an unquestioning acceptance of conventional wisdom and 'expert' advice and cast a more critical and objective eye over the facts.

In an extreme example, Ioannidis (2020) outlines how early studies during the COVID-19 pandemic could have potentially misled and shaped poor decision-making. While it is acknowledged that policy-makers had to use 'best evidence' at the time, it is claimed that early research was perhaps exaggerated and that the peer-review process was arguably flawed given those reviewing the work may have had strong opinions on the topic without sufficient expertise in the field. Ioannidis (2020) claimed that opinion-based peer review may have even solidified a literature of spurious statements that may have had the potential to impact on political decision-making.

SYSTEMATIC REVIEWS

Systematic reviews attempt to address the shortcomings of commentary reviews by bringing together all the published and unpublished material on a particular issue and drawing objective conclusions. Well-conceived and executed reviews can be one of the most efficient ways to become familiar with research and practice (Brownson et al., 2009) – although some argue they are biased towards 'Western' health issues, which often means that systematic reviews are perhaps used less frequently in lower-income countries

(Owusu-Addo et al., 2017; Woodall and Rowlands, 2021). Both the selection of studies and extraction of data should conform to explicit criteria so that the process is rigorous, transparent and essentially replicable. Evidence reviews, which have been in vogue in some health promotion circles, are also helpful in highlighting the literature on a given topic – see Woodall et al.'s (2010) review on empowerment – but a systematic review goes much further in systematically bringing together and assessing the validity of evidence (Thorogood, 2010).

Systematic reviews have a prominent place in assembling and evaluating evidence of effectiveness in health promotion, although historically the development of systematic review methodology took place within medical research (Shepherd, 2013; South and Lorenc, 2020). Studies suggest that they are not always well utilized by health promotion practitioners (Owusu-Addo et al., 2017) and that barriers exist to their utilization, including: a limited number of systematic reviews available on certain public health topics (such as the wider determinants of health) and that the narrow focus of reviews are not reflective of the complexity needed for effective public health decision-making (South and Lorenc, 2020). The development of the methodology for conducting systematic reviews has been focused particularly on healthcare interventions, pioneered by the Cochrane Collaboration. In an attempt to apply similar evidence-based principles to the development of social policy, the Campbell Collaboration has been established more recently. Within the UK, the NHS Centre for Reviews and Dissemination and the Evidence for Policy and Practice Information and Coordinating Centre (EPPI-Centre) have also been involved in the development of systematic reviews.

The process of conducting a systematic review involves a number of stages. An overview of the stages identified by the NHS Centre for Reviews and Dissemination is provided in Box 12.3.

BOX 12.3   STAGES IN THE SYSTEMATIC REVIEW PROCESS

Stage 1: Planning the review

Phase 0 Establishing the need for a review
Phase 1 Preparation of a proposal for a review
Phase 2 Development of a review protocol

Stage 2: Conducting a review

Phase 3 Identification of research
Phase 4 Selection of studies
Phase 5 Study quality assessment
Phase 6 Data extraction and monitoring progress
Phase 7 Data synthesis

(Continued)

> ## Stage 3: Reporting and dissemination
> Phase 8 The report and recommendations
> Phase 9 Getting evidence into practice
>
> *Source*: NHS Centre for Reviews and Dissemination (2001)

Ensuring that the selection of articles is free from bias and replicable is fundamental to the systematic review process. It is, therefore, important that written criteria for inclusion and exclusion are established at the outset. Guidance on undertaking systematic reviews developed by the NHS Centre for Reviews and Dissemination (2001) suggests that criteria for inclusion should be developed from consideration of the following key elements (referred to by the acronym PICOS):

- **P**opulation
- **I**nterventions
- **C**omparators
- **O**utcomes
- **S**tudy design

The Campbell Collaboration guidance lists questions that reviewers should consider in establishing criteria about which studies are relevant to the review (Campbell Collaboration, 2001: 4):

- What characteristics of studies will be used to determine whether or not a particular effort was relevant to the topic of interest?
- What characteristics of studies will lead to exclusion?
- Will relevance decisions be based on a reading of report titles, abstracts, full reports?
- Who will make the relevance decisions?
- How will the reliability of relevance decisions be assessed?

The studies ultimately selected should meet all the inclusion and none of the exclusion criteria. Although decisions should be based on explicit criteria, there will inevitably be a certain amount of subjectivity. Reliability is enhanced if papers are independently assessed by more than one reviewer. A further stage in the selection may involve identifying those papers that would be included in a narrative review only and those that might be included in a meta-analysis.

Daykin et al.'s (2013) review on the impact of music-making on the health, well-being and behaviour of young offenders and those considered at risk of offending, found 559 titles and abstracts from their electronic search of 11 databases. However, only 11 papers finally met the inclusion criteria. Palmer et al.'s (2021) systematic review examining health promotion interventions for African Americans delivered in US barbershops and hair salons identified a potential 1227 studies, but only had 14 papers that made the final selection. Thus, commenting on the lack of methodologically sound evaluations for inclusion is a common feature of systematic reviews. Notwithstanding the explicit rational basis for rejecting papers, there are questions about the feasibility of drawing generalizable conclusions from the final batch of papers, which frequently, as we have seen, constitute only a minute proportion of the literature available.

Speller et al. (1997b) contend that inclusion tends to be based on the quality of the research only and overlooks the quality of the health promotion intervention. Speller et al. also refer to problems arising from 'pooling' dissimilar interventions.

Shepherd (2013: 248) notes that:

> Many health promotion and public health interventions are multifaceted, involving a range of people with different skills and backgrounds, occurring in multiple settings, and covering a range of activities. To be meaningful, systematic reviews need to adequately describe these interventions, assess their effects, and illuminate the factors contributing to success or failure.

There has been a tendency for systematic reviews in health promotion to focus on outcomes rather than on process and implementation factors (Woodall and Cross, 2021). However, there are some exceptions to this, as a recent systematic review on peer interventions in prison to maintain and improve offender health not only looked at the effectiveness of interventions but also specifically examined process issues such as the recruitment, training and support of peer deliverers as well as issues relating to organizational support. This evidence was principally gathered through qualitative studies (South et al., 2015). Indeed, there is increasing emphasis on the importance of including qualitative studies in systematic reviews. The Campbell Collaboration guidelines (2001: 6) suggest that qualitative research can:

- contribute to the development of a more robust intervention by helping to define an intervention more precisely
- assist in the choice of outcome measures and assist in the development of valid research questions
- help to understand heterogeneous results from studies of effects.

A number of appraisal tools are available for assessing the quality of qualitative research. Nonetheless, the guidance notes the considerable debate – even among qualitative researchers themselves – about the suitability and applicability of assessment criteria. The critical appraisal of papers is important, as practitioners should be able go beyond what the descriptive findings of the research state to a more critical understanding of the methodological rigour about how the research was designed and conducted. If research is poorly designed and implemented the findings themselves are untrustworthy, whatever findings are presented. Criteria and checklists to assess different types of evidence have been developed in order to provide systematic and consistent judgements to be made about the methodological quality of the research undergoing assessment (Woodall and Rowlands, 2021).

We have focused here particularly on the selection of papers for inclusion in systematic reviews. However, it is worth noting that subjectivity and human error can influence the data extraction process. Shepherd's (2013) research, for example, based on interviewing a purposive sample of 17 systematic reviewers of health promotion research, found that subjectivity was an inevitable factor when conducting reviews, particularly when judging methodological quality. Nevertheless, subjectivity can be minimized by using clear data extraction forms and more than one assessor (Khan and

Kleijnen, 2001). Synthesizing findings can also be problematic, particularly when there is a lack of consistency and a wide divergence in the findings. Pawson and Tilley (1997) refer to the much-quoted review by Martinson (1974) that provides a summary of all published reports on attempts at rehabilitation of offenders between 1945 and 1967 and yet was only able to reach equivocal conclusions. While acknowledging the importance of accumulating sound evidence, Pawson and Tilley contend that answers are both complicated and may lack uniformity.

Clearly, it is important that the reviews bring together robust evidence, which will inevitably be related to the quality of the study design. There has been concern that, despite increasing recognition of the value of qualitative studies, the criteria for inclusion of studies within systematic reviews of health promotion have tended to replicate those adopted by evidence-based medicine, with overemphasis on RCTs and experimental studies (see Table 5.3 in Chapter 5).

Dixon-Woods et al. (2006: 29) argue that the influential methodology promoted by the Cochrane movement, which they refer to as the 'rationalist' model of systematic review, 'focuses exclusively on questions concerned with effectiveness, and almost exclusively on RCTs as a means of answering the question of whether something "works"'. Baxter et al. (2010: 100) broadly agree and note that:

> These study design hierarchies, however, are problematic in areas of research such as public health, with its preponderance of nontribal evidence exploring wider issues such as how interventions work, patients' experiences, or how public health can be improved and health inequalities reduced.

Attention to qualitative research synthesis is beginning to emerge in the literature and is gaining traction, but compared to the synthesis of quantitative data for systematic reviews it is very much in its infancy (Bronson and Davis, 2011). Practitioners working in public health have highlighted the value of systematic reviews that address context through qualitative or realist methods to aid their decision-making processes (South and Lorenc, 2020). Dixon-Woods et al. recognize the risk that qualitative research may merely be used for enhancement or illumination and thus take on 'a complementary but subsidiary "unequal handmaiden" role to the quantitative research' (2006: 32). The authors consider the difficulties – both technical and epistemological – of attempting to properly integrate qualitative studies. For example, should the review questions be defined from the outset according to conventional practice or should they develop through an iterative process involving reflection on issues emerging from the selected studies – with implications for revisiting the search strategy? They also note problems with accessing qualitative studies arising from the indexing of databases and divergent views about what constitutes qualitative research. In relation to synthesis, they distinguish between two broad approaches:

- **aggregative synthesis** (sometimes referred to as integrative synthesis) that focuses on summarizing data when the concepts, categories and variables used for this are 'largely secure and well specified' (Dixon-Woods et al., 2006: 36)
- **interpretive synthesis** that is concerned with the development of concepts.

An overview of the respective merits of different approaches to synthesizing data is provided by Dixon-Woods et al. (2004). These include: narrative summary; thematic analysis; grounded theory; meta-ethnography; content analysis; case survey; qualitative comparative analysis; Bayesian meta-analysis and other forms of meta-analysis. (See also NHS Centre for Reviews and Dissemination, 1999; Thomas and Harden, 2008.)

Although systematic reviews aspire to seek out and provide an objective and transparent synthesis of all evidence, we have noted a number of limitations. We might add that the search for evidence is frequently restricted to one language – usually English – which clearly inhibits the international exchange of information and cross-fertilization of ideas. Moreover, reviews can be time-consuming – both to obtain funding and to produce the reviews themselves. The complexity of the methods necessary for systematic reviewing, along with higher expectations of their quality, results in a situation whereby reviews conducted using limited resources may fall short of the mark by current standards (Shepherd, 2013).

The utility of reviews to professional, organizational and policy decisions will necessarily be dependent on the reliability of the review process and its relevance to practice. The NHS Centre for Reviews and Dissemination (2009: 170) notes that because of the complexity of public health interventions, 'traditional criteria for producing systematic reviews only partially fulfil the requirements for public health interventions' and a more iterative process may be needed.

Pawson (2002) is critical of the way in which systematic reviews look at the evidence on widely dissimilar interventions and their potential contribution to achieving broad health outcomes. For example, a review of initiatives to prevent injury might include interventions ranging from the distribution of free smoke alarms to school road safety education. In line with realistic evaluation, he argues that rather than identifying what works or does not work, the key issue is to understand generative mechanisms. Furthermore, the extent to which change takes place will be heavily influenced by the context. A realist synthesis would, therefore, be concerned with what works, for whom and in what circumstances. Instead of looking at simple cause–effect relationships, a realist synthesis would be reoriented towards identifying generative themes and their applicability in different situations. For example, it might focus on the use of incentives or 'giveaways' such as smoke alarms to establish for what purposes, which groups and in what contexts this type of approach would work.

EVIDENCE INTO PRACTICE

Crucial to the processes of evidence-based decision-making is communication of existing evidence to practitioners (Woodall and Rowlands, 2021). If evidence is to be useful it must be accessible: 'Simply making research available does not ensure that those that need to know about it get to know about it or can make sense of the findings' (NHS Centre for Reviews and Dissemination, 2009: 90). This is particularly crucial as studies have shown the difficulties of public health and health promotion practitioners being able to access research evidence easily (Homer et al., 2022; Owusu-Addo et al., 2017). Attention should, therefore, be given to planning the dissemination process to facilitate 'the transfer of research into practice'. On the one hand, this is dependent on the quality and relevance of the evidence and, on the other hand, the dissemination strategy used. We have already commented in Chapter 5 on the way in which practitioners use evidence. Clearly, it is essential that evidence meets the needs of practitioners and due attention is given to the dissemination of evidence of effectiveness.

The term 'knowledge transfer' has become a popular and catch-all concept for translating academic knowledge into a format that can be of use in non-academic environments. Davies et al. (2008) describe three types of activity that constitute knowledge transfer:

- knowledge push – information from researchers to potential users
- knowledge pull – demand for knowledge from the users of research
- linkage and exchange – a more productive and interactive engagement of knowledge between researchers and users.

Although simplified above, knowledge transfer is a complex process of interactions between researchers and potential users. This complexity was shown by Graham et al. (2006), who mapped the literature and identified over 60 models of knowledge transfer! How knowledge (evidence) is used varies: instrumental use of knowledge is where scientific evidence is used to take a decision or make concrete changes to practice; conceptual use of knowledge refers to changing users' frame of reference or ways of thinking; and persuasive use of knowledge is exemplified when decision-makers and professionals use knowledge to legitimize decisions or actions already undertaken (Dagenais et al., 2013).

Dixon-Woods et al. (2006: 30) draw attention to a key criticism of the evidence-based movement – that 'it results in reductionist and standardized models that fail to acknowledge individual variability or the influence of context' and contrast 'the orderly series of events, decisions and outcomes implied by "the evidence" and the inherently contingent, intuitive and fuzzy realities of practice and experience'. It is important, therefore, that evidence incorporates practitioner experience and expertise along with understanding of contextual factors:

> To determine whether an intervention, even one well founded in evidence, is likely to be successful requires an understanding of local contexts and circumstances, of local professionals' knowledge bases, commitment and engagement, and detailed assessment of the population at whom the intervention is aimed. (Kelly et al., 2004: 5)

Furthermore, as we have already argued, the evidence should incorporate theoretical perspectives that allow the implications for different circumstances to be drawn out.

Green and South (2006) identify a number of concerns about the mismatch between the evidence available and both the current health agenda and the needs of practitioners:

The evidence base is dominated by simple interventions which focus on changing individual behaviour rather than the more complex 'upstream determinants' of health and health action.

1. Interventions focus on a small range of risk behaviours.
2. Programme failures are rarely reported.
3. The emphasis of published reviews tends to be on outcomes rather than process and context.

There are clearly many variables that would determine the success of knowledge transfer efforts. These may vary from the applicability of the evidence for practitioners, to the credibility of the researcher or institution disseminating the evidence. A comprehensive set of issues related to the conditions that encourage research use are listed in Table 12.1 (taken from Dagenais et al., 2013).

Table 12.1   Conditions encouraging research

Characteristics of the users	• Receptivity and positive attitude towards research • Perceived utility of the research • Expertise with respect to the knowledge produced by the research
Organizational context	• Organizational culture that values research • Organization's level of involvement in the transfer process • Strong leadership from management • Consensus on the nature of the needs for knowledge • Common and shared vision of the results to be achieved • Resources dedicated to knowledge transfer activities
Characteristics of the knowledge	• Good fit with the users' values and needs • Applicability • Users' level of involvement in producing the knowledge • Accessibility of the information • Appropriate production schedule
Strategies for knowledge transfer and support	• Should take into account the characteristics of the target groups and their needs • Should be based on a relationship of trust with users • Exchange mechanisms (formal and informal) • Common language • Activities conducted at the right time • Adaptation of the format in which the knowledge is presented • Support and regular follow-up (systematic measurement of progress)
Characteristics of the researchers and of their settings	• Researchers' attitude towards collaboration • Researchers' skill in adapting knowledge (or ability to surround themselves with people to do this) • Researchers' credibility in the eyes of the users • Researchers' ability to relate to other people • Funding dedicated to knowledge transfer activities • Recognition of the value of knowledge transfer activities by the university establishment

Clearly, it is helpful to facilitate access to evidence of effectiveness. In the UK, the National Institute for Health and Clinical Excellence (NICE) regularly publishes guidance on public health issues – both in full and as a quick reference version. Research suggests that public health practitioners often do not have the time to examine evidence in detail and like 'byte-sized' pieces of evidence that are easier to consume (Homer et al., 2022). Health promotion practitioners themselves are generally reluctant – for various reasons, namely time and insufficient resources – to disseminate the evidence that they themselves generate through their practice (Fleming and Baldwin, 2020). Research demonstrates that practitioners either felt that the organizational culture they were working in was unsupportive to a dissemination and publishing culture or practitioners did not have the necessary skills to know how to disseminate effectively (Reilly et al., 2016).

Building on this, Martin-Fernandez et al. (2021) suggest that a favourable professional environment in practice contexts is critical for knowledge transfer within health promotion and moreover activities to support evidence dissemination – such as training and seminars and support infrastructure to develop skills – are fundamental. As Wilson et al. (2001) suggest, it is naive to suppose that if information is made available to practitioners, it will automatically be accessed, appraised and integrated into practice. Indeed, it is hardly surprising that the forces of inertia affecting changes in professional practice are not dissimilar to those influencing changes in individual behaviour. This resistance to change has been graphically encapsulated by Tyrrell (1951):

> The human mind is in the grip of an unconscious urge which makes it cling desperately to the world of familiar things and resists all that threatens to tear it away from its moorings.

Some time ago, Gibson (undated) developed a checklist, based on his personal experience, of some 50 ploys used to avoid change in the school curriculum (see Box 12.4).

BOX 12.4 HOW TO AVOID CURRICULUM CHANGE!

- It has been done before.
- It has never been done before.
- The parents wouldn't like it.
- It doesn't fit into any syllabus.
- It's too vague and I haven't got time anyway.
- We don't have suitable staff.
- The Head wouldn't go along with it.
- I am personally in favour, but the Unions you know ...
- It's not a multidisciplinary thing, is it?
- Not if it means another committee.
- Only if we can have another committee.
- I don't have the power to implement it.
- You don't have the right to suggest it.
- Who are you anyway?
- Have you had any experience of this sort of thing?
- etc.
- etc.

Source: Gibson (undated)
   Plus ça change!!

Various levels of pressure can be applied to encourage professionals to adopt improved practice – including guidance and codes of practice. However, as we noted in relation to individual behaviour change, voluntary adaptation is likely to secure greatest commitment and avoid a subversive backlash. Kelly et al. (2004: 7) draw on the work of Stacey to suggest that the appropriate time to introduce 'planning and control mechanisms such as guidance, application of standards of practice, and performance management' is when there is both:

- a high level of certainty about interventions based on the availability and strength of evidence, and
- a high level of agreement among practitioners about proposed change.

In our earlier consideration of the factors influencing behaviour change in Chapters 3 and 7, we made the important distinction between increasing awareness and actually changing behaviour. Dissemination of information, however effective, cannot be expected in itself to achieve changes in practice. A review of strategies for getting knowledge into practice and improving the quality of healthcare (NHS Centre for Reviews and Dissemination, 1999) concluded that:

- routine mechanisms are essential for achieving individual and organizational change
- individual beliefs, attitudes and knowledge influence professional behaviour, together with other important factors, such as the organizational, economic and community environments in which practitioners are working
- attempts to achieve change should be based on a 'diagnostic analysis' to identify factors that will affect the proposed change
- multifaceted interventions that tackle different barriers to change are more likely to be successful than single interventions
- adequate resources are needed along with people with appropriate knowledge and skills
- systematic strategies for achieving change should include monitoring and evaluation, along with plans to consolidate change.

Evidence-based health promotion holds out the promise of ensuring that energy and resources are directed to maximum effect by enabling effective interventions to be identified. It can also support practitioners' attempts to resist pressure to adopt ill-conceived, although politically appealing, stratagems or programmes. Middleton et al. (2001), for example, made their concerns known to the Home Office about the introduction into the UK of the 'Scared Straight' programme from the USA. They based their objection on the fact that systematic reviews of the programme had shown adverse outcomes. Furthermore, rather than being the cost-cutting exercise that some feared, evidence-based practice enables a realistic assessment to be made of the scope of the intervention necessary to achieve desired effects. It can, therefore, be used to generate arguments to secure sufficient funding, as highlighted by recent research, which showed how health promotion practitioners used evidence to obtain support for proposed strategies from management, partners and funding bodies (Li et al., 2015). However, whether or not these potential benefits are realized will ultimately be dependent on the quality of the evidence base and in particular:

- its relevance to practitioners
- identification of appropriate outcomes

- attention to process and context as well as outcomes
- recognition of the need for methodological pluralism
- consistency with the core values of health promotion
- effective dissemination.

KEY POINTS

- Efforts should be made to actively disseminate evaluation findings along with attention to the factors associated with the uptake of innovations and new ways of working.
- Practitioners are more likely to make use of evidence if it is relevant to their needs and current priorities.
- Evidence should include practitioners' perspectives and theoretical principles as well as research and evaluation studies.
- Systematic reviews are an important device for summarizing research evidence but need also to pay attention to the quality of interventions and include qualitative as well as quantitative studies.
- The findings of evaluation should inform the further development and refinement of health promotion theory.

CHAPTER 12: INTERNATIONAL CASE STUDIES

The following case studies on the online resources website are relevant to the content of this chapter: 3, 6 and 7.

CRITICAL REFLECTION AND APPLICATION TO PRACTICE

This chapter has shown the challenges faced in generating evidence of effectiveness for health promotion interventions. To what extent do you gather evidence of your own practice? How do you use evidence to make decisions in your practice? What type of evidence do you value the most? What can the research community do to improve the translation of research for practice?

ONLINE RESOURCES

Please visit https://study.sagepub.com/greentones5e for all the online resources for the book, including recommended further reading on each chapter subject, useful weblinks (both introduced by the authors), as well as the abovementioned case study material.

REFERENCES

Abbas, S., Isaac, N., Zia, M., Zakar, R. and Fischer, F. (2021) 'Determinants of women's empowerment in Pakistan: evidence from Demographic and Health Surveys, 2012–12 and 2017–18', *BMC Public Health*, *21*: 1328. doi: 10.1186/s12889-021-11276-6

Abbasi, K. (1999) 'The World Bank and world health under fire', *British Medical Journal*, *318*: 1003–6.

Abel, T. (2007) 'Cultural capital in health promotion', in D.V. McQueen and I. Kickbusch, *Health and Modernity: The Role of Theory in Health Promotion*. New York: Springer.

Abraham, C. and Sheeran, P. (2015) 'The health belief model', in M. Conner and P. Norman (eds), *Predicting and Changing Health Behaviour: Research and Practice with Social Cognition Models* (3rd edn). Maidenhead: Open University Press.

Abrahams, D. (2021) 'Land is now the biggest gun: climate change and conflict in Karamoja, Uganda', *Climate and Development*, *13*: 748–60.

Abramson, L.Y., Seligman, M.E.P. and Teasdale, J.D. (1978) 'Learned helplessness in humans: critique and reformulation', *Journal of Abnormal Psychology*, *87*: 49–74.

Abroms, L.C., Gold, R.S. and Allegrante, J.P. (2019) 'Promoting health on social media: the way forward', *Health Education & Behavior*, *46* (2S): 9S–11S.

Acheson, D. (1998) *Independent Inquiry into Inequalities in Health: Recommendations*. London: Department of Health.

ActKnowledge (undated a) *Theory of Change: Origins*. New York: ActKnowledge. (*Website*: www.theoryofchange. org/what-is-theory-of-change/toc-background/toc-origins).

ActKnowledge (undated b) *Theory of Change: Process*. New York: ActKnowledge. (*Website*: www.theoryofchange. org/what-is-theory-of-change/how-does-theory-of-change-work/when-to-use).

Adams, L. and Armstrong, E. (1995) *From Analysis to Synthesis II: The Revenge,* Report of the Penrith Symposium. Sheffield: Sheffield Health.

Ader, M., Berensson, K., Carlsson, P., Granath, M. and Urwitz, V. (2001) 'Quality indicators for health promotion programmes', *Health Promotion International*, *16* (2): 187–97.

Afful-Dadzie, E., Afful-Dadzie, A. and Egala, S.B. (2023) 'Social media in health communication: a literature review of information quality', *Health Information Management Journal*, *52* (1): 3–17.

Agampodi, T.C., Agampodi, S.B., Glozier, N. and Siribaddana, S. (2015) 'Measurement of social capital in relation to health in low and middle income countries (LMIC): a systematic review', *Social Science and Medicine*, *128*: 95–104.

Agha, S. and Meekers, D. (2019) 'Impact of an advertising campaign on condom use in urban Pakistan', *BMC Public Health*, *10*: 450. doi: 10.1186/1471-2458-10-450

Agustin, D.A. and Murti, B. (2018) 'A Precede-Proceed model on the determinants of adherence to HIV treatment: a path analysis of evidence from Indonesia', *Asian Journal of Pharmaceutical and Clinical Research*, *11* (11): 198–203.

Ahmad, A.R. and Murad, H.R. (2020) 'The impact of social media on panic during the COVID-19 pandemic in Iraqi Kurdistan: online questionnaire study', *Journal of Medical Internet Research*, *22* (5). doi: 10.2196/19556

Ahmad, O.B., Boschi-Pinto, C., Lopez, A.D., Murray, C.J.L., Kozano, R. and Inoue, M. (2001) *Age Standardization of Rates: A New WHO Standard*. GPE Discussion Paper Series, No. 31. Geneva: WHO.

Ajzen, I. (1991) 'The theory of planned behavior', *Organizational Behavior and Human Decision Processes*, *50*: 179–211.

Al-Rousan, T., Schwabkey, Z., Jirmanus, L. and Nelson, B.D. (2018) 'Health needs and priorities of Syrian refugees in camps and urban settings in Jordan: perspectives of refugees and health care providers', *Eastern Mediterranean Health Journal*, *24*: 243–53.

Aldoory, L. and Bonzo, S. (2005) 'Using communication theory in injury prevention campaigns', *Injury Prevention*, *11*: 260–3.

Aldridge Foundation and Johnson, M. (2008) *The User Voice of the Criminal Justice System*. London: The Aldridge Foundation.

Alinsky, S. (1969) *Reveille for Radicals*. New York: Vintage Books.

Alinsky, S.D. (1972) *Rules for Radicals*. New York: Random House.

Allara, E., Ferri, M., Bo, A., Gasparrini, A. and Faggiano, F. (2015) 'Are mass-media campaigns effective in preventing drug use? A Cochrane systematic review and meta-analysis', *BMJ Open*. doi: 10.1136/bmjopen-2014-007449

Allern, S. and Pollack, E. (2020) 'The role of think tanks in the Swedish political landscape', *Scandinavian Political Studies*, *43*: 145–69.

Allmark, P.J. and Tod, A. (2006) 'How should public health professionals engage with lay epidemiology?', *Journal of Medical Ethics*, *32* (8): 460–3.

Alshammari, A.S., Piko, B.F. and Fitzpatrick, K.M. (2021) 'Social support and adolescent mental heatlh and well-being among Jordanian students', *International Journal of Adolescence and Youth*, *26* (1): 211–23.

American Heritage Dictionary of the English Language (2000, 4th edn). New York: Houghton Mifflin.

Amuyunzu-Nyamongo, M., Jones, C. and McQueen, D. (2009) 'Repositioning health promotion in Africa', in M. Amuyunzu-Nyamongo and D. Nyamwaya (eds), *Evidence of Health Promotion Effectiveness in Africa*. Nairobi: African Institute for Health.

Anderson, D.S. and Miller, R.E. (2016) *Health and Safety Communication: A Practical Guide Forward*. London: Taylor & Francis.

Anderson, J. (1975) *The HEA Health Skills Dissemination Project: A Whole School Approach to Life Skills and Health Education*. Leeds: Counselling and Career Development Unit.

Anderson, J. (undated) *The HEA Health Skills Dissemination Project: A Whole School Approach to Life Skills and Health Education*. Leeds: Counselling and Career Development Unit.

Angus, J. (2002) *A Review of Evaluation in Community-Based Art for Health Activity in the UK*. Health Development Agency, NHS, CAHHM, University of Durham, UK.

Annett, H. and Rifkin, S. (1990) *Improving Urban Health*. Geneva: WHO.

Ansari, W.E. (1998) 'Partnerships in health: how's it going to work?', *Target*, 29 July: 18.

Antonovsky, A. (1979) *Health, Stress and Coping*. San Francisco, CA: Jossey-Bass.

Antonovsky, A. (1984) 'The sense of coherence as a determinant of health', in J.D. Matarazzo, S.M. Weiss, J.A. Herd, N.E. Miller and S.M. Weiss (eds), *Behavioural Health: A Handbook of Health Enhancement and Disease Prevention*. New York: John Wiley.

Antonovsky, A. (1987) *Unraveling the Mystery of Health*. San Francisco, CA: Jossey-Bass.

Antonovsky, A. (1996) 'The salutogenic model as a theory to guide health promotion', *Health Promotion International*, *11* (1): 11–18.

Aoki, N.J., Enticott, J.C. and Phillips, L.E. (2013) 'Searching the literature: four simple steps', *Transfusion*, *53*: 14–17.

Argyle, M. (1978) *The Psychology of Interpersonal Behaviour* (3rd edn). Harmondsworth: Penguin.

Argyle, M. and Kendon, A. (1967) 'The experimental analysis of social performance', *Advances in Experimental Social Psychology*, *3*: 35–98.

Armstrong, R., Waters, E., Crockett, B. and Keleher, H. (2007) 'The nature of evidence resources and knowledge translation for health promotion practitioners', *Health Promotion International*, *22*: 254–60.

Arnoldi, J. (2009) *Risk*. Cambridge: Polity Press.

Arnstein, S.R. (1969) 'A ladder of citizen participation', *Journal of the American Planning Association*, *35* (4): 216–24.

Aronson, E. (1976) *The Social Animal*. San Francisco, CA: W.H. Freeman.

Arshed, N. (2017) 'The origins of policy ideas: the importance of think tanks in the enterprise policy process in the UK', *Journal of Business Research*, *71*: 74–83.

ASH (2013) *ASH Briefing: UK Tobacco Control Policy and Expenditure*. (*Website*: http://ash.org.uk/information-and-resources/briefings/uk-tobacco-control-policy-and-expenditure-an-overview).

Ashton, J. (2007) 'Grasping defeat: health promotion is a doing word not a proper noun', *Journal of the Royal Society of Health*, *127* (5): 207–10.

Ashton, J. and Seymour, H. (1988) *The New Public Health*. Buckingham: Open University Press.

Atkin, C.K. and Rice, R.E. (2013) 'Strategies and principles for using mass, online, and mobile media in health communication campaigns', in K. Kim, A. Singhal and G. Kreps (eds), *Global Health Communication Strategies in the 21st Century: Design, Implementation and Evaluation*. New York: Peter Lang.

Atkins, L., Smith, J.A., Kelly, M.P. and Michie, S. (2013) 'The process of developing evidence-based guidance in medicine and public health: a qualitative study of views from the inside', *Implementation Science*, *8*: 1–12.

Atkinson, A.M., Sumnall, H. and Measham, F. (2011) 'Depictions of alcohol use in a UK Government partnered online social marketing campaign: Hollyoaks "The Morning after the night before"', *Drugs: Education, Prevention and Policy*, *18* (6): 454–67.

Australian Bureau of Statistics (ABS) (2012) 2049.0.55.001 *Information Paper –Methodology for Estimating Homelessness from the Census of Population and Housing, 2012*. (*Website*: www.abs.gov.au/ausstats/abs@.nsf/mf/2049.0.55.001).

Aveyard, H. and Sharp, P. (2012) *A Beginner's Guide to Evidence Based Practice in Health and Social Care*. Maidenhead: Open University Press.

Ayo, N. (2012) 'Understanding health promotion in a neoliberal climate and the making of health conscious citizens', *Critical Public Health*, *22*: 99–105.

Babb, P. (2005) *Measurement of Social Capital in the UK National Statistics*. London: Office for National Statistics. (*Website*: www.ons.gov.uk/ons/guide-method/user-guidance/social-capital-guide/the-social-capital-project/measurement-of-social-capital-in-the-uk-2005.pdf).

Babb, P., Martin, J. and Haezewindt, P. (2004) *Focus on Social Inequalities*. London: ONS. (*Website*: www.ons.gov.uk/ons/rel/social-inequalities/focus-on-social-inequalities/2004-edition/a-summary-of-focus-on-social-inequalities.pdf).

Bachrach, P. and Baratz, M.S. (1970) *Power and Poverty: Theory and Practice*. New York: Oxford University Press.

Backett-Milburn, K. and Wilson, S. (2000) 'Understanding peer education: insights from a process evaluation', *Health Education Research*, *15* (1): 85–96.

Baelz, P.R. (1979) 'Philosophy of health education', in I. Sutherland (ed.), *Health Education: Perspectives and Choices*. London: Allen & Unwin.

Bagnall, A., South, J., Hulme, C., Woodall, J., Vinall-Collier, K., Raine, G., Kinsella, K., Dixey, R., Harris, L. and Wright, N.M.J. (2015) 'A systematic review of the effectiveness and cost-effectiveness of peer education and peer support in prisons', *BMC Public Health*, *15*: 290. doi: 10.1186/s12889-015-1584-x

Bakewell, O. and Garbutt, A. (2005) *The Use and Abuse of the Logical Framework Approach and Outcomes Mapping*. OM Ideas Paper No. 1. (*Website*: www.pm4dev.com/resources/documents-and-articles/96-the-use-and-abuse-of-the-logical-framework-approach-sida/file.html).

Baldwin, L. (2020) 'Planning and implementing health promotion programs', in M. Fleming and L. Baldwin (eds), *Health Promotion in the 21st Century: New Approaches for Achieving Health for All*. London: Allen & Unwin.

Balkaran, S. and Lukman, Y. (2021) 'Covid-19 and the impact of public policy in compulsory mask-wearing in South Africa', *Journal of Public Administration*, *56* (3): 576–94.

Bambra, C., Gibson, M., Sowden, A., Wright, K., Whitehead, M. and Pettigrew, M. (2010) 'Tackling the wider social determinants of health and health inequalities: evidence from systematic reviews', *Journal of Epidemiology and Community Health*, *64* (4): 284–91.

Bandenburg, U. (2012) 'Volkswagen: a comprehensive approach to health promotion in the workplace', in A. Scriven and M. Hodgins (eds), *Health Promotion Settings: Principles and Practice*. London: Sage.

Bandura, A. (1977) 'Self-efficacy toward a unifying theory of behavioural change', *Psychological Review*, *64* (2): 191–225.

Bandura, A. (1982) 'Self-efficacy mechanism in human agency', *American Psychologist*, *37* (2): 122–47.

Bandura, A. (1986) *Social Foundations of Thought and Action: A Social Cognitive Theory*. Englewood Cliffs, NJ: Prentice-Hall.

Bandura, A. (1989) 'Human agency in social cognitive theory', *American Psychologist*, *44* (9): 1175–84.

Bandura, A. (1992) 'Exercise of personal agency through the self-efficacy mechanism', in R. Schwarzer (ed.), *Self-Efficacy: Thought Control of Action*. Washington, DC: Hemisphere Publishing.

Banken, R. (2001) *Strategies for Institutionalizing HIA*. ECHP Health Impact Assessment Discussion Papers, No. 1. Brussels: European Centre for Health Policy.

Barić, L. (1969) 'Recognition of the "at-risk" role', *International Journal of Health Education*, *12* (1): 2–12.

Barić, L. (1993) 'The settings approach – implications for policy and strategy', *Journal of the Institute of Health Education*, *31*: 17–24.

Barić, L. (1998) *People in Settings*. Altrincham: Barns Publications.

Baringhorst, S., Kneip, V. and Niesyto, J. (2009) *Political Campaigning on the Web*. Piscataway, NJ: Transaction Publishers.

Barker, A.B., Britton, J., Thomson, E. and Murray, R.L. (2021) 'Tobacco and alcohol content in soap operas broadcast on UK television: a content analysis and population exposure.' *Journal of Public Health*, *43* (3): 595–603.

Barker, D.J.P. and Rose, G. (1984) *Epidemiology in Medical Practice* (3rd edn). Edinburgh: Churchill Livingstone.

Barnekow Rasmussen, V. (2005) 'The European network of health promoting schools – from Iceland to Kyrgyzstan', *Promotion & Education*, *12* (3–4): 169–72.

Barnes, M. (ed.), Allan, D., Coad, J., Fielding, A., Hansen, K., Mathers, J., McCabe, A., Morris, K., Parry, J., Plewis, I., Prior, D. and Sullivan, A. (2004) *Assessing the Impact of the Children's Fund: The Role of Indicators. National Evaluation of the Children's Fund*. Birmingham: NECF.

Barnes, R. and Scott-Samuel, A. (2000) *Health Impact Assessment – A Ten Minute Guide*. Liverpool: Liverpool Public Health Observatory.

Barragan, N.C., Noller, A.J., Robles, B., Gase, L.N., Leighs, M.S., Bogert, S., Simon, P.A. and Kuo, T. (2014) 'The "Sugar Pack" health marketing campaign in Los Angeles County, 2011–2012', *Health Promotion Practice*, *15*: 208–16.

Barrett-Lennard, G.T. (1998) *Carl Rogers' Helping System: Journey and Substance*. London: Sage.

Barry, M.M. (2022) Foreword. in M.B. Mittelmark, G.F. Bauer, L. Vaandrager, J.M. Pelikan, S. Sagy, M. Eriksson, B. Lindström and C.M. Magistretti (eds), *The Handbook of Salutogenesis* (2nd edn). Zurich: Springer.

Barry, M.M., Allegrante, J.P., Lamarre, M.-C., Auld, M.E. and Taub, A. (2009) 'The Galway Consensus Conference: international collaboration on the development of core competencies for health promotion and health education', *Global Health Promotion*, *16*: 5–11.

Barry, M., Battel-Kirk, B. and Dempsey, C. (2012) 'The CompHP core competencies framework for health promotion in Europe', *Health Education Behaviour*, *39* (6): 648–62.

Bartholomew, L.K., Parcel, G.S., Kok, G. and Gottlieb, N.H. (2001) *Intervention Mapping: Designing Theory and Evidence-based Health Promotion Programs*. New York: McGraw Hill.

Bartholomew, L.K., Parcel, G.S., Kok, G., Gottlieb, N.H. and Fernandez, M.E. (2011) *Planning Health Promotion Programs: An Intervention Mapping Approach*. San Francisco, CA: Jossey-Bass.

Bartlett, R. (2013) 'The emergent modes of dementia activism', *Ageing and Society*, *1*: 1–22.

Basch, C.E. and Gold, R.S. (1986) 'Type V errors in hypothesis testing', *Health Education Research, 1* (4): 299–305.

Battel-Kirk, B., Barry, M.M., Taub, A. and Lysoby, L. (2009) 'A review of the international literature on health promotion competencies: identifying frameworks and core competencies', *Global Health Promotion, 16*: 12–21.

Bauer, G. F. (2022) Salutogenesis in health promoting settings: a synthesis across organizations, communities, and environments', in M. B. Mittelmark, G.F. Bauer, L. Vaandrager, J.M. Pelikan, S. Sagy, M. Eriksson, B. Lindström and C.M. Magistretti (eds), *The Handbook of Salutogenesis*. Cham: Springer.

Bauld, L. and Judge, K. (2000) 'Strong theory flexible methods: emergent approaches to health promotion evaluation', British Heart Foundation Health Promotion Research Group Workshop, '*Evaluating Health Promotion Interventions: Beyond the Dialogue*', Ilkley, 8–9 May.

Bauld, L., McNeill, A., Hajek, P., Britton, J. and Dockrell, M. (2016) 'E-cigarette use in public places: striking the right balance', *Tobacco Control, 26* (e1): e5–e6.

Baum, F. (2001) 'Healthy public policy', in T. Heller, R. Muston, M. Sidell and C. Lloyd (eds), *Working for Health*. London: Sage.

Baxter, S., Killoran, A., Kelly, M. and Goyder, E. (2010) 'Synthesizing diverse evidence: the use of primary qualitative data analysis methods and logic models in public health reviews', *Public Health, 124*: 99–106.

Baybutt, M. and Chemlal, K. (2016) 'Health-promoting prisons: theory to practice', *Global Health Promotion, 23* (Suppl): 66–74.

Baybutt, M., Dooris, M.T. and Farrier, A. (2019) 'Growing health in UK prison settings', *Health Promotion International, 34*: 792–802.

Baybutt, M., Hayton, P. and Dooris, M. (2010) 'Prisons in England and Wales: an important public health opportunity?', in J. Douglas, S. Earle, S. Handsley, L. Jones, C. Lloyd and S. Spurr (eds), *A Reader in Promoting Public Health: Challenge and Controversy* (2nd edn). Milton Keynes: Open University Press.

Beattie, A. (1991) 'Knowledge and control in health promotion: a test case for social policy and social theory', in J. Gabe, M. Calnan and M. Bury (eds), *The Sociology of the Health Service*. London: Routledge.

Beattie, A. (1993) 'The changing boundaries of health', in A. Beattie, M. Gott, L. Jones and M. Sidell (eds), *Health and Wellbeing: A Reader*. London: Macmillan.

Beauchamp, D.E. (1976) 'Public health as social justice', *Inquiry, 13*: 3–14.

Beauchamp, D.E. and Steinbock, B. (eds) (1999) *New Ethics for the Public's Health*. New York: Oxford University Press.

Beauchamp, T.L. (1978) 'The regulation of hazards and hazardous behaviors', *Health Education Monographs, 6* (2): 242–56.

Beauchamp, T.L. and Childress, J.F. (2019) *Principles of Biomedical Ethics* (8th edn). Oxford: Oxford University Press.

Becker, M.H. (ed.) (1984) *The Health Belief Model and Personal Health Behavior*. Thorofare, NJ: Charles B. Slack.

Beckwith, J. (2020) 'Knowledge, attitudes, and practices in reproductive and sexual health', *McGill Journal of Medicine, 9* (2): 119–25.

Begeny, J.C. and Greene, D.J. (2014) 'Can readability formulas be used to successfully gauge difficulty of reading materials?', *Psychology in the Schools, 51* (2). doi: 10.1002/pits.21740

Belbin, E., Downs, S. and Perry, P. (1981) 'How do I learn?', in J. Anderson, *The HEA Health Skills Dissemination Project: A Whole School Approach to Life Skills and Health Education*. Leeds: Counselling and Career Development Unit.

Bell, S. (2001) *LogFrames: Improved NRSP Research Project Planning and Monitoring*. Hemel Hempstead: DFID, NRSP.

Bennett, P. and Calman, K. (2001) *Risk Communication and Public Health*. Oxford: Oxford University Press.

Bennett, P. and Murphy, S. (1997) *Psychology and Health Promotion*. Buckingham: Open University Press.

Bennett, S., Corluka, A., Doherty, J., Tangcharoensathien, V., Patcharanarumol, W., Jesani, A., Kyabaggu, J., Namaganda, G., Hussain, A.Z. and Aikins, A. (2012) 'Influencing policy change: the experience of health think tanks in low- and middle-income countries', *Health Policy and Planning, 27*: 194–203.

Benson, D. and Russel, D. (2015) 'Patterns of EU energy policy outputs: incrementalism or punctuated equilibrium?', *West European Politics*, *38* (1): 185–205.

Bentley, C. (2008) *Systematically Addressing Health Inequalities*. London: Department of Health.

Berensson, M.K., Carlsson, P., Granath, M. and Urwitz, V. (2001) 'Quality indicators for health promotion programmes', *Health Promotion International*, *16* (2): 187–95.

Berger, A.A. (1991) *Media Analysis Techniques*. Newbury Park, CA: Sage.

Berkman, L.F., Glass, T., Brissette, I., Teresa, E. and Seeman, T.E. (2000) 'From social integration to health: Durkheim in the new millennium', *Social Science and Medicine*, *51*: 843–57.

Berkman, N.D., Davis, T.C. and McCormack, L. (2010) 'Health literacy: what is it?', *Journal of Health Communication*, *15* (Suppl 2): 9–19.

Berne, E. (1964) *Games that People Play*. New York: Grove Press.

Bernhard, J. (2001) *Health Education Research: Special Issue on Health Education and the Internet*, *16* (6): 643–5.

Birley, M. (2011) *Health Impact Assessment: Principles and Practice*. London: Earthscan.

Bivins, E.C. (1979) 'Community organisation – an old but reliable health education technique', in P.M. Lazes (ed.), *Handbook of Health Education*. New York: Aspen.

Blackwell, S. and Kosky, M. (2000) *The Role of 'Citizens' Juries' in Decisions about Equity in Health Care*. Perth, Australia: Medical Council.

Blaikie, N.W.H. (1991) 'A critique of the use of triangulation in social research', *Quality and Quantity*, *25*: 115–36.

Blake, G., Diamond, J., Foot, J., Gidley, B., Mayo, M., Shukra, K. and Yarnit, M. (2008) *Community Engagement and Community Cohesion*. York: Joseph Rowntree Foundation. (*Website*: www.jrf.org.uk/report/community-engagement-and-community-cohesion).

Blane, D., Brunner, E. and Wilkinson, R. (1996) *Health and Social Organization: Towards a Health Policy for the 21st Century*. London: Routledge.

Blaxter, M. (2007) 'How is health experienced?', in J. Douglas, S. Earle, S. Hansley, C.E. Lloyd and S. Spurr (eds), *A Reader in Promoting Public Health*. London: Sage.

Blaxter, M. (2010) *Health* (2nd edn). Cambridge: Polity.

Blaxter, M. and Patterson, S. (1982) *Mothers and Daughters: A Three-Generational Study of Health Attitudes and Behaviour*. London: Heinemann.

Bögemann, H. (2007) 'Promoting health and managing stress among prison employees', in L. Möller, H. Stöver, R. Jurgens, A. Gatherer and H. Nikogosian (eds), *Health in Prisons*. Copenhagen: WHO.

Bolam, B.L. (2005) 'Public participation in tackling health inequalities: implications from recent qualitative research', *European Journal of Public Health*, *15* (5): 447.

Bolam, B., Hodgetts, D., Chamberlain, K., Murphy, S. and Gleeson, K. (2003) '"Just do it": an analysis of accounts of control over health amongst lower socioeconomic status groups', *Critical Public Health*, *13*: 15–31.

Bonita, R., Beaglehole, R. and Kjellström, T. (2006) *Basic Epidemiology* (2nd edn). Geneva: WHO.

Borghesi, S. and Vercelli, A. (2010) 'Happiness and health: two paradoxes', *Journal of Economic Surveys*, *26* (2): 203–33.

Bosworth, M. (2002) *The US Federal Prison System*. Thousand Oaks, CA: Sage.

Botvin, G.J. (1984) 'The life skills training model: a broad spectrum approach to the prevention of cigarette smoking', in G. Campbell (ed.), *Health Education and Youth: A Review of Research and Developments*. Lewes, East Sussex: Falmer Press.

Boufides, C.H., Corcoran, E., Matthews, G.W., Herrick, J and Baker, E.L. (2019) 'Millennials as new messengers for public health', *Journal of Public Health Management and Practice*, *25* (2): 197–200.

Bourdieu, P. (1980) *Questions de Sociologie*. Paris: Les Editions des Minuit.

Boutilier, M., Cleverly, S. and Labonte, R. (2000) 'Community as a setting for health promotion', in B.D. Poland, L.W. Green and I. Rootman (eds), *Settings for Health Promotion: Linking Theory & Practice*. Thousand Oaks, CA: Sage.

Bowe, M., Wakefield, J.R.H., Kellezi, B., Stevenson, C., McNamara, N., Jones, B.A., Sumich, A. and Heym, N. (2022) 'The mental health benefits of community helping during crisis: coordinated helping, community identification and sense of unity during the COVID-19 pandemic', *Journal of Community & Applied Social Psychology, 32*: 521–35.

Bowling, A. (1997a) *Measuring Health: A Review of Quality of Life Measurement Scales* (2nd edn). Buckingham: Open University Press.

Bowling, A. (1997b) *Research Methods in Health*. Buckingham: Open University Press.

Bracht, N., Kingsbury, L. and Rissel, C. (1999) 'A five-stage community organization model for health promotion', in N. Bracht (ed.), *Health Promotion at the Community Level: New Advances*. Thousand Oaks, CA: Sage.

Bradley, E.H., Curry, L.A., Ramanadhan, S., Rowe, L., Nembhard, I.M. and Krumholz, H.M. (2009) 'Research in action: using positive deviance to improve quality of health care', *Implementation Science, 4* (1): 25–36.

Bradshaw, J. (1972) 'The concept of social need', *New Society*, 30 March.

Bradshaw, J. (1994) 'The conceptualization and measurement of need: a social policy perspective', in J. Popay and G. Williams (eds), *Researching the People's Health*. London: Routledge.

Brager, C. and Specht, H. (1973) *Community Organizing*. New York: Columbia University Press.

Brandenberger, L., Ingold, K., Fischer, M., Schläpfer, I. and Leifeld, P. (2022) 'Boundary spanning through engagement of policy actors in multiple issues', *Policy Studies Journal, 50*: 35–64.

Brandes, D. and Ginnis, P. (1986) 'A guide to student-centred learning', in J. Ryder and C. Campbell, *Balancing Acts in Personal, Social and Health Education*. London: Routledge.

Brandstetter, R., Bruijin, H., Byrne, M., Deslauriers, M., Förschner, M., Machačová, J., Orologa, J. and Scoppetta, A. (eds) (2006) *Successful Partnerships: A Guide*. Vienna: Forum on Partnerships and Local Governance as ZSI (Centre for Social Innovation).

Brann, M., Bute, J.J., Keeley, M., Petronio, S., Pines, R. and Watson, B. (2022) 'Interpersonal health communication theories', in T.L. Thompson and P.J. Schulz (eds), *Health Communication Theory*. Hoboken, NJ: John Wiley & Sons.

Braunack-Mayer, A. and Louise, J. (2008) 'The ethics of community empowerment: tensions in health promotion theory and practice', *Promotion & Education, 15* (3): 5–8.

Breakwell, G.M. (2007) *The Psychology of Risk*. Cambridge: Cambridge University Press.

Brehm, J.W. (1966) *A Theory of Psychological Reactance*. New York: Academic Press.

Brehm, S.S. and Brehm, J.W. (1981) *Psychological Reactance: A Theory of Freedom and Control*. New York: Academic Press.

Brennan, L., Klassen, K., Weng, E., Chin, S., Molenaar, A., Reid, M., Truby, H. and McCaffrey, T.A. (2020) 'A social marketing perspective of young adults concepts of eating for health: is it a question of morality?', *International Journal of Behavioral Nutrition and Physical Activity, 17*. doi: 10.1186/s12966-020-00946-3

Brennan, R.J. and Rimba, K. (2005) 'Rapid health assessment in Aceh Jaya District, Indonesia, following the December 26 tsunami', *Emergency Medicine Australasia, 17*: 341–50.

Breslow, L. (1999) 'From disease prevention to health promotion', *JAMA, 281*: 1030–3.

Breslow, L. (2004) 'Perspectives: the third revolution in health', *Annual Review of Public Health, 25* (April): xiii–xviii.

Breslow, L. (2006) 'Health measurement in the third era of health', *American Journal of Public Health, 96*: 17–19.

Breton, E. and de Leeuw, E. (2011) 'Theories of the policy process in health promotion research: a review', *Health Promotion International, 26*: 82–90.

Breuer, E., Comas-Herrera, A., Freeman, E., Albanese, E., Alladi, S., Amour, R., Evans-Lacko, S., Ferri, C.P., Govia, I., Iveth Astudillo García, C., Knapp, M., Lefevre, M., López-Ortega, M., Lund, C., Musyimi, C., Ndetei, D., Oliveira, D., Palmer, T., Pattabiraman, M., Sani, T.P., Taylor, D., Taylor, E., Theresia, I., Thomas, P.T., Turana, Y., Weidner, W. and Schneider, M. (2022) 'Beyond the project: building a strategic theory of change to address dementia care, treatment and support gaps across seven middle-income countries', *Dementia, 21*: 114–35.

Breunig, C. and Koski, C. (2018) 'Interest groups and policy volatility', *Governance, 31*: 279–97.

Bridgen, P. (2007) 'Evaluating the empowering potential of community-based health schemes: the case of community health policies in the UK since 1997', in J. Douglas, S. Earle, S. Handsley, C.E. Lloyd, and S. Spurr (eds), *A Reader in Promoting Public Health: Challenge and Controversy*. London: Sage.

Brint, S. (2001) 'Gemeinschaft revisited: a critique and reconstruction of the community concept', *Sociological Theory, 19*: 1–23.

British Standards Institute (1978) 'BS 4778 British Standard quality vocabulary', in Society of Health Education and Health Promotion Specialists, *Developing Quality in Health Education and Health Promotion. Society of Health Education and Health Promotion Specialists*.

Britton, A. (2010) 'Evaluating interventions: experimental study designs in health promotion', in M. Thorogood and Y. Coombes (eds), *Evaluating Health Promotion: Practice and Methods*. Oxford: Oxford University Press.

Broadcast Committee of Advertising Practice (2011) *Television Advertising Standards Code*. London: BCAP.

Brocklehurst, P.R., Morris, P. and Tickle, M. (2012) 'Social marketing: an appropriate strategy to reduce oral health inequalities?', *International Journal of Health Promotion and Education, 50* (2): 81–91.

Bronfenbrenner, U. (1977) 'Toward an experimental ecology of human development', *American Psychologist, 32*: 513–31.

Bronson, D.E. and Davis, T.S. (2011) *Finding and Evaluating Evidence: Systematic Reviews and Evidence-Based Practice*. New York: Oxford University Press.

Brook, R.H. and Lohr, K.N. (1985) 'Efficacy, effectiveness, variations, and quality: boundary-crossing research', *Medical Care, 23* (5): 710–22.

Brooks, F. and Kendall, S. (2013) 'Making sense of assets: what can an assets based approach offer public health?', *Critical Public Health, 23*: 127–30.

Broughton, B. (2001) *How LogFrame Approaches Could Facilitate the Planning and Management of Humanitarian Approaches* (*Website*: http://pdf2.hegoa.efaber.net/entry/content/942/How_logframe_approaches.pdf).

Brown, E.M., Smith, D.M., Epton, T. and Armitage, C. (2018) 'Do self-incentives and self-rewards change behavior? A systematic review and meta-analysis', *Behavior Therapy, 49*: 113–23.

Brown, L.D., Redelfs, A.H. Taylor, T.J. and Messer, R.L. (2015) 'Comparing the functioning of youth and adult partnerships for health promotion', *American Journal of Community Psychology, 56*: 25–35.

Brown, P. and Zavestoski, S. (2004) 'Social movements in health: an introduction', *Sociology of Health and Illness, 26*: 679–94.

Brown, R.C.H. (2018) 'Resisting moralisation in health promotion', *Ethical Theory and Moral Practice, 21*: 997–1011

Brown, R.C.H., Maslen, H. and Savulescu, J. (2019) 'Responsibility, prudence and health promotion', *Journal of Public Health, 41*: 561–5.

Brown, S.L. and Richardson, M. (2012) 'The effect of distressing imagery on attention to and persuasiveness of an antialcohol message: a gaze-tracking approach', *Health Education & Behavior, 39*: 8–17.

Brown, S.L. and Whiting, D. (2014) 'The ethics of distress: toward a framework for determining the ethical acceptability of distressing health promotion advertising', *International Journal of Psychology, 49*: 89–97.

Brownson, R.C., Fielding, J.E. and Maylahn, C.M. (2009) 'Evidence-based public health: a fundamental concept for public health practice', *Annual Review of Public Health, 30*: 175–201.

Bruner, J.S. (1971) *The Relevance of Education*. New York: Norton and Co.

Brunner, E. (1996) 'The social and biological basis of cardiovascular disease in office workers', in D. Blane, E. Brunner and R. Wilkinson (eds), *Health and Social Organization: Towards a Health Policy for the 21st Century*. London: Routledge.

Brunton, G., Thomas, J., O'Mara-Eves, A., Jamal, F., Oliver, S. and Kavanagh, J. (2017) 'Narratives of community engagement: a systematic review-derived conceptual framework for public health interventions', *BMC Public Health, 17* (1): 944–59.

Buchanan, D.R. (1994) 'Reflections on the relationship between theory and practice', *Health Education Research*, *9* (3): 273–83.

Buchanan, D.R. (2006) 'A new ethic for health promotion: reflections on a philosophy of health education for the 21st century', *Health Education and Behaviour*, *33*: 290–304.

Buck, D. and Frosini, F. (2012) *Clustering of Unhealthy Behaviours over Time: Implications for Policy and Practice.* London: The King's Fund.

Bull, T., Riggs, E. and Nchogu, S.N. (2012) 'Does health promotion need a Code of Ethics? Results from an IUHPE mixed method survey', *Global Health Promotion*, *19* (3): 8–20.

Bulmer, M. (1982) *The Use of Social Research: Social Investigations in Public Policy Making.* London: Allen & Unwin.

Bungay, H. and Vella-Burrows, T. (2013) 'The effects of participating in creative activities on the health and well-being of children and young people: a rapid review of the literature', *Perspectives in Public Health*, *133*: 44–52.

Bungay, H., Hughes, S., Jacobs, C. and Zhang, J. (2022) '*Dance for Health*: the impact of creative dance sessions on older people in an acute hospital setting', *Arts & Health*, *14* (1), 1–13.

Bunting, M. (2007) 'Capital ideas: Robert Putnam discusses the implications of his latest research into community, identity and trust', *The Guardian*, 18 July.

Bunton, R. (1992) 'Health promotion as social policy', in R. Bunton and G. Macdonald (eds), *Health Promotion: Disciplines and Diversity.* London: Routledge.

Bunton, R. and Macdonald, G. (eds) (2002) *Health Promotion: Disciplines and Diversity* (2nd edn). London: Routledge.

Burns, S.T., Amobi, N., Chen, J.V., O'Brien, M. and Haber, L.A. (2021) 'Readability of patient discharge instructions', *Journal of General Internal Medicine*, *37* (7): 1797–8.

Burton, P., Goodlad, R., Croft, J., Abbott, J., Hasting, A., Macdonald, G. and Slater, T. (2004) *What Works in Community Involvement in Area-Based Initiatives? A Systematic Review of the Literature.* Home Office Online Reports 53/04.

Buse, K., Mays, N. and Walt, G. (2012) *Making Health Policy.* Maidenhead: Open University Press.

Butterfoss, F.D., Goodman, R.M. and Wandersman, A. (1993) 'Community coalitions for prevention and health promotion', *Health Education Research*, *8* (3): 315–30.

Cabanero-Verzosa, C. (1996) *Communication for Behavior Change.* Washington, DC: World Bank.

Caley, M.J., O'Leary, R.A., Fisher, R., Low-Choy, S., Johnson, S. and Mengersen, K. (2014) 'What is an expert? A systems perspective on expertise', *Ecology and Evolution*, *4* (3): 231–42.

Callister, M., Coyne, S.M., Stern, L.A., Stockdale, L., Miller, M.J. and Wells, B.M. (2012) 'A content analysis of the prevalence and portrayal of sexual activity in adolescent literature', *Journal of Sex Research*, *49* (5): 477–86.

Calnan, M. (1987) *Health and Illness.* London: Tavistock.

Calouste Gulbenkian Foundation (1984) *A National Centre for Community Development* (Report of a Working Party). London: Gulbenkian Foundation.

Caltabiano, M.L. and Caltabiano, N.J. (2006) *Resilience and Health Outcomes in the Elderly.* Proceedings of the 39th Annual Conference of the Australian Association of Gerontology, Sydney, NSW, Australia, 22–24 November, pp. 1–11.

Campbell, C. (2003) *Letting Them Die: Why HIV/AIDS Prevention Programmes Often Fail.* Oxford: James Currey; Bloomington: Indiana University Press; and Cape Town: Juta.

Campbell, C. (2011) 'Embracing complexity: towards more nuanced understandings of social capital and health', *Global Health Action*, *4*: 5964. doi: 10.3402/gha.v4i0.5964

Campbell, C., Wood, R. and Kelly, M. (1999) *Social Capital and Health.* London: Health Development Agency.

Campbell Collaboration (2001) *Campbell Systematic Reviews: Guidelines for the Preparation of Review Protocols.* (*Website*: www.campbellcollaboration.org/images/pdf/plain-language/C2_Protocols_guidelines_v1.pdf).

Campbell, D. and Stanley, J. (1963) *Experimental and Quasi-Experimental Evaluations in Social Research*. Chicago, IL: Rand McNally.

Campbell, P.A. (2021) 'Lay participation with medical expertise in online self-care practices: social knowledge (co) productiong in the *Running Mania* injury forum', *Social Science & Medicine*, *277*. doi: 10.1016/j.socscimed.2021.113880

Campus, B., Fafard, P., St. Pierre, J. and Hoffman, S.J. (2021) 'Comparing the regulation and incentivization of e-cigarettes across 97 countries', *Social Science & Medicine*, *291*: 114187.

Canadian Council on Social Development (2001) *Defining and Redefining Poverty: A CCSD Perspective*. Position Paper. Ottawa, Ontario: CCSD.

Candela, A.G. (2019) 'Exploring the function of member checking', *The Qualitative Report*, *24*, 619-628.

Caplan, R. and Holland, J. (1990) 'Rethinking health education theory', *Health Education Journal*, *49*: 10–12.

Carcary, M. (2020) 'The research audit trail: methodological guidance for application in practice', *Electronic Journal of Business Research Methods*, *18*: 166–77.

Carlin, J.B., Taylor, P. and Nolan, T. (1998) 'School-based bicycle safety education and bicycle injuries in children: a case-control study', *Injury Prevention*, *4*: 22–7.

Carpenter, C.J. (2010) 'A meta-analysis of the effectiveness of health belief model variables in predicting behaviour', *Health Communication*, *25* (8): 661–9.

Carr-Hill, R. and Chalmers-Dixon, P. (2002) *A Review of Methods for Monitoring and Measuring Social Inequality, Deprivation and Health Inequalities*. Oxford: South East Public Health Observatory.

Carr-Hill, R. and Chalmers-Dixon, P. (2005) *The Public Health Observatory Handbook of Health Inequalities Measurement*. Oxford: SEPHO.

Carter, A.O., Saadi, H.F., Reed, R.L. and Dunn, E.V. (2011a) 'Assessment of obesity, lifestyle, and reproductive health needs of female citizens of Al Ain, United Arab Emirates', *Journal of Health, Population and Nutrition*, *22*: 75–83.

Carter, B. and Ford, K. (2013) 'Researching children's health experiences: the place for participatory, child-centered, arts-based approaches', *Research in Nursing and Health*, *36*: 95–107.

Carter, S.M. (2012) 'What is health promotion ethics?', *Health Promotion Journal of Australia*, *23* (1): 1-4.

Carter, S.M., Rychetnik, L., Lloyd, B., Kerridge, I.H., Baur, L., Bauman, A., Hooker, C. and Zask, A. (2011b) 'Evidence, ethics, and values: a framework for health promotion', *American Journal of Public Health*, *101* (3): 465–72.

Cassetti, V., Powell, K., Barnes, A. and Sanders, T. (2020) 'A systematic scoping review of asset-based approaches to promote health in communities: development of a framework', *Global Health Promotion*, *27*: 15–23.

Catalani, C.E., Veneziale, A., Campbell, L., Herbst, S., Butler, B., Springgate, B. and Minkler, M. (2012) 'Videovoice community assessment in post-Katrina New Orleans', *Health Promotion Practice*, *13*: 18–28.

Catelan, R.F., de Azevedo, F., Sbicigo, J.B., Vilanova, F., de Silva, L., Zanella, G.I., Ramos, M.L., Costa, A.B. and Nardi, H.N. (2022) 'Anticipated HIV stigma and delays in HIV testing among Brazilian heterosexual male soldiers', *Psychology & Sexuality*, *13* (2): 317–30.

Catford, J. (1983) 'Positive health indicators – towards a new information base for health promotion', *Community Medicine*, *5*: 125–32.

Catford, J. (1993) 'Auditing health promotion: what are the vital signs of quality?', *Health Promotion International*, *8* (2): 67–8.

Catford, J. (2010) 'Editorial: implementing the Nairobi Call to Action: Africa's opportunity to light the way', *Health Promotion International*, *25* (1). doi: 10.1093/heapro/daq018

Cattan, M. and Tilford, S. (2006) *Mental Health Promotion: A Lifespan Approach*. Maidenhead: McGraw Hill.

Caussy, D., Kumar, P. and Than Sein, U. (2003) 'Health impact assessment needs in South-East Asian countries', *Bulletin of the World Health Organization*, *81*: 439–43.

Cavanagh, S. and Chadwick, K. (2005) *Health Needs Assessment: A Practical Guide*. London: NICE.

Centers for Disease Control and Prevention (CDC) (2009) *Simply Put: A Guide for Creating Easy-to-Understand Materials* (3rd edn). Atlanta, GA: CDC.

Centers for Disease Control and Prevention (CDC) (2020) *Key Characteristics of Data Quality in Public Health Surveillance.* (*Website*: www.cdc.gov/ncbddd/birthdefects/surveillancemanual/chapters/chapter-7/chapter7.5.html#:~:text=Three%20basic%20characteristics%20of%20high,variables%20for%20cases%20are%20entered.)

Centre for Research on the Epidemiology of Disasters (2017) *The Human Cost of Natural Disasters: A Global Perspective.* Geneva: CRED.

Centre for Social Justice (2009) *Breakthrough Britain: Locked up Potential.* London: Centre for Social Justice.

Centre for Tobacco Control Research (2008) *Point of Sale Display of Tobacco Products.* Stirling: Centre for Tobacco Control Research, University of Stirling and The Open University.

Chambers, A., Damone, E., Chan, Y.T., Nyrop, K., Deal, A., Muss, H. and Carlot, M. (2022) 'Social support and outcomes in older adults with lung cancer', *Journal of Geriatric Oncology, 13*: 214–19.

Chandra, A., Williams, M., Plough, A., Stayton, A., Wells, K.B., Horta, M. and Tang, J. (2013) 'Getting actionable about community resilience: the Los Angeles County Community Disaster Resilience Project', *American Journal of Public Health, 103* (7): 1181–9.

Chapman, S. (1994) 'The A–Z of public health advocacy', in S. Chapman and D. Lupton (eds), *The Fight for Public Health: Principles and Practice of Media Advocacy.* London: BMJ Publishing Group.

Chapman, S. and Egger, G. (1983) 'Myth in cigarette advertising and health promotion', in S. Chapman and D. Lupton (1994), *The Fight for the Public Health: Principles and Practice of Media Advocacy.* London: BMJ Publishing Group.

Chapman, S. and Lupton, D. (1994) The Fight for Public Health: Principles and Practice of Media Advocacy. London: BMJ Publishing Group.

Chapman, S. and Wakefield, M. (2001) 'Tobacco control advocacy in Australia: reflections on 30 years of progress', *Health Education and Behavior, 28* (3): 274–89.

Charlton, B.G. (1991) 'Medical practice and the double-blind, randomized controlled trial: Editorial', *British Journal of General Practice, 42* (350): 355–6.

Charnofsky, S. (1971) *Educating the Powerless.* Belmont, CA: Wordsworth Publishers.

Chave, S.P.W. (1958) 'John Snow, the Broad Street pump and after', in J. Ashton, *The Epidemiological Imagination.* Buckingham: Open University Press.

Chen, F.-L. and Lee, A. (2016) 'Health-promoting educational settings in Taiwan: development and evaluation of the Health-Promoting School Accreditation System', *Global Health Promotion, 23* (Suppl): 18–25.

Chen, J. and Wang, Y. (2021) 'Social media use for health purposes: a systematic review', *Journal of Medical Internet Research, 23* (5). doi: 10.2196/17917

Cheng, C. and Dunn, M. (2015) 'Health literacy and the Internet: a study on the readability of Australian online health information', *Australian and New Zealand Journal of Public Health, 39* (4): 309–14.

Cheng, C., Cheung, S., Chio, J.H. and Chan, M.S. (2013) 'Cultural meaning of perceived control: a meta-analysis of locus of control and psychological symptoms across 18 cultural regions', *Psychological Bulletin, 139* (1): 152–88.

Chesterfield-Evans, A. and O'Connor, B. (1986) 'Billboard utilizing graffitists against unhealthy promotions (BUGA UP) – its philosophy and rationale and their application in health promotion', in D.S. Leathar, G.B. Hastings and J.K. Davies (eds), *Health Education and the Media.* London: Pergamon Press.

Cheung, R. (2018) *International Comparisons of Health and Wellbeing in Early Childhood.* London: Nuffield Trust.

Chien, Y. (2011) 'Use of message framing and color in vaccine information to increase willingness to be vaccinated', *Social Behaviour and Personality, 39* (8): 1063–72.

Chouinard, J.A. and Cousins, J.B. (2015) 'The journey from rhetoric to reality: participatory evaluation in a development context', *Educational Assessment, Evaluation and Accountability, 27*: 5–39.

Christakis, N.A. and Fowler, J.H. (2007) 'The spread of obesity in a large social network over 32 years', *New England Journal of Medicine, 358*: 2249–58.

Christens, B.D. (2013) 'In search of powerful empowerment', *Health Education Research, 28* (3): 371–4.

Christens, B.D. (2019) *Community Power and Empowerment.* Oxford: Oxford University Press.

Christens, B.D., Winn, L.T. and Duke, A.M. (2016) 'Empowerment and critical consciousness: a conceptual cross-fertilization', *Adolescent Research Review*, *1*: 15–27.

Chua, P.Y.S., Lee, S.L., Tow, Z.J., Mantok, R., Nor, M.K.H.M., Dorairaja, L., Jack, J., Rusly, N.F., Hanafi, N.M. and Zin, T. (2013) 'Rapid rural appraisal of a rural village in Sabah', *International Journal of Public Health Research*, *3*: 223–31.

Chung, J.E. (2017) 'Retweeting in health promotion: analysis of tweets about Breast Cancer Awareness Month', *Computers in Human Behavior*, *74*: 112–19.

Cicero, D.C. (2020) 'Measurement invariance of the Self-Concept Clarity Scale across race and sex', *Journal of Psychopathology and Behavioural Assessment*, *42* (2): 296–305.

Clark, A., Flèche, S., Layard, R., Powdthavee, N. and Ward, G. (2017) *The Key Determinants of Happiness and Misery*. CEP Discussion Papers, CEPDP1485. London: Centre for Economic Performance, London School of Economics and Political Science.

Clark, N. (2018) 'Exploring community capacity: Karen refugee women's mental health', *International Journal of Human Rights in Healthcare*, *11*: 244–56.

Clark, N.M., Lachance, L., Doctor, L.J., Gilmore, L., Kelly, C., Krieger, J., Lara, M., Meurer, J., Friedman Milanovich, A. and Nicholas, E. (2010) 'Policy and system change and community coalitions: outcomes from allies against asthma', *American Journal of Public Health*, *100*: 904–12.

Clarke, B., Swinburn, B. and Sacks, G. (2016) 'The application of theories of the policy process to obesity prevention: a systematic review and meta-synthesis', *BMC Public Health*, *16* (1): 1084–2003.

Clift, S. (2012) 'Creative arts as a public health resource: moving from practice-based research to evidence-based practice', *Perspectives in Public Health*, *132* (3): 120–7.

Coan, S., Woodward, J., South, J., Bagnall, A-M, Southby, K., Button, D. and Trigwell, J. (2020) 'Can a community empowerment intervention improve health and wellbeing in a post-industrial UK town?', *European Journal of Public Health*, *30* (s5): v88.

Cochrane Collaboration (2002) *Cochrane Collaboration Disclaimer about Cochrane Reviews*. Oxford: Cochrane Collaboration.

Coffe, H. and Bolzendahl, C. (2011) 'Gender gaps in political participation across sub-Saharan African nations', *Social Indicators Research*, *102* (2): 245–64.

Cohen, A.K. (1955) *Delinquent Boys: The Culture of the Gang*. New York: Free Press.

Cohen, B. (1963) *The Press and Foreign Policy*. Princeton, NJ: Princeton University Press.

Cohen, J.M. and Cohen, M.J. (1960) *The Penguin Dictionary of Quotations*. Harmondsworth: Penguin.

Cole, B., DeGabriele, G., Ho, G. and Anda, M. (2015) 'Exploring the utility of diffusion theory to evaluate social marketing approaches to improve urban sanitation in Malawi'. *Journal of Water, Sanitation and Hygiene for Development*, *5* (2): 289–300.

Colebatch, H.K. (1998) *Policy*. Buckingham: Open University Press.

Coleman, C.H., Bouëssaeu, M. and Reis, A. (2008) 'The contribution of ethics to public health', *Bulletin of the World Health Organization*, *86* (8): 577–578.

Coleman, J. (1988) 'Social capital in the creation of human capital', *American Journal of Sociology*, *94* (Suppl): S25–S120.

Coleman, J. (1990) *Foundations of Social Theory*. New York: Free Press.

Collins, R.L., Wong, E.C., Breslau, J., Burnam, M.A., Cefalu, M. and Roth, E. (2019) 'Social marketing of mental health treatment: California's mental illness stigma reduction campaign', *American Journal of Public Health*, *109* (S3): S228–S35.

Commission on Social Determinants of Health (CSDH) (2007) *Achieving Health Equity: From Root Causes to Fair Outcomes: Interim Statement*. Geneva: WHO. (*Website*: www.who.int/social_determinants/resources/interim_statement/en/index.html).

Commission on Social Determinants for Health (CSDH) (2008) *Closing the Gap in a Generation: Health Equity through Action on the Social Determinants of Health*. Geneva: WHO. (*Website*: www.who.int/social_determinants/final_report/en/).

COMMIT Research Group (1991) 'Community intervention trial for smoking cessation (COMMIT): summary of design and intervention', *Journal of the National Cancer Institute*, *83*(22): 1620–8.

Communication Evaluation Expert Panel (2007) 'Guidance for evaluating mass media communication health initiatives: summary of an expert panel discussion sponsored by the Centers for Disease Control and Prevention', *Evaluation and the Health Professions*, *30* (3): 229–53.

Communities Scotland (2005) *National Standards for Community Engagement*. (*Website*: www.voicescotland.org.uk/media/resources/NSfCE%20online_October.pdf).

Community Development Project (1977) *Gilding the Ghetto*. London: Community Development Project.

Condran, B., Gahagan, J. and Isfeld-Kiely, H. (2017) 'A scoping review of social media as a platform for multilevel sexual health promotion interventions', *Canadian Journal of Human Sexuality*, *26* (1): 26–37.

Connell, J.P. and Kubisch, A.C. (1998) 'Applying a theory of change approach to the evaluation of comprehensive community initiatives: progress, prospects and problems', in K. Fulbright-Anderson, A.C. Kubisch and J.P. Connell (eds), *New Approaches to Evaluating Community Initiatives, Vol. 2: Theory, Measurement and Analysis*. Washington, DC: Aspen Institute.

Connell, J.P., Kubisch, A.C., Schorr, L.B. and Weiss, C.H. (eds) (1995) *New Approaches to Evaluating Community Initiatives, Vol. 1: Concepts, Methods and Contexts*. Washington, DC: Aspen Institute.

Connelly, J. (2001) 'Critical realism and health promotion: effective practice needs an effective theory: Editorial', *Health Education Research*, *16* (2): 115–19.

Conner, M. and Norman, P. (eds) (2015) *Predicting and Changing Health Behaviour* (3rd edn). Maidenhead: Open University Press.

Conner, M. and Sparks, P. (2005) 'Theory of planned behaviour and health behaviour', in M. Conner and P. Norman (eds), *Predicting Health Behaviour* (2nd edn). Maidenhead: Open University Press.

Constantino-David, K. (1982) 'Issues in community organization', *Community Development Journal*, *17*: 190–201.

Cook, C. (2012) *Primary, Secondary, Tertiary and Quaternary Prevention*. Powerpoint Presentation. Walsh University, North Canton, Ohio. (*Website*: www.orthopt.org/uploads/content_files/CSM_2013/Handouts/Part_1_Cook.pdf).

Cook, T.D. and Campbell, D.T. (1979) *Quasi-Experimentation*. Chicago, IL: Rand McNally.

Cooper, H., Arber, S., Fee, L. and Ginn, J. (1999) *The Influence of Social Support and Social Capital on Health*. London: Health Development Agency.

Corcoran, N. and Ahmad, F. (2016) 'The readability and suitability of sexual health promotion leaflets', *Patient Education and Counselling*, *99*: 284–6.

Corcoran, N. and Bone, A. (2007) 'Using settings to communicate health promotion', in N. Corcoran (ed.), *Communicating Health: Strategies for Health Promotion*. London: Sage.

Cornacchione, J. and Smith, S.W. (2012) 'The effects of message framing within the stages of change on smoking cessation intentions and behaviors', *Health Communication*, *27* (6): 612–22.

Cornwall, A. and Pratt, G. (2011) 'The use and abuse of participatory rural appraisal: reflections from practice', *Agriculture and Human Values*, *28*: 263–72.

Cornwell, J. (1984) *Hard-Earned Lives*. London: Tavistock.

Coulthard, M., Walker, A. and Morgan, A. (2002) *People's Perceptions of their Neighbourhood and Community Involvement: Results from the Social Capital Module of the General Household Survey 2000*. London: The Stationery Office.

Coutts, A. and Fouad, F.M. (2013) 'Response to Syria's health crisis: poor and uncoordinated', *The Lancet*, *381*: 2242–3.

Coveney, J. (2010) 'Analyzing public health policy: three approaches', *Health Promotion Practice*, *11*: 515–21.

Craig, R.L., Felix, H.C., Walker, J.F. and Phillips, M.M. (2010) 'Public health professionals as policy entrepreneurs: Arkansas's childhood obesity policy experience', *American Journal of Public Health*, *100* (11): 2047–52.

Crawford, R. (1980) 'Healthism and the medicalization of everyday life', *International Journal of Health Services*, *10* (3): 365–88.

Crawshaw, P. and Newlove, C. (2011) 'Men's understandings of social marketing and health: neo-liberalism and health governance', *International Journal of Men's Health*, *10* (2): 136–52.

Cross, R. (2013) 'Young women's constructions of risky health practices: a Q-methodological study', *Psychology of Women Section Review*, *15* (2): 29–39.

Cross, R. and O'Neil, I. (2021) 'Health communication', in R. Cross, L. Warwick-Booth, S. Rowlands, J. Woodall, I. O'Neil and S. Foster, *Health Promotion: Global Principles and Practice* (2nd edn). Wallingford: CABI

Cross, R., Davis, S. and O'Neil, I. (2017a) *Health Communication: Theoretical and Critical Perspectives, Cambridge, Polity*.

Cross, R, Rowlands, S. and Foster, S. (2021) 'The foundations of health promotion', in R. Cross, L. Warwick-Booth, S. Rowlands, J. Woodall, I. O'Neil and S. Foster, *Health Promotion: Global Principles and Practice* (2nd edn). Wallingford: CABI

Cross, R., Woodall, J. and Warwick-Booth, L. (2017b) 'Empowerment: challenges in measurement', *Global Health Promotion*. *26*(2):93-96 doi: 10.1177/1757975917703304

Crossley, M.L. (2002) 'Introduction to the symposium on "health resistance": the limits of contemporary health promotion', *Health Education Journal*, *61* (2): 101–12.

Culyer, A.J. (1977) 'Need, values and health status measurement', in A.J. Culyer and K.G. Wright (eds), *Economic Aspects of Health Services*. London: Martin Robertson.

Cummins, S. and MacIntyre, S. (2002) '"Food deserts" – evidence and assumption in policy-making', *British Medical Journal*, *325*: 436–8.

Cunningham, G. (1963) 'Policy and practice', *Public Administration*, 41.

Curle, A. (1972) *Education for Liberation*. New York: John Wiley.

Dagenais, C., Queuille, L. and Ridde, V. (2013) 'Evaluation of a knowledge transfer strategy from a user fee exemption program for vulnerable populations in Burkina Faso', *Global Health Promotion*, *20*: 70–9.

Daghio, M.M., Fattori, G. and Ciardullo, A. (2006) 'Evaluation of easy-to-read information material on healthy life-styles written with the help of citizens' collaboration through networking', *Promotion & Education*, *XIII* (3): 191–6.

Dahlgren, G. and Whitehead, M. (1991) *Policies and Strategies to Promote Social Equity in Health*. Stockholm: Institute of Futures Studies.

Dale, R. and Hanbury, A. (2010) 'A simple methodology for piloting and evaluating mass media interventions: an exploratory study', *Psychology, Health & Medicine*, *15* (2): 231–42.

Daniel, P. and Dearden, P.N. (2001) *Integrating a Logical Framework Approach to Planning into the Health Action Zone Initiative*. Hull: HAZNET, Hull and East Riding Community Health NHS Trust.

Davey Smith, G. (1996) 'Income inequality and mortality: why are they related?', *British Medical Journal*, *312*: 987–8.

Davidoff, F., Haynes, B., Sackett, D.L. and Smith, R. (1995) 'Evidence-based medicine: a new journal to help doctors identify the information they need', *British Medical Journal*, *310*: 1085–6.

Davies, H., Nutley, S. and Walter, I. (2008) 'Why "knowledge transfer" is misconceived for applied social research', *Journal of Health Services Research and Policy*, *13*: 188–90.

Day, I. (2002) '"Putting yourself in other people's shoes": the use of forum theatre to explore refugee and homeless issues in schools', *Journal of Moral Education*, *31* (1): 21–34.

Daykin, N. (2019) 'Social movements and boundary work in arts, health and wellbeing: a research agenda', *Nordic Journal of Arts, Culture and Health*, *1*: 9–20.

Daykin, N., de Viggiani, N., Pilkington, P. and Moriarty, Y. (2013) 'Music-making for health, well-being and behaviour change in youth justice settings: a systematic review', *Health Promotion International*, *28*: 197–210.

De Andrade, M. (2016) 'Tackling health inequalities through asset-based approaches, co-production and empowerment: ticking consultation boxes or meaningful engagement with diverse, disadvantaged communities?', *Journal of Poverty and Social Justice*, *24* (2): 127–41.

de Greef, M. and Van den Broek, K. (2004) *Making the Case for Workplace Health Promotion: Analysis of the Effects of WHP*. Essen: ENWHP (*Website*: www.enwhp.org/fileadmin/downloads/report_business_case.pdf).

de Kadt, E. (1982) 'Ideology, social policy, health and health services: a field of complex interactions', *Social Science and Medicine*, *16*: 741–52.

de Leeuw, E. (2000) 'Commentary – beyond community action: communication arrangements and policy networks', in B. Poland, L.W. Green and I. Rootman (eds), *Settings for Health Promotion*. Thousand Oaks, CA: Sage.

de Leeuw, E. and Breton, E. (2013) 'Policy change theories in health promotion research: a review', in C. Clavier and E. De Leeuw (eds), *Health Promotion and the Policy Process*. Oxford: Oxford University Press.

de Leeuw, E., Green, G., Spanswick, L. and Palmer, N. (2015) 'Policymaking in European healthy cities', *Health Promotion International, 30* (Suppl): i18–i31.

de Saussure, F. (1915) *Course in General Linguistics*. London: Peter Owen. (English translation, 1960.)

de Silva, A.M., Martin-Kerry, J.M., Van, K., Hegde, S. and Heilbrunn-Lang, A. (2017) 'Developing a practical readability tool for assessing oral health promotion material for people with low literacy', *Health Education Journal, 76* (7): 809–17.

de Viggiani, N. (2006a) 'Surviving prison: exploring prison social life as a determinant of health', *International Journal of Prisoner Health, 2*: 71–89.

de Viggiani, N. (2006b) 'A new approach to prison public health? Challenging and advancing the agenda for prison health', *Critical Public Health, 16*: 307–16.

Deane, J. (2018) 'Health effects of mass-media interventions', *The Lancet, 6*: e960.

Deehan, A. and Wylie, A. (2010) 'Health promotion: the challenges, the questions of definition, discipline status and evidence base', in A. Wylie, T. Holt and A. Howe (eds), *Health Promotion in Medical Education: From Rhetoric to Action*. Oxford: Radcliffe Publishing, 10–22.

Defoe, J.R. and Breed, W.R. (1989) 'Consulting to change media contents: two cases in alcohol education', *International Quarterly of Community Health Education, 9*: 257–72.

Delaney, F. (1994a) 'Muddling through the middle ground: theoretical concerns in intersectoral collaboration and health promotion', *Health Promotion International, 9* (3): 217–25.

Delaney, F. (1994b) 'Making connections: research into intersectoral collaboration', *Health Education Journal, 53*: 474–85.

Delaney, F. (1994c) 'Policy and health promotion', *Journal of the Institute of Health Education, 32* (1): 5–9.

Deloitte (2010) *2010 Survey of Health Care Consumers: Key Findings, Strategic Implications*. Washington, DC: Deloitte Center for Health Solutions.

Denison, J., Tsui, S., Bratt, J., Torpey, K., Weaver, M. and Kabaso, M. (2012) 'Do peer educators make a difference? An evaluation of a youth-led HIV prevention model in Zambian schools', *Health Education Research, 27*: 237–47.

Denman, S., Moon, A., Parsons, C. and Stears, D. (2002) *The Health Promoting School: Policy Research and Practice*. London: Routledge Falmer.

Denzin, N.K. (1970) *The Research Act in Sociology*. London: Butterworths.

Denzin, N.K. (1994) 'The art and politics of interpretation', in N.K. Denzin and Y.S. Lincoln (eds), *Handbook of Qualitative Research*. Thousand Oaks, CA: Sage.

Department of Health (1988) *Public Health in England: The Report of the Committee of Inquiry into the Future Development of the Public Health Function, The Acheson Report. Cm. 289*. London: HMSO.

Department of Health (1992) *The Health of the Nation*. London: HMSO.

Department of Health (2003) *Health Equity Audit: A Guide for the NHS*. (*Website*: https://webarchive.nationalarchives.gov.uk/20070403001525/http://www.dh.gov.uk/en/Publicationsandstatistics/Publications/PublicationsPolicyAndGuidance/DH_4084138).

Department of Health (2004) *Choosing Health: Making Healthy Choices Easier. Cm. 6374*. London: The Stationery Office. (*Website*: http://webarchive.nationalarchives.gov.uk/+/http://www.dh.gov.uk/en/Publicationsandstatistics/Publications/PublicationsPolicyAndGuidance/DH_4094550).

Department of Health (2007a) *Health Survey for England: Introduction*. London: Department of Health.

Department of Health (2007b) *Health Impact Assessment*. London: Department of Health. (*Website*: http://webarchive.nationalarchives.gov.uk/+/http://www.dh.gov.uk/en/Publicationsandstatistics/Legislation/Healthassessment/index.htm)

Department of Health (2008) *Ambitions for Health*. London: Department of Health.

Department of Health (2012) *The Structure of Public Health England*. London: Department of Health.

Department of Health and Social Security (DHSS) (1980) *Inequalities in Health: Report of a Research Working Group Chaired by Sir Douglas Black*. London: DHSS.

Department of the Environment, Transport and the Regions (DETR) (2001) *Local Strategic Partnerships: Government Guidance*. London: DETR.

Department of Health and Social Care (DHSC) *What the Office for Health Improvement and Disparities does*. (*Website*: www.gov.uk/government/organisations/office-for-health-improvement-and-disparities)

Deviren, F. and Babb, P. (2005) *Young People and Social Capital*. London: National Statistics.

Dignan, M.B. and Carr, P.A. (1992) *Program Planning for Health* (2nd edn). Malvern, PA: Lee & Febiger.

Dijkstra, A. and de Vries, H. (2000) 'Subtypes of pre-contemplating smokers defined by different long-term plans to change their smoking behavior', *Health Education Research*, 15 (4): 423–34.

Dixey, R., Woodall, J. and Lowcock, D. (2013) 'Practising health promotion', in R. Dixey (ed.), *Health Promotion: Global Principles and Practice*. Wallingford: CABI.

Dixon, J. (1989) 'The limits and potential of community development for personal and social change', *Community Health Studies*, 12 (1): 82–92.

Dixon-Woods, M., Agarwal, S., Young, B., Jones, D. and Sutton, A. (2004) *Integrative Approaches to Qualitative and Quantitative Evidence*. London: Health Development Agency.

Dixon-Woods, M., Bonas, S., Booth, A., Jones, D.R., Miller, T., Sutton, A.J., Shaw, R.L., Smith, J.A. and Young, B. (2006) 'How can systematic reviews incorporate qualitative research? A critical perspective', *Qualitative Research*, 6 (1): 27–44.

Djian, A., Guignard, R., Gallopel-Morvan, K., Smadja, O., Davies, J., Blanc, A., Mercier, A., Walmsley, M. and Nguyen-Thanh, V. (2019) 'From "Stopober" to "Moi(S) Sans Tabac": how to import a social marketing campaign, *Journal of Social Marketing*, 9 (4): 345–56.

Do, M., Figueroa, M.E. and Kincaid, D.L. (2016) 'HIV testing among young people aged 16–24 in South Africa: impact of mass media communication programs', *AIDS Behaviour*, 20: 2033–44.

Donald, A. (2001) 'What is quality of life?', *What is … series*, 1 (9): 1–4.

Donaldson, I. and Rutter, P.D. (2017) *Donaldson's Essential Public Health* (4th edn). London: Routledge.

Donaldson, L. (1999) *Ten Tips for Better Health*. London: The Stationery Office.

Dooris, M. (2004) 'Joining up settings for health: a valuable investment for strategic partnerships?', *Critical Public Health*, 14: 37–49.

Dooris, M. (2006) 'Health promoting settings: future directions', *Promotion & Education*, 13 (1): 2–4.

Dooris, M. (2013) 'Expert voices for change: bridging the silos: towards healthy and sustainable settings for the 21st century', *Health and Place*, 20: 39–50.

Dooris, M. and Baybutt, M. (2021) 'The centrality of the settings approach in building back better and fairer', *International Journal of Health Promotion and Education*, 59: 195–7.

Dorfman, L. and Krasnow, I.D. (2014) 'Public health and media advocacy', *Annual Review of Public Health*, 35: 293–306.

Dorling, D., Rigby, J., Wheeler, B., Ballas, D., Thomas, B., Fahmy, E., Gordon, D. and Lupton, R. (2007) *Poverty Wealth and Place in Britain 1968–2005*. Bristol: Policy Press in association with Joseph Rowntree Foundation.

Douglas, M.J., Conway, L., Gorman, D., Gavin, S. and Hanlon, P. (2001) 'Developing principles for health impact assessment', *Journal of Public Health Medicine*, 23 (2): 148–54.

Dowd, E.T. (2002) 'Psychological reactance in health education and promotion', *Health Education Journal*, 61(2): 113–24.

Downie, R.S., Tannahill, C. and Tannahill, A. (1996) *Health Promotion Models and Values* (2nd edn). Oxford: Oxford University Press.

Doyal, L. and Gough, I. (1991) *A Theory of Human Need*. London: Macmillan.

Doyal, L. and Pennell, I. (1979) *The Political Economy of Health*. London: Pluto.

Draper, R. (1988) 'Healthy public policy: a new political challenge', *Health Promotion, 2* (3): 217–18.

Duan, K. I., Rodriguez Garza, F., Flores, H., Palazuelos, D., Maza, J., Martinez-Juarez, L.A., Elliott, P.F., Moreno Lázaro, E., Enriquez Rios, N., Nigenda, G., Palazuelos, L. and McBain, R.K. (2021) 'Economic evaluation of a novel community-based diabetes care model in rural Mexico: a cost and cost-effectiveness study', *BMJ Open, 11*: e046826.

Dubos, R. (1979) *The Mirage of Health.* New York: Harper Colophon.

Duncan, P. (2007) *Critical Perspectives on Health.* Basingstoke: Palgrave Macmillan.

Duncan, P. (2013) 'Failing to professionalise, struggling to specialise: the rise and fall of health promotion as a putative specialism in England, 1980–2000', *Medical History, 57* (3): 377–96.

Durfee, W. and Chase, T. (1999) *Brief Tutorial on Gantt Charts.* Minneapolis, MN: University of Minnesota.

Duryea, E.J. (1991) 'Principles of non-verbal communication in efforts to reduce peer and social pressure', *Journal of School Health, 61*: 5–10.

Dutta, M.J. (2020) *Communication, Culture and Social Change: Meaning, Co-option and Resistance.* London: Routledge.

Dworkin, G. (1972) 'Paternalism', *Monist, 56* (1): 64–84.

Dymond-Green, N. (2020) *How Can We Calculate Levels of Deprivation or Poverty in the UK? (Part 1). Data Impact Blog.* (*Website*: www.blog.ukdataservice.ac.uk)

Eagleton, T. (1991) *An Introduction to Ideology.* London: Verso.

Eakin, J., Robertson, A., Poland, B., Coburn, D. and Edwards, R. (1996) 'Towards a critical social science perspective on health promotion research', *Health Promotion International, 11* (2): 157–65.

Edgar, A., Salek, S., Shickle, D. and Cohen, D. (1998) *The Ethical QALY: Ethical Issues in Healthcare Resource Allocations.* Haslemere: Euromed Communications Ltd.

Educe Ltd and GFA Consulting (undated) *Five Vital Lessons: Successful Partnerships with Business.* (*Website*: www.educe.co.uk/?p=141).

Egan, M., Acharya, A., Sounderajah, V., Xu, Y., Mottershaw, A., Phillips, R., Ashrafian, H. and Darzi, A. (2021) 'Evaluating the effect of infographics on public recall, sentiment and willingness to use face masks during the COVID-19 pandemic: a randomised internet-based questionnaire study', *BMC Public Health, 21*: 367.

Ehrenreich, B. and English, D. (1979) *For Her Own Good: 150 Years of Experts' Advice to Women.* London: Pluto Press.

Ehsan, A., Klaas, H.S., Bastianen, A. and Spini, D. (2019) 'Social capital and health: a systematic review of systematic reviews', *Population Health, 8*. doi: 10.1016/j.ssmph.2019.110425

Eiser, J.R. and Eiser, C. (1996) *Effectiveness of Video for Health Education: A Review.* London: HEA.

EPPI-Centre (1999) *A Review of the Effectiveness and Appropriateness of Peer-Delivered Health Promotion Interventions for Young People.* London: Institute of Education, University of London.

Epstein, N.E., Bluethenthal, A., Visser, D., Pinsky, C. and Minklet, M. (2021) 'Leveraging arts for justice, equity, and public health: the Skywatchers Program and its implications for community-based health promotion practice and research', *Health Promotion Practice, 22* (Suppl 1): 91S–100S.

Erikson, R. and Torssander, J. (2008) 'Social class and cause of death', *European Journal of Public Health, 18* (5): 473–8.

Eriksson, B.M. (2010) *The Hitchhiker's Guide to Salutogenesis: Salutogenic Pathways to Health Promotion.* Folkhälsan Research Report: 2.

Eriksson, M. (2011) 'Social capital and health – implications for health promotion', *Global Health Action, 4*. doi: 10.3402/gha.v4i0.5611

Errington, G. and Towner, E. (2005) 'Injury prevention', in L. Ewles (ed.), *Key Topics in Public Health: Essential Briefings on Prevention and Health Promotion.* London: Elsevier.

Etzioni, A. (1967) 'Mixed scanning: a third approach to decision making', *Public Administration Review, 27*: 385–92.

European Centre for Health Policy (1999) *Gothenburg Consensus Paper: Health Impact Assessment.* Copenhagen: WHO Regional Office for Europe.

European Commission (2004) *Joint Report on Social Inclusion*. Brussels: Council of the European Union.

European Network of Workplace Health Promotion (ENWHP) (2007) *Luxembourg Declaration*. (*Website*: www. enwhp.org/fileadmin/rs-dokumente/dateien/Luxembourg_Declaration.pdf).

EuroQol (undated) *EuroQol EQ-5D*. (*Website*: https://euroqol.org).

Evans, D., Head, M.J. and Speller, V. (1994) *Assuring Quality in Health Promotion: How to Develop Standards of Good Practice*. London: HEA.

Evans, D.W. and McCormack, L. (2008) 'Applying social marketing in health care: communicating evidence to change consumer behaviour', *Medical Decision Making*, *28*: 718–31.

Evans, M. and Fisher, E.B. (2022) 'Social isolation and mental health: the role of nondirective and directive social support', *Community Mental Health Journal*, *58*: 20–40.

Ewert, B. (2017) 'Promoting health in schools: theoretical reflections on the settings approach versus nudge tactics', *Social Theory & Health*, *15* (4): 430–47.

Faden, R.R. and Faden, A.I. (1978) 'The ethics of health education as public health policy', *Health Education Monographs*, *6* (2): 180–97.

Fairbrother, P., Tyler, M., Hart, A., Mees, B., Phillips, R., Stratford, J. and Toh, K. (2013) 'Creating "community"? Preparing for bushfire in rural Victoria', *Rural Sociology*, *78*: 186–209.

Farrelly, M.C., Davis, K.C., Duke, J. and Messeri, P. (2008) 'Sustaining "truth": changes in youth tobacco attitudes and smoking intentions after 3 years of a national antismoking campaign', *Health Education Research*, Epub, 17 January.

Farrelly, M.C., Davis, K.C., Haviland, M.L., Messeri, P. and Healton, C.G. (2005) 'Evidence of a dose-response relationship between "truth" anti-smoking ads and youth smoking prevalence', *American Journal of Public Health*, *95* (3): 425–31.

Fauth, B., Renton, Z. and Solomon, E. (2013) *Tackling Child Poverty and Promoting Children's Well-Being: Lessons from Abroad*. London: National Children's Bureau.

Feighery, E. and Rogers, T. (1989) 'Building and maintaining effective coalitions', in F.D. Butterfoss, R.M. Goodman and A. Wandersman, 'Community coalitions for prevention and health promotion', *Health Education Research*, *8* (3): 315–30.

Felix, M., Chavis, D. and Florin, P. (1989) 'Enabling community development: language, concepts and strategies', presentation sponsored by Health Promotion Branch, Ontario Ministry of Health, Toronto, 16–18 May 1989.

Ferro, M.A. and Boyle, M.H. (2013) 'Self-concept among youth with a chronic illness: a meta-analytic review', *Health Psychology*, *32* (8): 839–48.

Festinger, L. (1957) *A Theory of Cognitive Dissonance*. Stanford, CA: Stanford University Press.

Fien, J. (1994) 'Critical theory, critical pedagogy and critical praxis in environmental education', in B.B. Jensen and K. Schnack (eds), *Action and Action Competence as Key Concepts in Critical Pedagogy*. Copenhagen: Royal Danish School of Educational Studies.

Fien, J. (2000) 'Education for sustainable consumption: towards a framework for curriculum and pedagogy', in B.B. Jensen, K. Schnack and V. Simovska (eds), *Critical Environmental and Health Education*. Copenhagen: Research Centre for Environmental and Health Education, Danish University of Education.

Fien, J. and Trainer, T. (1993) 'Education for sustainability', in J. Fien (ed.), *Environmental Education: A Pathway to Sustainability*. Geelong, Australia: Deakin University Press.

Fischer, C.B., Adrien, N., Silguero, J.J., Hopper, J.J., Chowdhury, A.I. and Werler, M.M. (2021) 'Mask adherence and rate of COVID-19 across the United States', *PLOS ONE*, *16*: e0249891.

Fishbein, M. (1976) 'Persuasive communication', in A.E. Bennett (ed.), *Communication between Doctors and Patients*. London: Oxford University Press for Nuffield Provincial Hospitals Trust.

Fishbein, M. and Ajzen, I. (1975) *Belief, Attitude, Intention and Behavior: An Introduction to Theory and Research*. Reading, MA: Addison-Wesley.

Fisher, R. (1949) *The Design of Experiments* (5th edn). Edinburgh: Oliver & Boyd.

Fisher, R. and Fisher, P. (2018) 'Peer education and empowerment: perspectives from young women working as peer educators with Home-Start', *Studies in the Education of Adults*, 50 (1): 74–91.

Fleming, M.-L. and Baldwin, L. (2020) *Health Promotion in the 21st Century: New Approaches to Achieving Health for All*. Abingdon: Routledge.

Fletcher, C.M. (1973) *Communication in Medicine: The Rock Carling Fellowship, 1972*. London: Nuffield Provincial Hospitals Trust.

Fletcher, J.R. (2021) 'Destigmatising dementia: the dangers of felt stigma and benevolent othering', *Dementia*, 20: 417–26.

Flynn, B.S., Worden, J.K., Yanushka Bunn, J., Connolly, S.W. and Dorwaldt, A.L. (2011) 'Evaluation of smoking prevention television messages based on the elaboration likelihood model', *Health Education Research*, 26 (6): 976–87.

Foot, J. (2012) *What Makes Us Healthy? The Asset Approach in Practice: Evidence, Action, Evaluation*. (*Website*: www.janefoot.co.uk).

Frank, R.H. (2000) 'Why living in a rich society makes us feel poor', *New York Times Magazine*, 15 October.

Frankel, S., Davison, C. and Davey Smith, G. (1991) 'Lay epidemiology and the rationality of responses to health education', *British Journal of General Practice*, 41: 428–30.

Frankena, W.K. (1970) 'A model for analyzing a philosophy of education', in J.R. Martin (ed.), *Readings in Philosophy of Education: A Study in Curriculum*. Boston, MA: Allyn & Bacon.

Frankham, J. (1998) 'Peer education: the unauthorised version', *British Educational Research Journal*, 24 (2): 179–93.

Freedman, A.M., Simmons, S., Lloyd, L.M., Redd, T.R., Alperin, M., Salek, S.S., Swier, L. and Miner, K.R. (2014) 'Public health training center evaluation: a framework for using logic models to improve practice and educate the public health workforce', *Health Promotion Practice*, 15: 80S–88S.

Freedom Organisation for the Right to Enjoy Smoking Tobacco (FOREST) (2008) *How Forest Works*. (*Website*: www.forestonline.org/about-forest/how-forest-works).

Freeman, B.M. (2019) 'Promoting global health and well-being of Indigenous youth through the connection of land and culture-based activism', *Global Health Promotion*, 26: 17–25.

Freidson, E. (1961) *Patients' Views of Medical Practice*. New York: Russell Sage.

Freire, P. (1972) *Pedagogy of the Oppressed*. Harmondsworth: Penguin.

French, J. (2000) *Understanding Health Promotion Through its Fault Lines*. PhD thesis, Leeds Metropolitan University, Leeds.

French, J. and Blair-Stevens, C. (2007) *Big Pocket Guide to Social Marketing* (2nd edn). London: National Consumer Council.

French, J. and Milner, S. (1993) 'Should we accept the status quo?', *Health Education Journal*, 52 (2): 98–101.

French, J.R.P. and Raven, B.H. (1959) 'The bases of social power', in D. Cartwright (ed.), *Studies in Social Power*. Ann Arbor, MI: University of Michigan Press.

Freudenberg, N. (1978) 'Shaping the future of health education: from behavior change to social change', *Health Education Monographs*, 6 (4): 372–7.

Freudenberg, N. (1981) 'Health education for social change: a strategy for public health in the US', *International Journal of Health Education*, 24 (3): 1–7.

Freudenberg, N. (1984) 'Training health educators for social change', *International Quarterly of Community Health Education*, 5 (1): 37–52.

Freudenberg, N. (2005) 'Public health advocacy to change corporate practices: implications for health education practice and research', *Health Education and Behavior*, 32: 298–319.

Friedli, L. (2013) 'What we've tried, hasn't worked: the politics of assets based public health 1', *Critical Public Health*, 23(2): 131–45.

Friedman, M. and Rosenman, R.H. (1974) *Type A Behavior and Your Heart*. New York: Knopf.

Fugelli, P. (2006) 'The zero-vision: potential side effects of communicating health perfection and zero risk', *Patient Education and Counselling*, 60: 267–71.

Fujita, N. (2010) *Beyond Logframe: Using Systems Concepts in Evaluation*. Japan: FASID.

Fukuyama, F. (1999) *Social Capital and Civil Society*. IMF Conference of Second Generation Reforms, Fairfax, VA: Institute of Public Policy, George Mason University. (*Website*: www.imf.org/external/pubs/ft/seminar/1999/reforms/fukuyama.htm).

Fulbright-Anderson, K., Kubisch, A.C. and Connell, J.P. (1998) *New Approaches to Evaluating Community Initiatives, Vol. 2: Theory, Measurement, and Analysis*. Washington, DC: Aspen Institute.

Gagne, R.M. (1985) *The Conditions of Learning and Theory of Instruction* (4th edn). New York: Holt Saunders.

Gagnon, M., Jacob, J.D. and Holmes, D. (2010) 'Governing through (in) security: a critical analysis of a fear-based public health campaign', *Critical Public Health, 20*: 245–56.

Galante, J., Friedrich, C., Dawson, A.F., Modrego-Alarcón, M., Gebbing, P., Delgado-Suárez, I., Gupta, R., Dean, L., Dalgleish, T., White, I.R. and Jones, P.B. (2021) 'Mindfulness-based programmes for mental health promotion in adults in nonclinical settings: a systematic review and meta-analysis of randomised controlled trials', *PLOS Medicine, 18*: e1003481.

Galbraith, J. (1973) *Economics and the Public Purpose*. New York: Mentor.

Gallie, W.B. (1955) 'Essentially contested concepts', *Proceedings of the Aristotelian Society, 56*: 167–98.

Garcia, L.B., Hernandez, K.E. and Mata, H. (2015) 'Professional development through policy advocacy: communicating and advocating for health and health equity', *Health Promotion Practice, 16* (2): 162–5.

Gardner, J. (2014) 'Ethical issues in public health promotion', *SAJBL, 7* (1): 30–3.

Gardner, L.A., Champion, K.E., Chapman, C., Newton, N.C., Slade, T., Smout, S. et al. (2023) 'Multiple lifestyle risk behaviours and hierarchical dimensions of psychopathology in 6640 Australian adolescents', *Australian & New Zealand Journal of Psychiatry, 57* (2): 241–51.

Garneau, A.B., Browne, A.J. and Varcoe, C. (2019) 'Understanding competing discourses as a basis for promoting equity in primary health care', *BMC Health Services Research, 19*. doi: 10.1186/s12913-019-4602-3

Garthwaite, K. and Bambra, C. (2017) '"How the other half live": Lay perspectives on health inequalities in an age of austerity', *Social Science & Medicine, 187*: 268–75.

Gatherer, A. and Møller, L. (2009) 'Social justice, public health and the vulnerable: health in prisons raises key public health issues', *Public Health, 123*: 407–9.

Gatherer, A., Møller, L. and Hayton, P. (2009) 'Achieving sustainable improvement in the health of women in prisons: the approach of the WHO Health in Prisons Project', in D.C. Hatton and A. Fisher (eds), *Women Prisoners and Health Justice*. Oxford: Radcliffe.

GDB 2019 *Risk Factor Collaborators* (2019) 'Global burden of 87 risk factors in 204 countries and territories, 1990-2019: a systematic analysis for the Global Burden of Disease Study 2019', *The Lancet, 369*: 1223–49.

Geekiyanage, D., Fernando, T. and Keraminiyage, K. (2020) 'Assessing the state of the art in community engagement for participatory decision-making in disaster risk-sensitive urban development', *International Journal of Disaster Risk Reduction, 51*: 101847.

Gerend, M.A. and Maner, J.K. (2011) 'Fear, anger, fruits, and veggies: interactive effects of emotion and message framing on health behaviour', *Health Psychology, 30* (4): 420–3.

Getachew-Smith, H., King, A.J. and Scherr, C.L. (2022) 'Process evaluation in health communication/media campaigns: A systematic review', *American Journal of Health Promotion, 36* (2). doi: 10.1177/08901171211052279

Ghaderi, A., Tabatabaei, S.M., Nedjatm S. Javadi, M. and Larijani, B. (2018) 'Explanatory definition of the concept of spiritual health: a qualitative study in Iran', *J Med Ethics Hist Med, 11*: 3. PMID: 30258553; PMCID: PMC6150917.

Gibson, M. (undated) 'How to avoid curriculum change', *personal communication*.

Giddens, A. (1991) *Modernity and Self Identity: Self and Society in the Late Modern Age*. Cambridge: Polity Press.

Giddens, A. and Sutton, P.W. (2021) *Sociology* (9th edn.). Cambridge: Polity.

Gilchrist, A. (2000) 'Community work in the UK – an overview', *Talking Point (Association of Community Workers), 191* (October–November): 1–4.

Gillies, P. (1998) 'Effectiveness of alliances and partnerships for health promotion', *Health Promotion International*, *13* (2): 99–120.

Ginn Daugherty, H. and Kammeyer, K.C.W. (1995) *An Introduction to Population* (2nd edn). New York: Guilford.

Glasgow Centre for Population Health (2011) *Asset-Based Approaches for Health Improvement: Redressing the Balance*. Briefing Paper Concept Series 9. Glasgow Centre for Population Health. (*Website*: www. gcph.co.uk/resilience_and_empowerment/asset_based_approaches/asset_based_approaches_for_health_ improvement).

Glasgow Centre for Population Health (2012) *Putting Asset-Based Approaches into Action: Identification, Mobilisation and Measurement of Assets*. Briefing Paper Concept Series 10. Glasgow Centre for Population Health.

Glasgow City Council (undated) *Commonwealth Games Health Impact Assessment Report*. Glasgow: Glasgow City Council.

Godfrey, C. (2001) 'Economic evaluation of health promotion', in I. Rootman, M. Goodstadt, B. Hyndman, D.V. McQueen, L. Potvin, J. Springett and E. Ziglio (eds), *Evaluation in Health Promotion: Principles and Perspectives*. Copenhagen: WHO.

Godin, G., Gagnon, H., Alary, M., Levy, J.J. and Otis, J. (2007) 'The degree of planning: an indicator of the potential success of health education programs', *Promotion & Education*, *14* (3): 138–42.

Gold, J., Aitken, C., Dixon, H., Gouillou, M., Spelman, T., Wakefield, M. and Hellard, M. (2011) 'A randomised controlled trial using mobile advertising to promote safer sex and sun safety to young people', *Health Education Research*, *26*: 782–94.

Golombok, S. (2015) *Modern Families: Parents and Children in New Family Forms*. Cambridge: Cambridge University Press.

González-Sanguino, C., Potts, L.C., Milenova, M. and Henderson, C. (2019) 'Time to Change's social marketing campaign for a new target population: results from 2017 to 2019', *BMC Psychiatry*, *19* (1): 417.

Goodman, R.M., Steckler, A. and Kegler, M.C. (1997) 'Mobilizing organizations for health enhancement: theories of organizational change', in K. Glanz, F.M. Lewis and B.K. Rimer (eds), *Health Behavior and Health Education: Theory, Research, and Practice* (2nd edn). San Francisco, CA: Jossey-Bass.

Goodyear, M. and Malhotra, N. (2007) *Sources of Routine Mortality and Morbidity Data, Including Primary Care Data, and How They Are Collected and Published at International, National, Regional and District Levels*. Buckinghamshire: PHAST, Department of Health. (*Website*: www.healthknowledge.org.uk/public-health-text-book/health-information/3b-sickness-health/collection-routine-ad-hoc-data).

Gordon, D. (1999) 'An alternative ten tips for staying healthy', in D. Raphael, 'The question of evidence in health promotion', *Health Promotion International*, *15* (4): 355–67.

Gordon, D., Mack, J., Lansley, S., Main, G., Nandy, S., Patsios, D. and Pomati, M. (2013) *The Impoverishment of the UK*. London: ESRC.

Gordon, R. (2013) 'Unlocking the potential of upstream social marketing', *European Journal of Marketing*, *47* (9): 1525–47.

Gostin, L.O. (2017) '2016: the year of the soda tax', *The Milbank Quarterly*, *95*: 19–23.

Gottlieb, N.H., Brink, S.G. and Levenson Gingis, P.L. (1993) 'Correlates of coalition effectiveness: the "Smoke Free Class of 2000" program', *Health Education Research*, *8* (3): 375–84.

Gough, I. (1992) 'What are human needs?', in J. Percy-Smith and I. Sanderson (eds), *Understanding Local Needs*. London: Institute for Public Policy Research.

Graham, I.D., Logan, J., Harrison, M.B., Straus, S.E., Tetroe, J., Caswell, W. and Robinson, N. (2006) 'Lost in knowledge translation: time for a map?', *Journal of Continuing Education in the Health Professions*, *26*: 13–24.

Granner, M.L. and Sharpe, P.A. (2004) 'Evaluating community characteristics and functioning: a summary of measurement tools', *Health Education Research*, *19* (5): 514–32.

Grazia Monaci, M., Scacchi, L., Posa, M. and Trentin, R. (2013) 'Peer pressure and alcohol consumption among university students: the moderating effect of emotional intelligence', *Bollettino di Psicologia Applicata*, *267*: 17–31.

Green, J. (2000) 'The role of theory in evidence-based health promotion practice: Editorial', *Health Education Research*, *15* (2): 125–9.

Green, J. (2008) 'Health education – the case for rehabilitation', *Critical Public Health*, *18* (4): 447–56.

Green, J. and South, J. (2006) *Evaluation*. Maidenhead: Open University Press.

Green, J. and Tones, K. (1999) 'Towards a secure evidence base for health promotion', *Journal of Public Health Medicine*, *21* (2): 133–9.

Green, J. and Tones, K. (2000) 'The health promoting school, general practice and the creative arts: an example of inter-sectoral collaboration', *Health Education*, *100* (3): 124–30.

Green, J., Ayrton, R., Woodall, J., Woodward, J., Newell, C., Cattan, M. and Cross, R. (2007) *Child Parent Interaction in Relation to Road Safety Education*. London: Department for Transport.

Green, L., Ashton, K., Azam, S., Dyakova, M., Clemens, T. and Bellis, M.A. (2021) 'Using health impact assessment (HIA) to understand the wider health and well-being implications of policy decisions: the COVID-19 "staying at home and social distancing policy" in Wales', *BMC Public Health*, *21*: 1456.

Green, L.W. (1996) 'Bringing people back to health', *Promotion & Education*, *III* (1): 23–6.

Green, L.W. and Kreuter, M.W. (1991) *Health Promotion Planning: An Educational and Environmental Approach*. Mountain View, CA: Mayfield.

Green, L.W. and Kreuter, M.W. (1999) *Health Promotion Planning: An Educational and Ecological Approach* (3rd edn). Mountain View, CA: Mayfield.

Green, L.W. and Kreuter, M.W. (2005) *Health Program Planning: An Educational and Ecological Approach* (4th edn). London: McGraw-Hill.

Green, L.W. and Lewis, F.M. (1986) *Measurement and Evaluation in Health Education and Health Promotion*. Palo Alto, CA: Mayfield.

Green, L.W., Glanz, K., Hochbaum, G.M., Kok, G., Kreuter, M.W., Lewis, F.M., Lorig, K., Morisky, D., Rimer, B.K. and Rosenstock, I.M. (1994) 'Can we build models on, or must we replace, the theories and models in health education?', *Health Education Research*, *9* (3): 397–404.

Green, L.W., Poland, B. and Rootman, I. (2000) 'The settings approach to health promotion', in B. Poland, L.W. Green and I. Rootman (eds), *Settings for Health Promotion: Linking Theory and Practice*. Thousand Oaks, CA: Sage.

Green, L.W., Simons-Morton, D.G. and Potvin, L. (1997) 'Education and life-style determinants of health and disease', in R. Detels, W.W. Holland, J. McEwen and G.S. Omenn (eds), *Oxford Textbook of Public Health, Vol. 1* (3rd edn). Oxford: Oxford University Press.

Greene, J.A., Choudhry, N.K., Kilabuk, E. and Shrank, W.H. (2011) 'Online social networking by patients with diabetes: a qualitative evaluation of communication with Facebook', *Journal of General Internal Medicine*, *26*: 287–92.

Greenwood, N., Amor, S., Boswell, J., Joliffe, D. and Middleton, B. (1999) *Scottish Needs Assessment Programme: Health Promotion in Prisons*. Glasgow: Office for Public Health in Scotland.

Gregg, R., Patel, A., Patel, S. and O'Connor, L. (2017) 'Public reaction to the UK government strategy on childhood obesity in England: a qualitative and quantitative summary of online reaction to media reports', *Health Policy*, *121* (4): 450–7.

Grier, S. and Bryant, C.A. (2005) 'Social marketing in public health', *Annual Review of Public Health*, *26*: 319–39.

Griffiths, J. and Dark, P. (2005) *Shaping the Future of Public Health: Promoting Health in the NHS*. Cardiff: Department of Health and Welsh Assembly Government.

Griffiths, J., Blair-Stevens, C. and Thorpe, A. (2008) *Social Marketing for Health and Specialised Health Promotion: Stronger Together – Weaker Apart: A Paper for Debate*. London: Shaping the Future of Health Promotion, Royal Society of Public Health, National Social Marketing Centre.

Griggs, S. and Howarth, D. (2018) 'The airports commission, the dilemmas of political leadership and the third runway at Heathrow airport', *The Political Quarterly*, *89*: 434–45.

Grimani, A., Aboagye, E. and Kwak, L. (2019) 'The effectiveness of workplace nutrition and physical activity interventions in improving productivity, work performance and workability: a systematic review', *BMC Public Health*, *19*: 1676.

Groene, O. (2006) *Implementing Health Promotion in Hospitals: Manual and Self- Assessment Forms*. Copenhagen: WHO Regional Office for Europe.

Groot, E. (2011) 'Use of evidence in WHO health promotion declarations: overview, critical analysis, and personal reflection', *Reflective Practice, 12*: 507–13.

Grossmeier, J., Fabius, R., Flynn, J.P., Noeldner, S.P., Fabius, D., Goetzel, R.Z. and Anderson, D.R. (2016) 'Linking workplace health promotion best practices and organizational financial performance: tracking market performance of companies with highest scores on the HERO scorecard', *Journal of Occupational and Environmental Medicine, 58* (1): 16–23.

Guan, M. and Monahan, J.L. (2017) 'Positive affect related to health and risk messaging', *Oxford Research Encyclopaedia of Communication*. doi: 10.1093/acrefore/9780190228613.013.268

Guba, E.G. and Lincoln, Y.S. (1989) *Fourth Generation Evaluation*. Newbury Park, CA: Sage.

Gugglberger, L. (2021) 'A brief overview of a wide framework – Health promoting schools: a curated collection', *Health Promotion International, 36*: 297–302.

Guli, V.M.E. and Geda, N.R. (2021) 'Maternal empowerment indicators predict health care seeking behavior during pregnancy: evidence from Ethiopian national data', *Journal of Human Ecology, 74* (1–3): 20–9.

Gundewar, A. and Chin, N.P. (2020) 'Social capital, gender, and health: an ethnographic analysis of women in a Mumbai slum', *Global Health Promotion, 27* (4): 42–9.

Guntzviller, L.M., King, A.J., Jensen, J.D. and Davis, L.A. (2017) 'Self-efficacy, health literacy, and nutrition and exercise behaviors in a low-income, Hispanic population', *Journal of Immigrant and Minority Health, 19* (2): 489–93.

Guttman, N. (2000) *Public Health Communication Interventions: Values and Ethical Dilemmas*. Thousand Oaks, CA: Sage.

Guttman, N. (2017) 'Ethical issues in health promotion and communication interventions', *Oxford Research Encyclopaedias: Communication*. doi: 10.1093/acrefore/9780190228613.013.118

Hagard, S. (2000) 'Benchmarking to promote better health', *Promotion & Education, 7* (2): 2–3.

Haglund, B., Weisbrod, R.R. and Bracht, N. (1990) 'Assessing the community: its services, needs, leadership, and readiness', in N. Bracht (ed.), *Health Promotion at the Community Level*. London: Sage.

Haglund, B.J.A., Jansson, B., Pettersson, B. and Tillgren, P. (1998) 'A quality assurance instrument for practitioners', in J.K. Davies and G. Macdonald (eds), *Quality, Evidence and Effectiveness in Health Promotion*. London: Routledge.

Haglund, B.J.A., Pettersson, B., Finer, B. and Tillgren, P. (1993) *The Sundsvall Handbook, 'We Can Do It!'*. Third International Conference on Health Promotion, Sundsvall, Sweden, 9–15 June.

Hagman, W., Andersson, D., Västfjäll, D. and Tinghög, G. (2015) 'Public views on policies involving nudges', *Review of Philosophy and Psychology, 6* (3): 439–53.

Haldane, V., Chuah, F.L.H., Srivastava, A., Singh, S.R., Koh, G.C.H., Seng, C.K. and Legido-Quigley, H. (2019) 'Community participation in health services development, implementation, and evaluation: a systematic review of empowerment, health, community, and process outcomes', *PLOS ONE, 14*: e0216112.

Hammerman, E.J., Aggalwal, A. and Poupis, L.M. (2021) 'Generalized self-efficacy and compliance with health behaviors related to COVID-19 in the US', *Psychology and Health*. doi: 10.1080/08870446.2021.1994969

Hammond, D., Fong, G.T., Borland, R., Cummings, K.M., McNeill, A. and Driezen, P. (2007) 'Text and graphic warnings on cigarette packages: findings from the ITC Four Country Survey', *American Journal of Preventive Medicine, 32* (3): 210–17.

Hancock, T. (1998) 'Caveat partner: reflections on partnership with the private sector', *Health Promotion International, 13* (3): 193–5.

Handy, C. (1993) *Understanding Organizations* (4th edn). Harmondsworth: Penguin.

Handyside, L., Warren, R., Devine, S. and Drovandi, A. (2021) 'Health needs assessment in a regional community pharmacy using the PRECEDE-PROCEED model', *Research in Social and Administrative Pharmacy, 17*: 1151–8.

Hanewinkel, R., Sargent, J.D., Poelen. E.A.P, Scholte, R., Florek, E., Sweeting, H., Hunt, K., Karlsdottir, S., Jonsson, S.H., Mathis, F., Faggiano, F. and Morgenstern, M. (2012) 'Alcohol consumption in movies and adolescent binge drinking in 6 European countries', *Pediatrics*, *129*: 709–20.

Hanley, T., Sefi, A., Grauberg, J., Prescott, J. and Etchebarne, A. (2021) 'A theory of change for web-based therapy and support services for children and young people: collaborative qualitative exploration', *JMIR Pediatrics and Parenting*, *4*: e23193.

Hanrieder, T. (2017) 'The public valuation of religion in global health governance: spiritual health and the faith factor', *Contemporary Politics*, *23* (1): 81–99.

Hanson, C., West, J., Beiger, B., Thackeray, R., Barnes, M. and McIntyre, E. (2011) 'Use and acceptance of social media among health educators', *American Journal of Health Education*, *42* (4): 197–204.

Harden, A. (2001) 'Peer-delivered health promotion for young people: a systematic review of different study designs', *Health Education Journal*, *60* (4): 339–53.

Harpham, T., Grant, E. and Thomas, E. (2002) 'Measuring social capital within health surveys: key issues', *Health Policy Planning*, *17* (1): 106–11.

Harris, A. and Harris, T. (1986) *Staying OK*. London: Pan.

Harrison, D., Wilson, R., Graham, A., Brown, K., Hesselgreaves, H. and Ciesielska, M. (2022) 'Making every contact count with seldom-heard groups? A qualitative evaluation of voluntary and community sector (VCS) implementation of a public health behaviour change programme in England', *Health & Social Care in the Community*, *30* (5): e3193–e206

Hart, J.T. (1971) 'The inverse care law', *Lancet, i*: 405–12.

Hastings, G. (2007) *Social Marketing: Why Should the Devil Have All the Best Tunes?* Oxford: Butterworth-Heinemann.

Hastings, G.B., Stead, M., Whitehead, M., Lowry, R., MacFadyen, L., McVey, D., Owen, L. and Tones, K. (1998) 'Using the media to tackle the health divide: future directions', *Social Marketing Quarterly*, *4* (3): 41–67.

Hattie, J. (1992) *Self Concept*. Hillsdale, NJ: Erlbaum.

Hawkins, B. and McCambridge, J. (2020) 'Policy windows and multiple streams: an analysis of alcohol pricing policy in England', *Policy & Politics*, *48*: 315–33.

Hayden, J. (2022) *Introduction to Health Behavior Theory* (4th edn). Burlington, MA: Jones and Bartlett Learning.

Health Communication Unit (2000) *Media Advocacy Workbook*. Toronto: Health Communication Unit.

Health Communication Unit (2001) *Logic Models Workbook Version 6.1*. Toronto: Health Communication Unit.

Health Education Authority (HEA) (1999a) *Art for Health: A Review of Good Practice in Community-Based Arts Projects and Interventions which Impact on Health and Well-Being: Report*. London: Health Development Agency.

Health Education Authority (HEA) (1999b) *Art for Health: A Review of Good Practice in Community-Based Arts Projects and Interventions which Impact on Health and Well-Being: Summary Bulletin*. London: Health Development Agency.

Heaver, R. (1992) 'Participatory rural appraisal: potential application in family planning, health and nutrition programmes', *RRA Notes Number 16: Special Issue on Applications for Health*: 13–21.

Helliwell, J.F., Layard, R., Sachs, J.D., De Neve, J., Aknin, L.B. and Wang, S. (2022) *Overview on Our Tenth Anniversary*. World Happiness Report. (*Website*: www.worldhappiness.report/ed/2022).

Henderson, J. (2010) 'Expert and lay knowledge: a sociological perspective', *Nutrition and Dietetics*, *67*: 4–5.

Henderson, P., Summer, S. and Raj, T. (2004) *Developing Healthier Communities*. London: Health Development Agency.

Hennink, M., Hutter, I. and Bailey, A. (2011) *Qualitative Research Methods*. London: Sage.

Herzlich, C. (1973) *Health and Illness*. London: Academic Press.

Hill-Dixon, A. (2019) 'Taking a community development approach to health', in C. Naylor (ed.), *Creating Healthy Places: Perspectives from NHS England's Healthy New Towns Programme*. London: The King's Fund.

Hillsdon, M. (2006) 'Motivational interviewing in health promotion', in W. MacDowall, C. Bonell and M. Davies, M. (eds), *Health Promotion Practice*. Maidenhead: Open University Press.

Hilton, D. (1988) 'Community-based or oriented: the vital difference', *Contact*, *106* (December): 1–4.

Hirst, P. (1969) 'The logic of the curriculum', *Journal of Curriculum Studies*, *1* (2): 142–58.

HM Government (2022) *Levelling up the United Kingdom*. London: Crown.

Hochbaum, G.M. (1958) *Public Participation in Medical Screening Programs: A Socio-Psychological Study*. Public Health Service Publication No. 572. Washington, DC: US Government Printing Office.

Hoernke, K., Djellouli, N., Andrews, L., Lewis-Jackson, S., Manby, L., Martin, S., Vanderslott, S. and Vindrola-Padros, C. (2021) 'Frontline healthcare workers' experiences with personal protective equipment during the COVID-19 pandemic in the UK: a rapid qualitative appraisal', *BMJ Open*, *11*: e046199.

Hogwood, B.W. and Gunn, L.A. (1984) *Policy Analysis for the Real World*. Oxford: Oxford University Press.

Hogwood, B.W. and Gunn, L.A. (1997) 'Why "perfect implementation" is unattainable', in M. Hill (ed.), *The Policy Process: A Reader*. London: Prentice Hall/Harvester Wheatsheaf.

Holloway, I. (1997) *Basic Concepts for Qualitative Research*. Oxford: Blackwell.

Holt, C.L., Clark, E.M., Kreuter, M.W. and Scharff, D.P. (2000) 'Does locus of control moderate the effects of tailored health education materials?', *Health Education Research*, *15* (4): 393–403.

Holt-White, E. (2019) *Public Opinion on the Determinants of, and Responsibility for, Health*. The Health Foundation. (*Website*: www.health.org.uk).

Home Office Community Cohesion Review Team (2001) *Community Cohesion*. London: Home Office.

Homer, C., Woodall, J., Freeman, C., South, J., Cooke, J., Holliday, J., Hartley, A. and Mullen, S. (2022) 'Changing the culture: a qualitative study exploring research capacity in local government', *BMC Public Health*, *22* (1341): 1–10.

Hopson, B. and Scally, M. (1980–2) *Lifeskills Teaching Programmes 1–5*. Leeds: Lifeskills Associates.

Hopson, B. and Scally, M. (1981) *Lifeskills Teaching*. Maidenhead: McGraw-Hill.

Horrobin, D.F. (1978) *Medical Hubris: A Reply to Ivan Illich*. Edinburgh: Churchill Livingstone.

Hospers, H.J., Kok, G.J. and Strecher, V.J. (1990) 'Attributions for previous failures and subsequent outcomes in a weight reduction program', *Health Education Quarterly*, *17*: 409–15.

Hovland, C.I., Janis, I.L. and Kelley, H.H. (1953) *Communication and Persuasion*. New Haven, CT: Yale University Press.

Hu, S.C. and Kuo, H.-W. (2016) 'The development and achievement of a healthy cities network in Taiwan: sharing leadership and partnership building', *Global Health Promotion*, 23 (Suppl): 8–17.

Hu, X., Wang, T., Huang, D., Wang, Y. and Li, Q. (2021) 'Impact of social class on health: the mediating role of health self-management', *PLOS ONE*, *16* (7). doi: 10.1371/journal.pone.0254692

Hubley, J. (2004) *Communicating Health: An Action Guide to Health Education and Health Promotion* (2nd edn). Oxford: Macmillan.

Hubley, J., Copeman, J. and Woodall, J. (2021) *Practical Health Promotion* (3rd edn). Cambridge: Polity.

Hughes, J. (1976) *Sociological Analysis: Methods of Discovery*. London: Nelson.

Hughner, R.S. and Kleine, S.S. (2004) 'Views of health in the lay sector: a compilation and review of how individuals think about health', *Health: An Interdisciplinary Journal for the Social Study of Health, Illness and Medicine*, *8*: 395–422.

Huitt, W. (1999) 'Conation as an important factor of mind', *Educational Psychology Interactive*. (*Website*: www.edpsycinteractive.org/topics/conation/conation.html).

Hummelbrunner, R. (2010) 'Beyond logframe: critique, variations and alternatives', in N. Fujita (ed.), *Beyond the Logframe: Using Systems Concepts in Evaluation*. Tokyo: Foundation for Advanced Studies on International Development.

Hunt, K., Brown, A., Eadie, D., McMeekin, N., Boyd, K., Bauld, L., Conaglen, P., Craig, P., Demou, E. and Leyland, A. (2022) 'Process and impact of implementing a smoke-free policy in prisons in Scotland: TIPs mixed-methods study', *Public Health Research*, *10*: 1–137.

Huter, K., Dubas-Jakóbczyk, K., Kocot, E., Kissimova-Skarbek, K. and Rothgang, H. (2018) 'Economic evaluation of health promotion interventions for older people: do applied economic studies meet the methodological challenges?', *Cost Effectiveness and Resource Allocation*, *16*: 14: 1–11.

Ige-Elegbede, J., Pilkington, P., Bird, E.L., Gray, S., Mindell, J.S., Chang, M., Stimpson, A., Gallagher, D. and Petrokofsky, C. (2021) 'Exploring the views of planners and public health practitioners on integrating health evidence into spatial planning in England: a mixed-methods study', *Journal of Public Health*, *43*: 664–72.

Ike, V. (2020) 'The impact of veto players on incremental and drastic policy making: Australia's carbon tax policy and its repeal', *Politics & Policy*, *48*: 232–64.

Illich, I. (1976) *The Limits to Medicine–Medical Nemesis: The Expropriation of Health*. Harmondsworth: Penguin.

Institute for Health Metrics and Evaluation (2013) *The Global Burden of Disease: Generating Evidence, Guiding Policy*. Seattle, WA: IHME.

International Institute for Global Health (2018) 'People, planet and participation: the Kuching statement on healthy, just and sustainable urban development', *Health Promotion International*, *33*: 149–51.

International Union for Health Education (1992) *Advocacy for Health*. Paris: International Union for Health Education.

International Union for Health Promotion and Education (IUPHE) (2016) *Core Competencies and Professional Standards for Health Promotion*. (*Website*: www.ukphr.org/wp-content/uploads/2017/02/Core_Competencies_ Standards_linkE.pdf).

Ioannidis, J.P.A. (2020) 'Coronavirus disease 2019: the harms of exaggerated information and non-evidence-based measures', *European Journal of Clinical Investigation*, *50*: e13222.

Ioannou, S. (2005) 'Health logic and health-related behaviours', *Critical Public Health*, *15*: 263–273.

Iriarte, L. and Musikanski, L. (2019) 'Bridging the gap between the sustainable development goals and happiness metrics', *International Journal of Community Well-Being*, *1* (2): 115–35.

Islam, S.N. and Winkel, J. (2017) *Climate Change and Social Inequality*. DESA Working Paper No. 152. New York: Department of Economic & Social Affairs.

Issel, L.M. (2009) *Health Program Planning and Evaluation: A Practical, Systematic Approach for Community Health*. Sudbury, MA: Jones & Bartlett Publishers.

Issel, L.M. (2014) *Health Program Planning and Evaluation: A Practical, Systematic Approach for Community Health* (3rd edn). Burlington, MA: Jones & Bartlett Learning.

Jaberi, A., Momennasab, M., Yektatalab, S., Ebadi, A. and Cheraghi, M.A. (2019) 'Spiritual health: a concept analysis', *Journal of Religion and Health*, *58* (5): 1537–60.

Jack, S.M., Brooks, S., Furgal, C.M. and Dobbins, M. (2010) 'Knowledge transfer and exchange processes for environmental health issues in Canadian aboriginal communities', *International Journal of Environmental Research and Public Health*, *7*: 651–74.

Jacobs-Lawson, J.M., Waddell, E.L. and Webb, A.K. (2011) 'Predictors of health locus of control in older adults', *Current Psychology*, *30*: 173–83.

Jacobson, L.D., Edwards, A.G.K., Granier, S.K. and Butler, C.C. (1997) 'Evidence-based medicine and general practice', *British Journal of General Practice*, *47*: 449–52.

James, S.L., Abate, D., Abate, K.H., Abay, S.M., Abbafati, C., Abbasi, N. et al. (2018) 'Global, regional, and national incidence, prevalence, and years lived with disability for 354 diseases and injuries for 195 countries and territories, 1990-2017: a systematic analysis for the Global Burden of Disease Study 2017', *The Lancet*, *392*: 1789–1859.

Janis, I.L. and Feshbach, S. (1953) 'Effects of fear-arousing communications', *Journal of Abnormal and Social Psychology*, *48* (1): 78–92.

Janis, I.L. and Mann, L. (1977) *Decision Making: A Psychological Analysis of Conflict, Choice, and Commitment*. New York: Free Press.

Jenkins, W.I. (1978) *Policy Analysis: A Political and Organisational Perspective*. London: Martin Robertson.

Jensen, B.B. (1991) *The Action Perspective in School Health Education*. Proceedings from Satellite Congress in Copenhagen, Research Centre for Environmental and Health Education, Copenhagen, 13–14 June 1991.

Jensen, B.B. (2000) 'Health knowledge and health education in the democratic health- promoting school', *Health Education*, *100* (4): 146–53.

Jensen, B.B. and Schnack, K. (1997) 'The action competence approach in environmental education', *Environmental Education Research*, *3* (2): 163–78.

Jochelson, K. (2005) *Nanny or Steward? The Role of Government in Public Health*. London: The King's Fund. (*Website*: www.kingsfund.org.uk/publications/nanny-or-steward).

John, P. (1998) *Analysing Public Policy*. London: Continuum.

Johns Hopkins Center for Communication Programs (undated) *'A' Frame for Advocacy*. Baltimore, MA: Johns Hopkins Bloomberg School of Public Health, Center for Communication Programs.

Johnson, A. and Baum, F. (2001) 'Health promoting hospitals: a typology of different organizational approaches to health promotion', *Health Promotion International*, *16*: 281–7.

Johnson, C.V., Bartgis, J., Worley, J.A., Hellman, C.M. and Burkhart, R. (2010) 'Urban Indian voices: a community-based participatory research health and needs assessment', *American Indian and Alaska Native Mental Health Research: The Journal of the National Center*, *17*: 49–70.

Johnson, J.L., Moser, L. and Garwood, C.L. (2013) 'Health literacy: a primer for pharmacists', *American Journal of Health-System Pharmacists*, *70*: 949–57.

Johnson, S., Van Hoye, A., Donaldson, A., Lemonnier, F., Rostan, F. and Vuillemin, A. (2020) 'Building health-promoting sports clubs: a participative concept mapping approach', *Public Health*, *188*: 8–17.

Jones, C. (2017) *Urban Deprivation and the Inner City*. London: Routledge.

Jones, L. and Sidell, M. (1997) *The Challenge of Promoting Health*. London: Macmillan.

Jordan, S., Töppich, J., Hamouda, O., von Rüden, U., Mensink, G.B. and Hölling, H. (2011) 'Monitoring and quality assurance of prevention and health promotion at the federal level', *Bundesgesundheitsblatt Gesundheitsforschung Gesundheitsschutz*, *54* (6): 745–51.

Joseph Rowntree Foundation (2008) *A Minimum Income Standard for Britain*. (*Website*: www.jrf.org.uk/book-shop/eBooks/2226-income-poverty-standards.pdf).

Joseph Rowntree Foundation (2022) *UK Poverty 2022: The Essential Guide to Understanding Poverty in the UK*. York: Joseph Rowntree Foundation.

Judge, K. (2000) 'Testing evaluation to the limits: the case of English Health Action Zones', *Journal of Health Services Research and Policy*, *5* (1): 3–5.

Judge, K. and Bauld, L. (2006) 'Learning from policy failure? Health action zones in England', *European Journal of Public Health*, *16* (4): 341–4.

Juneau, C.E., Jones, C.M., McQueen, D.V. and Potvin, L. (2011) 'Evidence-based health promotion: an emerging field', *Global Health Promotion*, *18*: 79–89.

Juneau, M. (2021) *Why Do the Japanese Have the Highest Life Expectancy in the World?* Montréal: Institut de Cardiologie de Montréal. (*Website*: www.observatoireprevention.org).

Kahneman, D. and Tversky, A. (1979) 'Prospect theory: an analysis of decisions under risk', *Econometrica*, *47*: 263–91.

Kanfer, F.H. and Karoly, P. (1972) 'Self-control: a behavioristic excursion into the lion's den', *Behavior Therapy*, *3*: 398–416.

Kannappan, S. and Shanmugam, K. (2019) 'Peer educators as change leaders – effectiveness of peer education process in creating awareness on reproductive health among women workers in textile industry', *Indian Journal of Community Medicine*, *44*: 252–5.

Kansiime, M.K., Tambo, J.A., Mugambi, I., Bundi, M., Kara, A. and Owuor, C. (2021) 'COVID-19 implications on household income and food security in Kenya and Uganda: findings from a rapid assessment', *World Development*, *137*: 105199.

Kaveh, M.H., Layeghiasl, M., Nazari, M., Ghahremani, L. and Karimi, M. (2021) 'What are the determinants of a workplace health promotion? Application of physical activity in the workplace (a qualitative study)', *Front Public Health*, *14* (8). doi: 10.3389/fpubh.2020.614631

Kashefi, E. and Mort, M. (2004) 'Grounded citizens' juries: a tool for health activism?', *Health Expectations*, *7*: 290–302.

Kasperson, J.X. and Kasperson, R.E. (2005) *The Social Contours of Risk*. London: Earthscan.

Kasperson, R.E. (1992) 'The social amplification of risk: progress in developing an integrative framework', in S. Kirimsky and D. Golding (eds), *Social Theories of Risk*. London: Praeger.

Kasperson, R.E., Renn, O., Slovic, P. and Brown, H.S. (1988) 'The social amplification of risk: a conceptual framework', *Risk Analysis, 8*: 177–87.

Katainen, A. (2006) 'Challenging the imperative of health: smoking and justifications of risk-taking', *Critical Public Health, 16*: 295–305.

Katz, E. and Lazarsfeld, P. (1955) *Personal Influence: The Part Played by People in the Flow of Mass Communication*. Glencoe, IL: Free Press.

Kawachi, I. (1997) 'Long live community', *American Prospect, 8* (35).

Kehl, K.A. and McCarty, K.N. (2012) 'Readability of hospice materials to prepare families for caregiving at the time of death', *Research in Nursing & Health, 35*: 242–9.

Keith, L.K. and Bracken, B.A. (1996) 'Self-concept instrumentation: a historical and evaluative review', in B.A. Bracken (ed.), *Handbook of Self-Concept: Developmental, Social and Clinical Considerations*. New York: Wiley.

Kelleher, D., Gabe, J. and Williams, G. (1994) 'Understanding medical dominance in the modern world', in J. Gabe, D. Kelleher and G. Williams (eds), *Challenging Medicine*. London: Routledge.

Kelly, M., Morgan, A., Ellis, S., Younger, T., Huntley, J. and Swann, C. (2010) 'Evidence-based public health: a review of the experience of the National Institute of Health and Clinical Excellence (NICE) of developing public health guidance in England', *Social Science and Medicine, 71*: 1056–62.

Kelly, M., Speller, V. and Meyrick, J. (2004) *Getting Evidence into Practice in Public Health*. London: Health Development Agency.

Kelly, M.P. and Barker, M. (2016) 'Why is changing health-related behaviour so difficult?', *Public Health, 136*: 109–16.

Kelly, M.P. and Charlton, B. (1995) 'The modern and the postmodern in health promotion', in R. Bunton, S. Nettleton and R. Burrows (eds), *The Sociology of Health Promotion*. London: Routledge.

Kemm, J.R. (1993) 'Towards an epidemiology of positive health', *Health Promotion International, 8* (2): 129–34.

Kemm, J. (2001) 'Health impact assessment: a tool for healthy public policy', *Health Promotion International, 16* (1): 79–85.

Kemm, J. (2007) *More than a Statement of the Crushingly Obvious: A Critical Guide to HIA*. West Midlands Public Health Observatory. (*Website*: http://webarchive.nationalarchives.gov.uk/20170106084411/http://www.apho.org.uk/resource/item.aspx?RID=44422).

Kemm, J. (2012a) 'Health impact assessment of policy', in J. Kemm, *Health Impact Assessment: Past Achievement, Current Understanding, and Future Progress*. Oxford: Oxford University Press.

Kemm, J. (2012b) 'Qualitative assessment: lay and civic knowledge', in J. Kemm, *Health Impact Assessment: Past Achievement, Current Understanding, and Future Progress*. Oxford: Oxford University Press.

Kerrison, S. and Macfarlane, A. (2000) *Official Health Statistics: An Unofficial Guide*. London: Arnold.

Khan, K.S. and Kleijnen, J. (2001) 'Phase 6: data extraction and monitoring progress', in *Undertaking Systematic Reviews of Research Effectiveness*. York: NHS Centre for Reviews and Dissemination.

Khomenko, S., Cirach, M., Pereira-Barboza, E., Mueller, N., Barrera-Gómez, J., Rojas-Rueda, D., de Hoogh, K., Hoek, G. and Nieuwenhuijsen, M. (2021) 'Premature mortality due to air pollution in European cities: a health impact assessment', *The Lancet Planetary Health, 5*: e121–e134.

Kickbusch, I. (1996) 'Tribute to Aaron Antonovsky – what creates health', *Health Promotion International, 11*: 5–6.

Kickbusch, I. (1997) '*Think health: what makes the difference?* Address at the Fourth International Conference on Health Promotion, 21–25 July, Jakarta, in E. Ziglio, S. Hagard, L. McMahon, S. Harvey and L. Levin, 'Principles methodology and practices of investment for health', Promotion & Education, 7 (2): 4–12.

Kickbusch, I. (1998) 'Health promotion in the 21st century: an era of partnerships to achieve health for all', Press Release, WHO/47. Geneva: WHO.

Kickbusch, I. (2007) 'The move towards a new public health', *Promotion & Education, Suppl 2*: 9.

Kickbusch, I. and Gleicher, D. (2012) *Governance for Health in the 21st Century*. Geneva: WHO.

Kidd, R. and Kumar, K. (1981) 'A critical analysis of pseudo-Freirean adult education', *Economic and Political Weekly*, 3–10 January: 27–36.

Kidder, J.L. (2022) 'Reconsidering edgework theory: practices, experiences and structures', *International Review for the Sociology of Sport, 57* (2): 183–200.

Kieffer, C. (1984) 'Citizen empowerment: a developmental perspective', in J. Rappaport, C. Swift and R. Hess (eds), *Empowerment: Steps Toward Understanding and Action*. New York: Haworth Press.

Kienzler, H. (2019) 'Mental health in all policies in contexts of war and conflict', *The Lancet Public Health, 4*: e547–e548.

Kim, C.R. and Free, C. (2008) 'Recent evaluations of the peer-led approach in adolescent sexual health education: a systematic review', *Perspectives on Sexual and Reproductive Health, 40*: 144–51.

Kim, S., Robbertz, A., Goodrum, N.M., Armisted, L.P., Cohen, L.L., Schulte, M.T. and Murphy, D.A. (2021) 'Maternal HIV stigma and child adjustment: qualitative and quantitative perspectives', *Journal of Child and Family Studies, 30* (10): 2402–12.

Kindervatter, S. (1979) *Non-Formal Education as an Empowering Process*. Amherst, MA: University of Massachusetts, Center for International Education.

King, G., Heaney, D.J., Boddy, D., O'Donnell, C.A., Clark, J.S. and Mair, F.S. (2011) 'Exploring public perspectives on e-health: findings from two citizen juries', *Health Expectations, 14*: 351–60.

King's Fund (2004) *Public Attitudes to Public Health Policy: Summary*. London: The King's Fund.

Kirklin, M.J. and Franzen, L.E. (1974) *Community Organization Bibliography*. Chicago, IL: Institute on the Church in Urban Industrial Society.

Kirscht, J.P. (1972) 'Perceptions of control and health beliefs', *Canadian Journal of Behavioral Science, 4*: 225–37.

Kitchen, P.J., Kerr, G., Schultz, D.E., McColl, R. and Pals, H. (2014) 'The elaboration likelihood model: review, critique and research agenda', *European Journal of Marketing, 48* (11/12): 2033–50.

Klapper, J.T. (1995) 'The effects of mass communication', in O. Boyd-Barrett and C. Newbold (eds), *Approaches to Media: A Reader*. London: Arnold.

Klocke, A. and Stadtmüller, S. (2019) 'Social capital in the health development of children', *Child Indicators Research, 12*: 1167–85.

Knowles, M.S., Holton, E.F., Swanson, R.A. and Robinson, P.A. (2020) *The Adult Learner: The Definitive Classic in Adult Education and Human Resource Development* (9th edn). Abingdon: Routledge.

Kobasa, S.C. (1979) 'Stressful life events, personality and health: an inquiry into hardiness', *Journal of Personality and Social Psychology, 37*: 1–11.

Kochuvilayil, T., Fernandez, R.S., Moxham, L.J., Lord, H., Alomari, A., Hunt, L., Middleton, R. and Halcombe, E.J. (2020) 'COVID-19: Knowledge, anxiety, academic concerns and preventative behaviours among Australian and Indian undergraduate nursing students: A cross-sectional study', *Journal of Clinical Nursing, 30*: 882–91.

Kocot, E., Kotarba, P. and Dubas-Jakóbczyk, K. (2021) 'The application of the QALY measure in the assessment of effects of health interventions on an older population: a systematic scoping review', *Archives of Public Health, 79*: 201. doi: 10.1186/s13690-021-00729-7

Kok, G., Den Broer, D.-J., de Vries, H., Gerards, F., Hospers, H.J. and Mudde, A.N. (1992) 'Self-efficacy and attribution theory in health education', in R. Schwarzer (ed.), *Self-Efficacy: Thought Control of Action*. Washington, DC: Hemisphere Publishing.

Kokko, S., Donaldson, A., Geidne, S., Seghers, J., Scheerder, J., Meganck, J., Lane, A., Kelly, B., Casey, M. and Eime, R. (2016) 'Piecing the puzzle together: case studies of international research in health-promoting sports clubs', *Global Health Promotion, 23* (Suppl): 75–84.

Kokko, S., Green, L.W. and Kannas, L. (2014) 'A review of settings-based health promotion with applications to sports clubs', *Health Promotion International, 29*: 494–509.

Kolb, D.A., Rubin, I.M. and McIntyre, J.M. (1971) *Organisational Psychology: An Experiential Approach*. London: Prentice-Hall.

Komduur, R.H., Korthals, M. and Molder, H. (2009) 'The good life: living for health and a life without risks? On a prominent script of nutrigenomics', *British Journal of Nutrition*, *101* (3): 307–16.

Korenik, D. and Węgrzyn, M. (2020) 'Public policy timing in a sustainable approach to shaping public policy', *Sustainability*, *12*: 2677.

Korp, P. (2008) 'The symbolic power of "healthy lifestyles"', *Health Sociology Review*, *1*: 18–26.

Kotler, P. and Zaltman, G. (1971) 'Social marketing and public health intervention', *Journal of Marketing*, *45* (2): 3–12.

Kotler, P., Roberto, N. and Lee, N. (2002) *Social Marketing: Improving the Quality of Life*. Thousand Oaks, CA: Sage.

Kreuter, M.W. and Skinner, C.S. (2000) 'Tailoring: what's in a name? Editorial', *Health Education Research*, *15* (1): 1–4.

Kreuter, M.W., Oswald, D.L., Bull, F.C. and Clark, E. (2000) 'Are tailored health education materials always more effective than non-tailored materials?', *Health Education Research*, *15* (3): 305–15.

Krieger, N. (1990) 'On becoming a public health professional: reflections on democracy, leadership, and accountability', *Journal of Public Health Policy*, *11*: 412–19.

Krieger, N. (2001) 'A glossary for social epidemiology', *Journal of Epidemiology and Community Health*, *55*: 693–700.

Krisberg, K. (2005) 'Anti-smoking campaign lowers youth smoking rates with "truth": funding threatened', *The Nation's Health*, *35* (3). (*Website*: www.medscape.com/viewarticle/502009).

Krisher, H.P., Darley, S.A. and Darley, J.M. (1973) 'Fear-provoking recommendations, intentions to take preventive actions, and actual preventive actions', *Journal of Personality and Social Psychology*, *26* (2): 301–18.

Kroeger, A. (1997) *The Use of Epidemiology in Local Health Planning: A Training Manual*. London: Zed Books.

Kubheka, B., Carter, V. and Mwaura, J. (2020) 'Social media health promotion in South Africa: opportunities and challenges', *African Journal of Primary Health Care & Family Medicine*, *12* (1): e1-e7.

Kulovesi, K. and Oberthür, S. (2020) 'Assessing the EU's 2030 climate and energy policy framework: incremental change toward radical transformation?', *Review of European, Comparative & International Environmental Law*, *29*: 151–66.

Laakso, M., Welling, P., Bukvova, H., Nyman, L., Björk, B.-C. and Hedlund, T. (2011) 'The development of open access journal publishing from 1993 to 2009', *PLOS ONE*, *6*: e20961.

Labonte, R. (1993) 'Community development and partnerships', in L. Jones and M. Sidell (eds), *The Challenge of Promoting Health*. London: Macmillan.

Labonte, R. and Laverack, G. (2001a) 'Capacity building for health promotion, Part 1: for whom? And for what purpose?', *Critical Public Health*, *11* (2): 112–27.

Labonte, R. and Laverack, G. (2001b) 'Capacity building in health promotion, Part 2: whose use? And with what measurement?', *Critical Public Health*, *11* (2): 129–38.

Lalonde, M. (1974) *A New Perspective on the Health of Canadians*. Ottawa: Ministry of National Health and Welfare..

Lane, A., Murphy, N., Donohoe, A. and Regan, C. (2017) 'Health promotion orientation of GAA sports clubs in Ireland', *Sport in Society*, *20* (2): 235–43.

Laplante-Lévesque, A., Brännström, Andersson, G. and Lunner, T. (2012) 'Quality and readability of English-language internet information for adults with hearing impairment and their significant others', *International Journal of Audiology*, *51*: 618–26.

Lardier, D.T., Jr, Bergeson, C., Bermea, A.M., Herr, K.G., Forenza, B., Garcia-Reid, P. and Reid, R.J. (2019) 'Community coalitions as spaces for collective voice, action, and the sharing of resources', *Journal of Community Psychology*, *47*: 21–33.

Larkey, L.K., Alatorre, C., Buller, D.B., Morrill, C., Klein Buller, M., Taren, D. and Sennott-Miller, L. (1999) 'Communication strategies for dietary change in a worksite peer educator intervention', *Health Education Research*, *14* (6): 777–90.

Lasswell, H.D. (1948) 'The structure and function of communication in society', in L. Bryson (ed.), *Communication of Ideas*. New York: Harper.

Last, J.M. (1963) 'The iceberg: completing the clinical picture in general practice', *Lancet*: 28–31; reprinted in J. Ashton (1994), *The Epidemiological Imagination*. Buckingham: Open University Press.

Latimer, A.E., Rench, T.A., Rivers, S.E., Katulak, N.A., Materese, S.A., Cadmus, L., Hicks, A., Hodorowski, J.K. and Salovey, P. (2008) 'Promoting participation in physical activity using framed messages: an application of prospect theory', *British Journal of Health Psychology*, *13*: 659–81.

Laverack, G. (2004) *Health Promotion Practice: Power and Empowerment*. London: Sage.

Laverack, G. (2006) 'Improving health outcomes through community empowerment: a review of the literature', *Journal of Health, Population and Nutrition*, *24*: 113–20.

Laverack, G. (2007) *Health Promotion Practice*. Maidenhead: Open University Press/McGraw Hill Education.

Laverack, G. (2009) *Public Health: Power, Empowerment and Professional Practice* (2nd edn). Basingstoke: Palgrave Macmillan.

Laverack, G. (2013) *Health Activism: Foundations and Strategies*. London: Sage.

Laverack, G. (2014) *A–Z of Health Promotion*. Basingstoke: Palgrave Macmillan.

Laverack, G. and Labonte, R. (2000) 'A planning framework for community empowerment goals within health promotion', *Health Policy and Planning*, *15* (3): 255–62.

Laverack, G. and Manoncourt, E. (2016) 'Key experiences of community engagement and social mobilization in the Ebola response', *Global Health Promotion*, *23* (1): 79–82.

Laverack, G. and Wallerstein, N. (2001) 'Measuring community empowerment: a fresh look at organizational domains', *Health Promotion International*, *16*: 179–85.

Lazarsfeld, P.F. and Merton, R.K. (1955) 'Mass communication, popular taste and organized social action', in W. Schramm (ed.), *Mass Communications*. Urbana, IL: University of Illinois Press.

Lazenbatt, A. and McMurray, F. (2004) 'Using participatory rapid appraisal as a tool to assess women's psycho-social health needs in Northern Ireland', *Health Education*, *104* (3): 174–87.

Le Gouais, A., Foley, L., Ogilvie, D. and Guell, C. (2019) 'Decision-making for active living infrastructure in new communities: a qualitative study in England', *Journal of Public Health*, *42*: e249–e258.

Leal, C.C., Branco-Illodo, I., Oliveira, B.M.N. and Esteban-Salvador, L. (2022) 'Nudging and choice architecture: perspectives and challenges', *Revista de Administração Contemparneá*, *26* (5). doi: 10.1590/1982-7849rac2022220098.en

Ledwith, M. (2007) 'Reclaiming the radical agenda: a critical approach to community development', *Concept*, *17* (2): 8–12.

Ledwith, M. (2020) *Community Development: A Critical Approach*. London: Policy Press.

Lee, B. (2019) *Violence: An Interdisciplinary Approach to Causes, Consequences and Cures*. Chichester: John Wiley & Sons. [Open Access – available online at: onlinelibrary.wiley.com/doi/book/10.10029781119240716].

Lefebvre, R.C. and Flora, J.A. (1988) 'Social marketing and public health intervention', *Health Education and Behavior*, *15* (3): 299–315.

Leichter, H.M. (1979) 'A comparative approach to policy analysis: healthcare policy in four nations', in G. Walt, *Health Policy: An Introduction to Process and Power*. London: Zed Books.

Leon, D.A., Walt, G. and Gilson, L. (2001) 'International perspectives on health inequalities and policy', *British Medical Journal*, *322*: 591–4.

Leppo, K., Ollila, E., Peña, S., Wismar, M. and Cook, S. (2013) *Health in All Policies: Seizing Opportunities, Implementing Policies*. Finland: Ministry of Social Affairs and Health.

LePrevost, C.E., Storm, J.F., Blanchard, M.R., Asuaje, C.R. and Cope, W.G. (2013) 'Engaging Latino farmworkers in the development of symbols to improve pesticide safety and health education and risk communication', *Journal of Immigrant Minority Health*, *15*: 975–81.

Lerer, L.B. (1999) 'How to do (or not to do) … health impact assessment', *Health Policy and Planning*, *14* (2): 198–203.

Lester, R.T., Ritco, P., Mills, E.J., Kariri, A., Karanja, S., Chung, M.H., Jack, W., Habyarimana, J., Sadatsafavi, M. and Najafzadeh, M. (2010) 'Effects of a mobile phone short message service on antiretroviral treatment adherence in Kenya (WelTel Kenya1): a randomised trial', *The Lancet, 376* (9755): 1838–45.

Leventhal, H. (1980) 'The common sense representation of illness danger', in S. Rachman (ed.), *Contribution to Medical Psychology, Vol. 2.* London: Pergamon.

Levin, L. and Ziglio, E. (1997) 'Health promotion as an investment strategy: a perspective for the 21st century', in M. Sidell, L. Jones, J. Katz and A. Peberdy (eds), *Debates and Dilemmas in Promoting Health.* London: Macmillan.

Lewin, R.W. (1951) *Field Theory in Social Science.* New York: Harper.

Lewis, F.M. (1987) 'The concept of control: a typology and health-related variables', *Advances in Health Education and Promotion, 2*: 277–309.

Lewis, J. (2001) 'Reflections on evaluation in practice', *Evaluation, 7* (3): 387–94.

LGpartnerships – Smarter Partnerships (undated) *Eight Tests of a Healthy Partnership.* (*Website*: www.lgpartnerships.com/howhealthy.asp).

Li, C. (2012) 'Persuasive messages on information system acceptance: a theoretical extension of elaboration likelihood model and social influence theory', *Computers in Human Behavior, 29*: 264–75.

Li, G., Wang, C., Song, B., Zhang, R., Zhang, D., He, X. and Cao, Y. (2021) 'Knowledge, attitudes, and practice patterns relating to female sexual health among obstetricians and gynecologists in China', *JAMA Network Open, 4* (5). doi: 10.1001/jamanetworkopen.2021.10695

Li, L., Guan, J., Liang, L, Lin, C. and Wu, Z. (2013) 'Popular opinion leader intervention for HIV stigma reduction in health care settings', *AIDS Education and Prevention, 25* (4): 327–35.

Li, V., Carter, S.M. and Rychetnik, L. (2015) 'Evidence valued and used by health promotion practitioners', *Health Education Research, 30* (2): 193–205.

Liamputtong, P. (2016) 'Qualitative research methodology and evidence-based practice in public health', in P. Liamputtong, *Public Health: Local and Global Perspectives.* Cambridge: Cambridge University Press.

Lichtenstein, S., Slovic, P., Fischoff, B., Layman, M. and Combs, B. (1978) 'Judged frequency of lethal events', *Journal of Experimental Psychology: Human Learning and Memory, 4* (6): 551–78.

Lincoln, Y.S. and Guba, E.G. (1985) *Naturalistic Inquiry.* Beverly Hills, CA: Sage.

Lindblom, C.E. (1979) 'Still muddling, not yet through', *Public Administration Review, 39*: 517–25.

Lindblom, C.E. and Woodhouse, E.J. (1993) *The Policy-Making Process* (3rd edn). Englewood Cliffs, NJ: Prentice Hall.

Lindquist, E.F. (1940) *Statistical Analysis in Educational Research.* New York: Houghton Mifflin.

Lindridge, A., MacAskill, S., Gnich, W., Eadie, D. and Holme, I. (2013) 'Applying an ecological model to social marketing communications', *European Journal of Marketing, 47* (9): 1399–420.

Linkenbach, J. and D'Atri, G. (1998) *The Montana Model.* Unpublished training manual for the Montana Social Norms Project.

Linnan, L.A. and Owens Ferguson, Y. (2007) 'Beauty salons: a promising health promotion setting for reaching and promoting health among African American women', *Health Education and Behavior, 34*: 517–30.

Linton, L. (2022) *STATIN To Roll Out National Population and Housing Census in April.* (*Website*: www.jis.gov.jm).

Lippmann, W. (1965) *Public Opinion.* New York: Free Press. (Originally published 1922.)

Lipsky, M. (1997) 'Street-level bureaucracy: an introduction', in M. Hill (ed.), *The Policy Process: A Reader* (2nd edn). Hemel Hempstead: Prentice-Hall/Harvester Wheatsheaf.

Liss, P.-E. (1990) *Health Care Need: Meaning and Measurement.* Linkoping Studies in Arts and Science 53. Linkoping: Linkoping University.

Litosseliti, L. (2006) *Gender and Language: Theory and Practice.* London: Hodder Arnold.

Liu, J., Schatzkin, E., Omoluabi, E., Fajemisin, M., Onuoha, C., Erinfolami, T., Ayodeji, K., Ogunmola, S., Shen, J., Diamond-Smith, N. and Sieverding, M. (2018) 'Introducing the subcutaneous depot medroxyprogesterone acetate injectable contraceptive via social marketing: lessons learned from Nigeria's private sector', *Contraception, 98* (5): 438–48.

Lo, A., King, B. and Mackenzie, M. (2020) 'Segmenting Chinese millennial restaurant customers: a lifestyle and health and environmental consciousness approach', *Journal of China Tourism Research*, *16* (2): 183–213.

Local Government Data Unit – Wales (2003) *Updating and Revising the Welsh Index of Multiple Deprivation*. (*Website*: https://gov.wales/statistics-and-research/welsh-index-multiple-deprivation-indicator-data/?lang=en).

Loch, M.R., Tanno de Souza, R.K., Mesas, A.E., Martinez-Gómez, D. and Rodríguez-Artalejo, F. (2015) 'Relationship between social capital indicators and lifestyle in Brazilian adults', *Cadernos de Saúde Pública*, *31* (8): 1636–47.

Lock, A. and Strong, T. (2010) *Social Constructionism: Sources and Stirrings in Theory and Practice*. Cambridge: Cambridge University Press.

London Health Economics Consortium (1996) *Local Health and the Vocal Community*. London: London Primary Health Care Forum.

London School of Economics (LSE) (2016) *Relationships and Good Health the Key to Happiness, not Income*. (*Website*: www.lse.ac.uk/website-archive/newsAndMedia/newsArchives/2016/12/Relationships-and-happiness. aspx).

Loney, M. (1981) 'The British community development projects: questioning the state', *Community Development Journal*, *16*: 55–67.

Loss, J., Lindacher, V. and Curbach, J. (2014) 'Online social networking sites – a novel setting for health promotion?', *Health & Place*, *26*: 161–70.

Ludbrook, A., Bird, S. and van Teijlingen, E. (2005) *International Review of the Health and Economic Impact of the Regulation of Smoking in Public Places: Summary Report*. Edinburgh: Health Scotland.

Lukes, S. (2021) *Power: A Radical View* (3rd edn). London: Red Globe Press.

Lupton, D. (1992) 'Discourse analysis: a new methodology for understanding the ideologies of health and illness', *Australian Journal of Public Health*, *16*: 145–50.

Lupton, D. (2006) 'Sociology and risk', in G. Mythen and S. Walklate (eds), *Beyond the Risk Society*. Maidenhead: Open University Press.

Lupton, D. (2012) Medicine as Culture: Illness, Disease and the Body (3rd edn). London: Sage.

Lupton, D. (2015) 'The pedagogy of disgust: the ethical, moral and political implications of using disgust in public health campaigns', *Critical Public Health*, *25* (1): 1–14.

Luque, J.S., Rivers, B.M., Gwede, C.K., Kambon, M., Green, B.L. and Meade, C.D. (2011) 'Barbershop communications on prostate cancer screening using barber health advisers', *American Journal of Men's Health*, *5*: 129–39.

Luque, J.S., Ross, L. and Gwede, C.K. (2014) 'Qualitative systematic review of barber-administered health education, promotion, screening and outreach programs in African-American communities', *Journal of Community Health*, *39* (1): 181–90.

Lustria, M.L.A., Noar, S., Cortese, J., Van Stee, S.K., Glueckauf, R.L. and Lee, J. (2013) 'A meta-analysis of web-delivered tailored health behavior change interventions', *Journal of Health Communication*, *18*: 1039–69.

Luthar, S. (ed.) (2003) *Resilience and Vulnerability*. Cambridge: Cambridge University Press.

Lutz, N., Taeymans, J., Ballmer, C., Verhaeghe, N., Clarys, P. and Deliens, T. (2019) 'Cost-effectiveness and cost-benefit of worksite health promotion programs in Europe: a systematic review', *European Journal of Public Health*, *29*: 540–6.

Lynch, E.A., Mudge, A., Knowles, S., Kitson, A.L., Hunter, S.C. and Harvey, G. (2018) '"There is nothing so practical as a good theory": a pragmatic guide for selecting theoretical approaches for implementation projects', *BMC Health Services Research*, *18*: 857.

Lynch, J., Davey Smith, G., Kaplan, G.A. and House, J.S. (2000) 'Income inequality and mortality: importance to health of individual income, psycho-social environment, or material conditions', *British Medical Journal*, *320*: 1200–4.

Lyng, S. (1990) 'Edgework: a social psychological analysis of voluntary risk-taking', *American Journal of Sociology*, *95* (4): 851–86.

Lyng, S. (2005) *Edgework: The Sociology of Risk-Taking*. New York: Routledge.

Lyons, A. and Heywood, W. (2016) 'Collective resilience as a protective factor for the mental health and well-being of HIV-positive gay men', *Psychology of Sexual Orientation and Gender Diversity*, 3 (4): 473–9.

Lyons, A., Fletcher, G. and Bariola, E. (2016) 'Assessing the well-being benefits of belonging to resilient groups and communities: development and testing of the Fletcher-Lyons Collective Resilience Scale (FLCRS)', *Group Dynamics*, 20: 65–77.

Ma, L.C., Chang, H.J., Liu, Y.M., Hsieh, H.L., Lo, L., Lin, M.Y. and Lu, K.C. (2013) 'The relationship between health-promoting behaviours and resilience in patients with chronic kidney disease', *Scientific World Journal*, *2013*: 124973.

Macdonald, G. and Bunton, R. (2002) 'Health promotion: discipline or disciplines?', in R. Bunton and G. Macdonald (eds), *Health Promotion: Disciplines and Diversity* (2nd edn). London: Routledge.

Macdonald, J.U. and Warren, W.G. (1991) 'Primary health care as an educational process: a model and a Freirean perspective', *International Quarterly of Community Health Education*, *12* (1): 35–50.

MacDonald, M.A. and Green, L.W. (2001) 'Reconciling concept and context: the dilemma of implementation in school-based health promotion', *Health Education and Behavior*, *28* (6): 749–68.

Macdonald, S. (2011) *An Exploration of Lay Epidemiology and Cancer*. PhD thesis, University of Glasgow, Glasgow. (*Website*: http://theses.gla.ac.uk/2583).

MacIntyre, S. and Pettigrew, M. (2000) 'Good intentions and received wisdom are not enough', *Journal of Epidemiology and Community Health*, *54*: 802–3.

Mackenbach, J. (1997) *Beyond the RCT? CIT! Report of the Expert Meeting Beyond the RCT – Towards Evidence-Based Public Health*. Rotterdam: GGD.

Macnab, A.J. and Mukisa, R. (2018) 'Celebrity endorsed music videos: innovation to foster youth health promotion', *Health Promotion International*, *34*: 716–25.

Mager, R.F. (1975) *Preparing Instructional Objectives*. Belmont, CA: Fearon.

Magura, S., Kang, S.Y. and Shapiro, J.L. (1994) 'Outcomes of intensive AIDS education for male adolescent drug users in jail', *Journal of Adolescent Health*, *15*: 457–63.

Mahdavi, A., Ahmadi, M., Nadermohamadi, M. and Adham, D. (2013) 'The relationship between mental health and self-esteem in students of medical sciences', *Health Med*, *7* (1): 150–63.

Manderson, L. and Aaby, P. (1992) 'An epidemic in the field? Rapid assessment procedures and health research', *Social Science and Medicine*, *35*: 839–50.

Mann, M., Hosman, C.M.H., Schaalma, H.P. and de Vries, N.K. (2004) 'Self-esteem in a broad-spectrum approach for mental health promotion', *Health Education Research*, *19* (4): 357–72.

Mantoura, P. and Potvin, L. (2013) 'A realist-constructionist perspective on participatory research in health promotion', *Health Promotion International*, *28*: 61–72.

Mappes, T.A. and Zembary, J.S. (1991) *Biomedical Ethics* (3rd edn). New York: McGraw Hill.

Marmot, M. (2005) 'Social determinants of health inequalities', *The Lancet*, *365*: 1099–104.

Marmot, M. (2006) 'Harveian Oration: health in an unequal world', *The Lancet*, *368*: 2081–94.

Marmot, M. (2010) *Fair Society, Healthy Lives. Executive Summary. The Marmot Review*. (*Website*: www.instituteofhealthequity.org/resources-reports/fair-society-healthy-lives-the-marmot-review).

Marmot, M., Allen, J., Boyce, T., Goldblatt, P. and Morrison, J. (2020) *Health Equity in England: The Marmot Review 10 Years on*. London: Institute of Health Equity.

Marmot Review Team (2011) *The Health Impacts of Cold Homes and Fuel Poverty*. London, Friends of the Earth & The Marmot Review Team.

Marrow, A.J. (1969) *The Practical Theorist: The Life and Work of Kurt Lewin*. New York: Basic Books.

Marsh, A. and Matheson, J. (1983) *Smoking Attitudes and Behaviour*. London: HMSO.

Marsh, D.R., Schroeder, D.G., Dearden, K.A., Sternin, J. and Sternin, M. (2004) 'The power of positive deviance', *British Medical Journal*, *329* (7475): 1177–9.

Marsh, J.M., Dobbs, T.D. and Hutchings, H.A. (2020) 'The readability of online health resources for phenylketonuria', *Journal of Community Genetics*, *11*: 451–9.

Marteau, T.M., Oglivie, D., Roland, M. and Suhrcke, M. (2011) 'Judging nudging: can nudging improve population health?', *British Medical Journal*, *342*: 263–5.

Martin, R.E., Murphy, K., Chan, R., Ramsden, V.R., Granger-Brown, A., Macaulay, A.C., Kahlon, R., Ogilvie, G. and Hislop, T.G. (2009) 'Primary health care: applying the principles within a community-based participatory health research project that began in a Canadian women's prison', *Global Health Promotion*, *16*: 43–53.

Martin, T.G., Burgman, M.A., Fidler, F., Kuhnert, P.M., Low Choy, S., McBride, M. and Mengersen, K. (2012) 'Eliciting expert knowledge in conservation science', *Conservation Biology*, *26* (1): 29–38.

Martin-Fernandez, J., Aromatario, O., Prigent, O., Porcherie, M., Ridde, V. and Cambon, L. (2021) 'Evaluation of a knowledge translation strategy to improve policymaking and practices in health promotion and disease prevention setting in French regions: TC-REG, a realist study', *BMJ Open*, *11*: e045936.

Maslow, A.H. (1954) *Motivation and Personality*. New York: Harper.

Maslow, A.H. (1970) *Motivation and Personality* (2nd edn). New York: Harper & Row.

Mason, P. and Barnes, M. (2007) 'Constructing theories of change: methods and sources', *Evaluation*, *13* (2): 151–70.

Matarasso, F. (2001) 'The health and social impact of participation in the arts', in T. Heller, R. Muston, M. Siddell and C. Lloyd (eds), *Working for Health*. London: Sage.

Mathers, J., Parry, J. and Wright, J. (2005) 'Participation in health impact assessment: objectives, methods and core values', *Bulletin of the World Health Organization*, *83* (1): 58–64.

May, T. (1993) *Social Research: Issues, Methods and Processes*. Buckingham: Open University Press.

McCartan, J. and Palermo, C. (2017) 'The role of a food policy coalition in influencing a local food environment: an Australian case study', *Public Health Nutrition*, *20* (5): 917–26.

McCubbin, M., Labonte, R. and Dallaire, B. (2001) *Advocacy for Healthy Public Policy as a Health Promotion Technology. Centre for Health Promotion* (online archives). (*Website*: http://sites.utoronto.ca/chp/download/2ndSymposium/McCubbin,%20Labonte,%20Dallaire.doc).

McGovern, R. and McGovern, W. (2011) 'Voluntary risk-taking and heavy-end crack cocaine use: an edgework perspective', *Health, Risk and Society*, *13*: 487–500.

McGuire, G. (1989) 'Theoretical foundations of campaigns', in R.E. Rice and C.K. Atkin (eds), *Public Communication Campaigns* (2nd edn). Newbury Park, CA: Sage.

McKeown, T. (1979) *The Role of Medicine: Dream, Mirage or Nemesis? Oxford*: Blackwell.

McKeown, T. and Lowe, C.R. (1974) *An Introduction to Social Medicine*. London: Blackwell.

McKinlay, J.B. (1975) 'A case for refocusing upstream: the political economy of illness', in A.J. Enelow and J.B. Henderson (eds), *Applying Behavioral Science to Cardiovascular Risk*. Washington, DC: American Heart Association.

McLennan, D., Noble, S., Noble, M., Plunkett, E., Wright, G. and Gutacker, N. (2019) *English Indices of Deprivation 2019: Technical Report*. London: Ministry of Housing, Communities and Local Government.

McLeroy, K. (1992) 'Editorial: health education research: theory and practice – future directions', *Health Education Research*, *7*: 1–8.

McLeroy, K.R., Bibeau, D., Steckler, A. and Glanz, K. (1988) 'An ecological perspective on health promotion programs', *Health Education Quarterly*, *15*: 351–77.

McLeroy, K., Steckler, A.B., Simons-Morton, B., Goodman, R.M., Gotlieb, N. and Burdine, J.N. (1993) 'Editorial: social science theory in health education: time for a new model', *Health Education Research*, *8* (3): 305–11.

McPhail, P., Ungoed-Thomas, J.R. and Chapman, H. (1972) 'Moral education in the secondary school', in J. Ryder and C. Campbell (eds), *Balancing Acts in Personal, Social and Health Education*. London: Routledge.

McPherson, K. (1994) 'The best and the enemy of the good: randomised controlled trials, uncertainty, and assessing the role of patient choice in medical decision making', *Journal of Epidemiology and Community Health*, *48*: 6–15.

McQuail, D. (ed.) (1972) *Sociology of Mass Communications*. Harmondsworth: Penguin.

McQuail, D. (2010) *Mass Communication Theory* (6th edn). London: Sage.

McQueen, D.V. (2007) 'Evidence and theory: continuing debates on evidence and effectiveness', in D.V. McQueen and C.M. Jones (eds), *Global Perspectives on Health Promotion Effectiveness*. New York: Springer.

Meherali, S., Punjani, N.S. and Mevawala, A. (2020) 'Health literacy interventions to improve health outcomes in low- and middle-income countries', *Health Literacy Research and Practice, 4* (4): e250–e266.

Mehmet, M., Roberts, R. and Nayeem, T. (2020) 'Using digital and social medica for health promotion: A social marketing approach for addressing co-morbid physical and mental health', *The Australian Journal of Rural Health, 28*: 149–58.

Mendelsohn, H. (1968) 'Which shall it be? Mass education or mass persuasion for health?', *American Journal of Public Health, 58*: 131–7.

Merigó, J.M. and Núñez, A. (2016) 'Influential journals in health research: a bibliometric study', *Globalization and Health, 12* (1): 46–58.

Michell, L. (1997) 'Loud, sad or bad: young people's perceptions of peer groups and smoking', *Health Education Research, 12* (1): 1–14.

Middleton, J., Reeves, E., Lilford, R., Howie, F. and Hyde, C. (2001) 'Collaboration with the Campbell Collaboration', *British Medical Journal, 323*: 1252.

Miilunpalo, S., Nupponen, R., Laitakari, J., Martila, J. and Paronen, O. (2000) 'Stages of change in two modes of health-enhancing physical activity: methodological aspects and promotional implications', *Health Education Research, 15* (4): 435–48.

Milburn, K. (1995) 'A critical review of peer education with young people with special reference to sexual health', *Health Education Research, 10* (4): 407–20.

Milio, N. (1981) *Promoting Health through Public Policy*. Philadelphia, PA: F.A. Davis.

Milio, N. (1988) 'Making healthy public policy: developing the science by learning the art: an ecological framework for policy studies', *Health Promotion, 2* (3): 263–74.

Milio, N. (2001) 'Glossary: healthy public policy', *Journal of Epidemiology and Community Health, 55*: 622–3.

Mill, J.S. (1961) *On Liberty, reprinted in Essential Works of John Stuart Mill*. New York: Bantam Books.

Miller, I. and Norman, W. (1979) 'Learned helplessness in humans: a review and attribution theory model', *Psychological Bulletin, 86*: 93–118.

Mills, C.W. (1959) *The Sociological Imagination*. New York: Oxford University Press.

Mimas (2001) *Health Survey for England*. Manchester: Mimas, University of Manchester.

Mindell, J., Hansell, A., Morrison, D., Douglas, M. and Joffe, M. (2001) 'What do we need for robust, quantitative health impact assessment?', *Journal of Public Health Medicine, 23* (3): 173–8.

Minkler, M. and Wallerstein, N. (1997) 'Improving health through community organization and community building', in K. Glanz, F.M. Lewis and B.K. Rimer (eds), *Health Behavior and Health Education: Theory, Research, and Practice* (2nd edn). San Francisco, CA: Jossey-Bass.

Minkler, M., Breckwich Vasquez, V., Rains Warner, J., Steusey, H. and Facente, S. (2006) 'Sowing the seeds for sustainable change: a community-based participatory research partnership for health promotion in Indiana, USA and its aftermath', *Health Promotion International, 21* (4): 293–300.

Mitchell Turner, M., Jang, Y. and Turner, S. (2021) 'Information-processing and cognitive theories', in T.L. Thompson and P.J. Schulz (eds.), *Health Communication Theory*. Hoboken, NJ: John Wiley & Sons.

Mitchinson, L., Dowrick, A., Buck, C., Hoernke, K., Martin, S., Vanderslott, S., Robinson, H., Rankl, F., Manby, L., Lewis-Jackson, S. and Vindrola-Padros, C. (2021) 'Missing the human connection: a rapid appraisal of healthcare workers' perceptions and experiences of providing palliative care during the COVID-19 pandemic', *Palliative Medicine, 35*: 852–61.

Mittelmark, M.B. (1999) 'Social ties and health promotion: suggestions for population-based research: Editorial', *Health Education Research, 14* (4): 447–51.

Mittelmark, M.B. (2001) 'Promoting social responsibility for health: health impact assessment and healthy public policy at the community level', *Health Promotion International, 16* (3): 269–74.

Mittelmark, M.B. and Bauer, G.F. (2022) 'Salutogenesis as a theory, as an orientation and as the sense of coherence', in M.B. Mittelmark, G.F. Bauer, L. Vaandrager, J.M. Pelikan, S. Sagy, M. Eriksson, B. Lindström and C.M. Magistretti (eds), *The Handbook of Salutogenesis* (2nd edn). Zurich, Springer.

Mittelmark, M.B. and Bull, T. (2013) 'The salutogenic model of health in health promotion research', *Global Health Promotion*, 20: 30–8.

Mittelmark, M.B., Bauer, G.F., Vaandrager, L., Pelikan, J.M., Sagy, S., Eriksson, M., Lindström, B. and Magistretti, C.M. (eds) (2022) *The Handbook of Salutogenesis* (2nd edn). Zurich: Springer.

Mogensen, F. (1997) 'Critical thinking: a central element in developing action competence in health and environmental education', *Health Education Research*, 12 (4): 429–36.

Molina-Betancur, J.C., Agudelo-Suárez, A.A. and Martínez-Herrera, E. (2021) 'Community health assets mapping in a slum in Medellin (Columbia)', *Gaceta Sanitaria*, 35 (4): 333–38.

Molleman, G.R.M., Ploeg, M.A., Hosman, C.M.H. and Peters, L.H.M. (2006) 'Preffi 2.0 – a quality assessment tool', *Promotion & Education*, 13 (1): 9–14.

Monahan, J.L. (1995) 'Using positive affect when designing health messages', in E. Maibach and R.L. Parrott (eds), *Designing Health Messages*. Thousand Oaks, CA: Sage.

Moon, G. and Gould, M. (2000) *Epidemiology: An Introduction*. Buckingham: Open University Press.

Mooney, G. and Leeder, S.R. (1997) 'Measuring health needs', in R. Detels, W.W. Holland, J. McEwen and G.S. Omenn (eds), *Oxford Textbook of Public Health, Vol. 3* (3rd edn). Oxford: Oxford University Press.

Moore, A. (2021) 'From education to empowerment: redesigning the role of students in college health promotion', *Journal of American College Health*. doi: 10.1080/07448481.2021.1920603

Morgan, A. (2006) 'Determinants of health', in M. Davies and W. Macdowall (eds), *Health Promotion Theory*. Maidenhead: Open University Press.

Morgan, A. and Ziglio, E. (2007) 'Revitalising the evidence base for public health: an assets model', *Promotion & Education*, 14: 17–23.

Morley, B., Niven, P., Dixon, H., Swanson, M., Szybiak, M., Shilton, T., Pratt, I.S., Slevin, T., Hill, D. and Wakefield, M. (2016) 'Population-based evaluation of the "LighterLife" health weight and lifestyle mass media campaign', *Health Education Research*, 31 (2): 121–35.

Morris, H., Larsen, J., Catterall, E., Moss, A.C. and Domborwski, U. (2020) 'Peer pressure and alcohol consumption in adults living in the UK: a systematic qualitative review', *BMC Public Health*, 20: 1014. doi: 10.1186/s12889-020-09060-2

Morris, S., Devlin, N. and Parkin, D. (2007) *Economic Analysis in Health Care*. Chichester: Wiley.

Morris, T. and Morris, P. (1963) *Pentonville: A Sociological Study of an English Prison*. London: Routledge.

Morton, K.L., Atkin, A.J., Corder, K., Suhrcke, M., Turner, D. and van Sluijs, E.M.F. (2017) 'Engaging stakeholders and target groups in prioritising a public health intervention: the Creating Active School Environments (CASE) online Delphi study', *BMJ Open*, 7. doi: 10.1136.bmjopen-2016-013340

Mosendz, P. and Randall, T. (2017) 'Trump hires three men for every woman'. (*Website*: www.bloomberg.com/news/articles/2017-03-09/trump-s-gender-gap-27-percent-of-appointees-are-women-so-far).

Mueller, J., Alie, C., Jonas, B., Brown, E. and Sherr, L. (2011) 'A quasi-experimental evaluation of a community-based art therapy intervention exploring the psychosocial health of children affected by HIV in South Africa', *Tropical Medicine and International Health*, 16 (1): 57–66.

Mulcahy, H. and Downey, J. (2021) *Community Profiling and Health Needs Assessment: A Practical Guide for Public Health Nurses*. Cork: UCC and NMPDU.

Munro, G. (2006) 'A decade of failure: self-regulation of alcohol advertising in Australia', *The Globe*, 3: 15–18.

Murphy, A., Chikovani, I., Uchaneishvili, M., Makhashvili, N. and Roberts, B. (2018) 'Barriers to mental health care utilization among internally displaced persons in the republic of Georgia: a rapid appraisal study', *BMC Health Services Research*, 18: 306.

Murphy, S. and Bennett, P. (2004) 'Health psychology and public health: theoretical possibilities', *Journal of Health Psychology*, 9: 13–27.

Murphy, S.T. and Zajonc, R.B. (1993) 'Affect, cognition, and awareness: affective priming with suboptimal and optimal stimulus', *Journal of Personality and Social Psychology, 64* (5): 723–39.

Murray, C.J.L., Vos, T., Lozano, R., Naghavi, M., Flaxman, A.D. et al. (2012) 'Disability-adjusted life years (DALYs) for 291 diseases and injuries in 21 regions, 1990–2010: a systematic analysis for the Global Burden of Disease Study 2010', *The Lancet, 380*: 2197–224.

Murray, S.A. (1999) 'Experiences with "rapid appraisal" in primary care: involving the public in assessing health needs, orienting staff, and education medical students', *British Medical Journal, 318*: 440–4.

Musa, A.S., Azmi, M.N.L. and Ismail, N.S. (2015) 'Exploring the uses and gratifications theory in the use of social media among the students of Mass Communication in Nigeria', *Malaysian Journal of Distance Education, 17* (2): 83–93.

Nabi, R.L. (2021) 'Theories of affective impact', in T.L. Thompson and P.J. Schulz (eds), *Health Communication Theory*. Hoboken, NJ: John Wiley & Sons.

Nabyonga-Orem, J., Dovlo, D., Kwamie, A., Nadege, A., Guangya, W. and Kirigia, J.M. (2016) 'Policy dialogue to improve health outcomes in low income countries: what are the issues and way forward?', *BMC Health Services Research, 16* (4): 217.

Naidoo, J. and Wills, J. (2000) *Health Promotion: Foundations for Practice*. London: Bailliere Tindall.

Naidoo, J. and Wills, J. (2016) *Foundations for Health Promotion* (4th edn). London: Elsevier.

Nair, Y. and Campbell, C. (2008) 'Building partnerships to support community-led HIV/AIDS management: a case study from rural South Africa', *African Journal of AIDS Research, 7* (1): 45–53.

Nam, V. (2013) *Population Census Topics Included in the 2011 Population and Housing Census for Jamaica*. New York: United Nations Secretariat, ESA/STAT/AC.277/6.

Nancholas, S. (1998) 'How to do (or not to do) … a logical framework', *Health Policy and Planning, 13* (2): 189–93.

National Assembly for Wales (1999) *Developing Health Impact Assessment in Wales*. Cardiff: National Assembly for Wales.

National Cancer Institute (1997) *Theory at a Glance: A Guide for Health Promotion Practice*. Bethesda, MD: National Cancer Institute.

National Cancer Institute (1998) *Making Health Communication Programs Work: A Planners Guide*. Bethesda, MD: Information Project Branch Office.

National Cancer Institute (2005) *Theory at a Glance: A Guide for Health Promotion Practice* (2nd edn). Bethesda: NCI. (*Website*: www.sbccimplementationkits.org/demandrmnch/wp-content/uploads/2014/02/Theory-at-a-Glance-A-Guide-For-Health-Promotion-Practice.pdf).

National Cancer Institute (2007) *Designing Print Materials: A Communication Guide for Breast Cancer Screening*. NIH Publications No. 07–6100. Bethesda: NCI.

National Cancer Institute (undated) *Making Health Communication Programs Work*. National Cancer Institute. (*Website*: www.cancer.gov/pinkbook).

National Institute for Health and Care Excellence (NICE) (2005) *Public Health Guidance Methods Manual version 1*. London: NICE.

National Institute for Health and Care Excellence (NICE) (2008) *Community Engagement to Improve Health. NICE Public Health Guidance 9*. London: NICE.

National Institute for Health and Care Research (NICE) (2022) *Health Information: Are You Getting Your Message Across?* doi: 10.3310/nihrevidence_51109

National Social Marketing Centre (2005) *Social Marketing Pocket Guide*. London: National Social Marketing Centre.

National Social Marketing Centre (2006) *It's Our Health*. London: National Social Marketing Centre.

National Social Marketing Centre (2007) *Big Pocket Guide to Social Marketing* (2nd edn). London: National Social Marketing Centre.

National Statistics (2007) *National Statistics Socio-economic Classification*. (*Website*: www.ons.gov.uk).

Navarro, V. (1976) 'The underdevelopment of health of working America: causes, consequences and possible solutions', *American Journal of Public Health*, 66: 538–47.

Nayak, M. (2019) *Ten Facts about Life Expectancy in the Central African Republic.* The Borgen Project. (*Website*: www.borgen.org).

Ndubuisi, N.E. (2021) 'Noncommunicable diseases prevention in low- and middle-income countries: An overview of health in all policies (HiAP)', *INQUIRY: The Journal of Health Care Organization, Provision, and Financing*, 58: 1–6.

Nelson, J.D., Moore, J.B., Blake, C., Morris, S.F. and Kolbe, M.B. (2013) 'Characteristics of successful community partnerships to promote physical activity among young people', *Preventing Chronic Disease*, 10. doi: 10.5888/pcd10.130110

Nettleton, S. (2020) *The Sociology of Health and Illness* (4th edn). Cambridge: Polity Press.

Nettleton, S. and Burrows, R. (1997) 'If health promotion is everybody's business what is the fate of the health promotion specialist?', *Sociology of Health & Illness*, 19 (1): 23–47.

Neumann, P.J. and Cohen, J.T. (2018) 'QALYs in 2018 – Advantages and concerns', *JAMA*. doi: 10.1001/jama.2018.6072

New Zealand Ministry of Health (2003) *A Guide to Developing Health Promotion Programmes in Primary Health Care Settings.* Wellington, New Zealand: Ministry of Health. (*Website*: www.hauora.co.nz/assets/files/PHO%20Info/dvpinghealthpromotionprogs.pdf).

Newburn, T. (2001) 'What do we mean by evaluation?', *Children and Society*, 15 (1): 5–13.

Newcastle Healthy City Project (1997) 'Taking a whole systems approach or why elephants matter', *Whole Systems Newsletter*, 2.

Newman, D.L. and Brown, R.B. (1996) *Applied Ethics for Program Evaluation.* Thousand Oaks, CA: Sage.

Newman, L., Baum, F., Javanparast, S., O'Rourke, K. and Carlon, L. (2015) 'Addressing social determinants of health inequities through settings: a rapid review', *Health Promotion International*, 30 (Suppl): ii126–ii143.

Newman, T., Curtis, K. and Stephens, J. (2001) *Do Community-Based Arts Projects Result in Social Gains? A Review of the Literature.* Barnados. (*Website*: www.barnardos.org.uk/commarts.pdf).

Ngu-yen, J.G., Nanayakkara, S. and Holden, A.C.L. (2020) 'Knowledge, attitudes and practice behaviour of midwives concerning periodontal health of pregnant patients', *International Journal of Environmental Research and Public Health*, 17. doi: 10.3390/ijerph17072246

NHS (2022) *Health Survey for England – Health, Social Care and Lifestyles.* (*Website*: www.digital.nhs.uk)

NHS Centre for Reviews and Dissemination (1999) 'Getting evidence into practice', *Effective Health Care*, 5 (1): 1–16.

NHS Centre for Reviews and Dissemination (2001) *Undertaking Systematic Reviews of Research Effectiveness.* CRD Report No. 4 (2nd edn). York: NHS Centre for Reviews and Dissemination.

NHS Centre for Reviews and Dissemination (2009) *Systematic Reviews: CRD's Guidance for Undertaking Reviews in Healthcare.* York: CRD. (*Website*: www.york.ac.uk/media/crd/Systematic_Reviews.pdf).

NHS Scotland (2019) *Understanding Needs.* NHS Scotland. (*Website*: www.healthscotland.scot/reducing-health-inequalities/understanding-needs).

Nicholson, C. (2007) 'Framing science: advances in theory and technology are fuelling a new era in the science of persuasion', *APS Observer*, 20 (1): 16–21.

Nickel, S. and von dem Knesebeck, O. (2020) 'Effectiveness of community-based health promotion interventions in urban areas: a systematic review', *Journal of Community Health*, 45: 419–34.

Niederdeppe, J., Farrelly, M.C. and Wenter, D. (2007) 'Media advocacy, tobacco control policy change and teen smoking in Florida', *Tobacco Control*, 16 (1): 47–52.

Nielsen, L., Sorenson, B.B., Donovan, R.J., Tjornhoj-Thomsen, T. and Koushede, V. (2017) 'Mental health is what makes life worth living': an exploration of lay people's understanding of mental health in Denmark', *International Journal of Mental Health Promotion*, 19 (1), 26–37.

Niemietz, K. (2011) *A New Understanding of Poverty: Poverty Measurement and Policy Implications.* London: Institute of Economic Affairs.

Nikku, N. (1997) *Informative Paternalism: Studies in the Ethics of Promoting and Predicting Health*. Linkoping: University of Linkoping.

Nishtar, S., Akerman, M., Amuyunzu-Nyamongo, M. Becker, D. Carroll, S. Goepel, E., Hills, M., Lamarre, M.-C., Mukhopadhyay, A., Perry, M. and Ritchie, J. (2006) 'The statement of the Global Consortium on Community Health Promotion', *Promotion & Education*, *13* (1): 7–8.

Niveau, G. (2007) 'Relevance and limits of the principle of "equivalence of care" in prison medicine', *Journal of Medical Ethics*, *33*: 610–13.

Noar, S.M. and Zimmerman, R.S. (2005) 'Health behaviour theory and cumulative knowledge regarding health behaviours: are we moving in the right direction?', *Health Education Research*, *20* (3): 275–90.

Noar, S.M., Benac, C.N. and Harris, M.S. (2007) 'Does tailoring matter? Meta-analytic review of tailored print health behaviour change interventions', *Pyschological Bulletin*, *133* (4): 673–93.

Noble, H. and Heale, R. (2019) 'Triangulation in research, with examples', *Evidence Based Nursing*, *22*: 67–8.

Nomura, Y., Matsuyama, T., Fukai, K., Okada, A., Ida, M., Yamauchi, N. et al. (2019) 'PRECEDE-PROCEED model based questionnaire and saliva tests for oral health check-up in adults', *Journal of Oral Science*, *61* (4): 544–8.

Norman, C.D. (2012) 'Social media and health promotion', *Global Health Promotion*, *19* (4): 3–6.

Norman, P. and Bennett, P. (1996) 'Health locus of control', in P. Conner and M. Norman (eds), *Predicting Health Behaviour*. Buckingham: Open University Press.

Novilla, M.L.B., Barnes, M.D., Natalie, G., Williams, P.N. and Rogers, J. (2006) 'Public health perspectives on the family: an ecological approach to promoting health in the family and community', *Family & Community Health*, *29* (1): 28–42.

Novillo-Ortiz, D. and Hernández-Pérez, T. (2017) 'Social media in public health: an analysis of national health authorities and leading causes of death in Spanish- speaking Latin American and Caribbean countries', *BMC Medical Informatics and Decision Making*, *17*: 16. doi: 10.1186/s12911-017-0411-y

Nuffield Council on Bioethics (2007) *Public Health: Ethical Issues*. (*Website*: nuffieldbioethics.org/assets/pdfs/ Public-health-ethical-issues.pdf).

Nunes, S., Fernandes, H., Fisher, J. and Fernandes, M.G. (2018) 'Psychometric properties of the Brazilian version of the lived experience component of the Spiritual Health and Life-Orientation Measure (SHALOM)', *Psicologia: Reflexão e Critica*, *31* (2). doi: 10.1186/s4115-018-0083-2

Nutbeam, D. (1996) 'Achieving "best practice" in health promotion: improving the fit between research and practice', *Health Education Research*, *11* (3): 317–26.

Nutbeam, D. (1998a) *Health Promotion Glossary*. Geneva: WHO.

Nutbeam, D. (1998b) 'Evaluating health promotion – progress, problems and solutions', *Health Promotion International*, *13* (1): 27–43.

Nutbeam, D. (1999) 'The challenge to provide "evidence" in health promotion', *Health Promotion International*, *14* (2): 99–101.

Nutbeam, D. (2000a) 'Health literacy as a public health goal: a challenge for contemporary health education and communication strategies into the 21st century', *Health Promotion International*, *15* (3): 259–67.

Nutbeam, D. (2000b) 'Health promotion effectiveness – the questions to be answered', in *The Evidence of Health Promotion Effectiveness: Shaping Public Health in a New Europe*. Paris: International Union for Health Promotion and Education (IUHPE).

Nutbeam, D. and Muscat, D.M. (2021) 'Health promotion glossary 2021', *Health Promotion International*, *36*: 1578–98.

Nutbeam, D., Harris, E. and Wise, M. (2010) *Theory in a Nutshell: A Practical Guide to Health Promotion Theories* (3rd edn). London: McGraw Hill.

Nutbeam, D., Smith, C., Murphy, S. and Catford, J. (1993) 'Maintaining evaluation designs in long-term community-based health promotion programmes', *Journal of Epidemiology and Public Health*, *47*: 127–33.

Nykiforuk, C.I. and Flaman, L.M. (2011) 'Geographic information systems (GIS) for health promotion and public health: a review', *Health Promotion Practice*, *12*: 63–73.

O'Brien, M.O. (1995) 'Health and lifestyle: a critical mess?', in R. Bunton, S. Nettleton and R. Burrows (eds), *The Sociology of Health Promotion*. London: Routledge.

Office of the Deputy Prime Minister (ODPM) and Department of Health (2005) *Creating Healthier Communities: A Resource Pack for Local Partnerships*. Wetherby: ODPM Publications.

Office of the High Commissioner for Human Rights (OHCHR) (1966) *International Covenant on Social, Economic and Cultural Rights*. Geneva: OHCHR. (*Website*: www.ohchr.org/en/professionalinterest/pages/cescr.aspx).

Office for National Statistics (ONS) (2005) *Summary of Main Topics Included in GHS Questionnaires: 1971–2005*. (*Website*: www.ons.gov.uk/ons/rel/ghs/general-household-survey/2005-report/rep-appendix-f.pdf).

Office for National Statistics (ONS) (2012) *2011 Census Coverage Survey Summary*. (*Website*: www.ons.gov.uk/ons/rel/ghs/general-household-survey/2005-report/rep-appendix-f.pdf).

Office for National Statistics (ONS) (2016) *Integrated Household Survey*. (*Website*: www.ons.gov.uk/peoplepopulationandcommunity/culturalidentity/sexuality/methodologies/integratedhouseholdsurvey).

Office for National Statistics (ONS) (2021) *Digital Take up of Census 2021 Beats Targets*. (*Website*: https://census.gov.uk/news/digital-take-up-of-census-2021-beats-targets).

O'Hara, L., Taylor, J. and Barnes, M. (2015) 'The extent to which the public health "war on obesity" reflects the ethical values and principles of critical health promotion: a multimedia critical discourse analysis', *Health Promotion Journal of Australia*, 26: 246–54.

Ojo, A. and Akinsola, E. (2012) 'Assessment of self-concept in Nigerian children using an indigenous children's self-concept scale', *IFE Psychology*, 20 (2): 46–55.

Oldenburg, B., Hardcastle, D.M. and Kok, G. (1997) 'Diffusion of innovations', in K. Glanz, F.M. Lewis and B.K. Rimer (eds), *Health Behavior and Health Education: Theory, Research, and Practice* (2nd edn). San Francisco, CA: Jossey-Bass.

Oleribe, O.O., Ukwedeh, O., Burstow, N.J., Gomaa, A.I., Sonderup, M.W., Cook, N., Waked, I., Spearman, W. and Taylor-Robinson, S.D. (2018) 'Health: redefined', *Pan African Medical Journal*, 30: 292. doi: 10.11604/pamj.2018.30.292.15436

O'Mara-Eves, A., Brunton, G., Oliver, S., Kavanagh, J., Jamal, F. and Thomas, J. (2015) 'The effectiveness of community engagement in public health interventions for disadvantaged groups: a meta-analysis', *BMC Public Health*, 15: 129. https://doi.org/10.1186/s12889-015-1352-y

O'Neill, A. (2022) *Infant Mortality in Japan 2009–2019*. (*Website*: www.statista.com/statistics/264717/countries-with-the-lowest-infant-mortality-rate/).

Onya, H. (2009) 'Health promotion capacity building in Africa: a call for action', *Global Health Promotion*, 16: 47–50.

Owusu-Addo, E., Cross, R. and Sarfo-Mensah, P. (2017) 'Evidence-based practice in local public health service in Ghana', *Critical Public Health*, 27 (1): 125–38.

Palmer, K.N.B., Rivers, P.S., Melton, F.L., McClelland, D.J., Hatcher, J., Marrero, D. G., Thomson, C.A. and Garcia, D.O. (2021) 'Health promotion interventions for African Americans delivered in U.S. barbershops and hair salons: a systematic review', *BMC Public Health*, 21: 1553.

Panter-Brick, C., Burgess, A., Eggerman, M., McAllister, F., Pruett, K. and Leckman, J.F. (2014) 'Engaging fathers – recommendations for a game change in parenting interventions based on a systematic review of the global evidence', *Journal of Child Psychology and Psychiatry*, 55 (11): 1187–212.

Parcel, G.S. and Meyer, M.P. (1978) 'Development of an instrument to measure children's health locus of control', *Health Education Monographs*, 6 (2): 149–59.

Parcel, G.S., Perry, C.L. and Taylor, W.C. (1990) 'Beyond demonstration: diffusion of health promotion innovations', in N. Bracht (ed.), *Health Promotion at the Community Level*. Newbury Park, CA: Sage.

Parker, E., Gould, T. and Fleming, M. (2007) 'Ethics in health promotion – reflections in practice', *Health Promotion Journal of Australia*, 18 (1): 69–72.

Parker, I. (2005) *Qualitative Psychology: Introducing Radical Research*. Maidenhead: Open University Press.

Parlett, M. and Hamilton, D. (1972) *Evaluation as Illumination: A New Approach to the Study of Innovatory Programmes*. Occasional Paper No. 9. Edinburgh: Centre for Research in the Educational Sciences, University of Edinburgh.

Parsons, T. (1958) 'Definitions of health and illness in the light of American values and social structure', in E. Jaco (ed.), *Patients, Physicians and Illness*. New York: Free Press.

Pasek, O., Michalska, J., Piechowicz, M., Stolinski, M. and Ganzcak, M. (2021) 'Effect of peer-education on the willingness to vaccinate against COVID-19 among high school students', *European Journal of Public Health, 31*: iii203. doi: 10.1093/eurpub/ckab164.536

Patrick, R., Armstrong, F., Hancock, T., Capon, A. and Smith, J.A. (2019) 'Climate change and health promotion in Australia: navigating political, policy, advocacy and research challenges', *Health Promotion Journal of Australia, 30*: 295–8.

Patton, M.Q. (1982) *Practical Evaluation*. Beverly Hills, CA: Sage.

Patton, M.Q. (1997) *Utilization Focused Evaluation*. Thousand Oaks, CA: Sage.

Pawson, R. (2002) 'Evidence-based policy: the promise of a "realist synthesis"', *Evaluation, 8* (3): 340–58.

Pawson, R. and Tilley, N. (1997) *Realistic Evaluation*. London: Sage.

Peker, A., Eroglu, Y. and Yildiz, M.N. (2021) 'Does high self-efficacy in adolescents minimize cyber bullying behaviour?', *Clinical and Experimental Health Sciences, 11*: 140–5.

Penţa, M.A. and Băban, A. (2018) 'Message framing in vaccine communication: a systematic review of published literature', *Health Communication, 33* (3): 299–314.

Percy-Smith, J. (2000) *Policy Responses to Social Exclusion: Towards Inclusion?* Buckingham: Open University Press.

Pérez, K., Olabarria, M., Rojas-Rueda, D., Santamariña-Rubio, E., Borrell, C. and Nieuwenhuijsen, M. (2017) 'The health and economic benefits of active transport policies in Barcelona', *Journal of Transport & Health, 4*: 316–24.

Performance and Innovation Unit (2002) *Social Capital: A Discussion Paper*. (*Website*: www.thinklocalactpersonal. org.uk/_assets/BCC/Social_Capital_PIU_Discussion_Paper.pdf).

Perkins, E.R., Simnett, I. and Wright, L. (1999) *Evidence-Based Health Promotion*. Chichester: John Wiley.

Perrett, S.E., Craddock, C., Dunseath, G., Shankar, G., Luzio, S. and Gray, B.J. (2022) 'Evaluating the impact of a prison smoking ban on the cardiovascular health of men in a UK prison', *International Journal of Prisoner Health*. doi: 10.1108/IJPH-02-2022-0012

Perth Charter for the Promotion of Mental Health and Wellbeing (2012) Coordinated by the Clifford Beers Foundation (UK) and Mentally Healthy (Western Australia). 3 December.

Peruga, A., López, M.J., Martinez, C. and Fernández, E. (2021) 'Tobacco control policies in the 21st century: achievements and open challenges', *Molecular Oncology, 15*: 744–52.

Petersen, A. and Lupton, D. (1996) *The New Public Health: Health and Self in the Age of Risk*. London: Sage.

Petersen, A., Davis, M., Fraser, F. and Lindsay, J. (2010) 'Healthy living and citizenship: an overview', *Critical Public Health, 20*: 391–400.

Petticrew, M. and Roberts, H. (2003) 'Evidence, hierarchies, and typologies: horses for courses', *Journal of Epidemiology and Community Health, 57*: 527–9.

Petticrew, M., Chalabi, Z. and Jones, D.R. (2012) 'To RCT or not to RCT: deciding when "more evidence is needed" for public health policy and practice', *Journal of Epidemiology and Community Health, 66*: 391–6.

Petty, R. and Cacioppo, J. (1986) 'The elaboration likelihood model of persuasion', in L. Berkowitz (ed.), *Advances in Experimental Social Psychology, Vol. 19*. Orlando, FL: Academic Press.

Pfau, M. (1995) 'Designing messages for behavioral inoculation', in E. Maibach and R.L. Parrott (eds), *Designing Health Messages*. Thousand Oaks, CA: Sage.

Pfau, M. and Van Bockern, S. (1994) 'The persistence of inoculation in conferring resistance to smoking initiation among adolescents: the second year', *Human Communication Research, 20*: 413–30.

Phi, G.T., Whitford, M. and Reid, S. (2018) 'What's in the black box? Evaluating anti-poverty tourism interventions utilizing theory of change', *Current Issues in Tourism, 21*: 1930–45.

Piaget, J. and Inhelder, B. (1969) *The Psychology of the Child*. London: Routledge & Kegan Paul.

Pidgeon, N., Kasperson, R.E. and Slovic, P. (2003) *The Social Amplification of Risk*. Cambridge: Cambridge University Press.

Plugge, E., Douglas, N. and Fitzpatrick, R. (2006) *The Health of Women in Prison*. Oxford: Department of Public Health, University of Oxford.

Poland, B. and Dooris, M. (2010) 'A green and healthy future: the settings approach to building health, equity and sustainability', *Critical Public Health, 20*: 281–98.

Poland, B., Green, L.W. and Rootman, I. (2000) 'Reflections on settings for health promotion', in B. Poland, L.W. Green and I. Rootman (eds), *Settings for Health Promotion: Linking Theory and Practice*. Thousand Oaks, CA: Sage.

Pollard, M.R. and Brennan, J.T. (1978) 'Disease prevention and health promotion initiatives: some legal considerations', *Health Education Monographs, 6* (2): 211–22.

Pop, O.M., Brînzainc, A., Sirlincan, E.O., Baba, C.O. and Chreches, R.M. (2013) 'Assessing health literacy in rural settings: a pilot study in rural areas of Cluj County, Romania', *Global Health Promotion, 20* (4): 35–43.

Popay, J. (2010) 'Community empowerment and health improvement: the English experience', in A. Morgan, M. Davies and E. Ziglio (eds), *Health Assets in a Global Context: Theory, Methods, Action*. New York: Springer.

Popay, J. (2021) 'Community empowerment and health equity', *Oxford Research Encyclopedias, Global Public Health*. doi: 10.1093/acrefore/9780190632366.013.1

Popham, W.J. (1978) 'Must all objectives be behavioural?', in D. Hamilton and M. Parlett (eds), *Beyond the Numbers Game*. London: Macmillan.

Popper, K. (1945) *The Open Society and its Enemies*. London: Routledge.

Popper, K. (1959) *The Logic of Scientific Discovery*. London: Hutchinson.

Porter, C. (2006) 'Ottawa to Bangkok: changing health promotion discourse', *Health Promotion International, 22* (1): 72–9.

Porter, C. (2016) 'Revisiting Precede-Proceed: a leading model for ecological and ethical health promotion', *Health Education Journal, 75* (6): 753–64.

Porter, E. and Coles, L. (2011) *Policy and Strategy for Improving Health and Wellbeing*. Exeter: Learning Matters.

Potvin, L. and McQueen, D. (2007) 'Modernity, public health and health promotion: a reflexive discourse', in D.V. McQueen and I. Kickbusch, *Health and Modernity: The Role of Theory in Health Promotion*. New York: Springer.

Pozo-Martin, F., Akazili, J., Der, R., Laar, A., Adler, A. J., Lamptey, P., Griffiths, U. K. and Vassall, A. (2021) 'Cost-effectiveness of a Community-based Hypertension Improvement Project (ComHIP) in Ghana: results from a modelling study', *BMJ Open, 11*: e039594.

Prashar, A., Abrahams, D., Taylor, D. and Scott-Samuel, A. (2004) *Merseytram Line 1: A Health Impact Assessment of the Proposed Scheme*. Liverpool: The International Health Impact Assessment Consortium. (*Website*: www.liverpool.ac.uk/media/livacuk/instituteofpsychology/researchgroups/impact/Merseytram_Line_1_HIA_-_Final.pdf).

Pressman, J. and Wildavsky, A. (1973) *Implementation: How Great Expectations in Washington are Dashed in Oakland*. Berkeley, CA: University of California Press.

Prestwich, A., Kenworthy, J. and Conner, M. (2017) *Health Behaviour Change: Theories, Methods and Interventions*. Abingdon: Routledge.

Preusting, L.C., Raadsen, M.P., Abourashed, A., Voeten, H.A.C.M., Wagener, M.N., de Wit, E. et al. (2021) 'COVID-19 related stigma and health-protective behaviours among adolescents in the Netherlands: an explorative study', *PLOS ONE, 16* (6). doi: 10.1371.journal.pone.0253342

Pringle, A., Zwolinsky, S., McKenna, J., Daly-Smith, A., Robertson, S. and White, A. (2013) 'Effect of a national programme of men's health delivered in English Premier League football clubs', *Public Health, 127* (1): 18–26.

Prochaska, J.O. and DiClemente, C.C. (1983) 'Stages and processes of self-change of smoking: toward an integrative model of change', *Journal of Consulting and Clinical Psychology, 51*: 390–5.

Prochaska, J.O. and DiClemente, C.C. (1984) *The Trans-theoretical Approach: Crossing Traditional Boundaries of Therapy*. Homewood, IL: Dow Jones Irwin.

Prochaska, J.O., Redding, C.A. and Evers, K.E. (1997) 'The transtheoretical model and stages of change', in K. Glanz, F.M. Lewis and B.K. Rimer (eds), *Health Behavior and Health Education: Theory, Research, and Practice* (2nd edn). San Francisco, CA: Jossey-Bass.

Pruger, R. and Specht, H. (1972) 'Assessing theoretical models of community organization practice: Alinsky as a case in point', in G. Zaltman, P. Kotler and I. Kaufman (eds), *Creating Social Change*. New York: Holt, Rinehart & Winston.

Public Health England (2015) *A Guide to Community-Centred Approaches for Health and Wellbeing*, London: Crown.

Public Health England (2016) *Public Health Skills and Knowledge Framework 2016*. London: Crown.

Public Health England (2018) *Health Matters: Community-Centred Approaches for Health and Wellbeing*. (*Website*: www.gov.uk/government/publications/health-matters-health-and-wellbeing-community-centred-approaches/health-matters-community-centred-approaches-for-health-and-wellbeing).

Puska, P. (2007) 'Health in all policies', *European Journal of Public Health*, *17* (4): 328.

Putnam, R.D. (1993) *Making Democracy Work: Civic Traditions in Modern Italy*. Princeton, NJ: Princeton University Press.

Putnam, R.D. (1995) 'Bowling alone: America's declining social capital', *Journal of Democracy*, *6* (1): 65–79.

Putnam, R.D. (1996) 'The strange disappearance of civic America', *The American Prospect*, *7* (24): 34–48.

Quick, B.L., Reynolds-Tylus, T., Gonzalez, A.M., Al-Ghaithi, S.H. and Mackert, M. (2021) 'Segmenting priority audiences employing individual difference variables to improve health promotion efforts', in T.L. Thompson and P.J. Schulz (eds), *Health Communication Theory*. Hoboken, NJ: John Wiley & Sons.

Quinn, S.C. (1999) 'Teaching community diagnosis: integrating community experience with meeting graduate standards for health educators', *Health Education Research*, *14* (5): 685–96.

Radius, S.M., Galer-Unti, R.A. and Tappe, M.K. (2009) 'Educating for advocacy: recommendations for professional preparation and development based on a needs and capacity assessment of health education faculty', *Health Promotion Practice*, *10* (1): 83–91.

Raeburn, J. and MacFarlane, S. (2003) 'Putting the public into public health: towards a more people-centred approach', in R. Beaglehole (ed.), *Global Public Health: A New Era*. Oxford: Oxford University Press.

Raeburn, J.M. and Rootman, I. (1989) 'Towards an expanded health field concept: conceptual and research issues in an era of health promotion', *Health Promotion*, *3* (4): 383–92.

Raeburn, J., Akerman, M., Chuengsatiansup, K., Mejia, F. and Oladepo, O. (2006) 'Community capacity building and health promotion in a globalized world', *Health Promotion International*, *21*: 84–90.

Rahman, M.A. (1995) 'Participatory development: toward liberation or co-optation', in G. Craig and M. Mayo (eds), *Community Empowerment*. London: Zed Books.

Rainey, R.C. and Harding, A.K. (2005) 'Acceptability of solar disinfection of drinking water treatment in Kathmandu Valley, Nepal', *International Journal of Environmental Health Research*, *15* (5): 361–72.

Rakow, L.F. (1989) 'Information and power: toward a critical theory of information campaigns', in C.T. Salmon (ed.), *Information Campaigns: Balancing Social Values and Social Change*. Newbury Park, CA: Sage.

Raleigh, V. (2021) *What is Happening to Life Expectancy in England?* London: The King's Fund. (*Website*: www.kingsfund.org.uk/publications/whats-happening-life-expectancy-england#:~:text=Compared%20with%20 2019%2C%20life%20expectancy,in%20the%20past%20two%20decades).

Ramaswamy, M. and Freudenberg, N.(2007) 'Health promotion in jails and prisons: an alternative paradigm for correctional health services', in R.B. Greifinger, J. Bick and J. Goldenson (eds), *Public Health Behind Bars: From Prisons to Communities*. New York: Springer.

Rana, I.A., Bhatti, S.S., Aslam, A.B., Jamshed, A., Ahmad, J. and Shah, A.A. (2021) 'COVID-19 risk perception and coping mechanisms: does gender make a difference?', *International Journal of Disaster Risk Reduction*. doi: 10.1016/j.ijdrr.2021.102096

Rangun, V.K., Karim, S. and Sandberg, S.K. (1996) 'Do better at doing good', *Harvard Business Review*, *74* (3): 42–54.

Rannamets, H. (2015) 'How movies influence our dietary behaviour', *Baltic Screen Media Review. 1*, 27–41.

Raphael, D. (2000) 'The question of evidence in health promotion', *Health Promotion International*, *15* (4): 355–67.

Raphael, D. (2001) *Inequality is Bad for Our Hearts: Why Low Income and Social Exclusion Are Major Causes of Heart Disease in Canada*. Toronto: North York Heart Health Network.

Rappaport, J. (1987) 'Terms of empowerment/exemplars of prevention: toward a policy for community psychology', *American Journal of Community Psychology*, *15* (2): 121–47.

Rashid, A.K. (2013) 'Efficacy of think tanks in influencing public policies: the case of Bangladesh', *Asian Journal of Political Science*, *21*: 62–79.

Rasmussen, S.R. (2013) 'The cost effectiveness of telephone counselling to aid smoking cessation in Denmark: a modelling study', *Scandinavian Journal of Public Health*, *41*: 4–10.

Ratzan, S.C. (2011) 'Our new "social" communication age in health', *Journal of Health Communication: International Perspectives*, *16* (8): 803–4.

Rawson, D. (1992) 'The growth of health promotion theory and its rational reconstruction', in R. Bunton and G. Macdonald (eds), *Health Promotion: Disciplines and Diversity*. London: Routledge.

Reardon, K.K. (1981) *Persuasion: Theory and Context*. Beverley Hills, CA: Sage.

Reason, P. and Rowan, J. (eds) (1981) *Human Enquiry: A Sourcebook of New Paradigm Research*. Chichester: Wiley.

Reed Johnson, F. (2009) 'Editorial: moving the QALY forward or just stuck in traffic?', *Value in Health*, *12* (Suppl 1): S38–S39.

Reich, M.R. (2002) *The Politics of Reforming Health Policies*. 5th European Conference on Effectiveness and Quality of Health Promotion, London, 11–13 June.

Reilly, T., Crawford, G., Lobo, R., Leavy, J. and Jancey, J. (2016) 'Ethics and health promotion practice: exploring attitudes and practices in Western Australian health organisations', *Health Promotion Journal of Australia*, *27* (1): 54–60.

Rencken, C.A., Harrison, A.D., Mtukushe, B., Bergam, S., Pather, A., Sher, R. et al. (2021) '"Those people motivate and inspire me to take my treatment." Peer support for adolescents living with HIV in Cape Town, South Africa', *Journal of the International Association of Providers of AIDS Care*, *20*: 1–9.

Rhodes, A. (1976) *Propaganda: The Art of Persuasion, World War II*. London: Angus & Robertson.

Ribera-Almandoz, O. and Clua-Losada, M. (2021) 'Health movements in the age of austerity: rescaling resistance in Spain and the United Kingdom', *Critical Public Health*, *31*: 182–92.

Rifkin, S. (1992) 'Rapid appraisals for health: an overview', *RRA Notes Number 16: Special Issue on Applications for Health*: 7–12.

Rippon, S. and South, J. (2017) *Promoting Asset Based Approaches for Health and Wellbeing: Exploring a Theory of Change and Challenges in Evaluation*. Leeds: Aligned Consultancy & Leeds Beckett University.

Risk, A. and Dzenowagis, J. (2001) 'Review of internet health information quality initiatives', *Journal of Medical Internet Research*, *3* (4): e28. doi: 10.2196/jmir.3.4.e28

Ritchie, D., Van den Broucke, S. and Van Hal, G. (2021) 'The health belief model and theory of planned behavior applied to mammography screening: a systematic review and meta-analysis', *Public Health Nursing*, *38*: 482–92.

Ritchie, J.E. (2007) 'Criteria and checkpoints for better community health promotion', *Promotion & Education*, *14* (2): 96–7.

Ritter, A. and McLauchlan, L. (2022) 'Citizens' juries and their role in improved alcohol policy: damp squib, or useful tool?', *Drugs: Education, Prevention and Policy*. doi: 10.1080/09687637.2022.2050185.

Robertson, S., Woodall, J., Henry, H., Hanna, E., Rowlands, S., Horrocks, J., Livesley, J. and Long, T. (2016) 'Evaluating a community-led project for improving fathers' and children's wellbeing in England', *Health Promotion International*, *33* (3): 410–21

Robson, C. (1993) *Real World Research*. Oxford: Blackwell.

Rodgers, J., Valuev, A.V., Hswen, Y. and Subramanian, S.V. (2019) 'Social capital and physical health: an updated review of the literature for 2007–2018', *Social Science & Medicine, 236*. doi: 10.1016/j.socscimed.2019.112360

Rogers, C. (1967) 'The interpersonal relationship in the facilitation of learning', in H. Kirschenbaum and V.L. Henderson (eds), *The Carl Rogers Reader* (1990 edn). London: Constable.

Rogers, C. (1983) 'Freedom to learn for the eighties', in J. Ryder and L. Campbell, *Balancing Acts in Personal, Social and Health Education: A Practical Guide for Teachers*. London: Routledge.

Rogers, E.M. (1995) *The Diffusion of Innovations* (4th edn). New York: Free Press.

Rogers, E.M. (2003) *Diffusion of Innovation Theory* (5th edn). New York: Free Press.

Rogers, E.M. (2010) *Diffusion of Innovations* (4th edn). New York: Free Press.

Rogers, E.M. and Shoemaker, F.F. (1971) *Communication of Innovations*. New York: Free Press.

Rojatz, D., Merchant, A. and Nitsch, M. (2016) 'Factors influencing workplace health promotion intervention: a qualitative systematic review', *Health Promotion International, 32* (5): 831–9.

Rokeach, M. (1973) *The Nature of Human Values*. New York: Free Press.

Rolfe, D.E., Ramsden, V.R., Banner, D. and Graham, I.D. (2018) 'Using qualitative health research methods to improve patient and public involvement and engagement in research', *Research Involvement and Engagement, 4*: 49. https://doi.org/10.1186/s40900-018-0129-8

Rollnick, S., Heather, N. and Bell, A. (1992) 'Negotiating behavior change in medical settings: the development of brief motivational interviewing', *Journal of Mental Health, 1*: 25–37.

Room, R. (2011) 'Addiction and personal responsibility as solutions to the contradictions of neoliberal consumerism', *Critical Public Health, 21*: 141–51.

Rose, G. (1992) *The Strategy of Preventive Medicine*. Oxford: Oxford Medical Publications.

Rosenstock, I.M. (1966) 'Why people use health services', *Milbank Memorial Fund Quarterly, 44*: 94–124.

Rosenstock, I.M. (1974) 'Historical origins of the health belief model', *Health Education Monographs, 2*: 1–8.

Ross, H.S. and Mico, P.R. (1980) *Theory and Practice in Health Education*. Palo Alto, CA: Mayfield.

Ross, M. (2013) *Health and Health Promotion in Prisons*. Abingdon: Routledge.

Rothman, A.J. and Salovey, P. (1997) 'Shaping perceptions to motivate healthy behavior: the role of message framing', *Psychological Bulletin, 121*: 3–19.

Rothman, J. (1979) 'Three models of community organization in practice', in F.M. Cox, J.L. Erlich, J. Rothman and J.E. Tropman (eds), *Strategies of Community Organization: A Book of Readings* (3rd edn). Itasca, IL: Peacock.

Rotter, J.B. (1966) 'Generalized expectancies for internal versus external control of reinforcement', *Psychological Monographs, 80* (1): 1–28.

Royle, J. and Speller, V. (1996) '*Assuring quality in health promotion*'. Paper presented at '*Quality Assessment in Health Promotion and Education*', Third European Conference on Effectiveness, September 1996, Turin, Italy; in V. Speller, L. Rogers and A. Rushmere, 'Quality assessment in health promotion settings', in J.K. Davies and G. Macdonald (eds), *Quality Evidence and Effectiveness in Health Promotion*. London: Routledge.

Ruggeri, K., Garcia-Garzon, E., Maguire, Á., Matz, S. and Huppert, F.A. (2020) 'Well-being is more than happiness and life satisfaction: a multidimensional analysis of 21 countries', *Health and Quality of Life Outcomes, 18* (192). doi: 10.1186/s12955-020-01423-y

Ruiter, R.A., Kessels, L.T., Peters, G.-J.Y. and Kok, G. (2014) 'Sixty years of fear appeal research: current state of the evidence', *International Journal of Psychology, 49*: 63–70.

Russell, L. and Moss, D. (2013) 'A meta-study of qualitative research into the experience of "symptoms" and "having a diagnosis" for people who have been given a diagnosis of bipolar disorder', *Europe's Journal of Psychology, 9* (3): 643–63.

Rutten, L.J.F., Blake, K.D., Greenberg-Worisek, A.J., Allen, S.V., Moser, R.P. and Hesse, B.W. (2019) 'Online health information seeking among US adults: measuring progress toward a Healthy People 2020 objective', *Public Health Reports, 134* (6): 617–25.

Ryan, W. (1976) *Blaming the Victim*. New York: Vintage Books.

Rychetnik, L., Hawe, P., Waters, E., Barratt, A. and Frommer, M. (2004) 'A glossary for evidence based public health', *Journal of Epidemiology and Community Health*, *58*: 538–45.

Ryder, J. and Campbell, L. (1988) *Balancing Acts in Personal, Social and Health Education: A Practical Guide for Teachers*. London: Routledge.

Sackett, D.L., Rosenberg, W.M.C., Gray, J.A.M., Haynes, R.B. and Richardson, W.S. (1996) 'Evidence-based medicine: what it is and what it isn't', *British Medical Journal*, *312*: 71–2.

Salomon, J.A., Wang, H., Freeman, M.K., Vos, T., Flaxman, A.D., Lopez, A.D. and Murray, C.J. (2012) 'Healthy life expectancy for 187 countries, 1990–2010: a systematic analysis for the Global Burden Disease Study 2010', *The Lancet*, *380* (9859): 2144–62.

Samuels, S. and Dale, S.K. (2022) 'Self-esteem, adverse life events, and mental health diagnoses among Black women living with HIV', *Ethnicity & Health*. doi: 10/1080/13557858.2022.2035690

Sarafino, E.P. and Smith, T.W. (2021) *Health Psychology: Biopsychosocial Interactions* (10th edn). San Francisco, CA: Wiley.

Sarbin, T.R. and Allen, V.L. (1968) 'Role theory', in G. Lindzey and E. Aronson (eds), *Handbook of Social Psychology, Vol. 1*. Reading, MA: Addison-Wesley.

Sardu, C., Mereu, A., Sotgiu, A. and Contu, P. (2012) 'A bottom-up art event gave birth to a process of community empowerment in an Italian village.' *Global Health Promotion*, *19*: 5–13.

Sarmiento, J.P. (2017) 'Healthy universities: mapping health-promotion interventions', *Health Education*, *117*: 162–75.

SAS (2008) *Return to Offender. Surfers Against Sewage*. (*Website*: www.sas.org.uk/campaign/return-to-offender).

Savage, M., Devine, F., Cunningham, N., Taylor, M., Li, Y., Hjellbrekke, J., Le Roux, B., Friedman, S. and Miles, A. (2013) 'A new model of social class? Findings from the BBC's *Great British Class Survey Experiment*', *Sociology*, *47*: 219–50.

Scala, K. (1996) *Health Promotion as Intervention in Social Settings*. Late European Summer School: Stratechniques for Health Promotion, Zeist, Netherlands, NIGZ, 6–11 October.

Scally, G. (2017) 'Whose behaviour needs to change? Key factors in an effective response to the burden of non-communicable disease', *Social Business*, *7* (3-4): 279–91.

Scally, G. (2021) 'England's new Office for Health Improvement and Disparities', *BMJ*, *374*: n2323. doi: 10.1136/bmj.n2323

Schillinger, D., Chittamuru, D. and Ramírez, S. (2020) 'From "infodemics" to health promotion: a novel framework for the role of social media in public health', *American Journal of Public Health*, *110* (9): 1393–6.

Schmidtke, D.J., Kubachi, K. and Rundle-Thiele, S. (2021) 'A review of social marketing interventions in low- and middle-income countries (2010–2019)', *Journal of Social Marketing*, *11* (3): 240–58.

Schnack, K. (2000) 'Action competence as a curriculum perspective', in B.B. Jensen, K. Schnack and V. Simovska (eds), *Critical Environmental and Health Education: Research Issues and Challenges*. Copenhagen: Danish University of Education.

Schwandt, T.A. (1994) 'Constructivist, interpretivist approaches to human inquiry', in N.K. Denzin and Y.S. Lincoln (eds), *Handbook of Qualitative Research*. Thousand Oaks, CA: Sage.

Schwarzman, J. (2019) Evaluation in Health Promotion: Gathering Evidence to Improve Effectiveness. PhD, Monash University.

Scott, K., Beckham, S.W., Gross, M., Pariyo, G., Rao, K.D., Cometto, G. and Perry, H.B. (2018) 'What do we know about community-based health worker programs? A systematic review of existing reviews on community health workers', *Human Resources for Health*, *16*: 39. doi: 10.1186/s12960-018-0304-x

Scott-Samuel, A. and O'Keefe, E. (2007) 'Health impact assessment, human rights and global public policy: a critical appraisal', *Bulletin of the World Health Organization*, *85* (3): 211–17.

Scott-Samuel, A. and Springett, J. (2007) 'Hegemony or health promotion? Prospects for reviving England's last discipline', *Journal of the Royal Society of Health*, *127* (5): 211–14.

Scriven, A. (2007) 'Guest editorial: shaping the future has become the rallying cry for health promoters in the first decade of the 21st century', *Journal of the Royal Society for the Promotion of Health*, *127* (5): 206.

Scriven, A. (2017) *Ewles and Simnett's Promoting Health: A Practical Guide* (7th edn). London: Elsevier.

Scriven, A. and Speller, V. (2007) 'Global issues and challenges beyond Ottawa: the way forward', *Promotion & Education*, *XIV* (4): 194–8.

Seedhouse, D. (1997) *Health Promotion: Philosophy, Prejudice and Practice*. New York: John Wiley & Sons.

Seligman, M.E.P. (1975) *Helplessness: On Depression, Development and Death*. San Francisco, CA: W.H. Freeman.

Selva, J. (2021) 'What is self-actualization?', *Positive Psychology*. (*Website*: positivepsychology.com)

Serrano-Garcia, I. (1984) 'The illusion of empowerment: community development within a colonial context', in J. Rappaport (ed.), *Studies in Empowerment: Steps Toward Understanding and Action*. New York: Howarth Press.

Settle, D. and Wise, C. (1986) 'Choices: materials and methods for personal and social education', in J. Ryder and C. Campbell, *Balancing Acts in Personal, Social and Health Education*. London: Routledge.

Shacklock Evans, E.G. (1962) 'The design of teaching experiments in education', *Educational Research*, *5* (1): 37–52.

Shareck, M., Frohlich, K.L. and Poland, B. (2013) 'Reducing social inequities in health through settings-related interventions: a conceptual framework', *Global Health Promotion*, *20*: 39–52.

Shavelson, R.J. and Marsh, H.W. (1986) 'On the structure of self concept', in R.T. Schwarzer (ed.), *Anxiety and Cognitions*. Hillsdale, NJ: Erlbaum.

Shaw, I. (2002) 'How lay are lay beliefs?', *Health*, *6*: 287–99.

Shaw, M. (2004) *Community Work: Policy, Politics and Practice*. Hull: Universities of Hull and Edinburgh.

Shaw, M., Dorling, D. and Davey Smith, G. (1999) 'Poverty, social exclusion and minorities', in M. Marmot and G. Wilkinson (eds), *Social Determinants of Health*. Oxford: Oxford University Press.

Shea, L. (2009) 'Using social media to get health care messages out: Facebook, Twitter and YouTube gets results', *Patient Education Management*, July: 76–8.

Shehata, W.M. and Abdeldaim, D.E. (2022) 'Social media and spreading panic among adults during the COVID-19 pandemic, Egypt', *Environmental Science and Pollution Research*, *29*: 23374–82.

Sheluchin, A., Johnston, R.M. and Linden, C. v. d. (2020) 'Public responses to policy reversals: the case of mask usage in Canada during COVID-19', *Canadian Public Policy*, *46*: S119–S126.

Shepherd, J. (2013) 'Judgment, resources, and complexity: a qualitative study of the experiences of systematic reviewers of health promotion', *Evaluation and the Health Professions*, *36*: 247–67.

Shilton, T., Howat, P., James, R., Burke, L., Hutchins, C. and Woodman, R. (2008) 'Health promotion competencies for Australia 2001–5: trends and their implications', *Promotion & Education*, *15* (2): 21–6.

Shirazi, M., Engelman, K.K., Mbah, O., Shirazi, A., Robbins, I., Bowie, J., Popal, R., Wahwasuck, A., Whalen-White, D., Greiner, A., Dobs, A. and Bloom, J. (2015) 'Targeting and tailoring health communications in breast screening interventions', *Progress in Community Health Partnerships: Research, Education and Action*, *9* (Special Issue): 83–9.

Sidell, M. (2010) 'Older people's health: applying Antonovsky's salutogenic paradigm', in J. Douglas, S. Earle, S. Handsley, S. Jones, C. Lloyd and S. Spurr (eds), *A Reader Promoting Public Health, Challenge and Controversy* (2nd edn). London: Sage.

Signal, L. (1998) 'The politics of health promotion: insights from political theory', *Health Promotion International*, *13* (3): 257–63.

Sim, J. (1990) *Medical Power in Prisons*. Milton Keynes: Open University Press.

Sindall, C. (2002) 'Does health promotion need a code of ethics?' *Health Promotion International*, *17* (3): 201–3.

Sinopoli, A., Saulle, R., Marino, M. De Belvis, A.G., Federici, A. and La Torre, G. (2018) 'The PRECEDE-PROCEED model as a tool for public health screening', *European Journal of Public Health*, *28* (Suppl 4): 20181101.

Skierkowski, D.D., Florin, P., Harlow, S., Machan, J. and Ye, Y. (2021) 'A readability analysis of online mental health resources', *American Psychologist, 74* (4): 474–83.

Skills for Health and Public Health Resource Unit (2009) *Public Health Skills and Career Framework Multidisciplinary/Multi-Agency/Multi-Professional.* (*Website*: www.healthcareers.nhs.uk/sites/default/files/documents/PHSCF%20March%202009.pdf).

Skinner, B.F. (1971) *Beyond Freedom and Dignity.* New York: Knopf.

Skinner, C. (2018) 'Issues and challenges in census taking', *Annual Review of Statistics and its Application, 5*: 49–63.

Slovic, P., Fischoff, B. and Lichtenstein, S. (1982) 'Why study risk perception?', *Risk Analysis, 2* (2): 89–93.

Smith, B.J., Rissel, C., Shilton, T. and Bauman, A. (2016) 'Advancing evaluation practice in health promotion', *Health Promotion Journal of Australia, 27* (3): 184–6.

Smith, C. (2000) '"Healthy prisons": a contradiction in terms?', *Howard Journal of Criminal Justice, 39*: 339–53.

Smith, G. (2001) 'Reflections on the limitations to epidemiology', *Journal of Clinical Epidemiology, 54*: 325–31.

Smith, J.A., Schmitt, D., Fereday, L. and Bonson, J. (2015) 'Ethics and health promotion within policy and practice contexts in a small jurisdiction: perspectives from the Northern Territory', *Health Promotion Journal of Australia, 26*: 231–4.

Smith, K.E. and Katikireddi, S.V. (2013) 'A glossary of theories for understanding policymaking', *Journal of Epidemiology and Community Health, 67*: 198–202.

Smith, M.K. (2016) *Community Work.* (*Website*: www.infed.org/community/b-comwrk.htm).

Smith, N., Littlejohns, L.B. and Thompson, D. (2001) 'Shaking out the cobwebs: insights into community capacity and its relation to health outcomes', *Community Development Journal, 36* (1): 30–41.

Smith, R. (2007) *Reducing Health Inequalities: Issues for London and Priorities for Action.* London: Greater London Authority.

Sobel, M.E. (1981) *Lifestyle and Social Structure: Concepts, Definition, Analyses.* New York: Academic Press.

Social Exclusion Unit (2002) *Reducing Re-offending by Ex-prisoners.* London: The Stationery Office.

Society for Public Health Education (SOPHE) (1976) *Code of Ethics.* Washington, DC: SOPHE.

Society of Health Education and Health Promotion Specialists (1997) *Code of Professional Conduct for Health Education and Health Promotion Specialists. Principles and Practice Standing Committee.* Society of Health Education and Health Promotion Specialists.

Solomon, D.S. (1989) 'A social marketing perspective on communication campaigns', in R.E. Rice and C.K. Atkin (eds), *Public Communication Campaigns* (2nd edn). Newbury Park, CA: Sage.

Song, I.S. and Hattie, J.A. (1984) 'Home environment, self-concept and academic achievement: a causal modeling approach', *Journal of Educational Psychology, 76*: 1269–81.

Soubhi, H. and Potvin, L. (2000) 'Homes and families as health promotion settings', in B.D. Poland, L.W. Green and I. Rootman (eds), *Settings for Health Promotion: Linking Theory and Practice.* Thousand Oaks, CA: Sage.

Soul City Institute (2008) *Soul Beat Africa.* Johannesburg: Soul City Institute Health and Development Communication. (*Website*: http://saapa.net/countries/south-africa/soul-city-institute-for-health-development-communication).

South, E. and Lorenc, T. (2020) 'Use and value of systematic reviews in English local authority public health: a qualitative study', *BMC Public Health, 20*: 1100.

South, J. and Tilford, S. (2000) 'Perceptions of research and evaluation in health promotion', *Health Education Research, 15* (6): 729–41.

South, J. and Woodall, J. (2010) *Empowerment and Health and Wellbeing: Evidence Summary.* Leeds: Centre for Health Promotion Research, Leeds Metropolitan University.

South, J., Bagnall, A.-M., Stansfield, J.A., Southby, K.J. and Mehta, P. (2019) 'An evidence-based framework on community-centred approaches for health: England, UK', *Health Promotion International, 34* (2): 356–66.

South, J., Bagnall, A. and Woodall, J. (2015) 'Developing a typology for peer education and peer support delivered by prisoners', *Journal of Correctional Health Care, 23* (2): 214–29.

South, J., White, J. and Gamsu, M. (2013) *People Centred Public Health.* Bristol: Policy Press.

South, J., White, J. and Raine, G. (2010) *Community Health Champions: Evidence Summary*. Leeds: Centre for Health Promotion Research, Leeds Metropolitan University.

South, J., Woodall, J., Kinsella, K., Dixey, R., Penson, B. and de Viggiani, N. (2012) *Peers in Prison Settings (PiPs) Expert Symposium – Conference Proceedings*. Leeds: Leeds Metropolitan University, Institute for Health and Wellbeing.

Sparks, M. (2011) 'Building healthy public policy: don't believe the misdirection', *Health Promotion International*, *26*: 259–62.

Speller, V., Evans, D. and Head, M.J. (1997a) 'Developing quality assurance standards for health promotion practice in the UK', *Health Promotion International*, *12* (3): 215–24.

Speller, V., Learmonth, A. and Harrison, D. (1997b) 'The search for evidence of effective health promotion', *British Medical Journal*, *315*: 361–3.

Speller, V., Parish, R., Davison, H. and Zilnyk, A. (2012) *CompHP Professional Standards for Health Promotion Handbook*. EAHC Project number 20081209.

Speller, V., Rogers, L. and Rushmere, A. (1998) 'Quality assessment in health promotion settings', in J.K. Davies and G. Macdonald (eds), *Quality, Evidence and Effectiveness in Health Promotion*. London: Routledge.

Springett, J. (1998) 'Quality measures and evaluation of healthy city policy initiatives', in J.K. Davies and G. Macdonald (eds), *Quality, Evidence and Effectiveness in Health Promotion*. London: Routledge.

Springett, J. (2001) 'Appropriate approaches to the evaluation of health promotion', *Critical Public Health*, *11* (2): 139–51.

Springett, J., Owens, C. and Callaghan, J. (2007) 'The challenge of combining "lay" knowledge with "evidence-based" practice in health promotion: Fag Ends Smoking Cessation Service', *Critical Public Health*, *17*: 243–56.

Sriranganathan, G., Jaworsky, D., Larkin, J., Flicker, S., Campbell, L., Flynn, S., Janssen, J. and Erlich, L. (2012) 'Peer sexual health education interventions for effective programme evaluation', *Health Education Journal*, *71*: 62–71.

St Leger, L. (1997) 'Health promoting settings: from Ottawa to Jakarta', *Health Promotion International*, *12*: 99–101.

Stacey, M. (1994) 'The power of lay knowledge', in J. Popay and J. Williams (eds), *Researching the People's Health*. London: Routledge.

Stainton Rogers, W. (1991) *Explaining Health and Illness: An Exploration of Diversity*. London: Harvester Wheatsheaf.

Standing Conference for Community Development (2001) *Strategic Framework for Community Development*. Sheffield: SCCD. (*Website*: www.changesfoundations.net/wp-content/uploads/2012/02/SCCD-Strategic-Framework.pdf).

Stansfield, S.A. (1999) 'Social support and social cohesion', in M. Marmot and R.G. Wilkinson (eds), *Social Determinants of Health*. Oxford: Oxford University Press.

Starfield, B., Hyde, J., Gérvas, J. and Heath, I. (2008) 'The concept of prevention: a good idea gone astray?', *Journal of Epidemiology and Community Health*, *62*: 580–3.

Stead, M., Angus, K., Langley, T., Katikireddi, S.V., Hinds, K., Hilton, S. et al. (2019) *Mass Media to Communicate Public Health Messages in Six Topic Areas: A Systematic Review and Other Reviews of the Evidence*. National Institute for Health and Care Research. doi: 10.3310/phr07080

Steele, M., Mialon, M., Browne, S., Campbell, N. and Finucane, F. (2021) 'Obesity, public health ethics and the nanny state', *Ethics, Medicine and Public Health*, *19*: 100724.

Stenhouse, L. (1975) 'A critique of the objectives model', in L. Stenhouse (ed.), *An Introduction to Curriculum Research and Development*. London: Heinemann.

Stephen, C. (2020) 'Expanding the concept of healthy public policy for animals, health, and society', in C. Stephen (ed.), *Animals, Health, and Society*. London: CRC Press.

Steury, E.E. (2013) 'Malaria prevention in Zambia: a practical application of the diffusion of innovations model', *Journal of Transcultural Nursing*, *24* (2): 189–94.

Stevens, N.H., Foote, S. and Wu, P. (2008) 'Education theatre program: promoting health', *Permanente Journal*, *12* (3): 90–2.

Stewart, D. (2008) *The Problems and Needs of Newly Sentenced Prisoners: Results from a National Survey.* London: Ministry of Justice.

Stoneham, M. and Edmunds, M. (2020) 'Policy, legislation and environmental change', in M.-L. Fleming and L. Baldwin (eds), *Health Promotion in the 21st Century: New Approaches to Achieving Health for All.* Abingdon: Routledge.

Stronks, K., Hoeymans, N., Haverkamp, B., den Hertog, F.R.J., van Bon-Martens, M.J.H., Galenkmap, H., Verweij, M. and van Oers, H.A.M. (2018) 'Do conceptualisations of health differ across social strata? A concept mapping among lay people', *BMJ*, *8* (4). doi: 10.1136/bmjopen-2017-020210

Sun, C.J., Nall, J.L. and Rhodes, S.D. (2019) 'Perceptions of needs, assets, and priorities among black men who have sex with men with HIV: community-driven actions and impacts of a participatory photovoice process', *American Journal of Men's Health*, *13*. doi: 10.1177/1557988318804901

Sutherland, E.H. and Cressy, D.R. (1960) *Principles of Criminology.* Philadelphia, PA: Lippincott.

Sutherland, I. (1979) *Health Education: Perspectives and Choices.* London: Allen & Unwin.

Swinburn, B.A. (2008) 'Obesity prevention: the role of policies, laws and regulations', *Australia and New Zealand Health Policy*, *5* (12). (*Website*: www.anzhealthpolicy.com/content/5/1/12).

Symvoulakis, E.K., Karagergiou, I., Linardakis, M., Papagiannis, D., Hatzoglou, C., Symeonidis, A. and Rachiotis, G. (2022) 'Knowledge, attitudes, and practices of primary care physicians towards COVID-19 in Greece: a cross-sectional study', *Healthcare*, *10*: 545. doi: 10.3390/healthcare10030545

Szczuka, Z., Banik, A., Abraham, C. Kulis, E. and Luszczynska, A. (2021) 'Associations between self-efficacy and sedentary behaviour: a meta-analysis', *Psychology & Health*, *36* (3): 271–89.

Taha Can Tuman (2022) 'The effect of type D personality on anxiety, depression and fear of COVID-19 disease in healthcare workers', *Archives of Environmental & Occupational Health*, *77* (3): 177–84.

Tannahill, A. (1992) 'Epidemiology and health promotion: a common understanding', in R. Bunton and G. Macdonald (eds), *Health Promotion Disciplines and Diversity.* London: Routledge.

Tannahill, A. (2008) 'Beyond evidence – to ethics: a decision-making framework for health promotion, public health and health improvement', *Health Promotion International*, *23* (4): 380–90.

Tanta, I., Mihovilović, M. and Sablić, Z. (2014) 'Uses and gratification theory – why adolescents use Facebook?', *Medij Istraž*, *20* (2): 85–110.

Tapper, K. (2021) *Health Psychology and Behaviour Change.* London: Macmillan Education.

Taylor, E.N. and Wallace, L.E. (2011) 'For shame: feminism, breastfeeding advocacy, and maternal guilt', *Hypatia*, *27* (1): 76–100.

Taylor, L. and Blair-Stevens, C. (2002) *Introducing Health Impact Assessment (HIA): Informing the Decision-Making Process.* London: Health Development Agency.

Taylor, M. (1995) 'Community work and the state: the changing context of UK practice', in G. Craig and M. Mayo (eds), *Community Empowerment: A Reader in Participation and Development.* London: Zed Books.

Tazerji, S.S., Shahabinejad, F., Tokasi, M., Rad, M.A., Khan, M.S., Safdar, M. et al. (2022) 'Global data analysis and risk factors associated with morbidity and mortality of COVID-19.', *Gene Reports*, *26*. doi: 10.1016/j,ge nrep.2022.101505

Te'eni-Harari, T., Lampert, S.I. and Lehman-Wilzig, S. (2007) 'Information processing of advertising among young people: the Elaboration Likelihood Model as applied to youth', *Journal of Advertising Research*, *47*: 326–40.

Tengland, P. (2012) 'Behavior change or empowerment: on the ethics of health- promotion strategies', *Public Health Ethics*, *5* (2): 140–53.

Tengland, P. (2016) 'Behavior change or empowerment: on the ethics of health- promotion goals', *Health Care Analysis*, *24* (1): 24–46.

Terris, M. (1983) 'The complex tasks of the second epidemiologic revolution', *Journal of Public Health Policy*, *4*(1): 8–24.

Terris, M. (1996) 'Concepts of health promotion: dualities in public health theory', in J. French, *'Understanding health promotion through its fault lines'*. PhD thesis, Leeds Metropolitan University, Leeds.

Tesh, S., Tuohy, C., Christoffel, T., Hancock, T., Norsigian, J., Nightingale, E. and Robertson, L. (1988) 'The meaning of healthy public policy', *Health Promotion*, *2* (3): 257–62.

Thaler, R.H. and Sunstein, C.R. (2008) *Nudge: Improving Decisions about Health, Wealth and Happiness*. London: Penguin.

Thesenvitz, J. (2003) *Conditions for Successful Workplace Health Promotion Initiatives*. Toronto, Canada: Centre for Health Promotion, University of Toronto.

Thomas, F. and Aggleton, P. (2016) 'A confluence of evidence: what lies behind a "whole school" approach to health education in schools?', *Health Education*, *116* (2): 154–76.

Thomas, J. and Harden, A. (2008) 'Methods for the thematic synthesis of qualitative research in systematic reviews', *BMC Medical Research Methodology*, *8*: 45.

Thomas, S.A. and González-Prendes, A.A. (2009) 'Powerlessness, anger, and stress in African American women: implications for physical and emotional health', *Health Care for Women International*, *30*: 93–113.

Thompson, C., Clary, C., Er, V., Adams, J., Boyland, E., Burgoine, T., Cornelsen, L., de Vocht, F., Egan, M., Lake, A.A., Lock, K., Mytton, O., Petticrew, M., White, M., Yau, A. and Cummins, S. (2021) 'Media representations of opposition to the "junk food advertising ban" on the Transport for London (TfL) network: a thematic content analysis of UK news and trade press', *SSM – Population Health*, *15*: 1–10.

Thompson, T.L. and Robinson, P.J. (2021) 'The basics of health communication theory', in T.L. Thompson and P.J. Schulz (eds), *Health Communication Theory*. Hoboken, NJ: John Wiley & Sons.

Thoresen, C.E. and Mahoney, M.J. (1974) *Behavioral Self-Control*. New York: Holt, Rinehart and Winston.

Thornton, L., Gardner, L.A., Osman, B., Green, O., Champion, K.E., Bryant, Z. et al. (2021) 'A multiple health behavior change, self-monitoring mobile app for adolescents: development and usability study of the Health4Life app', *JMIR Formative Research*, *5* (4): e25513. doi: 10.2196/25513

Thorogood, M. (2010) 'Using systematic reviews in health promotion', in M. Thorogood and Y. Coombes (eds), *Evaluating Health Promotion: Practice and Methods*. Oxford: Oxford University Press.

Thorogood, M. and Coombes, Y. (2010) *Evaluating Health Promotion: Practice and Methods*. Oxford: Oxford University Press.

Thrall, A.T., Lollio-Fakhreddine, J., Berent, J., Donnelly, L., Herrin, W., Paquette, Z., Wenglinski, R. and Wyatt, A. (2008) 'Star power: celebrity advocacy and the evolution of the public sphere', *International Journal of Press/ Politics*, *13*: 362–85.

Tilford, S. (2000) 'Evidence-based health promotion', *Health Education Research*, *15* (6): 659–63.

Tilford, S., Green, J. and Tones, K. (2003) *Values, Health Promotion and Public Health*. Leeds: Centre for Health Promotion Research, Leeds Metropolitan University.

Tobi, P. (2013) *Redesigning Joint Strategic Needs Assessment: An Asset-Based Approach*. UEL Research and Knowledge Exchange Conference, 2013, University of East London, London, 26 June.

Toll, B.A., Salovey, P., O'Malley, S.S., Mazure, C.M., Latimer, A. and McKee, S. (2008) 'Message-framing for smoking cessation: the interaction of risk perceptions and gender', *Nicotine & Tobacco Research*, *10* (1): 195–200.

Tones, B.K. (1979) 'Past achievement, future success', in I. Sutherland (ed.), *Health Education: Perspectives and Choices*. London: Allen & Unwin.

Tones, B.K. (1981) 'Affective education and health', in J. Cowley, K. David and T. Williams (eds), *Health Education in Schools*. London: Harper & Row.

Tones, B.K. (1987) 'Health promotion, affective education and the personal–social development of young people', in K. David and T. Williams (eds), *Health Education in Schools*. London: Harper & Row.

Tones, K. (1986) 'Preventing drug misuse: the case for breadth, balance and coherence', *Health Education Journal*, *45* (4): 223–30.

Tones, K. (1993) 'Changing theory and practice: trends in methods, strategies and settings in health education', *Health Education Journal*, *52* (3): 125–39.

Tones, K. (2001) 'Health promotion: the empowerment imperative', in A. Scriven and J. Orme (eds), *Health Promotion: Professional Perspectives* (2nd edn). London: Palgrave.

Tones, K. (2002) 'Health literacy: new wine in old bottles?', *Health Education Research*, *17* (3): 287–90.

Tones, K. and Delaney, F. (1995) *Commissioning Health Promotion: A Consultancy Document*. Cambridge: Cambridge and Huntingdon Health Commission.

Tones, K. and Green, J. (1999) *A Case Study of Withymoor Village Surgery – A Health Hive: Health Promotion and Creative Arts in General Practice*. Leeds: Health Promotion Design.

Tones, K. and Tilford, S. (1994) *Health Education: Effectiveness, Efficiency and Equity*. London: Chapman & Hall.

Tones, K. and Tilford, S. (2001) *Health Promotion: Effectiveness, Efficiency and Equity* (3rd edn). London: Nelson Thornes.

Topol, E. (2015) *The Patient Will See You Now: The Future of Medicine is in Your Hands*. New York: Basic Books.

Torp, S., Kokko, S. and Ringsberg, K.C. (2014) *Promoting Health in Everyday Settings: Opportunities and Challenges*. London: Sage

Torrance, H. (2012) 'Triangulation, respondent validation, and democratic participation in mixed methods research', *Journal of Mixed Methods Research*, 6: 111–23.

Torrissen, W. and Stickley, T. (2018) 'Participatory theatre and mental health recovery: a narrative inquiry', *Perspectives in Public Health*, *138* (1): 47–54.

Tracy, S.J. (2013) *Qualitative Research Methods: Collecting Evidence, Crafting Analysis, Communicating Impact*. Chichester: Wiley-Blackwell.

Tremblay, M.C. and Richard, L. (2014) 'Complexity: a potential paradigm for a health promotion discipline', *Health Promotion International*, *29* (2): 378–88.

Truth (undated) *Truth: About Us*. (*Website*: www.thetruth.com/aboutUs.cfm).

Tulloch, J. and Lupton, D. (2003) *Risk and Everyday Life*. London: Sage.

Turner, C.M. (1978) *Interpersonal Skills in Further Education*. Blagdon: Further Education Staff College, Coombe Lodge.

Turner, G. and Shepherd, J. (1999) 'A method in search of a theory: peer education and health promotion', *Health Education Research*, *14* (2): 235–47.

Tyrrell, G.N.M. (1951) *Homo Faber*. London: Methuen.

United Nations (UN) (1948) *Universal Declaration on Human Rights*. (*Website*: www.un.org/Overview/rights.html).

United Nations (UN) (1966) *International Covenant on Economic, Social and Cultural Rights*. Geneva: Office of the United Nations High Commissioner for Human Rights.

United Nations (UN) (1990) *Basic Principles for the Treatment of Prisoners. Adopted and Proclaimed by General Assembly Resolution 45/111 of* 14 December 1990. New York: United Nations.

United Nations (UN) (2011) *2011 High-Level Meeting on Prevention and Control of Non-Communicable Diseases*. New York: General Assembly, UN, 19–20 September 2011. (*Website*: www.un.org/en/ga/ncdmeeting2011).

United Nations Children's Fund (UNICEF) (2013) *Child Well-being in Rich Countries: A Comparative Overview*. (*Website*: www.unicef-irc.org/publications/pdf/rc11_eng.pdf)

United Nations Children's Fund (UNICEF) (2021) *Central African Republic: Key Demographic Indicators*. (*Website*: https://data.unicef.org/country/caf/).

United Nations Development Programme (UNDP) (2013) *Human Development Report 2013*. New York: UNDP.

United Nations Economic Commission for Europe and Statistical Office of the European Communities (undated) *Recommendations for the 2000 Censuses of Population and Housing in the ECE Region*. Statistical

Standards and Studies (No. 49). Geneva: United Nations. (*Website*: http://ec.europa.eu/eurostat/ramon/stat-manuals/files/2000_censuses_ECE_region_EN.pdf).

United Nations Population Division (UNPD) (2022) *Life Expectancy of the World Population*. (*Website*: www.worldometers.info)

United Nations Statistics Division (2002) *World Population Housing and Census Programme*. New York: United Nations Statistics Division.

Unwin, N., Carr, S., Leeson, J. and Pless-Mulloli, T. (1997) *An Introductory Study Guide to Public Health and Epidemiology*. Buckingham: Open University Press.

Upton, D. and Thirlaway, K. (2014) *Promoting Healthy Behaviour: A Practice Guide*. Abingdon: Routledge.

Usher, K., Jackson, D., Walker, R., Durkin, J., Smallwood, R., Robinson, M. et al. (2021) 'Indigenous resilience in Australia: a scoping review using a reflective decolonizing collective dialogue', *Frontiers in Public Health*. doi: 10.3389/fpubh.2021.630601

Van den Broucke, S. (2012) 'Theory-informed health promotion: seeing the bigger picture by looking at the details', *Health Promotion International*, 27: 143–7.

Van der Putten, M., Makone, A.S., Chiriseri, E.T. and Vichit-Vadakan, N. (2012) 'Fostering a paradigm shift in the roles of health promotion education in Southeast Asia', *Research on Humanities and Social Sciences*, 2 (3): 28–37.

Van Winkle, R. (2002) *Active Teaching – Active Learning: Teaching Techniques and Tools*. Corvallis, OR: Oregon State University. (*Website*: http://extension.oregonstate.edu/catalog/4h/4-H0259L.pdf).

Vassallo, A., Jones, A. and Freeman, B. (2022) 'Social media: frenemy of public health?', *Public Health Nutrition*, 25 (1): 61–4.

Vaughan, C. (2014) 'Participatory research with youth: idealising safe social spaces or building transformative links in difficult environments?', *Journal of Health Psychology*, 19: 184–92.

Vazquez, M.A. and Pastrana, N.A. (2022) 'Social marketing in Latin America: a historical overview', *Social Marketing Quarterly*, 28 (1): 8–27.

Verduyn, P., Ybarra, O., Résibois, M., Jonides, J. and Kross, E. (2017) 'Do social network sites enhance or undermine subjective well-being? A critical review', *Social Issues and Policy Review*, 11: 274–302.

Veronese, G., Dhaouadi, Y. and Afana, A. (2021) 'Rethinking sense of coherence: perceptions of comprehensibility, manageability, and meaningfulness in a group of Palestinian health care providers operating in the West Bank and Israel', *Transcultural Psychiatry*, 58 (1): 38–51.

Villalonga-Olives, E. and Kawachi, I. (2017) 'The dark side of social capital: a systematic review of the negative health effects of social capital', *Social Science & Medicine*, 194: 105–27.

Vindrola-Padros, C., Chisnall, G., Cooper, S., Dowrick, A., Djellouli, N., Symmons, S.M., Martin, S., Singleton, G., Vanderslott, S., Vera, N. and Johnson, G.A. (2020) 'Carrying out rapid qualitative research during a pandemic: emerging lessons from COVID-19', *Qualitative Health Research*, 30: 2192–204.

Visram, S., Carr, S.M. and Geddes, L. (2015) 'Can lay health trainers increase uptake of NHS health checks in hard-to-reach populations? A mixed-method pilot evaluation', *Journal of Public Health*, 37 (2): 226–33.

Vitoria, P., Pereira, S.E., Muinos, G., De Vries, H. and Lima, M.L. (2020) 'Parents modelling, peer influence and peer selection impact on adolescent smoking behavior: a longitudinal study in two age cohorts', *Addictive Behaviors*, 100. doi: 10.1016/j.addbeh.2019.106131

Vlassoff, C. and Tanner, M. (1992) 'The relevance of rapid assessment to health research and interventions', *Health Policy and Planning*, 7 (1): 1–9.

Vos, T., Lim, S. and Murray, C.J.L. (2020) 'Global burden of 369 diseases and injuries, 1990–2019: a systematic analysis of the Global Burden of Disease, 2019', *The Lancet*, 366 (10258): 1204–22. doi: 10.1016/S0140-6736(20)30925-9

Wakefield, M.A., Loken, B. and Hornik, R.C. (2010) 'Use of mass media campaigns to change health behaviour', *The Lancet*, 376: 1261–71.

Wallace, J., Nwosu, B. and Clarke, M. (2012) 'Barriers to the uptake of evidence from systematic reviews and meta-analyses: a systematic review of decision makers' perceptions', *BMJ Open*, 2 (5): e001220. doi: 10.1136/bmjopen-2012-001220

Wallack, L.M. (1980) *Mass Media Campaigns: The Odds Against Finding Behavior Change*. Berkeley, CA: University of California Social Research Group.

Wallack, L. (1998) 'Media advocacy: a strategy for empowering people and communities', in M. Minkler (ed.), *Community Organizing and Community Building for Health*. New Brunswick, NJ: Rutgers University Press.

Wallack, L., Dorfman, L., Jernigan, D. and Makani, T. (1993) *Media Advocacy and Public Health: Power for Prevention*. Thousand Oaks, CA: Sage.

Wallerstein, N. (2002) 'Empowerment to reduce health disparities', *Scandinavian Journal of Public Health, 30*: 72–7.

Wallerstein, N. (2006) *What Is the Evidence on Effectiveness of Empowerment to Improve Health?* Copenhagen: WHO.

Wallston, B.S., Wallston, K.A., Kaplan, G.D. and Maides, S.A. (1976) 'A development and validation of the health locus of control (HLC) scale', *Journal of Consulting and Clinical Psychology, 44*: 580–5.

Wallston, K.A. (1991) 'The importance of placing measures of health locus of control beliefs in a theoretical context', *Health Education Research, 6* (2): 251–2.

Wallston, K.A. and Wallston, B.S. (1982) 'Who is responsible for your health? The construct of health locus of control', in G.S. Sanders and J. Suls (eds), *Social Psychology of Health and Illness*. Hillsdale, NJ: Erlbaum.

Wallston, K.A., Malcarne, V.L., Flores, L., Hansdottir, I., Smith, C.A., Stein, M.J., Weisman, M.H. and Clements, P.J. (1999) 'Does God determine your health? The God locus of health control scale', *Cognitive Therapy and Research, 23* (2): 131–42.

Wals, A.E.J. and Jickling, B. (2000) 'Process-based environmental education seeking standards without standardizing', in B.B. Jensen, K. Schnack and V. Simovska (eds), *Critical Environmental and Health Education*. Copenhagen: Danish University of Education.

Walt, G. (1994) *Health Policy: An Introduction to Process and Power*. London: Zed Books.

Waluyo, A., Mansyur, M., Earnshaw, V.A., Steffen, A., Herawati, T., Riri, M. and Culbert, G.J. (2022) 'Exploring HIV stigma among future healthcare providers in Indonesia', *AIDS Care, 34* (1): 29–38.

Wang, C. and Burris, M.A. (1994) 'Empowerment through photo novella: portraits of participation', *Health Education Quarterly, 21* (2): 171–86.

Wang, C., Liu, J., Pu, R., Li, Z., Guo, W., Feng, Z. et al. (2020) 'Determinants of subjective health, happiness, and life satisfaction among young adults (18–24 years) in Guyana', *BioMed Research International*. doi: 10.1155/2020/9063808

Wang, D., Stewart, D., Yuan, Y. and Chang, C. (2015) 'Do health-promoting schools improve nutrition in China?', *Health Promotion International, 30* (2): 359–68.

Wang, H. and Singhal, A. (2016) 'East Los High: transmedia edutainment to promote the sexual and reproductive health of young Latina/o Americans', *American Journal of Public Health, 106* (6): 1001–10.

Wang, P., Wang, R., Tian, M., Sun, Y., Ma, J., Tu, Y. and Yan, Y. (2021) 'The pathways from Type A personality to physical and mental health amid COVID-19: a multiple-group path model of frontline anit-epidemic medical staff and ordinary people', *International Journal of Environmental and Public Health, 18*: 1874. doi: 10.3390/ijerph18041874

Warwick, D.P. and Kelman, H.C. (1973) 'Ethical issues in social intervention', in G. Zaltman (ed.), *Processes and Phenomena of Social Change*. New York: Wiley.

Warwick-Booth, L. and Foster, S. (2021) 'People, power and communities', in R. Cross, S. Foster, I. ONeil, S. Rowlands, L. Warwick-Booth and J. Woodall (eds.), *Health Promotion: Global Principles and Practice* (2nd edn). Wallingford: CABI.

Warwick-Booth, L. and Rowlands, S. (2021) 'Policies for health in the 21st century', in R. Cross, S. Foster, I O. Neil, S. Rowlands, L. Warwick-Booth and J. Woodall (eds.), *Health Promotion: Global Principles and Practice*. (2nd edn). Wallingford: CABI.

Warwick-Booth, L., Cross, R. and Lowcock, D. (2021) *Contemporary Health Studies: An Introduction* (2nd edn). Cambridge: Polity.

Warwick-Booth, L., Dixey, R. and South, J. (2013) 'Healthy public policy', in R. Dixey (ed.), *Health Promotion: Global Principles and Practice*. Wallingford: CABI.

Waters, E., Gibbs, L., Tadic, M., Ukoumunne, O.C., Magarey, A., Okely, A.D., Silva, A., Armit, C., Green, J. and O'Connor, T. (2017) 'Cluster randomised trial of a school-community child health promotion and obesity prevention intervention: findings from the evaluation of fun 'n healthy in Moreland!', *BMC Public Health, 18* (1): 92–108.

Watson, J., Speller, V., Markwell, S. and Platt, S. (2000) 'The Verona benchmark: applying evidence to improve the quality of partnership', *Promotion & Education, 7* (2): 16–23.

Watson, M.C. (2002) 'Normative needs assessment: is this an appropriate way in which to meet the new public health agenda?', *International Journal of Health Promotion and Education, 40* (1): 4–8.

Weaks, D., Wilkinson, H., Houston, A. and McKillop, J. (2012) *Perspectives on Ageing with Dementia*. York: Joseph Rowntree Foundation.

Weber, M. (1968) *Economy and Society, Vol. 1.* New York: Bedminster Press.

Webster, F.E. (1975) 'Social marketing: what makes it different?', *Management Science, 13* (1): 70–7.

Weil, A.R. (2018) 'Diffusion of innovation', *Health Affairs, 37* (2): 175.

Weinstein, N.D. (1982) 'Unrealistic optimism about susceptibility to health problems', *Journal of Behavioral Medicine, 5* (4): 441–60.

Weinstein, N.D. (1984) 'Why it won't happen to me: perceptions of risk factors and susceptibility', *Health Psychology, 3* (5): 431–57.

Wellings, K. and Macdowall, W. (2000) 'Evaluating mass media approaches to health promotion', *Health Education, 100* (1): 23–32.

Wells, R., Howarth, C. and Brand-Correa, L.I. (2021) 'Are citizen juries and assemblies on climate change driving democratic climate policymaking? An exploration of two case studies in the UK', *Climatic Change, 168*: 5.

Wenzel, E. (1997) 'A comment on settings in health promotion', *Internet Journal of Health Promotion.* (*Website*: http://ldb.org/setting.htm).

Werner, D. (1980) 'Health care and human dignity', in S.B. Rifkin (ed.), *Health, the Human Factor: Readings in Health, Development and Community Participation.* (CONTACT Special Series No. 3). Geneva: WCC.

Werner, E.E. (1987) 'Resilient children', in E.E. Fitzgerald and M.G. Walraven (eds), *Annual Editions Human Development 87/88.* Guilford, CT: Dushkin.

Wharf-Higgins, J. and Begoray, D. (2012) 'Expand the borderlands between media and health: conceptualizing "critical media health literacy"', *Journal of Media Literacy Education, 4* (2): 136–48.

Wharf-Higgins, J., Strange, K., Scarr, J., Pennock, M., Barr, V., Yew, A., Drummond, J. and Terpstra, J. (2011) '"It's a feel. That's what a lot of our evidence would consist of": public health practitioners' perspectives on evidence', *Evaluation and the Health Professions, 34*: 278–96.

Whitehead, D. (2006) 'The health promoting prison (HPP) and its imperative for nursing', *International Journal of Nursing Studies, 43*: 123–31.

Whitehead, M. (1987) *The Health Divide.* London: Health Education Council.

Whitehead, M. (1992) Policies and Strategies to Promote Equity. Copenhagen: WHO.

Whitehead, M. and Tones, K. (1990) *Avoiding the Pitfalls: Notes on the Planning and Implementation of Health Education Strategies and the Special Role of the HEA.* London: Health Education Authority.

Whitehead, M., Taylor-Robinson, D. and Barr, B. (2021) 'Poverty, health, and covid-19', *BMJ, 372*: 367. doi: 10.1136/bmj.n376

Whitelaw, S., Baxendale, A., Bryce, C., MacHardy, L., Young, I. and Witney, E. (2001) '"Settings"-based health promotion: a review', *Health Promotion International, 16* (4): 339–53.

Whiting, L., Kendall, S. and Wills, W. (2012) 'An asset-based approach: an alternative health promotion strategy?', *Community Practitioner, 85* (1): 25–8.

WHO (1946) *Constitution.* Geneva: WHO.

WHO (1978) *Declaration of Alma Ata.* International Conference on Primary Health Care, 6–12 September, Alma Ata. Geneva: WHO.

WHO (1984) *Health Promotion: A Discussion Document on the Concepts and Principles.* Copenhagen: WHO.

WHO (1986) *Ottawa Charter for Health Promotion*. First International Conference on Health Promotion, 17–21 November, Ottawa. Copenhagen: WHO Regional Office for Europe.

WHO (1988) *The Adelaide Recommendations*. Geneva: WHO. (*Website*: www.who.int/healthpromotion/conferences/previous/adelaide/en).

WHO (1991) *Sundsvall Statement on Supportive Environments for Health*. Geneva: WHO.

WHO (1995) *Securing Investment in Health: Report of a Demonstration Project in the Provinces of Bolzano and Trento*. Copenhagen: WHO.

WHO (1997) *The Jakarta Declaration on Leading Health Promotion into the 21st Century*. Geneva: WHO. (*Website*: www/who.int/hpr/archive/docs/jakarta/english.html).

WHO (1998a) *Fifty-First World Health Assembly (WHA51.12): Health Promotion*. Copenhagen: WHO.

WHO (1998b) *Health for All in the Twenty-First Century (A51/5)*. Geneva: WHO.

WHO (1998c) *The WHO Approach to Health Promotion: Settings for Health*. Geneva: WHO.

WHO (1998e) *Health Promotion Evaluation: Recommendations to Policymakers: Report of the WHO European Working Group on Health Promotion Evaluation*. Copenhagen: WHO Regional Office for Europe.

WHO (1999) *Health21: The Health for All Policy Framework for the WHO European Region*. European Health for All Series, No. 6. Copenhagen: WHO Regional Office for Europe.

WHO (2000a) *Mexico Ministerial Statement for the Promotion of Health: From Ideas to Action*. Fifth Global Conference on Health Promotion: Bridging the Equity Gap, 5–9 June, Mexico. Geneva: WHO.

WHO (2000b) *Report of the Technical Programme*. Fifth Global Conference on Health Promotion: Bridging the Equity Gap, 5–9 June, Mexico. Geneva: WHO.

WHO (2002a) *World Health Report 2002 – Reducing Risks, Promoting Healthy Life, Chapter 3 – Perceiving Risks*. Geneva: WHO. (*Website*: www.who.int/whr/2002/en/).

WHO (2002b) *Community Participation in Local Health and Sustainable Development: Approaches and Techniques. European Sustainable Health and Development Series 4*. Copenhagen: WHO Regional Office for Europe. (*Website*: www.euro.who.int/document/e78652.pdf).

WHO (2005) *The Bangkok Charter for Health Promotion in a Globalised World*. Geneva: WHO. (*Website*: www.who.int/healthpromotion/conferences/6gchp/bangkok_charter/en/index.html).

WHO (2006a) *Constitution of the World Health Organization. Basic Documents*. 45th Edition. Geneva: WHO. (*Website*: www.who.int/governance/eb/who_constitution_en.pdf).

WHO (2006b) *A Guide to Healthy Food Markets*. Geneva: WHO.

WHO (2007a) *The Right to Health*. Geneva: WHO. (Website: www.who.int/mediacentre/factsheets/fs323/en/index.html).

WHO (2007b) *Global Climate Change: Implications for International Public Health Policy. Geneva: WHO*. (*Website*: www.who.int/bulletin/volumes/85/3/06-039503/en).

WHO (2008a) *WHO Framework Convention on Tobacco Control*. Geneva: WHO. (*Website*: http://apps.who.int/iris/bitstream/handle/10665/42811/9241591013.pdf;jsessionid=9E3D69F02106344FA91F8DE88B6B-5D07?sequence=1).

WHO (2008b) *Background Paper for Trenčín Statement on Prisons and Mental Health*. Copenhagen: WHO.

WHO (2009) *The Nairobi Call to Action*. Geneva: WHO.

WHO (2010) *Healthy Workplaces: A Model for Action*. Geneva: WHO.

WHO (2011) *10 Facts of Health Inequities and Their Causes*. (*Website*: www.who.int/features/factfiles/health_inequities/facts/en/).

WHO (2012) *Rio Political Declaration on Social Determinants of Health*. Geneva: WHO.

WHO (2013a) *International Classification of Diseases*. Geneva: WHO.

WHO (2013b) *Health Statistics and Health Information Systems*. Geneva: WHO.

WHO (2013c) *Global Health Observatory Data Repository*. Geneva: WHO.

WHO (2013d) *Metrics: Disability-Adjusted Life Year (DALY)*. Geneva: WHO. (*Website*: www.who.int/healthinfo/global_burden_disease/metrics_daly/en/).

WHO (2013e) *The Helsinki Statement on Health in All Policies*. Geneva: WHO.

WHO (2016a) *The Shanghai Declaration*. Geneva: WHO. (*Website*: www.who.int/healthpromotion/conferences/9gchp/shanghai-declaration.pdf).

WHO (2016b) *Healthy Workers, Healthy Future*. Geneva: WHO.

WHO (2018) *Infographics*. (*Website*: www.who.int/mediacentre/infographic/en).

WHO (2019) *Healthy Markets*. Geneva: WHO. (*Website*: www.who.int/healthy_settings/types/markets/en/).

WHO (2020) *The Impact of COVID-19 on Mental, Neurological and Substance Use Services*. Geneva: WHO.

WHO (2021a) *10th Global Conference on Health Promotion Charters a Path for Creating 'Well-Being' Societies*. Geneva: WHO. (*Website*: www.who.int/news/item/15-12-2021-10th-global-conference-on-health-promotion-charters-a-path-for-creating-well-being-societies).

WHO (2021b) *Noncommunicable Diseases. Factsheet*. (*Website*: www.who.int/news-room/fact-sheets/detail/non-communicable-diseases).

WHO (2021c) *The Geneva Charter for Well-Being*. Geneva: WHO.

WHO (2022) *Global Health Estimates: Leading Causes of DALYs Disease Burden 2000–2019*. (*Website*: www.who.int/gho).

WHR (2022) *World Happiness Report*. (*Website*: www.worldhappiness.report/ed/2022).

Whyte, W.F. (1943) *Street Corner Society*. Chicago, IL: Chicago University Press.

Whyte, W.F. (1991) *Social Theory for Action: How Individuals and Organizations Learn to Change*. Thousand Oaks, CA: Sage.

Whyte, W.F. (1997) *Creative Problem Solving in the Field: Reflections on a Career*. Walnut Creek, CA: Alta Mira Press.

Wiggers, J. and Sanson-Fisher, R. (1998) 'Evidence-based health promotion', in R. Scott and R. Weston (eds), *Evaluating Health Promotion*. Cheltenham: Stanley Thornes.

Wiley, L.F., Berman, M.L. and Blanke, D. (2013) 'Who's your nanny? Choice, paternalism and public health in the age of personal responsibility', *Journal of Law, Medicine and Ethics, 41*: 88–91.

Wilkinson, G. (1994) 'Divided we fall', *British Medical Journal, 308*: 1113–14.

Wilkinson, R. and Marmot, M. (2003) *The Solid Facts*. Copenhagen: WHO.

Wilkinson, R. and Pickett, K. (2009) *The Spirit Level: Why More Equal Societies Almost Always Do Better*. London: Allen Lane.

Wilkinson, R.G. (1997) 'Socio-economic determinants of health: health inequalities: relative or absolute material standards', *British Medical Journal, 314* (7080): 591–5.

Williams, A. and Kind, R. (1992) 'The present state of play about QALYS', in A. Hopkins (ed.), *Measure of the Quality of Life and the Uses to Which Such Measures May Be Put*. London: Royal College of Physicians.

Williams, E., Buck, D. and Babalola, G. (2020) *What Are Health Inequalities?* London: The King's Fund. (*Website*: www.kingsfund.org.uk/publications/what-are-health-inequalities)

Williams, G. and Popay, J. (1994) 'Lay knowledge and the privilege of experience', in J. Gabe, D. Kelleher and G. Williams (eds), *Challenging Medicine*. London: Routledge.

Williams, R.G.A. (1983) 'Concepts of health: an analysis of lay logic', *Sociology, 17* (2): 185–204.

Wills, J. (2023) *Foundations for Health Promotion* (5th edn). London: Elsevier.

Wills, J. and Rudolph, M. (2010) 'Health promotion capacity building in South Africa', *Global Health Promotion, 17*: 29–35.

Wilson, P., Richardson, R., Sowden, A.J. and Evans, D. (2001) 'PHASE 9: getting evidence into practice', in *Undertaking Systematic Reviews of Research Effectiveness. CRD Report, No. 4* (2nd edn). York: NHS Centre for Reviews and Dissemination.

Windahl, S., Suignitzer, B. and Olson, J.T. (2009) *Using Communication Theory: An Introduction to Planned Communication* (2nd edn). London: Sage.

Winkler, M.S., Krieger, G.R., Divall, M.J., Cissé, G., Wielga, M., Singer, B.H., Tanner, M. and Utzinger, J. (2013) 'Untapped potential of health impact assessment', *Bulletin of the World Health Organization, 91*: 298–305.

Winton, W.M. (1987) 'Do introductory textbooks present the Yerkes–Dodson law correctly?', *American Psychologist*, *42*: 202–3.

Wise, M. (2001) 'The role of advocacy in promoting health', *Promotion & Education*, *8* (2): 69–74.

Witte, K. and Allen, M. (2000) 'A meta-analysis of fear appeals: implications for effective public health campaigns', *Health Education and Behavior*, *27* (5): 591–615.

Wodak, R. (2001) 'What CDA is about – a summary of its history, important concepts and its developments', in R. Wodak and M. Meyer (eds), *Methods of Critical Discourse Analysis*. London: Sage.

Wodak, R. (2008) 'Introduction: discourse studies – important concepts and terms', in R. Wodak and M. Krzyanowski (eds), *Qualitative Discourse Analysis in the Social Sciences*. Basingstoke: Palgrave Macmillan.

Woelk, G., Daniels, K., Cliff, J., Lewin, S., Sevene, E., Fernandes, B., Mariano, A., Matinhure, S., Oxman, A.D. and Lavis, J.N. (2009) 'Translating research into policy: lessons learned from eclampsia treatment and malaria control in three southern African countries', Health Research Policy and Systems, *7* (1): 31. doi: 10.1186/1478-4505-7-31

Women's Health West (2010) *Developing Goals and Objectives Fact Sheet: A Guide to Health Promotion Action*. Victoria, Australia: Department of Health.

Wood, L.A. and Kroger, R.O. (2000) *Doing Discourse Analysis: Methods for Studying Action in Text and Talk*. London: Sage.

Woodall, J. (2010) *Control and Choice in Three Category-C English Prisons: Implications for the Concept and Practice of the Health Promoting Prison*. PhD thesis, Leeds Metropolitan University, Leeds.

Woodall, J. (2012a) 'Health promoting prisons: an overview and critique of the concept', *Prison Service Journal*, *202*: 6–12.

Woodall, J. (2012b) 'Social and environmental factors influencing in-prison drug use', *Health Education*, *1*: 31–46.

Woodall, J. (2013) 'Identifying health promotion needs among prison staff in three English prisons: results from a qualitative study', *Health Promotion Practice*, *14*, 256–62.

Woodall, J. (2016) 'A critical examination of the health promoting prison two decades on', *Critical Public Health*, *26* (5): 615–21.

Woodall, J. (2020a) 'COVID-19 and the role of health promoters and educators', *Emerald Open Research*, *2* (28). doi: https://doi.org/10.35241/emeraldopenres.13608.2

Woodall, J. (2020b) 'Health promotion co-existing in a high-security prison context: a documentary analysis', *International Journal of Prisoner Health*. *16* (3)@ 237-247.

Woodall, J. and Cross, R. (2021) *Essentials of Health Promotion*. London: Sage.

Woodall, J. and Freeman, C. (2020) 'Where have we been and where are we going? The state of contemporary health promotion', *Health Education Journal*, *79* (6): 621–32.

Woodall, J. and Rowlands, S. (2021) 'Professional practice', in R. Cross, S. Foster, I. O'Neil, S. Rowlands, L. Warwick-Booth and J. Woodall (eds), *Health Promotion: Global Principles and Practice*. Wallingford: CABI.

Woodall, J. and South, J. (2012) 'Health promoting prisons: dilemmas and challenges', in A. Scriven and M. Hodgins (eds), *Health Promotion Settings: Principles and Practice*. London: Sage.

Woodall, J. and Tattersfield, A. (2018) 'Perspectives on implementing smoke-free prison policies in England and Wales', *Health Promotion International*, *33* (6): 1066–73.

Woodall, J., de Viggiani, N., Dixey, R. and South, J. (2014) 'Moving prison health promotion along: toward an integrative framework for action to develop health promotion and tackle the social determinants of health', *Criminal Justice Studies*, *27* (1): 114–32.

Woodall, J., Dixey, R. and South, J. (2013a) 'Prisoners' perspectives on the transition from the prison to the community: implications for settings-based health promotion', *Critical Public Health*, *23*: 188–200.

Woodall, J., Dixey, R. and South, J. (2013b) 'Control and choice in English prisons: developing health-promoting prisons', *Health Promotion International*. *29* (3): 474–82. doi: 10.1093/heapro/dat019

Woodall, J., Freeman, C. and Warwick-Booth, L. (2021) 'Health-promoting prisons in the female estate: an analysis of prison inspection data', *BMC Public Health*, *21*: 1–8.

Woodall, J., Raine, G., South, J. and Warwick-Booth, L. (2010) *Empowerment and Health and Well-Being: Evidence Review*. Leeds: Centre for Health Promotion Research, Leeds Metropolitan University.

Woodall, J., South, J., Dixey, R., de Viggiani, N. and Penson, W. (2015) 'Expert views of peer-based interventions for prisoner health', *International Journal of Prisoner Health*, 11 (2): 87–97.

Woodall, J., Warwick-Booth, L. and Cross, R. (2012a) 'Has empowerment lost its power?', *Health Education Research*, 27 (4): 742–5.

Woodall, J., Warwick-Booth, L., South, J. and Cross, R. (2018) 'What makes health promotion research distinct?', *Scandinavian Journal of Public Health*, 46 (Suppl 20): 118–22.

Woodall, J., White, J. and South, J. (2012b) 'Improving health and well-being through community health champions: a thematic evaluation of a programme in Yorkshire and Humber', *Perspectives in Public Health*, 133: 96–103.

Woodall, J., Woodward, J., Witty, K. and McCulloch, S. (2013c) *An Evaluation of Calderdale's Toothbrushing in Schools Scheme*. Leeds: Institute for Health and Wellbeing.

Woolcock, M. (2001) 'The place of social capital in understanding social and economic outcomes', *Canadian Journal of Policy Research*, 2 (1): 11–17.

Workforce Council of Australia (2013) *TIP SHEET: Developing Goals and Objectives*. Australia, Queensland Government. (*Website*: www.checkup.org.au).

World Bank (1993) *World Development Report 1993*. New York: Oxford University Press.

Worley, C.G. and Jules, C. (2020) 'COVID-19's uncomfortable revelations about agile and sustainable organizations in a VUCA world', *The Journal of Applied Behavioral Science*, 56: 279–83.

Wren, B. (1977) *Education for Justice*. London: SCM Press.

Wright, M.T., Roche, B., von Unger, H., Block, M. and Gardner, B. (2010) 'A call for an international collaboration on participatory research for health', *Health Promotion International*, 25: 115–22.

Wright, N., Bleakley, A., Butt, C., Chadwick, O., Mahmood, K., Patel, K. and Salhi, A. (2011) 'Peer health promotion in prisons: a systematic review', *International Journal of Prisoner Health*, 7: 37–51.

Yadav, R. and Kobayashi, M. (2015) 'A systematic review: effectiveness of mass media campaigns for reducing alcohol-impaired driving and alcohol-related crashes', *BMC Public Health*, 15. doi: 10.1186/s12889-015-2088-4

Yanovitzky, I. and Stryker, J. (2001) 'Mass media, social norms, and health promotion efforts: a longitudinal study of media effects on youth binge drinking', *Communication Research*, 28 (2): 208–39.

Ye, Y., Wu, R., Wang, T., Yao, X., Yang, Y., Long, C. et al. (2021) 'Preventative behaviours and family inequalities during the COVID-19 pandemic: a cross-sectional study in China', *Infectious Diseases of Poverty*, 10. doi: 10.1186/s40349-021-00884-7

Yerkes, R.M. and Dodson, J.D. (1908) 'The relation of strength of stimulus to rapidity of habit formation', *Journal of Comparative Neurology and Psychology*, 18: 459–82.

Yiengprugsawan, V., Somboonsook, B., Seubsman, S. and Sleigh, A. (2012) 'Happiness, mental health, and socio-demographic associations among a national cohort of Thai adults', *Journal of Happiness Studies*, 13 (6): 1019–29.

Young, B., Lewis, S., Katikireddi, S.V., Bauld, L., Stead, M., Angus, K., Campbell, M., Hilton, S., Thomas, J., Hinds, K., Ashie, A. and Langley, T. (2018) 'Effectiveness of mass media campaigns to reduce alcohol consumption and harm: a systematic review', *Alcohol and Alcoholism*, 53 (3): 302–16

Young, I. and Williams, T. (1989) *The Healthy School*. Edinburgh: Scottish Health Education Group.

Yurt, S., Saglam Aksut, R. and Kadioglu, H. (2019) 'The effect of peer education on health beliefs about breast cancer screening', *International Nursing Review*, 66: 498–505.

Zacharakis-Jutz, J. (1988) 'Post-Freirean adult education: a question of empowerment and power', *Adult Education Quarterly*, 39 (1): 41–7.

Zack, B., Smith, C., Andrews, M.C. and May, J.P. (2013) 'Peer health education in Haiti's National Penitentiary: The "Health through Walls" experience', *Journal of Correctional Health Care*, 19: 65–8.

Zajonc, R.B. (1980) 'Feeling and thinking: preferences need no inferences', *American Psychologist*, *35*: 151–75.

Zalmanovitch, Y. and Cohen, N. (2015) 'The pursuit of political will: politicians' motivation and health promotion', *International Journal of Health Planning and Management*, *30* (1): 31–44.

Zeedyk, M.S. and Wallace, L. (2003) 'Tackling children's road safety through edutainment: an evaluation of effectiveness', *Health Education Research*, *18* (4): 493–505.

Ziglio, E., Hagard, S. and Griffiths, J. (2000a) 'Health promotion development in Europe: achievements and challenges', *Health Promotion International*, *15* (2): 143–54.

Ziglio, E., Hagard, S., McMahon, L., Harvey, S. and Levin, L. (2000b) 'Principles, methodology and practices of investment for health', *Promotion & Education*, *7* (2): 4–15.

Zlatanović, L. (2018) 'Self-efficacy and health behaviour: Some implications for medical anthropology', *Journal of the Anthropological Society of Serbia*, *51*: 17–25.

Zuckerman, M. (1990) 'The psychophysiology of sensation seeking', *Journal of Personality*, *58* (1): 313–45.

Zuckerman, M. and Kuhlman, D.M. (2000) 'Personality and risk-taking: common biosocial factors', *Journal of Personality*, *65*: 96–102.

INDEX

Page numbers followed by "f" indicate figures; those followed by "t" indicate tables.